HIV Infection
A Clinical Manual
Second Edition

C000143506

Howard Libman, M.D.
Associate Professor of Medicine, Boston University School of
Medicine; Associate Director, Clinical AIDS Program, Department of
Medicine, Boston City Hospital, Boston

Robert A. Witzburg, M.D.
Associate Professor of Medicine, Boston University School of
Medicine; Associate Director, Department of Medicine, Boston City
Hospital, Boston

Little, Brown and Company
Boston/Toronto/London

Sponsoring Editor: *Laurie Anello*
Production Editor: *Marie A. Salter*
Copyeditor: *Libby Dabrowski*
Indexer: *Dorothy Hoffman*
Production Supervisor: *F. David Bell*
Designer: *Peter Goodrich*
Cover Designer: *Jill Haber*

Library of Congress Cataloging-in-Publication Data
HIV infection : a clinical manual / [edited by] Howard Libman, Robert
   A. Witzburg.—2nd ed.
      p.   cm.
   Rev. ed of: Clinical manual for care of the adult patient with HIV
infection. 1990.
   Includes bibliographical references and index.
   ISBN 0-316-51162-5

   Second   Printing

   1. AIDS (Disease)   2. AIDS (Disease)—Patients—Care.   I. Libman,
Howard.   II. Witzburg, Robert A.   III. Clinical manual for care of
the adult patient with HIV infection.
   [DNLM: 1. HIV Infections.   2. HIV Infections—complications.
3. HIV Infections—therapy.   4. Opportunistic—therapy.   WD 308
H6752 1993]
RC607.A26C58   1993
616'.97'92—dc20
DNLM/DLC
for Library of Congress   93-3548
                                                                  CIP

Printed in the United States of America

EB-NC

To the patients and staff of Boston City Hospital

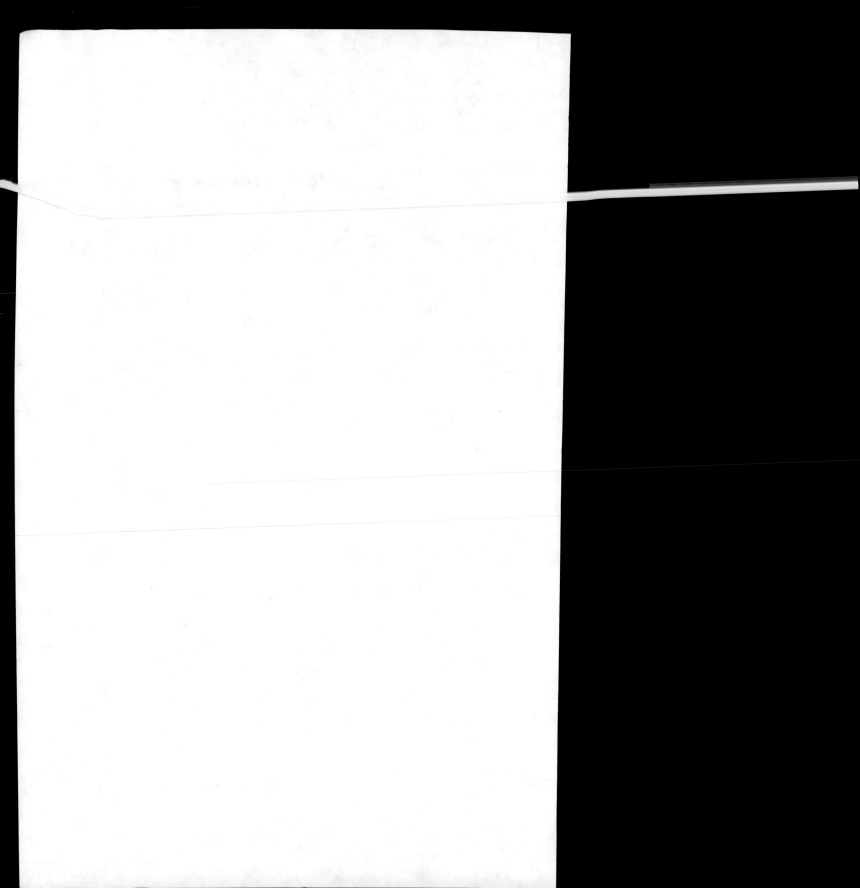

Contents

IV. Special Topics

Contributing Authors

Nezam H. Afdhal, M.D.
Assistant Professor of Medicine, Boston University School of Medicine; Chief of Gastroenterology and Hepatology, Boston City Hospital, Boston

Lawrence M. Barat, M.D.
Instructor in Medicine, Boston University School of Medicine; Attending Physician, Division of Infectious Diseases, Boston City Hospital, Boston

Thomas W. Barber, M.D.
Assistant Professor of Medicine, Boston University School of Medicine; Attending Physician, Division of Infectious Diseases, Boston City Hospital, Boston

David L. Battinelli, M.D.
Assistant Professor of Medicine, Boston University School of Medicine; Residency Program Director, Department of Medicine, Boston University Medical Center, Boston

Alexandra Beckett, M.D.
Assistant Professor of Psychiatry, Harvard Medical School; Director, HIV-Related Programs, Department of Psychiatry, Beth Israel Hospital, Boston

Paul E. Berard, M.D.
Assistant Professor of Medicine, Boston University School of Medicine; Attending Physician, Division of Hematology/Oncology, Boston City Hospital, Boston

Sheilah A. Bernard, M.D.
Assistant Professor of Medicine, Boston University School of Medicine; Director, Coronary Care Unit, Boston City Hospital, Boston

Steven C. Borkan, M.D.
Assistant Professor of Medicine, Boston University School of Medicine; Attending Physician, Renal Section, Boston City Hospital, Boston

Mariel Brittis, M.D.
Clinical Assistant Professor of Ophthalmology, Cornell University Medical College; Assistant Attending Ophthalmologist, New York Hospital–Cornell Medical Center, New York

Robert A. Burke, R.N., M.A., C.I.C.
Nurse Epidemiologist, Department of Hospital Epidemiology, Boston University Medical Center, Boston

Robert Carr, M. Ed.
Director, Counseling and Testing Services, AIDS Bureau, Massachusetts Department of Public Health, Boston

Timothy P. Cooley, M.D.
Assistant Professor of Medicine, Boston University School of Medicine; Attending Physician, Division of Hematology/Oncology, Boston City Hospital, Boston

Ellen R. Cooper, M.D.
Assistant Professor of Pediatrics, Boston University School of Medicine; Attending Physician, Division of Infectious Diseases, Boston City Hospital, Boston

Donald E. Craven, M.D.
Professor of Medicine and Microbiology, Boston University School of Medicine; Director, Clinical AIDS Program, Department of Medicine, Boston City Hospital, Boston

Bret E. Davis, M.D.
Instructor, Department of Dermatology, Boston University School of Medicine; Skin Oncology Fellow, Boston University Medical Center, Boston

Eileen Dunn, R.D.
Staff Dietician, Boston City Hospital, Boston

Maura A. Fagan, M.D.
Instructor in Medicine, Boston University School of Medicine; Fellow, Division of Infectious Diseases, Boston City Hospital, Boston

Harrison W. Farber, M.D.
Associate Professor of Medicine, Boston University School of Medicine; Director, Medical Intensive Care Unit, Boston City Hospital, Boston

Marshall Forstein, M.D.
Instructor in Psychiatry, Harvard Medical School; Director, HIV Mental Health Services, Department of Psychiatry, The Cambridge Hospital, Cambridge, Massachusetts

Jon D. Fuller, M.D.
Assistant Clinical Professor of Medicine, Boston University School of Medicine; Assistant Director, Clinical AIDS Program, Department of Medicine, Boston City Hospital, Boston

Gail M. Garvin, R.N., M.Ed.
Nurse Epidemiologist, Epidemiology Unit, Boston City Hospital, Boston

Gladys Gibbs, M.D.
Attending Physician, Department of Obstetrics and Gynecology, Grant Hospital, Columbus, Ohio

Leonard H. Glantz, J.D.
Professor of Health Law, Boston University Schools of Medicine and Public Health, Boston

Kevan L. Hartshorn, M.D.
Assistant Professor of Medicine, Boston University School of Medicine; Attending Physician, Division of Hematology/Oncology, Boston City Hospital, Boston

James J. Heffernan, M.D., M.P.H.
Associate Professor of Medicine, Boston University School of Medicine; Attending Physician and Director, General Medicine Consultation Service, Department of Medicine, Boston City Hospital, Boston

Douglas Hein
Coordinator of Counseling and Testing, Public Health AIDS Program, Department of Health and Hospitals, Boston

Howard K. Koh, M.D.
Associate Professor of Dermatology, Medicine, and Public Health, Boston University Schools of Medicine and Public Health; Attending Physician, Departments of Dermatology and Medicine, Boston University Medical Center, Boston

Howard Libman, M.D.
Associate Professor of Medicine, Boston University School of Medicine; Associate Director, Clinical AIDS Program, Department of Medicine, Boston City Hospital, Boston

Colleen Manning Osten, R.D.
Director of Nutrition Services, Greenery Rehabilitation and Skilled Nursing Center, Boston

Stephen I. Pelton, M.D.
Vice Chairman of Pediatrics, Boston University School of Medicine; Acting Chief of Pediatrics, Boston City Hospital, Boston

Edward S. Peters, D.M.D.
Clinical Instructor in Oral Pathology and Oral Medicine, Harvard School of Dental Medicine; Clinical Fellow, Division of Dentistry, Department of Surgery, Brigham and Women's Hospital, Boston

Anne Marie Regan, R.N., M.Ed.
Clinical Instructor in Pediatrics, Boston University School of Medicine; Research Coordinator, Pediatric AIDS Program, Boston City Hospital, Boston

John A. Rich, M.D., M.P.H.
Assistant Professor of Medicine, Boston University School of Medicine; Attending Physician, Department of Medicine, Boston City Hospital, Boston

Carol A. Saunders, R.N., B.S.N.
Director, Clinical Research Associates, Boston

Tina Schwartz, R.N., M.S.N.
Pediatric Clinical Nurse Specialist, Department of Nursing, and Coordinator, Pediatric AIDS Program, Boston City Hospital, Boston

Christopher Shanahan, M.D.
Clinical Instructor in Medicine, Boston University School of Medicine; Attending Physician, Department of Medicine, Boston City Hospital, Boston

Abby Shevitz, M.D.
Research Physician, Community Research Initiative of New England; Attending Physician, Immunodeficiency Clinic, Boston City Hospital, Boston

Robert W. Simms, M.D.
Assistant Professor of Medicine and Clinical Program Director, Arthritis Section, Boston University School of Medicine; Attending Physician, Boston City Hospital, Boston

Kathleen A. Steger, R.N., M.P.H.
Lecturer, Boston University School of Public Health; Associate Director, Clinical AIDS Program, Department of Medicine, Boston City Hospital, Boston

Judith L. Steinberg, M.D.
Assistant Professor of Medicine, Boston University School of Medicine; Attending Physician, Divisions of Infectious Diseases and General Internal Medicine, Boston City Hospital, Boston

Alan M. Sugar, M.D.
Associate Professor of Medicine, Boston University School of Medicine; Attending Physician, Boston City Hospital and Boston University Medical Center, Boston

Carol A. Sulis, M.D.
Assistant Professor of Medicine, Boston University School of Medicine; Attending Physician, Division of Infectious Diseases, Boston City Hospital, Boston

Nagagopal Venna, M.D., M.R.C.P.(I), M.R.C.P.(UK)
Associate Professor of Neurology, Boston University School of Medicine; Director, Clinical Neurology, Boston City Hospital, Boston

Brant L. Viner, M.D.
Assistant Professor of Medicine, Boston University School of Medicine; Attending Physician, Division of Infectious Diseases, Boston City Hospital, Boston

Randall P. Wagner, M.D.
Guest Researcher, Laboratory of Immunology, National Institute of Dental Research, National Institutes of Health, Bethesda, Maryland

Anna Wald, M.D.
Acting Instructor, University of Washington School of Medicine; Attending Physician, Harborview Medical Center, Seattle

Alan A. Wartenberg, M.D.
Assistant Professor of Medicine, Tufts University School of Medicine; Medical Director, Addiction Recovery Program, Faulkner Hospital, Boston

Robert A. Witzburg, M.D.
Associate Professor of Medicine, Boston University School of Medicine; Associate Director, Department of Medicine, Boston City Hospital, Boston

Beth Zeeman, M.D.
Clinical Instructor in Medicine, Boston University School of Medicine; Attending Physician, Department of Medicine, Boston City Hospital, Boston

Preface

As Sicknesse is the greatest misery,
so the greatest misery of sicknes is solitude;
when the infectiousnes of the disease
deterrs them who should assist, from comming . . .

John Donne, *Devotions Upon Emergent Occasions*

This manual is intended to support physicians, nurses, and other health care professionals in their efforts to provide high-quality care to adults infected with human immunodeficiency virus (HIV). The text originated in 1988 as a loose-leaf publication for the medical house officers and attending staff of the Department of Medicine at Boston City Hospital. In response to the success of the original effort, a revised and expanded version, *Clinical Manual for Care of the Adult Patient with HIV Infection*, was published in 1990 through the New England AIDS Education and Training Center, and a supplement followed in 1991. The current edition represents an entirely new and updated text.

We have attempted to organize this manual around practical management issues, which are accessible from an organ system or disease perspective. Part I provides an overview of HIV infection; Part II addresses its clinical manifestations; Part III describes associated opportunistic diseases; and Part IV covers a variety of special topics, including ambulatory management, risk reduction for health care workers, and HIV infection in specific populations.

The field of HIV-related research is in constant flux, and standards of clinical practice continue to evolve. There are many unresolved issues surrounding the care of patients with HIV infection. We have tried to indicate where uncertainty exists and to present a reasonable approach to management based on current literature. We hope that in areas where optimal therapy is not known, health care providers will make every effort to enroll patients in clinical research protocols.

We thank the authors for their informative and timely contributions. We are also indebted to Dr. Jon Fuller and Susan Libman for their editorial assistance, and to Nancy Connor and Ellen DiFiore for their administrative and secretarial support. Finally, we wish to acknowledge the house officers and faculty of Boston City Hospital and Boston University School of Medicine, whose commitment and professionalism continue to inspire us.

H.L.
R.A.W.

I/Overview of HIV Infection

Notice

The indications and dosages of all drugs in this book have been recommended in the medical literature and conform to the practices of the general medical community. The medications described do not necessarily have specific approval by the Food and Drug Administration for use in the diseases and dosages for which they are recommended. The package insert for each drug should be consulted for use and dosage as approved by the FDA. Because standards for usage change, it is advisable to keep abreast of revised recommendations, particularly those concerning new drugs.

1 /Epidemiology, Natural History, and Staging

Kathleen A. Steger

Acquired immunodeficiency syndrome (AIDS) was not recognized as a distinct clinical entity until May 1981, when the first cases of *Pneumocystis carinii* pneumonia (PCP) were noted in previously healthy, young homosexual men from Los Angeles [1, 2]. Since that time, human immunodeficiency virus (HIV) infection has become a global health problem of enormous magnitude. In 1988, it was estimated that 5 to 10 million persons worldwide were infected with HIV and that approximately 1 million new AIDS cases could be expected by 1993 [3]. The major route of HIV transmission in Africa and Asia is heterosexual behavior, and it is anticipated that by the year 2000, the majority of AIDS cases worldwide will be in women and children. Conversely, in the United States, the majority of cases have been acquired through homosexual behavior and injection drug use.

Historical Milestones

In the fall of 1982, a year after the first 100 cases of AIDS were reported, the Centers for Disease Control (CDC) established a case definition of this newly recognized syndrome [4] (Table 1-1). Since then, there have been several revisions of the AIDS case definition. The 1987 revision, which greatly increased the number of reportable AIDS cases, included HIV encephalopathy and wasting syndrome, and presumptive diagnoses made on the basis of laboratory evidence; it eliminated cases due to other causes of immunodeficiency [5, 6]. The CDC recently further expanded the AIDS case definition to include all HIV-infected patients with CD4 lymphocyte counts of less than 200/mm^3, regardless of clinical status.

Human immunodeficiency virus was first isolated in May 1983, but was not generally accepted as the cause of AIDS until 1984 [7–9]. The HIV enzyme-linked immunosorbent assay (ELISA) antibody test became available for clinical use and screening of blood donations in March 1985 [10]. In March 1987, azidothymidine (AZT; now known as zido-

Table 1-1 Milestones of the HIV epidemic

Date	Event
Fall 1982	First 100 cases of AIDS reported to CDC
May 1983	Human immunodeficiency virus (HIV), formerly LAV, HTLV-III, first isolated
March 1985	Routine screening of blood donations for antibody to HIV using the enzyme-linked immunosorbent assay (ELISA) begins
March 1987	Initial clinical trials of azidothymidine (AZT) as antiretroviral agent
July 1987	Food and Drug Administration approves AZT for treatment of AIDS/AIDS-related complex
August 1987	CDC broadens AIDS case definition by including patients with laboratory evidence of HIV plus wasting syndrome, encephalopathy, or one of a broader range of AIDS-indicative diseases
January 1989	First 100,000 AIDS cases reported in the United States
June 1989	CDC early intervention guidelines for HIV-infected persons based on CD4 lymphocyte counts issued
January 1993	Further expansion of the CDC case definition of AIDS

vudine, or ZDV) was made available as an investigational agent and approved by the Food and Drug Administration 4 months later based on promising initial results in AIDS patients [11]. Early intervention guidelines for HIV-infected adults were established in 1989; these included ZDV for patients with CD4 cell counts of less than $500/mm^3$ and prophylaxis against PCP for those with CD4 cell counts of less than $200/mm^3$ (or with a prior episode of PCP regardless of CD4 count) [12]. Zidovudine is believed to improve survival in patients with AIDS [13].

Epidemiology of HIV Infection and AIDS

There is wide geographic variation in AIDS case reporting and in HIV seroprevalence rates. Although AIDS cases have been reported from all 50 states, the majority continue to be identified in cities affected early in the epidemic [14]. The usefulness of AIDS case reports as a means of monitoring the epidemic is limited by the quality of surveillance activities and the substantial delay between acquisition of HIV infection and the development of AIDS. As of February 1, 1992, a total of 202,843

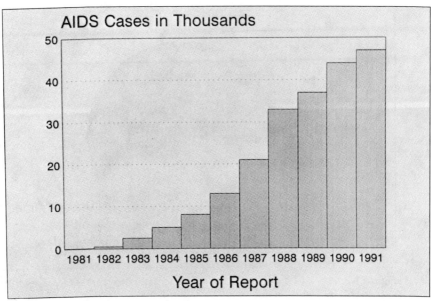

Figure 1-1. *The number of reported AIDS cases as of December 1991 in the United States by year of report. (Adapted from J Laurence, AIDS Statistics Update. The AIDS Reader 1:150, 1991.)*

AIDS cases had been reported in the US [15]. Projections made by the CDC in May 1988, using mathematical models, predicted that there would be 365,000 AIDS cases at that time [6]. These predictions are based on estimates of both the number of people currently infected with HIV and the rate at which those individuals progress to AIDS. Their accuracy may be compromised by limitations of HIV seroprevalence data and incomplete information on the efficacy of early medical intervention. However, despite some uncertainties, it is clear that HIV infection has spread rapidly. The doubling time for AIDS was only 6 months in 1982 and has increased to more than a year [16]. However, it took 8 years to accumulate the first 100,000 reported AIDS cases in the US and only 26 months for the second 100,000 [17] (Fig. 1-1).

Many important shifts in the epidemic have occurred over the past few years. While homosexual and bisexual men still account for a majority of nationally reported AIDS cases, cases attributable to injection drug use, either directly or through heterosexual exposure, have increased dramatically (Fig. 1-2). Women now account for 11 percent of total reported AIDS cases and represent the fastest growing risk group in the US [18]. The ratio of male-to-female AIDS cases has decreased from 15:1 in 1982 to 9:1 in 1990; in some populations of inner-city adoles-

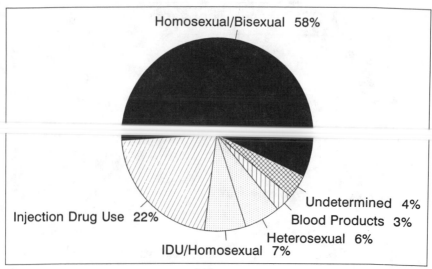

Figure 1-2. Pie chart depicting the percentage of reported US AIDS cases as of January 1, 1992, attributable to the various risk behaviors. (Data from the Massachusetts Department of Public Health, Massachusetts AIDS Surveillance Monthly Update, January 1, 1992.)

cents, the gender ratio for HIV infection is now 1:1 [18]. Potential expansion of the AIDS epidemic to involve the heterosexual population more generally depends on whether it follows the African model (in which spread is bidirectional) or the hepatitis B model [19]. In the latter scenario, infection is largely confined to major risk groups with relatively little spread outside of them.

The growth of the epidemic to include injection drug users (IDUs) and their sexual partners has had a disproportionate impact on communities of color, women, the indigent, and the homeless [20]. These populations have traditionally had limited access to health care, but more recently an effort has been made to facilitate their access to early treatment of HIV infection and clinical trials.

HIV-2

HIV-2 infection has been recognized particularly in West Africa and its previously Portuguese colonies [21]. Risk factors for HIV-2 appear to be the same as those for HIV, and HIV-2 can result in the clinical syndrome of AIDS. The relatively small number of cases reported in the US have all been associated with residence in or travel to West Africa, or sexual contact with a West African. While the majority of HIV-2 infections are identifiable by routine HIV antibody testing, the diagnostic laboratory should be alerted in cases in which HIV-2 is suspected.

Seroprevalence Data

Seroprevalence surveys of HIV infection have been ongoing for the past several years in military and Job Corps applicants, Red Cross blood donors, IDUs entering drug treatment, newborns, hospital inpatients, women seeking reproductive health care services, adolescents, and the homeless. While HIV seroprevalence rates for individual groups cannot be generalized to the entire population, they provide a means to measure the current and projected impact of HIV infection. The data derived from these surveys have demonstrated that HIV can spread rapidly in defined geographic areas [20].

Risk Group Trends: The Spreading Epidemic

Although the HIV epidemic has expanded into other populations, the majority of AIDS cases in the US (59%) continue to involve men reporting homosexuality or bisexuality as their risk behavior [22]. The overall prevalence of HIV among homosexual and bisexual men is not known because rates are based on nonrandom samples and vary widely in time and place [23]. In some cohorts of homosexual men, the new HIV infection rate has fallen to 0.5 to 3.0 percent per year [24]. While there appears to be a leveling of new AIDS cases in this risk group, there is concern over a possible rebound effect with a waning of adherence to safer sexual practices [25].

A decreasing number of new AIDS cases in coagulation factor recipients has been recognized, as well as a somewhat less dramatic decline in cases involving patients who have received blood transfusions [26]. Although the US blood supply is screened for HIV by serologic testing, about 1 in 153,000 units of blood remains infected [27]. If blood from an HIV-infected donor is transfused, the likelihood of transmission to the recipient increases with the number of units of blood received and the donor's stage of HIV disease [28].

Despite some slowing of the HIV epidemic among homosexual and bisexual men, transfusion recipients, and hemophiliacs, the rate of new AIDS cases continues to climb in women, blacks, Latinos, IDUs, and infants, especially in large metropolitan areas [18, 20, 29]. In Boston, the rate of HIV infection in IDUs entering a public drug treatment program increased from 15 percent in 1984 to 39 percent in 1988 [30]. However, one must be cautious in interpreting these trends, as program changes, such as admission policies prioritizing clients with symptomatic HIV disease, may bias seroprevalence results. Nonetheless, data collected from blinded seroprevalence surveys of drug treatment clients entering three Boston-area clinics since 1987 demonstrate increasing rates of HIV infection, with the highest occurring in clients of the inner-city program

[31]. Seroprevalence rates as high as 50 to 60 percent have been reported in IDUs in New York City and Newark, New Jersey [20].

Rates of HIV infection in women delivering babies at Boston City Hospital have been monitored for the past several years by blinded screening of cord blood samples for HIV antibody. The seroprevalence rate has increased from 1.6 percent in 1987 to 2.8 percent in 1990 [32]. These rates are double the overall rates for Massachusetts during the same time period.

Transmission of HIV

Numerous studies have focused on assessing the rate of transmission of HIV by various routes. Studies on heterosexual transmission of HIV have focused primarily on male-to-female transmission, which appears to be a more efficient route than from female to male. While Padian and associates [22] described a rate of male-to-female transmission of 23 percent in a cohort of female sexual partners of HIV-infected men, Clumeck and colleagues [33] reported a rate of 56 percent in 19 women heterosexually exposed to a single HIV-infected man in Belgium. In the former study, the number of sexual exposures and the practice of anal intercourse were associated with increased HIV transmission; in the latter, two instances of HIV infection followed a single sexual exposure to the male index case. This may indicate the presence of "hypertransmitters" of the virus and reemphasizes the importance of strict adherence to safe sexual practices.

The relative efficiency of male-to-female versus female-to-male HIV transmission remains controversial. The disproportionate number of cases in women, as opposed to men, who have acquired the virus heterosexually may be due to the larger pool of HIV-infected men in the US [34]. Peterman and associates [35] reported an HIV transmission rate of 8 percent in a cohort of male sexual partners of women infected with HIV via blood transfusion. Cameron and colleagues [36] described a higher rate of female-to-male transmission (23%) in an African cohort, in whom lack of circumcision, presence of genital ulcer disease, and more frequent contact with prostitutes were associated with increased risk of HIV infection.

Several studies have investigated the risk of HIV transmission associated with homosexual exposure. These rates appear to vary by the populations sampled and prevalence of higher-risk behaviors. Rates of transmission have ranged from 42 percent in partners of asymptomatic HIV-positive men in Boston to nearly 60 percent in partners of symptomatic HIV-positive men in Toronto [37, 38]. Factors that appear to increase the risk of HIV transmission in homosexual men include an increased number of unprotected sexual exposures, presence of other sexually transmitted diseases (STDs), engaging in receptive anal intercourse without a condom, and receptive "fisting" [37, 38]. The increased risk associated with the presence of STDs and receptive anal practices is probably due to mucosal breaks, which allow HIV-infected semen to enter the bloodstream. High rates of HIV infection have been described in urban STD clinics [39].

In addition to homosexual and heterosexual HIV transmission, many studies have assessed the risk of vertical transmission (mother to infant) of the virus [40, 41]. HIV can be transmitted transplacentally during gestation, labor and delivery, and postnatally through breast milk [29]. The proportion of perinatally acquired cases of HIV infection attributable to each of these mechanisms is unknown, as is the true frequency of vertical transmission. Estimates of the rate of vertical HIV transmission have decreased over time from approximately 60 percent in early studies to 12 percent currently [41, 42]. Recent data on the rates of vertical transmission are more reliable due to improved methods for diagnosing HIV infection in newborns, such as polymerase chain reaction testing, and the availability of outcome data from large, multicenter longitudinal studies of pregnant HIV-infected women.

Numerous behaviors associated with injection drug use appear to increase the risk of HIV transmission. These include increased number of injections per month, more cocaine injections per month, the use of "shooting galleries," reuse and sharing of needles, and a more recent history of drug use [20, 43]. Other factors may also play an important role in HIV transmission among IDUs and their sexual partners, including the number of heterosexual drug-using sex partners, low income, and being black or Latino [20, 43]. These racial differences are probably the result of increased involvement in high-risk behaviors rather than a genetic predisposition to infection.

Studies have also investigated HIV transmission among transfusion recipients, household contacts of HIV-infected persons, and health care workers [44–46].

Natural History of HIV Infection

Most of the information on the natural history of HIV infection has been derived from large cohort studies of homosexual and bisexual men. Unfortunately, there is a paucity of data from longitudinal cohorts of IDUs and even fewer studies in women. For this reason, we know little about the natural history of HIV disease in these specific risk groups.

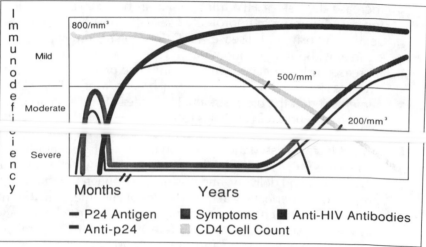

Figure 1-3. *Natural history of HIV infection. (Courtesy of Dr. Jon Fuller, Boston City Hospital.)*

There has been much discussion recently about possible gender differences in HIV disease. A correlation between HIV infection and more rapidly progressive cervical dysplasia has been suggested [47]. The applicability of the AIDS case definition to women has been challenged, as there is growing concern that the lack of gender-specific conditions has resulted in discrimination regarding disability and other social benefits. The mortality for women with AIDS quadrupled between 1985 and 1988, and AIDS is now the leading cause of death in black women of childbearing age in New York City [20, 48]. The fact that many HIV-infected women have children has had a dramatic social impact [18].

Spectrum of HIV Disease

Human immunodeficiency virus is one of the five known human retroviruses. The AIDS virus is from the lentivirus group, which establishes chronic, slowly progressive infections with long, asymptomatic latency periods [49]. AIDS is the end-stage result of a prolonged, chronic erosion of the immune system caused by HIV [50] (Fig. 1-3). The clinical manifestations of HIV disease are primarily infections or neoplasms that would normally be controlled by the immune system. While a clear definition exists for AIDS, the intermediate manifestations of HIV infection are poorly classified. The majority of individuals currently infected with HIV do not have AIDS. Overall, the rate at which AIDS develops in HIV-infected persons ranges from 4 to 10 percent per year; a majority will have clinical symptoms within 10 to 15 years of seroconversion.

Early HIV Infection and Prognosis

Primary infection with HIV is often asymptomatic. However, within days to weeks of the initial phase of viral replication, symptoms of the acute HIV syndrome may appear. These are nonspecific and may be attributed to mononucleosis, a severe cold, or the "flu" [51–53]. In addition to flu-like symptoms, additional manifestations have been described, including aseptic meningitis, peripheral neuropathy, encephalopathy, and splenomegaly with cytopenia [51, 54]. The diagnosis of primary HIV infection is made by demonstrating HIV antibody seroconversion. Following the acute HIV syndrome, the patient enters a prolonged asymptomatic or latent phase, during which measurable but low-level viral replication is seen. In adults, this asymptomatic phase lasts a median of 10 years before the development of AIDS, although it may be longer [55].

Within months after HIV infection, it is possible to detect a gradual reduction in the number of CD4 lymphocytes, but this does not generally lead to the emergence of opportunistic infections or malignancies until the count falls below 200/mm^3. While an average decrease in CD4 cell counts of 85/mm^3/year has been described in a homosexual cohort, this rate of decline may be slower in IDUs [56–58]. Early medical interventions have prolonged the time interval between acquisition of HIV infection and progression to AIDS and may also improve survival [59].

One of the earliest recognized syndromes, persistent generalized lymphadenopathy (PGL), is defined by the presence of unexplained adenopathy in two or more extrainguinal sites for 3 months or longer. Some people progress directly to AIDS without ever developing PGL; in approximately 38 percent of patients with PGL, AIDS develops within 6 years after presentation [56]. Data suggest that the prognosis for PGL is no different from that for asymptomatic HIV infection [57].

Factors that may influence the rate of disease progression include the strain of HIV, the disease status of the source of infection, and the age of the recipient. Other factors that appear to affect the natural history include antiretroviral therapy with ZDV and PCP prophylaxis. Controversies remain regarding the effects of race and gender on the natural history of HIV infection, and these require large-scale longitudinal studies of representative cohorts to be resolved. It is known that progression to AIDS is faster in persons at the extremes of age, with the youngest having the shortest latency phase. Several clinical and laboratory param-

Table 1-2 *Independent predictors of HIV disease progression*

Symptoms
Constitutional symptoms

Signs
Hairy leukoplakia
Oral candidiasis

Laboratory studies
CD4 cell count
CD4:CD8 ratio
Serum β_2-microglobulin
Serum and urine neopterin
p24 antigen
Serum and mononuclear cell HIV titer
HIV-related anemia
Erythrocyte sedimentation rate

eters have been identified as independent predictors of HIV disease progression (Table 1-2).

AIDS and Prognosis

Life expectancy with AIDS is improving because of earlier recognition of HIV infection, the use of antiretroviral and prophylactic medications, and better management of opportunistic infections. Recent data have shown that the vast majority of deaths in patients with HIV disease occur when the CD4 cell count falls below $50/mm^3$ [60]. Common causes of death include bacterial infections, PCP, Kaposi's sarcoma, wasting syndrome, and lymphoma [61].

Early survival data came from a large cohort study of 5,833 AIDS patients diagnosed before 1986 in New York City prior to the use of ZDV [62]. One-year survival was approximately 50 percent, and 2-year survival was 30 percent. Women, blacks, and IDUs had shorter survival than men, whites, and homosexuals, respectively. However, differences in survival rates may have been the result of delayed access to medical care or delayed diagnosis in the former groups. In more recent studies, no difference in the prognoses of these groups is discernible [63, 64]. The indicator disease with which the patient presented clearly affected life expectancy in the New York City cohort. Median survival for men with Kaposi's sarcoma alone was between 18 and 24 months. Survival for patients with PCP alone was 10.5 months, and in patients with other opportunistic infections, it was only 7 months.

Moore and associates [13] reported a longitudinal population-based study using data from the Maryland AIDS Registry in which median survival for patients with AIDS was 140 days longer for those diagnosed between 1987 and 1989 than for those diagnosed between 1983 and

1985. Other studies have also shown this trend, which may be attributable to the increased use of ZDV and prophylactic therapy against PCP [59, 65, 66].

Classification and Staging of HIV Infection

There are several reasons to stage or classify HIV infection, the most important of which is the management of patients. Staging helps determine appropriate medical therapy, intervals for follow-up study, eligibility for clinical trials, and prognosis. Other purposes of disease staging include the development of research protocols for new therapies, epidemiologic reporting and public health projections, and determination of disability.

Several terms and classification systems for HIV infection have been described. It is useful to think of HIV infection as a chronic disease resulting in a wide clinical spectrum that ranges from the asymptomatic (latency phase), to symptoms suggesting mild to moderate immunologic dysfunction, to complications indicating profound immunosuppression (AIDS) (see Fig. 1-3).

AIDS-related complex (ARC) is a term that originally referred to a specific HIV-related syndrome but has since been modified by many providers to identify any important disease manifestations that do not meet the CDC criteria for AIDS; others have chosen no longer to use the term ARC at all. As originally described, ARC is characterized by the gradual onset of fever, night sweats, fatigue, anorexia, weight loss, diarrhea, and/or generalized lymphadenopathy. Thrush, shingles and other skin infections, and refractory dermatitis may also be present. Skin tests to assess cell-mediated immunity are usually nonreactive. The CD4 cell count is generally below $500/mm^3$.

The original CDC case definition of AIDS antedated the availability of the HIV antibody test and was based on (1) the development of an opportunistic disease process indicating defective cell-mediated immunity (PCP, Kaposi's sarcoma, or other specified opportunistic infections) and (2) the lack of an established cause of profound immunosuppression [4]. These criteria were later modified to include additional opportunistic diseases in the context of serologic or virologic evidence of HIV infection.

Additional revisions in 1987 incorporated an algorithm based on the results of HIV antibody testing [67]. Recently the CDC case definition has been further expanded to include HIV-infected patients with any of the following conditions: (1) CD4 lymphocyte count of less than 200/mm^3 or CD4 percentage of less than 14, (2) pulmonary tuberculosis, (3) recurrent bacterial pneumonia, or (4) invasive cervical cancer. The current CDC AIDS case definition is presented in Table 1-3.

Table 1-3 CDC AIDS case definition

| | Definitive diagnosis | | | | | | Presumptive diagnosis | | | | |
Disease[a]	Symptoms or exam	Histology/ cytology	Endos- copy/ autopsy	Laboratory/ clinical test	R/O other causes	HIV testing required?	Clinical symp- toms	Physical exam	R/O other causes	Laboratory/ clinical test	HIV testing required?
Bacterial infection, recurrent (2 or more w/in 2 yrs) (pt age < 13 yr), excludes otitis media				culture		yes					NA
Candidiasis of esophagus		X/or	X			no	X	X/or		microscopy	yes
Candidiasis of trachea, bronchi, lungs		X/or	X			no					NA
CD4 lymphocyte count < 200 cells/mm³ or CD4% < 14%						**yes**					**NA**
Cervical cancer, invasive		**X**				**yes**					**NA**
Coccidiomycosis, disseminated (site other than lungs, cervical, or hilar lymph nodes)		X/or		culture or antigen		yes					NA
Cryptococcosis, extrapulmonary		X/or		culture or antigen		no					NA
Cryptosporidiosis (diarrhea > 1 mo)		X				no					NA
Cytomegalovirus (other than liver, spleen, or lymph nodes, pt age > 1 mo)		X				no					NA

Condition	Definitive dx		Definitive method					Presumptive
Cytomegalovirus retinitis	X				yes	X	X	yes
Herpes simplex virus (ulcer > 1 mo or bronchitis, pneumonitis, esophagitis in pt age > 1 mo)	X/or		culture		no			NA
Histoplasmosis (site other than lungs, cervical, or hilar lymph nodes)	X/or		culture or antigen		yes			NA
HIV encephalopathy	X		CSF & brain CT, MRI or autopsy	X	yes			NA
HIV wasting syndrome	X			X	yes			NA
Isosporiasis (diarrhea > 1 mo)	X				yes			yes
Kaposi's sarcoma (pt age < 60 yr)	X				no		X	yes
Kaposi's sarcoma (pt age > 60 yr)	X				yes		X	yes
Lymphoma of the brain (primary) (pt age < 60 yr)	X				no			NA
Lymphoma of the brain (primary) (pt age > 60 yr)	X				yes			NA
Lymphoid interstitial pneumonia or hyperplasia (pt age < 13 yr)	X	X, CXR[b]			no	X[b]		yes

Table 1-3 (continued)

Disease[a]	Definitive diagnosis						Presumptive diagnosis				
	Symptoms or exam	Histology/ cytology	Endos-copy/ autopsy	Laboratory/ clinical test	R/O other causes	HIV testing required?	Clinical symp-toms	Physical exam	R/O other causes	Laboratory/ clinical test	HIV testing required?
Lymphoma, non-Hodgkin's						yes					NA
Mycobacteria tuberculosis (extrapulmonary)				culture		yes				AFB (+)	yes
Mycobacteria tuberculosis (pulmonary)				**culture**		**yes**				**AFB (+)**	**yes**
Mycobacterium avium complex, M. kansasii (site other than lungs, cervical, or hilar lymph nodes)				culture		no					NA

16

					AFB (+)	yes
Mycobacterium, other species or unidentified (site other than lungs, cervical, or hilar lymph nodes)	culture	yes			AFB (+)	yes
Pneumocystis carinii pneumonia (PCP)		no	X	X	ABG/PFT & CXR or gallium scan	yes
Pneumonia, recurrent (twice w/in a 12-mo period)	**culture & CXR**	**yes**	X		[c]	**NA**
Progressive multifocal leukoencephalopathy (PML)		no	X			NA
Salmonella septicemia (recurrent, non-typhoid)	culture	yes	X			NA
Toxoplasmosis of brain (pt age > 1 mo)		no	X	X	X[d]	yes

[a] Boldfaced type indicates addition to case definition.
[b] No response to antibiotic treatment, infiltrates present 2 mo or more.
[c] Cases that do not have lab confirmation of a causative organism for one of the episodes of pneumonia may be presumptively diagnosed.
[d] Brain imaging or radiography with contrast and serum antibody or response to therapy.

Source: Courtesy of Massachusetts Department of Public Health. Data from Centers for Disease Control, Revision of the CDC surveillance case definition for acquired immunodeficiency syndrome, MMWR 36(15): 1–15, 1987; and from Centers for Disease Control, 1993 Revised classification system for HIV infection and expanded surveillance case definition for AIDS among adolescents and adults, MMWR 41 (RR-17):1–19, 1992.

Table 1-4 1993 Revised classification system for HIV infection

CD4 cell count categories	Clinical categories		
	(A) Asymptomatic, primary HIV infection, or PGL	(B) Symptomatic, not A or C conditions	(C) AIDS-indicator conditions
1. ≥ 500/mm³	A1	B1	C1
2. 200–499/mm³	A2	B2	C2
3. < 200/mm³	A3	B3	C3

PGL = persistent generalized lymphadenopathy.
Note: Categories A3, B3, C1, C2, and C3 comprise the expanded AIDS surveillance case definition.
Source: Adapted from Centers for Disease Control, 1993 Revised classification system for HIV infection and expanded surveillance case definition for AIDS among adolescents and adults, *MMWR* 41(RR-17):1–19, 1992.

Several general systems for categorizing HIV disease have been described. The revised CDC classification system stratifies patients according to their clinical status and CD4 lymphocyte count [67] (Table 1-4). The Walter Reed Army Institute of Research has published a classification system that stratifies HIV infection according to the level of immunodeficiency [68]. Patients are placed in one of six stages based on CD4 lymphocyte counts, anergy panel skin testing, and the presence or absence of opportunistic infections. A more recent staging system developed by the World Health Organization (WHO) in July 1990 also uses four clinical stages based on a variety of definitive or presumptive clinical parameters or the individual's activity level, or both [69] (Table 1-5).

A clinically useful way to classify HIV infection is based on the management implications of the patient's CD4 cell count (Table 1-6). Group I includes those patients with CD4 counts greater than or equal to 500/mm³; group II, those with CD4 counts between 200 and 500/mm³; and group III, those with CD4 counts of less than 200/mm³. Antiretroviral therapy and prophylactic therapy against PCP are indicated in group III patients, antiretroviral therapy alone in group II, and neither in group I.

Conclusion

The AIDS epidemic, although still relatively new, represents one of the greatest challenges in human history. Although much has been learned

Table 1-5 *WHO clinical stages for HIV infection*

Clinical stage 1: Infected, presymptomatic
1. Asymptomatic
2. Persistent generalized lymphadenopathy

Performance scale 1: asymptomatic, normal activity

Clinical stage 2: Early (mild) disease
3. Weight loss < 10% of body weight
4. Minor mucocutaneous manifestations (seborrheic dermatitis, prurigo, fungal nail infections, recurrent oral ulcerations, angular cheilitis)
5. Herpes zoster, within the last 5 yr
6. Recurrent upper respiratory tract infections (e.g., bacterial sinusitis)

And/or performance scale 2: symptomatic, normal activity

Clinical stage 3: Intermediate (moderate) disease
7. Weight loss > 10% of body weight
8. Unexplained chronic diarrhea, > 1 mo
9. Unexplained prolonged fever (intermittent or constant), > 1 mo
10. Oral candidiasis (thrush)
11. Oral hairy leukoplakia
12. Pulmonary tuberculosis, within the past year
13. Severe bacterial infections (e.g., pneumonia, pyomyositis)

And/or performance scale 3: bedridden < 50% of the day during the last month

Clinical stage 4: Late (severe) disease (essentially equivalent to AIDS)
14. HIV wasting syndrome, as defined by CDC[a]
15. *Pneumocystis carinii* pneumonia
16. Toxoplasmosis of the brain
17. Cryptosporidiosis with diarrhea, > 1 mo
18. Cryptococcosis, extrapulmonary
19. Cytomegalovirus disease of an organ other than liver, spleen, or lymph nodes
20. Herpes simplex virus infection, mucocutaneous, > 1 mo, or visceral of any duration
21. Progressive multifocal leukoencephalopathy
22. Any disseminated endemic mycosis (e.g., histoplasmosis, coccidioidomycosis)
23. Candidiasis of the esophagus, trachea, bronchi, or lungs
24. Atypical mycobacteriosis, disseminated
25. Nontyphoid *Salmonella* septicemia
26. Extrapulmonary tuberculosis
27. Lymphoma
28. Kaposi's sarcoma
29. HIV encephalopathy, as defined by CDC[b]

And/or performance scale 4: bedridden > 50% of the day during the last month

[a] HIV wasting syndrome: Weight loss > 10% of body weight, plus either unexplained chronic diarrhea (> 1 mo), or chronic weakness and unexplained prolonged fever (> 1 mo).

[b] HIV encephalopathy: Clinical findings of disabling cognitive and/or motor dysfunction that interferes with activities of daily living, progressing over weeks to months, in the absence of a concurrent illness or condition other than HIV infection that could explain the findings.

Source: Adapted from *Weekly Epidemic Record* 29:221–224, 1990.

Table 1-6 Clinical staging of HIV infection

Group	Clinical assessment	Management
I	CD4 cell count ≥ 500; symptoms generally absent	No specific treatment
II	CD4 cell count ≥ 200 but < 500; symptoms may be present or absent	Antiretroviral therapy
III	CD4 cell count < 200; symptoms are common	Antiretroviral therapy; prophylaxis against *Pneumocystis carinii* pneumonia

about HIV infection over the past decade, the epidemic remains unchecked. The accessibility of people of all nations to one another has set the stage for rapid international spread of this disease. This same "global neighborhood" must be used to our advantage. We must blend our scientific knowledge about HIV infection with social and educational strategies if this deadly epidemic is to be controlled.

References

1. Gottlieb MS, Schanker HM, Fan PT, et al. Pneumocystis pneumonia—Los Angeles. *MMWR* 30:250–252, 1981.
2. Gottlieb MS, Schroff R, Schanker HM, et al. *Pneumocystis carinii* pneumonia and mucosal candidiasis in previously healthy homosexual men: Evidence of a new acquired cellular immunodeficiency. *N Engl J Med* 305:1425–1431,1981.
3. Mann JM, Chin J. AIDS: A global perspective. *N Engl J Med* 319:302–303, 1988.
4. Centers for Disease Control. Update on acquired immunodeficiency syndrome (AIDS)—United States. *MMWR* 31:507–514, 1982.
5. Centers for Disease Control. Revision of the CDC surveillance case definition for acquired immunodeficiency syndrome. *MMWR* 36 (suppl 1):3–15, 1987.
6. Centers for Disease Control. AIDS and human immunodeficiency virus infection in the United States: 1988 update. *MMWR* 38:1–14, 1988.
7. Barre-Sinoussi F, Chermann JC, Rey F, et al. Isolation of a T-lymphotropic retrovirus from a patient at risk for acquired immune deficiency syndrome (AIDS). *Science* 220:868–871, 1983.
8. Gallo RC, Salahuddin SZ, Popovic M, et al. Frequent detection and isolation of cytopathic retroviruses (HTLV-III) from patients with AIDS and at risk for AIDS. *Science* 224:500–503, 1984.
9. Broder S, Gallo RC. A pathogenic retrovirus (HTLV-III) linked to AIDS. *N Engl J Med* 311:1292–1297, 1984.

10. Centers for Disease Control. Provisional Public Health Service inter-agency recommendations for screening donated blood and plasma for antibody to the virus causing acquired immunodeficiency syndrome. *MMWR* 34:1–5, 1985.
11. Fischl MA, Richman DD, Grieco MH, et al. The efficacy of azidothymidine (AZT) in the treatment of patients with AIDS and AIDS-related complex. *N Engl J Med* 317:185–191, 1987.
12. Centers for Disease Control. Recommendations for prophylaxis against *Pneumocystis carinii* pneumonia for adults and adolescents infected with human immunodeficiency virus. *MMWR* 41(RR-4):1–11, 1992.
13. Moore RD, Hildalgo J, Sugland BW, Chaisson RE. Zidovudine and the nat-ural history of the acquired immunodeficiency syndrome. *N Engl J Med* 324:1412–1416, 1991.
14. Osmond D. Growth of the Epidemic in the U.S.: Rates for Incidence and Mortality. In PT Cohen, MA Sande, PA Volberding (eds), *The AIDS Knowl-edge Base.* Waltham, MA: The Medical Publishing Group, 1990. (1.5) Pp 1–5.
15. Massachusetts Department of Public Health. *Massachusetts AIDS Surveil-lance Monthly Update,* January 1, 1992.
16. Centers for Disease Control. Update: Acquired immunodeficiency syn-drome—United States. *MMWR* 35:757, 1986.
17. Centers for Disease Control. The second 100,000 cases of acquired immunodeficiency syndrome—United States, June 1981–December 1991. *MMWR* 41:28–29, 1992.
18. Carpenter CCJ, Mayer KH, Stein MD, et al. Human immunodeficiency virus infection in North American women: Experience with 200 cases and a review of the literature. *Medicine* 70:307–325, 1991.
19. Osmond D. Prevalence of Infection and Projections for the Future. In PT Cohen, MA Sande, PA Volberding (eds), *The AIDS Knowledge Base.* Wal-tham, MA: The Medical Publishing Group, 1990. (1.7) Pp 1–8.
20. Friedland G. Parenteral Drug Users. In RA Kaslow, DP Francis (eds), *Epi-demiology of AIDS Expression, Occurrence and Control of Human Immu-nodeficiency Virus Type 1 Infection.* Oxford, UK: Oxford University Press, 1989. Pp 153–178.
21. DeCock KM, Brun-Vezinet F. Epidemiology of HIV-2 infection. *AIDS* 3 (suppl 1):S89–S95, 1989.
22. Padian N, Marquis L, Francis DP, et al. Male-to-female transmission of human immunodeficiency virus. *JAMA* 258:788–790, 1987.
23. Winkelstein W, Jr, Padian NS, Rutherford G, Jaffe HW. Homosexual Men. In RA Kaslow, DP Francis (eds), *Epidemiology of AIDS Expression, Occur-rence and Control of Human Immunodeficiency Virus Type 1 Infection.* Oxford, UK: Oxford University Press, 1989. Pp 117–135.
24. Hessol NA, O'Malley P, Lifson A, et al. Incidence and prevalence of HIV infection among homosexual and bisexual men, 1979–1988. Fifth Inter-national Conference on AIDS, Montreal, June 1989.
25. Berkelman R, Karon J, Thomas P, et al. Are AIDS cases among homosexual males leveling? Fifth International Conference on AIDS, Montreal, June 1989.

26. Centers for Disease Control. Update: Acquired immunodeficiency syndrome—United States, 1989. *MMWR* 39:81–86, 1990.

27. Cumming PD, Wallace EL, Schorr JB, Dodd RY. Exposure of patients to human immunodeficiency virus through the transfusion of blood components that test antibody negative. *N Engl J Med* 321:941–946, 1989.

28. Ward JW, Bush TJ, Perkins HA, et al. The natural history of transfusion-associated infection with human immunodeficiency virus: Factors influencing the rate of progression to disease. *N Engl J Med* 321:947–952, 1989.

29. Rogers M. Perinatal Infection. In RA Kaslow, DP Francis (eds), *Epidemiology of AIDS Expression, Occurrence and Control of Human Immunodeficiency Virus Type 1 Infection.* Oxford, UK: Oxford University Press, 1989. Pp 231–241.

30. Steger KA, Craven DE, Shea BF, et al. Use of paper-absorbed fingerstick blood samples for studies of antibody to human immunodeficiency virus type 1 in intravenous drug users. *J Infect Dis* 162:964–967, 1990.

31. Steger KA, Zawacki A, Allen D, et al. Antibody to HIV-1 in intravenous drug users (IVDU) entering methadone treatment programs (MTP) in Boston. Sixth International Conference on AIDS, San Francisco, June 1990.

32. Donegan SP, Steger KA, Recla L, et al. Seroprevalence of human immunodeficiency virus in parturients at Boston City Hospital: Implications for public health and obstetrical practice. *Am J Obstet Gynecol* 167:622–629, 1992.

33. Clumeck N, Taelman H, Hermans P, et al. A cluster of HIV among heterosexual people without apparent risk factors. *N Engl J Med* 321:1460–1462, 1989.

34. Osmond D. Heterosexual Transmission of HIV. In PT Cohen, MA Sande, PA Volberding (eds), *The AIDS Knowledge Base.* Waltham, MA: The Medical Publishing Group, 1990. (2.4) Pp 1–9.

35. Peterman TA, Stoneburner RL, Allen JR, et al. Risk of human immunodeficiency virus transmission from heterosexual adults with transfusion-associated infections. *JAMA* 259:55–58, 1988.

36. Cameron DW, Plummer FA, Simonsen JN, et al. Female to male heterosexual transmission of HIV infection in Nairobi. Third International Conference on AIDS, Washington, DC, June 1987.

37. Seage GR, Horsburg CR, Hardy AM, et al. Increased suppressor T cells in probable transmitters of HIV. *Am J Public Health* 79:1638–1642, 1989.

38. Coates RA, Calzavara L, Read SE, et al. Risk factors for HIV infection in male sexual contacts of men with AIDS or an AIDS related condition. *Am J Epidemiol* 128:729–739, 1988.

39. Quinn TC, et al. Evaluation of the human immunodeficiency virus epidemic among patients attending sexually transmitted disease clinics: A decade of experience. *J Infect Dis* 165:541–544, 1992.

40. Ryder RW, Wats N, Hassig SE, et al. Perinatal transmission of the human immunodeficiency virus type 1 to infants of seropositive women in Zaire. *N Engl J Med* 320:1637–1642, 1989.

41. Ades AE, Newell ML, Peckham CS, et al. Mother-to-child transmission of

HIV infection: The European Collaborative Study. *Lancet* 2:1039–1042, 1988.

42. Scott GB, Hutto C, Makuch RW, et al. Survival in children with perinatally acquired human immunodeficiency virus type 1 infection. *N Engl J Med* 321:1791–1796, 1989.

43. Schoenbaum EE, Hartel D, Selwyn PA, et al. Risk factors for human immunodeficiency virus infection in intravenous drug users. *N Engl J Med* 321:874–879, 1989.

44. Peterman T, Allen J. Recipients of Blood and Blood Products. In RA Kaslow, DP Francis (eds), *Epidemiology of AIDS Expression, Occurrence and Control of Human Immunodeficiency Virus Type 1 Infection*. Oxford, UK: Oxford University Press, 1989. Pp 179–193.

45. Fischl MA, Dickinson GM, Scott GB, et al. Evaluation of heterosexual partners, children, and household contacts of adults with AIDS. *JAMA* 257:640–644, 1987.

46. Centers for Disease Control. Public Health Service statement of management of occupational exposure to human immunodeficiency virus, including considerations regarding zidovudine postexposure use. *MMWR* 39:1–14, 1990.

47. Maiman M, Fruchter RG, Serur E, et al. Human immunodeficiency virus infection and cervical neoplasia. *Gynecol Oncol* 38:377–382, 1990.

48. Chu SY, Buchler JW, Berkelman R. Impact of the human immunodeficiency virus epidemic on mortality of women of reproductive age, United States. *JAMA* 264:225–229, 1990.

49. Varmus H. Retroviruses. *Science* 240:1427–1436, 1988.

50. Burke DS, Redfield RR. The Stages of HIV Infection: A Predictable Progressive Disease. In *HIV Infections and Disease: Monographs for Physicians and Other Health Care Workers*. Chicago: American Medical Association, 1989.

51. Cooper DA, Gold J, Maclean P, et al. Acute AIDS retrovirus infection: definition of a clinical illness associated with seroconversion. *Lancet* 1:537–540, 1985.

52. Ho DD, Sarngadharan MG, Resnick L, et al. Primary human T-lymphotropic virus type III infection. *Ann Intern Med* 103:880–883, 1985.

53. Eyster ME, Gail MH, Ballard JO. Natural history of human immunodeficiency virus infections in hemophiliacs: Effect on T-cell subsets, platelet count, and age. *Ann Intern Med* 107:1–6, 1987.

54. Piette AM, Tusseau F, Vignon D, et al. Acute neuropathy coincident with seroconversion for anti-LAV/HTLV-III. *Lancet* 1:852–853, 1986.

55. Bacchett P, Moss AR. Incubation period of AIDS in San Francisco. *Nature* 338:251–253, 1989.

56. Kaplan JE, Spira TJ, Fishbein DB, et al. A six-year follow-up of HIV-infected homosexual men with lymphadenopathy: Evidence for an increased risk for developing AIDS after the third year of lymphadenopathy. *JAMA* 260:2694–2697, 1988.

57. Moss AR, Bacchetti P, Osmond D, et al. Seropositivity for HIV and the development of AIDS or AIDS related condition: Three year follow up

of the San Francisco General Hospital cohort. *Br Med J* 296:745–750, 1988.

58. Margolick JB, et al. Changes in T-lymphocyte subsets in intravenous drug users with HIV-1 infection. *JAMA* 267:1631–1636, 1992.

59. Graham NMH, et al. The effects on survival of early treatment of human immunodeficiency virus infection. *N Engl J Med* 326:1037–1042, 1992.

60. Phillips AN, et al. Prognostic indicators for the development of AIDS among intravenous drug users. *JAMA* 268:2662–2666, 1992.

61. Stein M, et al. Causes of death in persons with human immunodeficiency virus infection. *Am J Med* 93:387–392, 1992.

62. Rothenberg R, Woelfel M, Stoneburner R, et al. Survival with the acquired immunodeficiency syndrome. *N Engl J Med* 317:1297–1302, 1987.

63. Creagh-Kirk T, Doi P, Andrews E, et al. Survival experience among patients with AIDS receiving zidovudine. *JAMA* 260:3009–3015, 1988.

64. Munoz A, et al. Prognostic indicators for the development of AIDS among intravenous drug users. *J AIDS* 5:694–700, 1992.

65. Lemp GF, Payne SF, Neal D, et al. Survival trends for patients with AIDS. *JAMA* 263:402–406, 1990.

66. Harris JE. Improved short term survival of AIDS patients initially diagnosed with *Pneumocystis carinii* pneumonia, 1984 through 1987. *JAMA* 263:397–401, 1990.

67. Centers for Disease Control. 1993 Revised classification system for HIV infection and expanded surveillance case definition for AIDS among adolescents and adults. *MMWR* 41(RR-17):1–19, 1992.

68. Redfield RR, Wright DC, Tramont EC. The Walter Reed staging classification for HTLV-III/LAV infection. *N Engl J Med* 314:131–132, 1986.

69. Laurence J. AIDS Statistics Update. *The AIDS Reader* 1:150, 1991.

2/HIV Diagnostic Testing

Donald E. Craven, Kathleen A. Steger

The isolation of human immunodeficiency virus (HIV), type 1, was first reported in 1983, and enzyme immunoassays (EIAs or ELISAs) to detect antibodies to HIV became available in March 1985 [1–3]. First-generation EIAs were derived from crude tissue culture lysates of HIV and were designed to screen blood donors. Second-generation EIAs, using HIV proteins produced by recombinant technology, have improved sensitivity and specificity. To increase specificity further, positive EIA results are confirmed by Western blot (WB) testing. In addition to EIAs and WB, a number of other tests are now available to diagnose HIV infection (Table 2-1).

Although the diagnosis of HIV infection is often made clinically, serologic tests are helpful for confirmation, and are particularly useful in asymptomatic patients and persons with atypical presentations (Table 2-2). The availability of antiretroviral therapy has increased demand for HIV testing, but numerous legal and ethical issues persist [1, 4–7].

This chapter provides an overview of the serologic tests used to detect the presence of HIV infection. These include p24 antigen, antibodies to the HIV core and surface antigens, HIV culture, and polymerase chain reaction (PCR) amplification to detect proviral DNA in peripheral blood mononuclear cells (PBMCs). HIV culture, PCR, and specific antibody to p24 (anti-p24) are not currently available to most clinicians. Readers are also referred to more detailed reviews of tests for diagnosing and staging of HIV infection [2, 8–10].

Recently a clinical syndrome similar to HIV disease, but without laboratory evidence of HIV infection, has been recognized in a limited number of patients [11]. The epidemiology and natural history of this condition—idiopathic CD4 lymphocytopenia—are currently under investigation by the Centers for Disease Control. The relationship of this syndrome to HIV infection is uncertain.

The Structure of HIV

Familiarity with the HIV genome and structure is essential to understanding serologic testing (Fig. 2-1). The major components of the HIV

25

Table 2-1 Diagnostic tests for HIV infection

HIV antibodies
   Enzyme immunoassay
   Latex agglutination
   Western blot
   Indirect immunofluorescent antibody
   Radioimmunoassays (anti-p24, anti-gp41, anti-gp120)*
Serologic tests for p24 antigen
HIV culture*
Polymerase chain reaction or gene amplification*

*Not readily available for clinical use.

Table 2-2 Clinical use of diagnostic tests for HIV

Diagnosis of HIV disease (HIV antibody tests)
   Acute infection (p24 appears before anti-HIV)
   Asymptomatic carrier; latent infection
   Persistent, generalized lymphadenopathy
   Unexplained fever and weight loss
   Unexplained neurologic disease
   Unusual or recurrent skin rashes
   Recurrent or unusual bacterial infections
   Opportunistic infections or malignancies
Progression of HIV disease (p24 antigen, CD4 cell count)
Response to antiretroviral therapy (p24 antigen, CD4 cell count)

RNA genome include the *gag* region, producing p17, p24, and p55 core proteins, and the *env* (envelope portion), which is responsible for the surface glycoproteins gp120 and gp41 [12, 13]. The *pol* portion of the HIV genome also produces the enzyme reverse transcriptase for integrating viral RNA into cellular DNA and the regulator genes *tat, rev, net* (*orf* B), and *vif.*

HIV Antibody Assays

Anti-HIV appears to be a good marker of active or latent infection and is presently the mainstay for clinical diagnosis of HIV infection. Enzyme immunoassay is the standard diagnostic screening test for HIV in the United States.

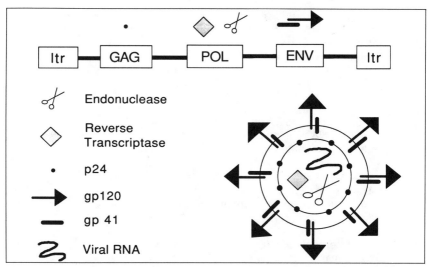

Figure 2-1. Schematic representation of HIV genome and virus with core and envelope proteins (ltr = long terminal repeat segment). (Courtesy of Dr. Jon Fuller, Boston City Hospital.)

Enzyme Immunoassay

There are seven commercially available EIA kits for the diagnosis of HIV infection, each with slightly different antigens and reagents [2, 8, 9, 14]. All EIA results are confirmed by WB or immunofluorescent antibody (IFA) testing. An EIA sample with very high absorbance, indicating high levels of antibody, generally indicates a true positive result, whereas a low titer is more difficult to interpret and may represent a false-positive test or early infection. Of note is the fact that many of the EIAs for HIV-1 also detect up to 90 percent of HIV-2 strains.

The EIA test is performed by incubating patient sera in the wells of microtiter plates coated with recombinant HIV antigens [2, 8, 9, 14]. If HIV antibodies (immunoglobulin G) are present, they will bind to the antigen-coated wall of the microtiter plate. After washing, an enzyme-linked goat anti-human antibody is added, incubated, and washed out. The amount of bound antibody is measured by spectrophotometric analysis of the color produced by cleavage of substrate added to the well. The absorbance values are compared to positive and negative control wells. All samples that are initially positive are repeated. Positive EIA results are routinely confirmed by WB or IFA testing before they are reported to patients.

Each of the seven EIA kits has a sensitivity and specificity greater than 98 percent, with many approaching 100 percent [2, 8, 9, 14]. Several factors may result in false-positive and false-negative EIAs (Table 2-3).

Table 2-3 Causes of false-positive and false-negative EIAs

False-positive EIA
Antibodies against class II leukocyte antigens
Antibodies against smooth-muscle, parietal cell, mitochondrial, nuclear, leukocyte, and T-cell antigens
Severe alcoholic liver disease, primary biliary cirrhosis
Heat inactivation or positive syphilis serology
Hematologic malignancies, lymphoma
Acute DNA viral infection, HIV-2 infection
Renal transplants, chronic renal failure
Stevens-Johnson syndrome
Passively acquired anti-HIV from hepatitis B immunoglobulin

False-negative EIA
Acute disease before seroconversion ("window period")
Malignancy
Intensive or long-term immunosuppressive therapy
Replacement transfusion
Bone marrow transplantation
EIAs that primarily detect antibody to p24
B-cell dysfunction

Source: Adapted from B Lo, RL Steinbrook, M Cooke, et al, Voluntary screening for HIV infection. *Ann Intern Med* 110:727–733, 1989.

In a high-risk population, the false-positive EIA rate will be low and the positive predictive value will be high. Conversely, in a low-risk population, the number of false-positive EIAs will be high and the predictive value will be low [8, 14, 15].

Western Blot

Commercially available kits for WB are licensed by the Food and Drug Administration to confirm positive EIAs. In comparison to the EIA, WB, which identifies antibodies to specific HIV proteins, is a poor screening test [2, 8, 9, 14]. Western blot is costly and labor intensive, and its reagents and interpretation are not standardized.

The WB procedure involves the separation of HIV proteins by molecular weight using gel electrophoresis. The proteins are then transferred or "blotted" to nitrocellulose paper. Next, serum is layered over the paper to allow antibodies to bind to specific HIV core and surface antigens. After washing, the specific bound antibodies are detected by goat anti-human globulins conjugated to an enzyme or radioactive probe. Although interpretation and scoring of the WB often vary between laboratories, standards for interpretation have been suggested [2, 8, 9, 14, 16]. A positive WB should contain antibodies against two of three major protein bands or a reaction with each of three gene products.

Western blot with protein markers that do not meet the diagnostic criteria for HIV is considered indeterminate. The number of indeterminate results varies with the population sampled and strictness of criteria used to define a positive test. Persons with an indeterminate WB should have their test repeated in 3 to 6 months. In one study, only 4 of 93 blood donors with a repeatedly reactive EIA and indeterminate WB (reactive to p24 only) eventually developed a positive WB [17]. The likelihood of indeterminate WBs later being identified as positive increases in patients who continue to practice high-risk behaviors for HIV transmission.

In one report false-positive HIV test results using EIA and WB were identified in fewer than 1 in 135,000 Army recruits [18]. Likewise, in a study of 630,190 units of blood from 290,110 donors, false-positive EIA and WB testing occurred in 6 of 10,000 samples [19]. False-positive rates are higher in inexperienced laboratories. In one study, 10 of 19 laboratories bidding to perform WB testing for the military failed proficiency testing at least once [20]. In addition to the characteristics of the population sampled, sensitivity and specificity vary by the criteria used to interpret the WB. False-positive tests can result from the presence of other serum proteins, proteins in the filter paper, antibodies to other retroviral antigens, and antibodies to mitochondrial, nuclear or leukocyte antigens, and class I or II HLA antigens [2, 8, 9, 14].

Immunofluorescent Antibody

Immunofluorescent antibody testing is an alternative to the WB for confirmation of EIA results; it has comparable sensitivity and specificity [2, 8, 9, 14]. IFA requires the use of an immunofluorescent microscope and a skilled technician, but is less costly and more rapid than WB. To perform IFA, a slide is prepared with crude HIV antigen, and serum is laid over the slide so that, if antibodies are present, they will bind to specific HIV antigens. The slide is then washed and goat anti-human fluorescent antibody is added. The level of fluorescence on the test slide is compared to control slides with uninfected tissue culture cells.

Rapid Tests

Because of the expense and equipment required for detection of HIV antibody by EIA, WB, and IFA, rapid and inexpensive screening tests, such as latex agglutination, red cell agglutination, or dipstick, are needed. Such assays would be particularly useful in developing countries [21–23]. The latex agglutination assay can be performed in minutes with a minimum of technical skill. Data obtained from screening high-risk populations indicate a sensitivity of greater than 99 percent and specificity of 100 percent. Further studies are needed in low-risk populations. Good quality control is required to perform these tests, and some states have prohibited them from use outside of licensed laboratories.

HIV Antigen Assays

Commercial assays are available for p24 antigen in serum, plasma, and cerebrospinal fluid [2, 8, 9, 24]. This antigen is a marker for viral replication and is present both in early HIV infection and in advanced symptomatic disease. Assays for p24 may be useful in monitoring disease activity and response to therapy [25–28]. HIV p24 antigenemia may be present as early as 2 weeks after primary HIV infection and persist for months before anti-HIV becomes detectable. Persistence of p24 antigenemia in primary HIV infection may be a poor prognostic sign [26, 28].

The assay is performed by coating microtiter plates or beads with anti-p24. If antigen is present it binds to the antibody; the well is washed, and a second anti-p24 antibody is added. This is followed with an enzyme-linked goat anti-human antibody. Levels of p24 antigen as low as 10 to 50 pg/ml can be reliably detected. Sensitivity of the assay may be improved by acid hydrolysis of serum to release p24 bound in antigen-antibody complexes [29]. The presence of antigen late in disease appears to correlate with the loss of p24 antibody, the presence of symptoms, and progression to AIDS [8, 24, 26, 28].

HIV Culture

Culture of HIV is difficult, expensive, and not routinely available for diagnostic use [2, 8, 9, 30]. HIV culture may be helpful in specific clinical settings, but special laboratory facilities are required for biohazard containment [30, 31]. It is useful for characterization of viral isolates, evaluating resistance to antiretroviral therapy, and diagnosis in neonates or patients with unusual manifestations of HIV disease. Culture is performed by incubating peripheral blood mononuclear cells in tissue culture. Assays for p24 antigen and reverse transcriptase can be used to establish the presence of the virus [2, 9, 30].

Using improved techniques for HIV culture, Coombs and associates [32] demonstrated that over 97 percent of 213 HIV-infected persons had positive HIV cultures of PBMCs regardless of CD4 count or clinical stage of infection. By comparison, plasma viremia was detected in 23 percent of patients with asymptomatic infection, 45 percent of patients with AIDS-related complex, and 82 percent of patients with AIDS. Plasma HIV titers ranged from 10^0 to $10^{4.3}$, were higher in patients with symptomatic disease, and were associated with a decline in CD4 lymphocytes. Ho and colleagues [33] reported the presence of HIV in 100 percent of the peripheral blood and plasma samples from HIV-positive patients. Plasma and PBMC titers of HIV were over 100-fold higher in symptomatic than in asymptomatic patients; approximately 1 in 400 circulating mononuclear cells harbored HIV in symptomatic individuals. Of note is the fact that treatment with zidovudine significantly lowered plasma but not PBMC titers of HIV, and levels in treated patients were 25-fold lower than those of untreated symptomatic patients.

Polymerase Chain Reaction

Polymerase chain reaction is a highly sensitive gene amplification technique that can detect fragments of HIV in the peripheral blood mononuclear cells of infected patients [34–39]. The PCR method is based on a repetition of three steps: denaturation, annealing of the extension primers (synthetic oligonucleotides of viral DNA), and primer extension or amplification [34]. Target sequences of the virus are identified, and DNA probes designed to attach to the target sequences are coupled to a proprietary detection system. PCR may be sensitive enough to detect one HIV sequence in 100,000 host cells.

Polymerase chain reaction can be used to identify patients with early or latent infection (no detectable antibody to HIV) and detect infection in newborns or children who have HIV immunoglobulin G (IgG) antibody from their mother [34, 35, 37, 40]. PCR can also be utilized to assess patients with a positive EIA and an indeterminate WB. Imgawa and associates used PCR to diagnose HIV infection several years before the development of a positive EIA, but this was a highly select group of patients who may have continued to practice high-risk behaviors [36, 41]. Others have been unable to corroborate these findings [42, 43]. Because of the high sensitivity of PCR, there is a concern over the risk of laboratory contamination, underscoring the need for good controls. Further data are needed to clarify the clinical role of PCR.

Clinical Use of HIV Diagnostic Tests

HIV Antibody Testing

The question of who should be tested for HIV and under what circumstances remains controversial. Persons for whom HIV antibody testing

Table 2-4 *Persons at risk for HIV infection*

Individuals who received a blood transfusion between 1978 and 1985
Homosexual/bisexual men and their sexual partners
Injection drug users
Persons with sexually transmitted diseases
Prostitutes
Prisoners
Women of childbearing age who are at risk through drug use, prostitution, unprotected sex
Children born to HIV-infected mothers
Persons born in endemic areas
Heterosexuals having "unsafe sex" or multiple sexual partners

Source: Adapted from Perspectives in disease prevention and health promotion: Public Health Service guidelines for counseling and antibody testing to prevent HIV infection and AIDS. *MMWR* 36:509–515, 1987.

should be considered are listed in Table 2-4. Voluntary testing should be offered to persons who are at risk for HIV infection [1]. Mandatory testing in the United States is currently performed on blood donors, military recruits, and some life and health insurance applicants. Routine, voluntary HIV testing of 15- to 54-year-old patients hospitalized in high prevalence areas has recently been proposed [44]. HIV antibody screening is used routinely in hospitals for the screening of donors of tissue for organ transplantation. Efforts have been made to institute HIV screening of high-risk patients before elective surgery, and recommendations were recently published for screening health care workers who perform "high-risk" procedures [45]. Referral sites for anonymous or mandatory HIV testing and counseling are available in most states [1]. These include "alternative test sites," hospital clinics, sexually transmitted disease clinics, drug clinics, and the American Red Cross.

Physician Responsibilities

The AIDS epidemic continues to grow, and physicians will be asked increasingly often about the risks and benefits of HIV testing. Potential risks include a false-positive test, anxiety and depression, loss of confidentiality, and discrimination. For some patients, depression may be severe enough to pose the risk of suicide. On the other hand, for those who are seropositive, testing can provide the opportunity for early medical intervention and improved quality of life.

After appropriate counseling, informed consent should be obtained before HIV testing. Specific responsibilities of the physician include educating patients, discussing the confidentiality of HIV test results, urging individuals who are seropositive to notify sexual partners, counseling them to reduce risky behaviors, and ensuring the availability of medical and psychological care [6, 7]. Confidentiality of test results should be strictly maintained in accordance with hospital and state regulations.

Serologic Response in HIV Disease

p24 antigen initially appears shortly after the acquisition of HIV, approximately 1 to 4 months before anti-HIV, and is present during the acute HIV infection [8, 46] (see Fig. 1-3). The decrease in p24 antigen is associated with the appearance of p24 antibody, which generally signals progression to the asymptomatic phase of HIV infection. Months to years after infection, antibody to p24 is lost and p24 antigen reappears, often in association with symptomatic HIV disease. HIV replication correlates with the presence of p24 antigen.

T-Lymphocyte Phenotyping

Positive diagnostic tests for HIV are usually followed by phenotypic analysis of lymphocytes to evaluate a patient's degree of immunosuppression related to HIV infection and appropriate clinical management. T lymphocytes express CD3 (T3) markers on their surface, and can be further subdivided into cells that express the helper/inducer phenotype (CD4 or T4) or suppressor/cytotoxic phenotype (CD8 or T8) [2]. Patients with HIV infection have a decline in both the absolute number and percentage of CD4 lymphocytes over time [47, 48]. This determination is usually made by staining peripheral blood leukocytes with antibody to CD3, CD4, and CD8, which are then analyzed by a fluorescence-activated cell sorter [49]. When the patient's CD4 count becomes less than 500/mm^3, antiretroviral therapy is indicated [50]. When the CD4 count becomes less than 200/mm^3 or following an episode of *Pneumocystis carinii* pneumonia (PCP), prophylaxis against PCP is instituted [51].

References

1. Perspectives in disease prevention and health promotion: Public Health Service guidelines for counseling and antibody testing to prevent HIV infection and AIDS. *MMWR* 36:509–515, 1987.

2. Davey RT, Lane HC. Laboratory methods in the diagnosis and prognostic staging of infection with human immunodeficiency virus type 1. *Rev Infect Dis* 12:912–930, 1990.
3. Barre-Sinoussi F, Chermann JC, Rey F, et al. Isolation of a T-lymphotropic retrovirus from a patient at risk for acquired immune deficiency syndrome (AIDS). *Science* 220:868–871, 1983.
4. Fischl MA, Richman DD, Hansen N, et al. Safety and efficacy of zidovudine (AZT) in the treatment of subjects with mildly symptomatic human immunodeficiency virus type 1 (HIV) infection. *Ann Intern Med* 112:727–737, 1990.
5. Drugs for AIDS and associated infections. *Med Lett Drugs Ther* 33:95–102, 1991.
6. Lo B, Steinbrook RL, Cooke M, et al. Voluntary screening for HIV infection. *Ann Intern Med* 110:727–733, 1989.
7. Volberding PA, Cohen PT. Indications for Use of HIV Antibody Testing. In PT Cohen, MA Sande, PA Volberding (eds), *The AIDS Knowledge Base*. Waltham, MA: The Medical Publishing Group, 1990. (2.1.1) Pp 1–9.
8. Schleupner CJ. Detection of HIV-1 Infection. In GL Mandell, RG Douglas, Jr, JE Bennett (eds), *Principles and Practice of Infectious Diseases* (3rd ed). New York: Churchill Livingstone, 1990. Pp 1092–1102.
9. Jackson JB, Balfour HH, Jr. Practical diagnostic testing for human immunodeficiency virus. *Clin Microbiol Rev* 1:124–138, 1988.
10. Steckelberg JM, Cockerill FR, III. Serologic testing for human immunodeficiency virus antibodies. *Mayo Clin Proc* 63:373–380, 1988.
11. Conference Summary Report. Eighth International Conference on AIDS, Amsterdam, July 1992.
12. Gallo RC, Wong-Staal F. Human T-lymphotropic retrovirus (HTLV-III) as the cause of the acquired immunodeficiency syndrome. *Ann Intern Med* 103:679–689, 1985.
13. Essex M, Allan J, Kanki P, et al. Antigens of human T-lymphocyte virus type III/lymphadenopathy-associated virus. *Ann Intern Med* 103:700–703, 1985.
14. Wilber J. HIV Antibody Testing: Methodology. In PT Cohen, MA Sande, PA Volberding (eds), *The AIDS Knowledge Base*. Waltham, MA: The Medical Publishing Group, 1990. (2.1.2) Pp 1–8.
15. Carlson JR, Bryant ML, Hinrichs SH, et al. AIDS serology testing in low and high risk groups. *JAMA* 253:3405–3408, 1985.
16. Centers for Disease Control. Interpretive criteria used to report Western blot results for HIV-1-antibody-testing—United States. *MMWR* 40:692–695, 1991.
17. Kleinman S, Fitzpatrick L, Secord K, Wilke D. Follow-up testing and notification of anti-HIV Western blot atypical (indeterminate) donors. *Transfusion* 28:280–282, 1988.
18. Burke DS, Brundage JF, Redfield RR, et al. Measurement of the false-positive rate in a screening program for human immunodeficiency virus infections. *N Engl J Med* 319:961–964, 1988.
19. MacDonald KL, Jackson JB, Bowman RJ, et al. Performance characteristics of serologic tests for human immunodeficiency virus type 1 (HIV-1) anti-

body among Minnesota blood donors. *Ann Intern Med* 110:617–621, 1989.

20. Centers for Disease Control. Update: Serologic testing for antibodies to human immunodeficiency virus. *MMWR* 36:833–845, 1988.

21. Quinn TC, Riggin CH, Kline RL, et al. Rapid latex agglutination assay using recombinant envelope polypeptide for the detection of antibody to the HIV. *JAMA* 260:510–513, 1988.

22. Kemp BE, Rylatt DB, Bundesen PG, et al. Autologous red cell agglutination assay for HIV-I antibodies: Simplified test with whole blood. *Science* 241:1352–1354, 1988.

23. Van de Perre P, Nzaramba D, Allen S, et al. Comparison of six serological assays for human immunodeficiency virus antibody detection in developing countries. *J Clin Microbiol* 26:552–556, 1988.

24. Crowe S, Mills J, McGrath M. HIV Antigen Testing. In PT Cohen, MA Sande, PA Volberding (eds), *The AIDS Knowledge Base*. Waltham, MA: The Medical Publishing Group, 1990. (2.1.3) Pp 1–4.

25. Chaisson RE, Allain JP, Leuther M, Volberding PA. Significant changes in HIV antigen level in the serum of patients treated with azidothymidine. *N Engl J Med* 315:1610–1611, 1986.

26. Lange JMA, Paul DA, Huisman H, et al. Persistent HIV antigenemia and decline of HIV core antibodies associated with transition to AIDS. *Br Med J* 293:1459–1462, 1986.

27. Goudsmit J, Paul DA, Lange JMA, et al. Expression of human immunodeficiency virus antigen (HIV-Ag) in serum and cerebrospinal fluid during acute and chronic infection. *Lancet* 2:177–180, 1986.

28. Goudsmit J, Lange JMA, Paul DA, Dawson GJ. Antigenemia and antibody titers to core and envelope antigens in AIDS, AIDS-related complex, and subclinical human immunodeficiency virus infection. *J Infect Dis* 155:558–560, 1987.

29. Bollinger RC, Kline R, Francis H, et al. Acid hydrolysis increases the sensitivity of p24 antigen detection for the evaluation of antiviral therapy in asymptomatic HIV-1 infected individuals. Seventh International Conference on AIDS, Florence, Italy, June 1991.

30. McGrath MS. HIV Isolation and Cultivation. In PT Cohen, MA Sande, PA Volberding (eds), *The AIDS Knowledge Base*. Waltham, MA: The Medical Publishing Group, 1990. (2.1.4) Pp 1–4.

31. Levy JA, Shimabukuro J. Recovery of AIDS-associated retroviruses from patients with AIDS related conditions and clinically healthy individuals. *J Infect Dis* 152:734–738, 1985.

32. Coombs RW, Collier AC, Allain JP, et al. Plasma viremia in human immunodeficiency virus infection. *N Engl J Med* 321:1626–1631, 1989.

33. Ho DD, Moudgil T, Alam M. Quantitation of human immunodeficiency virus type 1 in the blood of infected persons. *N Engl J Med* 321:1621–1625, 1989.

34. Cohen PT. Assays for HIV Nucleic Acid: The Polymerase Chain Reaction. In PT Cohen, MA Sande, PA Volberding (eds), *The AIDS Knowledge Base*. Waltham, MA: The Medical Publishing Group, 1990. (2.1.5) Pp 1–5.

35. Rogers MF, Ou CY, Rayfield M, et al. Use of PCR for early detection of

proviral sequences of HIV in infants born to seropositive mothers. *N Engl J Med* 320:1649–1654, 1989.

36. Imagawa DT, Lee MH, Wolinsky SM, et al. Human immunodeficiency virus type 1 infection in homosexual men who remain seronegative for prolonged periods. *N Engl J Med* 320:1458–1462, 1989.

37. Wolinsky SM, Rinaldo CR, Kwok S, et al. Human immunodeficiency virus type 1 (HIV-1) infection a median of 18 months before a diagnostic Western blot. *Ann Intern Med* 111:961–972, 1989.

38. Luce M, McCreedy B, Chimera J. Polymerase chain reaction amplification for the detection of human immunodeficiency virus. *Infect Med* 8:50–56, 1991.

39. Muul LM. Current status of polymerase chain reaction assays in clinical research of human immunodeficiency virus infection. *AIDS Updates* 3:1–19, 1990.

40. Katz SL, Wilfert CM. Human immunodeficiency virus infection of newborns. *N Engl J Med* 320:1687–1689, 1989.

41. Imagawa D, Detels R. HIV-1 in seronegative homosexual men. *N Engl J Med* 325:1250–1251, 1991.

42. Horsburgh CR, Jr, Ou CY, Jason J, et al. Concordance of polymerase chain reaction with human immunodeficiency virus antibody detection. *J Infect Dis* 162:542–545, 1990.

43. Horsburgh CR, Jr, Jason J, Longini IM, Jr, et al. Duration of human immunodeficiency virus infection before detection of antibody. *Lancet* 2:637–640, 1989.

44. Janssen RS, et al. HIV infection among patients in U.S. acute care hospitals: Strategies for counseling and testing of hospital patients. *N Engl J Med* 327:445–452, 1992.

45. Centers for Disease Control. Recommendations for preventing transmission of human immunodeficiency virus and hepatitis B virus to patients during exposure-prone invasive procedures. *MMWR* 40:1–9, 1991.

46. Allain JP, Laurian Y, Paul DA, et al. Long-term evaluation of HIV antigen and antibodies to p24 and gp41 in patients with hemophilia. *N Engl J Med* 317:1114–1121, 1987.

47. Lane HC, Fauci AS. Immunologic abnormalities in the acquired immunodeficiency syndrome. *Ann Rev Immunol* 3:477–500, 1985.

48. Masur H, Ognibene FP, Yarchoan R, et al. CD4 counts as predictors of opportunistic pneumonias in human immunodeficiency virus (HIV) infection. *Ann Intern Med* 111:223–231, 1989.

49. Taylor JM, Fahey JL, Detels R, Giorgi JV. CD4 percentage, CD4 number, and CD4:CD8 ratio in HIV infection: Which to choose and how to use. *J AIDS* 2:114–124, 1989.

50. Volberding PA, Lagakos SW, Koch MA, et al. Zidovudine in asymptomatic human immunodeficiency virus infection. *N Engl J Med* 322:941–949, 1990.

51. Centers for Disease Control. Recommendations for prophylaxis against *Pneumocystis carinii* pneumonia for adults and adolescents infected with human immunodeficiency virus. *MMWR* 41(RR-4):1–11, 1992.

3/Laboratory Evaluation

Abby Shevitz

As knowledge of HIV infection has increased, so has the availability and complexity of laboratory, radiologic, and invasive tests. Laboratory testing may be helpful in the management of HIV infection in a number of ways: (1) screening for common treatable processes, (2) staging and prognostication, (3) differential diagnosis, (4) supporting therapeutic decisions, and (5) clinical research. The utility of laboratory testing is limited by cost, availability, technical skill, and diagnostic yield. Laboratory tests used in the initial evaluation and health care maintenance of the HIV-infected patient are listed in Table 3-1.

Biochemistry and Urinalysis

Electrolytes and renal function often become abnormal in the course of HIV infection, especially at times of severe illness. Sodium wasting, physiologically appropriate water retention, or the syndrome of inappropriate antidiuretic hormone secretion associated with pulmonary or neurologic disease can induce hyponatremia. Potassium disorders can result from medications, intravascular volume disturbances, diarrhea, vomiting, or adrenal insufficiency. Abnormal magnesium, calcium, and phosphate values occur with renal disease, malnutrition, alcoholism, and medications (foscarnet). Acute renal insufficiency occurs in 3 to 13 percent of all AIDS patients at some time during their illness and is usually associated with medications, volume depletion, or sepsis [1–3]. Chronic renal failure is generally associated with advanced HIV disease and carries a dismal prognosis.

Urinalysis often reveals significant abnormalities. Pyuria, microscopic hematuria, and urinary tract infection are common [1]. Although up to 50 percent of HIV-infected patients excrete over 500 mg protein in 24 hours, only 7 to 10 percent have nephrotic-range proteinuria, and even fewer have the nephrotic syndrome [1–4].

Albumin determination is useful in the evaluation of nutritional status, hepatic function, and renal protein wasting. A low albumin value carries a poor prognosis. Although total protein measurement usually reveals a large globulin fraction, this is rarely of clinical importance and generally does not require further evaluation.

Table 3-1 *Laboratory evaluation of the HIV-infected patient*

Initial
    Electrolytes
    Renal function tests
    Urinalysis
    Liver function tests
    Complete blood and differential counts
    CD4 cell count
    Syphilis serology
    Viral hepatitis screen
    Toxoplasmosis serology
    Purified protein derivative (PPD)/anergy panel
    Chest radiograph
    Rectal exam/stool test for occult blood
    Pap smear in women

Health care maintenance
    CD4 cell count
    Syphilis serology
    PPD/anergy panel
    Stool test for occult blood
    Pap smear in women

Although hepatic failure is unusual in AIDS (5% of cases), liver function tests (LFTs) become abnormal in 60 to 70 percent of patients sometime during the course of the disease [5]. Icterus is rare, and serum bilirubin usually remains normal. An elevated bilirubin level has been associated with bacterial sepsis, chronic active hepatitis, and micronodular cirrhosis [6]. Serum transaminases often become abnormal but in no characteristic pattern. An elevated alkaline phosphatase (ALP) is often a marker of serious disease. In several series, a serum ALP of greater than 200 units per liter with a normal bilirubin was present in almost every case of hepatic *Mycobacterium avium* complex (MAC) infection, cytomegalovirus (CMV) infection, histoplasmosis, drug toxicity, or Kaposi's sarcoma (KS) diagnosed by liver biopsy or at autopsy [5, 7, 8]. A recent study described very elevated values in the absence of clinical evidence of opportunistic infection or obstruction, but 4 of 5 persons were demonstrated on postmortem examination to have had hepatic MAC [9].

Hepatic involvement with lymphoma is usually reflected by high ALP and bilirubin levels [6]. Sclerosing cholangitis, papillary stenosis, and bile duct strictures occur in AIDS patients and usually present as severe right upper quadrant pain, fever, high ALP, normal bilirubin, and variable transaminases. Serum lactate dehydrogenase (LDH) level, not in itself diagnostic of hepatic disease, is often elevated with *Pneumocystis carinii* pneumonia (PCP) and lymphoma [7].

Endocrinologic testing is discussed only briefly here. While all endocrine glands may be affected in the course of HIV infection, the adrenal glands, pancreas, and testicles are those most frequently found to be involved at autopsy. Clinical endocrinopathy is infrequent [10]. Marked adrenal insufficiency is unusual; when it occurs, CMV infection or ketoconazole is usually responsible. Impotence or decrease in libido may be due to testicular failure caused by infections (toxoplasmosis, *Mycobacterium tuberculosis*, CMV) or medications (ketoconazole, corticosteroids). Pancreatic disorders include asymptomatic infiltration (CMV, cryptosporidiosis, toxoplasmosis, KS, or lymphoma), and idiopathic and drug-associated pancreatitis (parenteral pentamidine, didanosine). Sick euthyroid syndrome has also been described [10].

Hematology

Complete Blood Count with Differential

A complete blood count (CBC) with differential frequently reveals abnormalities such as neutropenia, anemia, and thrombocytopenia [11]. Cytopenias result from primary HIV marrow suppression, peripheral destruction by antibodies, medications (zidovudine [ZDV], chemotherapeutic agents, ganciclovir, sulfonamides), marrow infection (mycobacterial), or marrow invasion by lymphoma.

CD4 Lymphocyte Count

The CD4 (T4) lymphocyte count or percentage is the most commonly used surrogate marker for assessing the degree of immunodeficiency. The CD4 count should be obtained in the initial evaluation of all HIV-infected persons for staging purposes and rechecked at least every 6 to 12 months if it is greater than 500/mm³. If the count is lower, falling rapidly, or near a critical value, more frequent retesting is advised. Because of variability in CD4 determinations, it is prudent to repeat the value before making any therapeutic interventions. Acute viral infections, such as herpes simplex or varicella-zoster, may transiently lower the CD4 count. While the effect of acute fungal, bacterial, and protozoal infections is less clear, CD4 counts are optimally obtained in the absence of acute illness.

When the CD4 count is less than 500/mm³, antiretroviral therapy is indicated. In two studies, ZDV slowed progression to AIDS, improved CD4 cell counts, and decreased p24 antigen compared to placebo in persons with counts between 200 and 500/mm³ [12, 13]. Before the availability of ZDV, a CD4 cell count of less than 200/mm³ in a person without AIDS indicated a 31 percent chance of development of AIDS within 1 year and an 87 percent chance in 3 years, but survival rates have improved in recent years [14–16]. Opportunistic infections are most common for persons with CD4 cell counts of less than 200/mm³, and PCP prophylaxis is recommended [17]. Values of less than 50 cells/mm³ in patients receiving ZDV are associated with increased mortality (median survival of 12 months) [18].

Other Surrogate Markers

p24 antigen (HIV viral core protein) measurements are not widely available in clinical laboratories. A positive antigen indicates a fourfold increased risk of progression to AIDS within 3 years (59 vs. 15%) [14]. β_2-microglobulin levels also increase with impending AIDS. Initial studies revealed that a level of over 5 μg/ml predicted AIDS in 69 percent of patients over 3 years; no patients with values of 2.6 μg/ml or less developed AIDS at a mean of 2 years follow-up study [14, 19]. More recently, however, this test has been shown to be elevated in injection drug users and, therefore, may not be a reliable surrogate marker in this population [20]. Quantitation of plasma viremia correlates with stage of disease and mortality, but its role in clinical practice has not been established [21]. HIV viral cultures are difficult and expensive to perform. Their greatest potential clinical use lies in identifying antiretroviral drug resistance [22].

Glucose 6-Phosphate Dehydrogenase

Patients being considered for PCP prophylaxis or treatment with dapsone should be screened for glucose 6-phosphate dehydrogenase (G6PD) deficiency because of the risk of severe drug-induced hemolysis.

Erythropoietin

Serum erythropoietin titers are inversely related to hemoglobin levels in anemic AIDS and AIDS-related complex (ARC) patients not receiving ZDV. Levels in patients on ZDV are less tightly correlated and should be assayed to predict potential response to erythropoietin administration [23]. Recombinant erythropoietin has been shown to significantly decrease transfusion dependence for persons receiving ZDV who have anemia and a serum erythropoietin level of less than 500 mU/ml [24].

Bone Marrow Examination

Bone marrow abnormalities occur throughout the spectrum of HIV infection, even in the absence of opportunistic diseases [11, 25]. Hypocellularity is the most frequent finding associated with peripheral cytopenias. Dysplasia is common, as are atypical lymphocytic aggregates. Bone marrow aspirate/biopsy may reveal granulomas or organisms, or both, permitting a rapid presumptive diagnosis of disseminated fungal or mycobacterial disease. Isolator blood cultures, which are more sensitive and less invasive, are also useful in this setting [26, 27].

Serologies

Syphilis

Syphilis serologic testing should be performed routinely in all patients who are HIV infected or at risk for HIV infection. All persons who are rapid plasma reagin (RPR) and treponemal antibody positive should be encouraged to undergo HIV testing. Because neurosyphilis may be asymptomatic, some authorities advocate that all HIV-infected individuals who have serologic evidence of syphilis should undergo lumbar puncture [28]. Most HIV-infected patients have a normal serologic response to syphilis infection, but some may have negative tests, and others may have extraordinarily high titers [29]. Close monitoring of HIV-infected patients with syphilis is essential because of the risk of treatment failure or relapse [28–30]. Nontreponemal testing (e.g., RPR) should be performed monthly for the first 3 months and at 3-month intervals thereafter [29].

Viral Hepatitis

The great majority (90%) of HIV-infected patients have serologic evidence of prior hepatitis B infection. Of all AIDS patients, 5 to 19 percent test positive for hepatitis B surface antigen, although chronic active hepatitis and cirrhosis are uncommon [5, 31]. HIV-infected persons who are negative for hepatitis B surface antigen (HBsAg) and hepatitis B core antibody (HBcAb) should receive hepatitis B vaccine. Antibody to hepatitis C is found in the majority of patients with non-A, non-B hepatitis

[32]. Rates of hepatitis C in drug users have been reported to be as high as 70 percent but are low in homosexual men with HIV infection [33, 34].

Toxoplasmosis Serology

Toxoplasmosis has been reported to occur in 24 percent of AIDS patients who carry toxoplasmic antibodies at baseline, but rarely in persons without them [35, 36]. The immunoglobulin G (IgG) antibody titer was thought to be almost always positive in patients with central nervous system (CNS) disease [37, 38]. However, a more recent study reports that about 20 percent of people with CNS toxoplasmosis have no detectable antibodies [39]. Serology can be used to identify those at greatest risk for toxoplasmosis for enrollment in prophylaxis trials.

Cryptococcal Antigen

Cryptococcal antigen level is almost always elevated in cerebrospinal fluid (CSF) from persons with meningitis [38]. Because of wide fluctuations in AIDS patients, it is not as useful for determining prognosis or response to therapy. However, persistently high CSF titers are associated with an increased risk of relapse [40, 41].

Pulmonary Studies

Purified Protein Derivative/Anergy Panel

As HIV-infected patients become progressively immunocompromised, they lose skin test reactivity to purified protein derivative (PPD) and control antigens. Nonetheless, 20 to 30 percent of HIV-infected patients are PPD positive. These patients are more likely to develop active disease than are PPD-positive persons without HIV infection [42–44]. Therefore, intermediate-strength (5TU) PPD testing with a control panel should be performed in HIV-infected individuals as part of initial screening (and on a regular basis thereafter in those who test negative) to detect PPD conversions or loss of skin test reactivity. Induration of 5 mm or more at 48 to 72 hours is significant in this population and requires preventive therapy with isoniazid [44]. Anergic patients who are at high risk for tuberculosis exposure should also receive prophylaxis. A chest x-ray (CXR) should be performed on anergic and PPD-positive individuals to rule out active TB.

Chest Roentgenography

It is reasonable to obtain a baseline CXR in HIV-infected patients (particularly injection drug users) so that comparison for subtle changes can be made in the event of new respiratory symptoms. PCP usually presents with an abnormal CXR, but up to 23 percent of radiographs will be unremarkable [45]. In PCP, the CXR usually demonstrates bilateral perihilar infiltrates, which progress to a diffuse interstitial pattern and later to alveolar infiltrates or consolidation with air bronchograms [45–48]. The interstitial markings may be reticular or finely nodular [49]. Other less common presentations include apical infiltrates, unilateral or unilobar infiltrates, nodules greater than 10 mm, cavitary lesions, and pneumothorax [45, 46, 49–51]. In persons who have been receiving aerosol pentamidine, localized upper-lobe infiltrates may develop. As intrathoracic adenopathy is very rare in PCP, this finding suggests other diseases, such as mycobacterial or cryptococcal infection, KS, or lymphoma [45, 46, 52, 53]. Pleural effusions are more likely to represent TB, KS, or bacterial or fungal infection than PCP [53, 54].

Pulmonary herpes simplex virus (HSV), CMV, nonspecific interstitial pneumonitis (NIP), and lymphocytic interstitial pneumonitis (LIP) usually present with a diffuse interstitial pattern on CXR indistinguishable from that of PCP [46, 53, 55]. MAC may show similar findings, but has an upper-lobe predilection, associated intrathoracic adenopathy, and a coarsely nodular pattern [45]. Pulmonary TB usually appears as unilateral or bilateral middle-/lower-lobe infiltrates, sometimes with hilar or mediastinal adenopathy or pleural effusions. Histoplasmosis, coccidioidomycosis, and histoplasmosis may be difficult to differentiate from other opportunistic infections, although calcifications and cavitation are frequent [56]. Cryptococcal infection presents with a nodular pattern, cavitation, adenopathy, and/or consolidation [45]. In evaluating pulmonary symptoms/signs and radiologic findings, it is important to remember that often more than one pathogen is present; for example, up to 27 percent of patients with PCP have coexistent infections [45–47, 54, 57]. Pulmonary KS may not be evident on CXR, but generally presents as large nodules, cavities, or a pleural effusion. Lymphoma may cause an interstitial pattern, intrathoracic adenopathy, mass effect, or pleural effusion [46, 48].

Arterial Blood Gases

In addition to CXR, arterial blood gases are an essential first step in the evaluation of respiratory symptoms in an HIV-infected individual. Because a change in the alveolar-arterial oxygen gradient is an important early indicator of active pulmonary disease, patients with a history of smoking or chronic lung disease should have a baseline blood gas analysis performed. Of patients with active PCP, 8 to 25 percent have a normal blood gas [54, 58].

Gallium Scan

The greatest utility of gallium-67 citrate scanning has been in the evaluation of pulmonary processes. Gallium scanning is 95 percent sensitive for PCP, and, when lung uptake is equal to or greater than hepatic uptake, specificity approaches 90 percent [58–61]. Because the predictive value of a positive scan is so high (85–95%), it may be useful in determining the need for bronchoscopic lavage or sputum examination in persons with respiratory symptoms but a normal blood gas and CXR. Gallium scanning may also be helpful in diagnosing recurrent PCP. Nodal gallium uptake suggests MAC, TB, lymphoma, toxoplasmosis, or generalized adenopathy [62, 63].

Gallium scanning is negative in KS, whether pulmonary, nodal, cutaneous, or visceral [59, 64]. Thallium-201 scintigraphy, however, may detect KS of the skin, mucous membranes, nodes, and viscera [65]. Therefore, nodal, pulmonary, and gastrointestinal lesions that are gallium negative but thallium avid are likely to reveal KS on biopsy.

Sputum Analysis

Sputum Gram's stain, acid-fast stain, and cultures should be performed on all HIV-infected patients with pneumonia. Many centers now have the capability to induce and evaluate sputum specimens for PCP by direct fluorescent antibody staining, but the sensitivity of this technique is variable [66, 67]. A positive sputum sample is diagnostic of PCP, but a negative examination does not exclude the diagnosis.

Bronchoscopy

While the diagnosis of PCP is sometimes made presumptively, bronchoscopy still has an important role. Bronchoalveolar lavage is diagnostic in 80 to 90 percent of patients with PCP, but, when performed on lobar or segmental bronchi or with biopsy, the yield approaches 95 to 100 percent [68, 69]. Patients with atypical CXR features or inadequate response to empiric PCP therapy may require bronchoscopy to identify other pathogens. The yield of bronchoscopic biopsy for TB or MAC is approximately 80 percent [61, 68]. Although KS lesions may be visible on bronchoscopy, biopsy yield is only 8 percent, whereas that of open thoracotomy is greater than 90 percent [68]. A diagnosis of NIP, LIP, or lymphoma may be supported by bronchoscopy, but open thoracotomy is sometimes necessary for definitive diagnosis. Thus, bronchoscopy is optimally used to diagnose first episodes of PCP when reliable induced sputum examination is unavailable or negative, and to determine the cause of an atypical CXR appearance or poor response to empiric PCP therapy.

Gastrointestinal/Hepatic Studies

Rectal Examination/Stool Occult Blood Test

Because of the increased risk of gastrointestinal KS and squamous cell carcinoma of the rectum in HIV-infected homosexual men, periodic rectal examinations and stool testing for occult blood are indicated.

Stool Studies

In the event of diarrhea, stool specimens should be cultured for bacterial pathogens and examined for ova and parasites. In advanced HIV disease, a modified acid-fast stain should also be performed to look for evidence of cryptosporidiosis or isosporosis. Patients who have recently received antibiotic therapy should have a *Clostridium difficile* titer assay performed.

Upper and Lower Endoscopy

Esophageal candidiasis can be diagnosed presumptively if thrush is present and the patient describes odynophagia or retrosternal pain with swallowing. If there is no response to empiric antifungal therapy, upper endoscopy is necessary for differentiation from CMV or HSV infection. The stomach is the least commonly involved portion of the gastrointestinal tract in AIDS, but KS, lymphoma, CMV, cryptosporidiosis, and occasionally TB may be found; the duodenum is the most frequently involved area and can harbor CMV, MAC, TB, KS, or lymphoma [64]. Biopsy of the small intestine in the context of diarrhea may reveal the causative organism. Alternatively, there may be diffuse cellular changes suggesting primary HIV enteropathy without other identifiable pathogens. Stool cultures and sigmoidoscopy may be useful in investigating diarrhea and other lower gastrointestinal symptoms [70].

Liver Biopsy

Liver function test results are frequently abnormal in the AIDS population, and liver biopsy may be indicated on occasion. Biopsy only rarely reveals fulminant hepatitis or cirrhosis, but opportunistic diseases and biliary tract abnormalities are sometimes identified. MAC is the most common opportunistic infection involving the liver [8]. In 60 percent or more of cases, the organism is also present in other tissues, and the sensitivity of isolator blood cultures is very high, reducing the need for liver biopsy [5, 6, 29]. Patients generally have hepatomegaly and fever, significantly elevated ALP, and normal bilirubin and coagulation studies [5–8]. Disseminated CMV involves the liver in 40 percent of cases and presents much like MAC [5]. Other less common causes of a high ALP with normal bilirubin include tuberculosis, histoplasmosis, coccidioidomycosis, cryptococcosis, and granulomatous drug reactions. Kaposi's sarcoma is associated with a similar LFT pattern but is rarely identifiable on biopsy. Cutaneous lesions are usually present in persons with hepatic KS [5, 6, 8]. Hepatic lymphoma is occasionally diagnosed by biopsy and can be visualized as a mass on abdominal computed tomographic (CT) scan or ultrasound. Alkaline phosphatase and bilirubin are generally elevated [6].

Endoscopic Retrograde Cholangiopancreatography

Sclerosing cholangitis, papillary stenosis, and bile duct strictures are characterized by the same LFT pattern described for MAC, but present with right upper quadrant abdominal pain [71]. Nuclear, abdominal ultrasound or CT scan may suggest these diagnoses, but endoscopic retrograde cholangiopancreatography (ERCP) or liver biopsy, or both, are necessary for confirmation.

Neurologic Studies

Computed Tomography and Magnetic Resonance Imaging

Computed tomography of the brain is an essential part of the evaluation of the HIV-infected patient with new central nervous system symptoms. Single or multiple contrast-enhancing nodules or rings in the white matter, corticomedullary junction, or basal ganglia are most commonly caused by toxoplasmosis [48, 72]. There is often mass effect and edema. Lesions usually show improvement after 10 to 14 days of therapy, with resolution occurring in 10 days to 6 months, but calcifications may persist [48, 72, 73]. Mycobacterial, fungal, and bacterial abscesses, as well as lymphoma, may also occasionally cause ring-enhancing lesions on head CT [74]. Lymphomatous lesions may be deeper, periventricular, or demonstrate irregular or meningeal enhancement [74, 75]. Cryptococcal infection and CMV cause nonspecific CT abnormalities [73]. Herpes simplex virus encephalitis may show unilateral or reduced attenuation in the temporal lobes [74]. Progressive multifocal leukoencephalopathy (PML) appears as low-density areas in white matter without mass effect or contrast enhancement [73, 75]. All of these neurologic diseases may be present with a negative head CT [37, 74, 76]. Magnetic resonance imaging is more sensitive for toxoplasmosis and PML and, therefore, should be obtained when intracerebral pathology is suspected in the context of a negative contrast-enhanced CT. The most common CNS radiologic abnormality in HIV-infected patients with neurologic symptoms is atrophy [38, 77].

Lumbar Puncture

Among asymptomatic HIV-infected persons who have CD4 lymphocyte counts over 400, 25 to 30 percent have a CSF white cell count of greater than $10/mm^3$, 6 to 8 percent have a CSF protein greater than 55 mg/dl, and 5 to 10 percent have a low CSF glucose [78]. With more advanced stages of the disease, neurologically asymptomatic individuals more often have a high protein, but the other changes in CSF profile are less clearly correlated. In acute aseptic meningitis associated with primary HIV infection, lumbar puncture usually reveals mononuclear pleocytosis, low CSF glucose, and high CSF protein [38]. Three quarters of people with HIV encephalopathy have an abnormal lumbar puncture, usually revealing mild mononuclear pleocytosis, hypoglycorrhachia, and protein elevation to 50 to 100 mg/dl [38, 75, 77].

Cryptococcal meningitis is characterized by CSF pleocytosis in 35 percent of patients, elevated CSF protein in 69 percent, and positive cryptococcal antigen in nearly 100 percent. India ink preparation reveals the fungus in 82 percent of cases, and fungal cultures are always positive [38]. In toxoplasmosis, the CSF protein is often elevated, but other findings are variable. Less common infections potentially diagnosed by CSF analysis include aspergillosis, coccidioidomycosis, histoplasmosis, candidiasis, TB, MAC, and bacterial meningitis [79]. A normal CSF is common with lymphoma, but occasionally mild pleocytosis, elevated protein, or suspicious cytology may be present [38, 75].

Although symptomatic neurosyphilis remains unusual in HIV-infected persons, syphilis progresses more rapidly with early neurologic involvement [28, 37, 38]. Therefore, a syphilis serology should be obtained on all CSF specimens, and lumbar puncture should be seriously considered in HIV-infected persons who are RPR and treponemal antibody positive. Any CSF abnormality in this context is considered indicative of possible neurosyphilis.

Neuropsychological Testing

HIV-infected patients without acute medical illness or evidence of neurologic disease frequently demonstrate subtle abnormalities on formal neuropsychological testing. Twelve percent of asymptomatic persons demonstrate significant impairments [76, 80]. Common abnormalities include slow information processing, impaired problem solving, visuospatial difficulty, poor abstraction ability, and impaired fine motor control and speed. A clinical diagnosis of HIV dementia is based on findings of psychomotor slowing, forgetfulness, personality change, and decreased knowledge acquisition. Whereas formal neuropsychological testing will reliably identify these abnormalities, the "mini-mental status examination" is much less sensitive [38]. Confirming the diagnosis of HIV dementia/encephalopathy is important because it qualifies as an "indicator disease" for AIDS and symptoms may improve when the patient receives high-dose ZDV therapy [81, 82].

Tissue Biopsy

Skin Biopsy

Dermatologic lesions are extremely common in HIV-infected patients. Viral, fungal, bacterial, parasitic, drug-related, malignant, and idiopathic conditions have been described. Therefore, biopsy with special stains and cultures is often necessary for lesions that are unusual in appearance or do not respond to empiric therapy. Because syphilis serologies may be falsely negative, lesions suggestive of this diagnosis should be biopsied. Although the diagnosis of KS may be made presumptively by experienced practitioners, an AIDS classification should generally be based on biopsy-proven KS, as should any decision to treat patients with chemotherapy or radiation therapy.

Lymph Node Biopsy

Because persistent generalized lymphadenopathy is commonly associated with HIV infection, it is not necessary to biopsy all persons with enlarged nodes. However, many other processes, including syphilis, TB, toxoplasmosis, lymphoma, and KS, may also cause adenopathy. Biopsy is appropriate for nodes that are asymmetric, rapidly growing, or associated with constitutional symptoms or cytopenia [83].

Pelvic Examination/Papanicolaou Smear

Regular pelvic examination and Pap smear are important in HIV-infected women because of their high rate of cervical dysplasia [84–86]. The Centers for Disease Control recommends that HIV-infected women have annual Pap smears, assuming this yields adequate cytology; others have suggested colposcopy if results are uninterpretable [86, 87]. Some clinicians perform routine Pap smears twice per year. More frequent pelvic examinations may be necessary because of the high incidence of vaginal candidiasis, pelvic inflammatory disease, and genital ulcer disease [87–90].

References

1. Kaplan MS, Wechsler M, Benson MC. Urologic manifestations of AIDS. *Urology* 30:441–443, 1987.
2. Rao TK, Friedman EA, Nicastri AD. The types of renal disease in the acquired immunodeficiency syndrome. *N Engl J Med* 316:1062–1068, 1987.
3. Pardo V, et al. Glomerular lesions in the acquired immunodeficiency syndrome. *Ann Intern Med* 101:429–434, 1984.
4. Rao TK, et al. Associated focal and segmental glomerulosclerosis in the acquired immunodeficiency syndrome. *N Engl J Med* 310:669–673, 1984.
5. Glasgow BJ, et al. Clinical and pathologic findings of the liver in the acquired immune deficiency syndrome (AIDS). *Am J Clin Pathol* 83:582–588, 1985.
6. Schneiderman DJ, et al. Hepatic disease in patients with the acquired immune deficiency syndrome (AIDS). *Hepatology* 7:925–930, 1987.
7. Kahn SA, et al. Hepatic disorders in the acquired immune deficiency syndrome: A clinical and pathological study. *Am J Gastroenterol* 81:1145–1148, 1986.
8. Rodgers VD, Kagnoff MF. Acquired immunodeficiency syndrome and disease of the gastrointestinal tract. *Immunol Allergy Clin North Am* 8:451–467, 1988.
9. Payne TH, et al. Marked elevations of serum alkaline phosphatase in patients with AIDS. *J AIDS* 4:238–243, 1991.
10. Aron DC. Endocrine complications of the acquired immunodeficiency syndrome. *Arch Intern Med* 149:330–333, 1989.
11. Zon LI, Arkin C, Groopman JE. Hematologic manifestations of the human immune deficiency virus (HIV). *Br J Haematol* 66:251–256, 1987.
12. Fischl MA, et al. The safety and efficacy of zidovudine (AZT) in the treatment of subjects with mildly symptomatic human immunodeficiency virus type 1 (HIV) infection. *Ann Intern Med* 112:727–737, 1990.
13. Volberding PA, et al. Zidovudine in asymptomatic human immunodeficiency virus infection. *N Engl J Med* 322:942–949, 1990.

14. Moss AR, Bacchetti P, Osmond D, et al. Seropositivity for HIV and the development of AIDS or AIDS related condition: Three year follow up of the San Francisco General Hospital cohort. *Br Med J* 296:745–750, 1988.
15. Kaplan JE, Spira TJ, Fishbein DB, et al. A six-year follow-up of HIV-infected homosexual men with lymphadenopathy: Evidence for an increased risk for developing AIDS after the third year of lymphadenopathy. *JAMA* 260:2694–2697, 1988.
16. Creagh-Kirk T, Doi P, Andrews E, et al. Survival experience among patients with AIDS receiving zidovudine. *JAMA* 260:3009–3015, 1988.
17. Centers for Disease Control. Recommendations for prophylaxis against *Pneumocystis carinii* pneumonia for adults and adolescents infected with human immunodeficiency virus. *MMWR* 41(RR-4):1–11, 1992.
18. Yarchoan R, et al. CD4 count and the risk for death in patients infected with HIV receiving antiretroviral therapy. *Ann Intern Med* 155:184–189, 1991.
19. Morfeldt-Manson J, et al. Elevated serum beta-2-microglobulin—a prognostic marker for development of AIDS among patients with persistent generalized lymphadenopathy. *Infection* 16:109–110, 1988.
20. Flegg PJ, et al. Beta-2-microglobulin levels in drug users: the influence of risk behaviour. *AIDS* 5:1021–1024, 1991.
21. Schnittman SM, et al. Increasing viral burden in CD4-positive T cells from patients with HIV infection reflects rapidly progressive immunosuppression and clinical disease. *Ann Intern Med* 113:438–443, 1990.
22. Schleupner CJ. Diagnostic Tests for HIV-1 Infection. In GL Mandell, RG Douglas, JE Bennett (eds), *Principles and Practice of Infectious Diseases*. New York: Churchill Livingstone, 1990. Pp 1092–1102.
23. Rarick MU, et al. Serum erythropoietin titers in patients with human immunodeficiency virus (HIV) infection and anemia. *J AIDS* 4:593–597, 1991.
24. Fischl M, et al. Recombinant human erythropoietin for patients with AIDS treated with zidovudine. *N Engl J Med* 322:1488, 1990.
25. Spivak JL, et al. Hematologic abnormalities in the acquired immune deficiency syndrome. *Am J Med* 77:224–228, 1984.
26. Northfelt DW, et al. The usefulness of diagnostic bone marrow examination in patients with human immunodeficiency virus (HIV) infection. *J AIDS* 4:659–666, 1991.
27. Young LS, et al. Mycobacterial infections in AIDS patients, with an emphasis on the *Mycobacterium avium* complex. *Rev Infect Dis* 8:1024–1033, 1986.
28. Johns DR, Tierney M, Felsenstein D. Alteration in the natural history of neurosyphilis by concurrent infection with the human immunodeficiency virus. *N Engl J Med* 316:1569–1572, 1987.
29. Centers for Disease Control. Recommendations for diagnosing and treating syphilis in HIV-infected patients. *MMWR* 37:600–608, 1988.
30. Berry CD, et al. Neurologic relapse after benzathine penicillin therapy for secondary syphilis in a patient with HIV infection. *N Engl J Med* 316:1587–1590, 1987.

31. Lebovics E, et al. The hepatobiliary manifestations of human immuno-deficiency virus infection. *Am J Gastroenterol* 83:1–7, 1988.
32. Alter HJ, et al. Detection of antibody to hepatitis C virus in prospectively followed transfusion recipients with acute and chronic non-A, non-B hepatitis. *N Engl J Med* 321:1494–1500, 1989.
33. Tor J, et al. Sexual transmission of hepatitis C virus and its relation with hepatitis B virus and HIV. *Br Med J* 301:1130–1133, 1990.
34. Esteban JI, et al. Hepatitis C virus antibodies among risk groups in Spain. *Lancet* 2:295–297, 1989.
35. Grant IH, et al. *Toxoplasma gondii* serology in HIV-infected patients: the development of central nervous system toxoplasmosis in AIDS. *AIDS* 4:519–521, 1990.
36. Luft BJ, Remington JS. Toxoplasmic encephalitis. *J Infect Dis* 157:1–6, 1988.
37. Levy RM, et al. Neurological manifestations of the acquired immunode-ficiency syndrome (AIDS): Experience at UCSF and review of the litera-ture. *J Neurosurg* 62:475–495, 1985.
38. McArthur JC. Neurologic manifestations of AIDS. *Medicine* 66:407–437, 1987.
39. Porter SB, Sande MA. Toxoplasmosis of the central nervous system in the acquired immunodeficiency syndrome. *N Engl J Med* 327:1643–1648, 1992.
40. Kovacs JA, et al. Cryptococcosis in the acquired immunodeficiency syn-drome. *Ann Intern Med* 103:533–538, 1985.
41. Zuger A, et al. Cryptococcal disease in patients with the acquired immu-nodeficiency syndrome: Diagnostic features and outcome of therapy. *Ann Intern Med* 104:234–240, 1985.
42. Stoneburner RL, et al. Tuberculosis and acquired immunodeficiency syn-drome—New York City. *MMWR* 36:785–795, 1987.
43. Selwyn PA, et al. A prospective study of the risk of tuberculosis among intravenous drug users with human immunodeficiency virus infection. *N Engl J Med* 320:545–550, 1989.
44. Centers for Disease Control. Tuberculosis and human immunodeficiency virus infection: Recommendations of the advisory committee for the elimination of tuberculosis (ACET). *MMWR* 38:236–250, 1989.
45. Suster B, et al. Pulmonary manifestations of AIDS: Review of 106 epi-sodes. *Radiology* 161:87–93, 1986.
46. Cohen BA, et al. Pulmonary complications of AIDS: Radiologic features. *Am J Radiol* 143:115–122, 1984.
47. McCauley DI, et al. Radiographic patterns of opportunistic lung infections and Kaposi sarcoma in homosexual men. *Am J Radiol* 139:653–658, 1982.
48. Barter S. Radiological features of AIDS. *Clin Immunol Allergy* 6:601–625, 1986.
49. DeLorenzo LJ, et al. Roentgenographic patterns of *Pneumocystis carinii* pneumonia in 104 patients with AIDS. *Chest* 91:323–327, 1987.
50. Milligan SA, et al. *Pneumocystis carinii* pneumonia radiographically sim-ulating tuberculosis. *Am Rev Respir Dis* 132:1124–1126. 1985.

51. Barrio JL, et al. *Pneumocystis carinii* pneumonia presenting as cavitating and noncavitating solitary pulmonary nodules in patients with the acquired immunodeficiency syndrome. *Am Rev Respir Dis* 134:1094–1096, 1986.
52. Afessa B, et al. *Pneumocystis carinii* pneumonia complicated by lymphadenopathy and pneumothorax. *Arch Intern Med* 148:2651–2654, 1988.
53. Frieco MH, Chinoy-Acharya P. Lymphocytic interstitial pneumonia associated with the acquired immune deficiency syndrome. *Am Rev Respir Dis* 131:952–955, 1985.
54. Stover DE, et al. Spectrum of pulmonary diseases associated with the acquired immune deficiency syndrome. *Am J Med* 78:429–437, 1985.
55. Morris JC, et al. Lymphocytic interstitial pneumonia in patients at risk for the acquired immune deficiency syndrome. *Chest* 91:63–67, 1987.
56. Goodman PC, Gamsu G. Radiographic findings in the acquired immunodeficiency syndrome. *Postgrad Radiol* 7:3–15, 1987.
57. Simmons JT, et al. Nonspecific interstitial pneumonitis in patients with AIDS: Radiologic features. *Am J Radiol* 149:265–268, 1987.
58. Murray JF, et al. Pulmonary complications of the acquired immunodeficiency syndrome. *N Engl J Med* 310:1682–1688, 1984.
59. Woolfenden JM, et al. Acquired immunodeficiency syndrome: Ga-67 citrate imaging. *Radiology* 162:383–387, 1987.
60. Kramer EL, et al. Diagnostic implications of Ga-67 chest-scan patterns in human immunodeficiency virus–positive patients. *Radiology* 170:671–676, 1989.
61. Tuazon CU, et al. Utility of gallium-67 scintigraphy and bronchial washings in the diagnosis and treatment of *Pneumocystis carinii* pneumonia in patients with the acquired immune deficiency syndrome. *Am Rev Respir Dis* 132:1087–1092, 1985.
62. Kramer EL, et al. Gallium-67 scans of the chest in patients with acquired immunodeficiency syndrome. *J Nucl Med* 28:1107–1114, 1987.
63. Bekerman C, Bitran J. Gallium-67 scanning in the clinical evaluation of human immunodeficiency virus infection: Indications and limitations. *Semin Nucl Med* 17:273–276, 1988.
64. Megibow AJ, Balthazar EJ, Hulnick DH. Radiology of nonneoplastic gastrointestinal disorders in acquired immune deficiency syndrome. *Semin Roentgenol* 22:31–41, 1987.
65. Lee VW, et al. AIDS-related Kaposi sarcoma: Findings on thallium-201 scintigraphy. *Am J Radiol* 151:1233–1235, 1988.
66. Kovacs JA, Ng VL, Masur H, et al. Diagnosis of *Pneumocystis carinii* pneumonia: Improved detection in sputum with use of monoclonal antibodies. *N Engl J Med* 318:589–593, 1988.
67. Pitchenik AE, Ganjei P, Torres A, et al. Sputum examination for the diagnosis of *Pneumocystis carinii* pneumonia in the acquired immunodeficiency syndrome. *Am Rev Respir Dis* 133:226–229, 1986.
68. Murray JF, et al. Pulmonary complications of the acquired immunodeficiency syndrome: Report of a National Heart, Lung, and Blood Institute workshop. *N Engl J Med* 310:1682–1688, 1984.

69. Ognibene FP, et al. The diagnosis of *Pneumocystis carinii* pneumonia in patients with the acquired immunodeficiency syndrome using subsegmental bronchoalveolar lavage. *Am Rev Respir Dis* 129:929–932, 1984.
70. Gazzard BG. HIV disease and the gastroenterologist. *Gut* 29:1497–1505, 1988.
71. Cello JP. Acquired immunodeficiency syndrome cholangiopathy: Spectrum of disease. *Am J Med* 86:539–546, 1989.
72. Levy RM, Rosenbloom S, Perrett LV. Neuroradiologic findings in AIDS: A review of 200 cases. *Am J Radiol* 147:977–983, 1986.
73. Elkin CM, et al. Intracranial lesions in the acquired immunodeficiency syndrome: Radiological (computed tomographic) features. *JAMA* 253:393–396, 1985.
74. Sze G, et al. The neuroradiology of AIDS. *Semin Roentgenol* 22:42–53, 1987.
75. Snider WD, et al. Neurological complications of acquired immune deficiency syndrome: Analysis of 50 patients. *Ann Neurol* 14:403–418, 1983.
76. Grant I, et al. Evidence for early central nervous system involvement in the acquired immunodeficiency syndrome (AIDS) and other human immunodeficiency virus (HIV) infections: Studies with neuropsychologic testing and magnetic resonance imaging. *Ann Intern Med* 107:828–836, 1987.
77. Navia BA, Price RW. The acquired immunodeficiency syndrome dementia complex as the presenting or sole manifestation of human immunodeficiency virus infection. *Arch Neurol* 44:65–69, 1987.
78. Marshall DW, et al. Spectrum of cerebrospinal fluid findings in various stages of human immunodeficiency virus infection. *Arch Neurol* 45:954–958, 1988.
79. Elder GA, Sever JL. Neurologic disorders associated with AIDS retroviral infection. *Rev Infect Dis* 10:286–302, 1988.
80. Tross S, et al. Neuropsychological characterization of the AIDS dementia complex: A preliminary report. *AIDS* 2:81–88, 1988.
81. Yarchoan R, et al. Response of human immunodeficiency-virus-associated neurological disease to 3'-azido-3'-deoxythymidine. *Lancet* 1:132–135, 1987.
82. Schmitt FA, et al. Neuropsychological outcome of zidovudine (AZT) treatment of patients with AIDS and AIDS-related complex. *N Engl J Med* 319:1573–1578, 1988.
83. Abrams DI. AIDS-related lymphadenopathy: The role of biopsy. *J Clin Oncol* 4:126–127, 1986.
84. Maiman M, et al. Colposcopic evaluation of human immunodeficiency virus seropositive women. *Obstet Gynecol* 78:84–88, 1991.
85. Maiman M, et al. Human immunodeficiency virus and cervical neoplasia. *Gynecol Obstet* 38:377–382, 1990.
86. Centers for Disease Control. Risk for cervical disease in HIV infected women—New York City. *MMWR* 39:846–849, 1990.
87. Minkoff HL, DeHovitz JA. Care of women infected with the human immunodeficiency virus. *JAMA* 266:2253–2258, 1991.

88. Rhoads JL, et al. Chronic vaginal candidiasis in women with human immunodeficiency virus infection. *JAMA* 257:3105–3107, 1987.
89. Imam W, et al. Hierarchical pattern of mucosal candida infections in HIV seropositive women. *Am J Med* 89:142–146, 1990.
90. Hoegsberg B, et al. Sexually transmitted diseases and human immunodeficiency virus infection among women with pelvic inflammatory diseases. *Am J Obstet Gynecol* 163:1135–1139, 1990.

II/Clinical Syndromes

4/Fever

Lawrence M. Barat, Thomas W. Barber, Robert A. Witzburg

The clinician confronted with a febrile HIV-infected patient may feel overwhelmed by the potentially large differential diagnosis. A rational approach to fever in this population requires an understanding of the patient's presenting symptoms and signs in the context of his or her stage of HIV disease. A systematic search for both infectious and non-infectious etiologies is warranted for all episodes of fever.

Fever and the Natural History of HIV Disease

A self-limited febrile illness associated with seroconversion is often the first clinical manifestation of HIV infection (Table 4-1). This syndrome (Centers for Disease Control [CDC] category A1: primary HIV infection) occurs 8 to 12 weeks after exposure to HIV and has been well charac-terized [1–4]. It may present as a "mononucleosis-like" syndrome con-sisting of fever, constitutional symptoms, sore throat, diffuse adenopa-thy, headache, diarrhea, and a maculopapular rash involving the trunk. In some patients, seroconversion is associated with an acute, transient meningoencephalitis or peripheral neuropathy, or both. The duration of this illness is usually 2 to 3 weeks. Primary HIV infection may also be asymptomatic or present as a nonspecific viral syndrome.

The progression of HIV disease after seroconversion is variable, but the patient generally remains asymptomatic for an extended period (CDC categories A2, A3: asymptomatic infection or persistently gener-alized lymphadenopathy). Despite the lack of clinical illness during these years, HIV continues to proliferate, causing damage to the immune system and resulting in a progressive decline in the CD4 lym-phocyte count. By definition, fever does not occur during this stage of disease.

Fever associated with recurrent conventional bacterial infection may be an early manifestation of HIV disease. Pneumonia, sinusitis, and skin infections are seen most frequently. The onset of symptomatic HIV dis-ease is usually heralded by high-grade viremia. Many patients experi-ence intermittent fevers, generalized adenopathy, diarrhea, and weight loss without other explanation. Previously classified as AIDS-related complex (ARC), the CDC now describes it as clinical category B. Febrile

Table 4-1 *Fever and the natural history of HIV disease*

CDC clinical category	Immune status	Causes of fever
A1	Acute illness: +p24 antigen, lymphopenia Recovery: +HIV antibody; decreased CD4:CD8 ratio	Acute HIV infection: "mononucleosis-like syndrome"
A2, A3	Variable: normal → lymphopenia with decreased CD4:CD8 ratio	Fever not characteristic
B1, B2, B3	Variable: lymphopenia with decreased CD4:CD8 ratio; increased immunoglobulins; impaired humoral immunity	Increased frequency of common bacterial infections, viral infections (HSV, VZV), and tuberculosis
C1, C2, C3	Variable: lymphopenia with decreased CD4:CD8 ratio; anergy to skin tests; increased immunoglobulins; increased immune complexes; increased p24 antigen; increased β_2-microglobulin	All of above listed under category B, plus opportunistic infections (PCP, cryptococcosis, toxoplasmosis) and neoplasms (lymphoma, visceral KS)

CDC = Centers for Disease Control; HSV = herpes simplex virus; VZV = varicella-zoster virus; PCP = *Pneumocystis carinii* pneumonia; KS = Kaposi's sarcoma.

illnesses occur commonly as patients progress to CDC category C, the causes of which include opportunistic infections, neoplastic diseases, and other manifestations diagnostic of AIDS. Febrile illnesses during advanced HIV disease may be multifactorial and require careful evaluation.

Differential Diagnosis of Fever in the HIV-Infected Patient

Infections

The first consideration in the differential diagnosis of fever in the HIV-positive patient should always be infection, as it remains the major cause of death among patients with AIDS [5]. Furthermore, many infectious complications of HIV disease respond well to appropriate antimicrobial therapy, making early, accurate diagnosis important. In two prospective case studies of febrile HIV-infected patients, infection proved to be the cause of fever in 63 and 81 percent of those in whom a source could be established [6, 7].

The list of potential infectious etiologies of fever is long and includes viral, bacterial, parasitic, and fungal pathogens. Susceptibility to these diverse infections varies with the individual patient's degree of immunosuppression. Infections with bacteria, such as *Streptococcus pneumoniae*, *Staphylococcus aureus*, nontyphoidal strains of *Salmonella*, and other enteric bacterial pathogens, may occur early in the course of HIV disease [8, 9]. *Mycobacterium tuberculosis* infection, including extrapulmonary involvement, may also be an early manifestation of HIV disease, as may reactivation of herpes simplex virus (HSV) and varicella-zoster virus (VZV) infections [10, 11].

As patients become more immunocompromised (CD4 cell count < 200/mm^3), infections such as *Pneumocystis carinii* pneumonia (PCP), cryptococcal meningitis, and toxoplasmic encephalitis must be considered in the differential diagnosis of fever [12]. Also at this stage, refractory mucocutaneous HSV and multidermatomal VZV infections may be seen. In patients who are severely immunocompromised (CD4 cell count < 50/mm^3), cytomegalovirus, *Mycobacterium avium* complex, and cryptosporidial infections must also be considered [10, 12, 13]. Patients with advanced HIV disease may be even more susceptible to bacterial infections, both community-acquired and nosocomial, than those with early disease. Except for conventional bacterial pathogens and *M. tuberculosis*, microbiologic cure of opportunistic infections is usually not possible, and relapse of symptomatic disease is common. In these instances, the goal of therapy becomes suppression of clinical disease [14–16].

HIV-infected patients are at increased risk for other sexually transmitted diseases, including syphilis, gonorrhea, intestinal parasites, and mucosal viral pathogens. Coinfection with other retroviruses (e.g., HIV-2, HTLV-1) and possibly, other, as yet unidentified, viral agents may contribute to fever in some individuals [17–19].

Neoplasms

HIV-infected patients are at significantly increased risk for certain neoplastic diseases, especially non-Hodgkin's lymphoma and Kaposi's sarcoma (KS) [20]. Fever is frequently part of the clinical presentation of lymphoma; it is less commonly associated with KS, occurring only with disseminated visceral disease [21]. The clinician should be hesitant to attribute fevers to lymphoma or KS until a full evaluation has been completed to rule out concurrent infection.

Other Causes

Reactions to prescribed or illicit drugs are sometimes responsible for fever. HIV-positive patients appear to have increased sensitivity to many medications, especially antibiotics, and are often prescribed an assortment of drugs to manage their diverse medical problems. The presence of pruritus, rash, or eosinophilia may support the diagnosis of drug fever. Injection drug users (IDUs) may present with febrile reactions to self-injected pyrogens and other non–HIV-related infectious complications [22].

Both lymphoid and nonspecific interstitial pneumonitis have been reported to cause fever in HIV-infected individuals. Although rare, autoimmune vasculitis has been described in HIV-positive individuals and represents another possible noninfectious cause of fever [23].

Evaluation of Fever in the HIV-Infected Patient

Given an understanding of the natural history of HIV infection and the evolving differential diagnosis of fever as immunodeficiency progresses, a rational plan for evaluation of the patient can be developed (Table 4-2). Any persistent temperature greater than 100.4°F (38°C) should be considered significant. It is important to review the past medical history, list of current medications, and available baseline laboratory data. Particular attention should be given to the CD4 lymphocyte count. Recent purified protein derivative (PPD) skin test and anergy panel status, as well as prior syphilis and hepatitis serology, may also aid in the diagnostic evaluation.

The primary data collected in the history and physical examination are of critical importance in evaluating the febrile patient. The clinician should elicit from the patient a history of the duration, degree, and pattern of fever, as well as any associated symptoms. A complete review of symptoms, focusing particular attention on the respiratory, gastrointestinal, dermatologic, and neurologic systems, is also warranted. An assessment of past and current risk behaviors contributes important diagnostic clues. Whereas opportunistic infections were reported to be the most common cause of fever in a group of predominantly homosexual men, a study of a largely IDU population found that over 50 percent of observed fevers were caused by infection with common bacterial pathogens [6, 7]. Finally, travel history, geographic region of origin,

Table 4-2 *Evaluation of fever in the HIV-infected patient*

History
    Symptoms of present illness
    Exposure to tuberculosis
    Exposure to sexually transmitted diseases
    Exposure to viral hepatitis
    Travel/hobbies
    Drug use

Physical examination
    Signs of present illness
    Focus on fundi, pharynx, lungs, abdomen, skin, and neurologic examinations

Laboratory evaluation
    Complete blood and differential counts
    Liver function tests
    Urinalysis
    Blood cultures (including isolator tubes in advanced HIV disease)
    Chest x-ray
    Purified protein derivative and anergy panel
    Syphilis serology
    Viral hepatitis serologies
    Other studies as determined by clinical presentation

sexual practices, exposure to animals and animal products, and unusual hobbies may lead the clinician to investigate specific causes of fever.

A complete physical examination should be performed in the febrile patient, with particular attention given to the systems mentioned previously, including examination of the fundi, the oral cavity, and the skin. A dilated ophthalmologic examination is indicated in severely immunocompromised individuals to assess for CMV infection. Laboratory investigation is directed by clues obtained in the history and physical examination, but should generally include complete blood and differential counts, liver function tests, urinalysis, blood cultures, and chest x-ray. If not previously available, baseline PPD and anergy panel, as well as syphilis and viral hepatitis serologies, are indicated. In significantly immunocompromised patients, serum cryptococcal antigen and lysis-centrifugation (isolator) blood cultures for mycobacteria and fungi should also be obtained, particularly if history and physical examination fail to reveal a cause of fever.

The performance of other studies should be based on presenting symptoms and signs (e.g., arterial blood gas in the patient with dyspnea). Computed tomography (CT) or magnetic resonance imaging (MRI) scan of the head and lumbar puncture are indicated in patients with new neurologic symptoms. Isotope studies, such as gallium, thallium, and indium-labeled leukocyte scans, may be useful in the diagnostic evaluation for PCP, lymphoma, and visceral KS, but should not be considered as screening tests [24, 25].

The pace of the evaluation is determined by the severity of the clinical illness, the likely diagnoses, the degree of immunodeficiency, and the likelihood of finding a condition that is amenable to treatment. Empiric therapy should be initiated in acutely ill patients for the most likely diagnosis(es) and/or those that carry the highest risk of morbidity or mortality if treatment is delayed. Final diagnosis sometimes rests on the examination of specimens obtained by invasive procedures. In individuals with advanced HIV disease, often more than one active pathologic process can be identified at a given time. Although mucosal surfaces may be colonized with many potential pathogens, any organism identified in tissue or in normally sterile body fluid is considered pathologic, even in the absence of an inflammatory response by the host.

In patients with advanced HIV disease, new symptoms associated with fever must be aggressively pursued. Mild dyspnea or cough may portend an episode of PCP and should lead to a pulmonary evaluation. Subtle complaints of headache or altered mental status/behavior should prompt the clinician to perform appropriate neurologic tests. The development of or change in degree of adenopathy in one or more regions associated with constitutional symptoms may reflect the presence of lymphoma or extrapulmonary mycobacterial disease and may necessitate a lymph node biopsy.

Despite careful attention to findings on history, physical examination, and laboratory studies, some febrile HIV-infected patients defy diagnosis, even after days or weeks of intensive evaluation. A diagnosis may ultimately be made by obtaining tissue via bone marrow, liver, lymph node, or other organ biopsy, or by careful serologic evaluation for organisms that are difficult to culture. In some cases, no diagnosis can be made, and the fever is attributed to HIV infection itself. In these instances, the evaluation can be stopped and the patient closely observed.

Conclusion

Evaluation of fever in the HIV-infected patient is based on a knowledge of the natural history of the clinical and immunologic features of HIV disease and the presenting symptoms and signs of the illness. Identification of treatable infection is the first priority. Malignancy, drug reaction, and autoimmune phenomena are other potential causes of fever. Because the prevalence of opportunistic diseases is high and the clinical manifestations are often subtle early in the course, prompt evaluation of all febrile episodes is warranted.

References

1. Centers for Disease Control. 1993 Revised classification system for HIV infection and expanded case definition for AIDS among adolescents and adults. *MMWR* 41(RR-17):1–19, 1992.
2. Cooper DA, Gold JW, MacLean P, et al. Acute AIDS retrovirus infection: Definition of a clinical illness associated with seroconversion. *Lancet* 1:537–540, 1985.
3. Ho DD, Sarngadharan MC, Resnick L, et al. Primary human T-lymphotropic virus type III infection. *Ann Intern Med* 103:880–883, 1985.
4. Tindall B, Bavar S, Donovan B, et al. Characterization of the acute clinical illness associated with human immunodeficiency virus infection. *Arch Intern Med* 148:945–949, 1988.
5. Grant IH, Armstrong D. Management of infectious complications in acquired immunodeficiency syndrome. *Am J Med* 81 (suppl 1A):59–72, 1986.
6. Sepkowitz K, Telzak EE, Armstrong D. A prospective study of fever among outpatients with advanced HIV infection. Seventh International Conference on AIDS, Florence, Italy, June 1991.
7. Barat LM, Craven DE, Steinberg JL, et al. A prospective study of fever among outpatients with advanced HIV infection. Seventh International Conference on AIDS, Florence, Italy, June 1991.
8. Witt DJ, Craven DE, McCabe WR. Bacterial infections in adults with acquired immune deficiency syndrome (AIDS) and AIDS-related complex. *Am J Med* 82:900–906, 1987.
9. Sperber SJ, Schleupner CJ. Salmonellosis during infection with human immunodeficiency virus. *Rev Infect Dis* 9:925–934, 1987.
10. Modilevsky T, Sattler FR, Barnes PF. Mycobacterial disease in patients with human immunodeficiency virus infection. *Arch Intern Med* 149:2201–2205, 1989.
11. Melbye M, Grossman RJ, Goedert JJ, et al. Risk of AIDS after herpes zoster. *Lancet* 1:728–731, 1987.
12. Masur H, Ognibene FP, Yarchoan R, et al. CD4 counts as predictors of opportunistic pneumonias in human immunodeficiency virus infection. *Ann Intern Med* 111:223–231, 1989.
13. Palestine AG, Polis MA, De Smet MD, et al. A randomized controlled trial of foscarnet in the treatment of cytomegalovirus retinitis in patients with AIDS. *Ann Intern Med* 115:665–673, 1991.
14. Armstrong D, Gold JW, Dryjanski J, et al. Treatment of infections in patients with the acquired immunodeficiency syndrome. *Ann Intern Med* 103:738–743, 1985.
15. Kaplan LD, Wofsky CB, Volberding PA. Treatment of patients with acquired immunodeficiency syndrome and associated manifestations. *JAMA* 257:1367–1374, 1987.
16. Glatt AE, Chirgwin K, Landesman SH. Treatment of infections associated with human immunodeficiency virus. *N Engl J Med* 318:1439–1448, 1988.
17. Robert-Guroff M, Weiss SH, Giron JA, et al. Prevalence of antibodies to

HTLV-I, -II, and -III in intravenous drug abusers from an AIDS endemic region. *JAMA* 255:3133–3137, 1986.
18. Centers for Disease Control. AIDS due to HIV-2 infection—New Jersey. *MMWR* 37:33–35, 1988.
19. Cortes E, Detels R, Aboulafia D, et al. HIV-1, HIV-2, and HTLV-1 infection in high-risk groups in Brazil. *N Engl J Med* 320:953–958, 1989.
20. Kaplan MH, Susin M, Pahwa S, et al. Neoplastic complications of HTLV-III infection: Lymphomas and solid tumors. *Am J Med* 82:389–396, 1987.
21. Bach MC, Bagwell SG, Fanning JP. Primary pulmonary Kaposi's sarcoma in the acquired immune deficiency syndrome: A cause of persistent pyrexia. *Am J Med* 85:274–275, 1988.
22. Marantz PR, Linzer M, Feiner CJ, et al. Inability to predict diagnosis in febrile intravenous drug abusers. *Ann Intern Med* 106:823–828, 1987.
23. Kopelman RG, Zolla-Panzer S. Association of human immuno-deficiency virus infection and autoimmune phenomena. *Am J Med* 84:82–88, 1988.
24. Fineman DS, Palestro CJ, Kim CK, et al. Detection of abnormalities in febrile AIDS patients with In-III-labeled leukocyte and Ga-67 scintigraphy. *Radiology* 170:677–680, 1989.
25. Kramer EL, Sanger JJ, Garay SM, et al. Gallium-67 scans of the chest in patients with acquired immunodeficiency syndrome. *J Nucl Med* 28:1107, 1987.

5/Weight Loss and Malnutrition

James J. Heffernan, Colleen Manning Osten, Eileen Dunn

Clinical Manifestations

Substantial weight loss, generally regarded as a reduction from baseline of greater than 10 percent, occurs in an overwhelming majority (62–79%) of patients with AIDS [1, 2]. In one series, the mean weight loss among 50 men with AIDS who did not receive enteral intubation or parenteral support was 11.8 kg [3]. Primary HIV infection has been associated with some degree of weight loss in 46 percent of cases; non-AIDS symptomatic HIV disease is often characterized by tissue wasting, although the pattern and magnitude are less well characterized [4]. Recognition of the frequency and importance of weight loss in AIDS resulted in the inclusion of the "HIV wasting syndrome" in the revised Centers for Disease Control surveillance case definition in 1987. This syndrome consists of serologic evidence of HIV infection and "findings of profound involuntary weight loss > 10% of baseline body weight plus either chronic diarrhea (at least two loose stools per day for > 30 days) or chronic weakness and documented fever (intermittent or constant for > 30 days) in the absence of a concurrent illness that could explain the findings" [5]. Patients with AIDS are commonly malnourished on admission to the hospital, and their weight drops an average of 16 percent during hospitalization. Early in the course of the epidemic, nutritional interventions were rarely implemented [1]. While more recent data suggest better attention to nutritional support, fewer than 20 percent of major AIDS treatment centers in the United States currently have standard nutrition protocols [6].

In otherwise normal individuals, malnutrition is associated with a number of immunologic defects: lymphopenia (especially affecting CD4 cell count), depressed cell-mediated immunity, diminished killer cell function, reduced levels of complement and secretory immunoglobulins, and depressed phagocytosis. However, it remains unclear whether malnutrition or its treatment in an HIV-infected patient alters progression of the underlying disease. Nutritional therapy clearly has beneficial effects on the clinical course and immunologic status of critically ill patients with other conditions, and most authorities consider such support to be an integral part of the management of AIDS patients [7].

Laboratory Data

The pattern of weight loss in most patients with AIDS is that of protein-calorie malnutrition, with evidence of more profound body cell mass depletion than weight reduction alone would suggest. Significant reductions in total body potassium, retinol-binding protein concentration, iron binding capacity, and serum albumin concentration have been demonstrated in AIDS patients compared to healthy homosexual control subjects [2]. Body fat content may remain normal. Patients with AIDS also have relative overhydration in the extracellular space despite an overall decrease in body water. These findings are similar to the pattern of wasting noted in the clinical settings of burn, sepsis, trauma, and surgery. A subset of patients with AIDS, generally those with restricted protein-calorie intake but without concurrent diarrheal illness, may show a more typical pattern of starvation, with utilization of fat stores and better maintenance of body cell mass [2]. Cachectin/tumor necrosis factor (TNF) suppresses lipoprotein lipase in adipocytes in vitro and causes weight loss under experimental conditions. Levels of TNF have been found to be uniformly elevated in patients with AIDS, normal in those with asymptomatic HIV infection, and variably elevated in those with intermediate stages of HIV disease [8]. It is not known whether the elevated level of TNF in those with symptomatic HIV disease represents a response to HIV infection per se or a response to secondary infections or malignancies, or both. It is likely, although not yet proven, that other cytokines such as interleukin-1 and interferon play a role in the anorexia and tissue wasting associated with HIV infection [9].

Differential Diagnosis

The causes of weight loss in an HIV-infected individual are legion [10–12]. The problem is generally multifactorial (Table 5-1); identified causes of weight loss often respond to specific interventions or to the application of directed nutrition management, or both. Chronic diarrhea is quite common among patients with AIDS in the US; not surprisingly, given broader exposure to potential gastrointestinal pathogens, severe diarrhea or wasting, or both, are even more prevalent among patients with AIDS from Haiti and Africa, contributing to the syndrome of "slim disease" [13]. North American patients with AIDS and chronic diarrhea have demonstrated more profound reductions in body cell mass and shorter survival than AIDS patients without diarrhea; preliminary data suggest that the magnitude of depletion is more important than the cause itself in determining prognosis. The search for the cause of chronic diarrhea in patients with advanced HIV infection should proceed beyond repeated stool examinations; endoscopy with small bowel

Table 5-1 Factors contributing to weight loss in HIV infection

Problem	Etiology	Management
Food not accessible or preparation difficulties	Social or health causes	Social service Homemaker
Anorexia	Intercurrent illness HIV infection Depression	Treat Megestrol acetate Antidepressant therapy
Nausea/vomiting	Medications HIV gastroparesis	Discontinue Metoclopramide
Dysphagia/odynophagia	Gingivitis/periodontitis Opportunistic diseases	Dental referral Specific Rx
Diarrhea/malabsorption	Opportunistic diseases HIV infection	Specific Rx Antiretroviral therapy

biopsy, light and electron microscopic examination, and morphometric studies have identified occult pathogens in up to 50 percent of such cases [14].

Patients with AIDS, wasting syndrome, and disseminated infection with cytomegalovirus (CMV) or *Mycobacterium avium* complex (MAC), or both, have been noted to succumb when body weight drops one third below ideal values [15]. A recently developed prognostic staging system for AIDS has suggested that persistent diarrhea and serum albumin less than 2.0 gm/dl are more sensitive predictors of short-term survival than is a 10 percent loss of body weight [16].

Evaluation

A complete nutritional assessment is indicated in an HIV-infected patient whenever malnutrition is suspected, especially when the individual has had an involuntary 20-lb or 10 percent reduction from usual weight. The cornerstone of nutritional assessment is an accurate diet history to evaluate and quantify the patient's past and present oral intake; to identify any difficulties with obtaining, eating, or tolerating foods; and to determine whether the patient is following nutritionally sound practices. A detailed list of medications must be obtained: Zidovudine may cause profound dysgeusia or myopathy with muscle wasting; trimethoprim-sulfamethoxazole, sulfadiazine, ketoconazole, and antimycobacterial agents commonly produce anorexia; the use of anticancer chemotherapeutic agents may be attended by severe nausea, anorexia, or mucositis; and pentamidine rarely causes diabetes mellitus. Nutritional assessment should include both anthropometric measure-

Table 5-2 Calculation of patient's basal caloric requirements[a]

BEE (male) = 66 + (13.7 × wt) + (5 × ht) − (6.8 × age)[b]
BEE (female) = 655 + (9.6 × wt) + (1.7 × ht) − (4.7 × age)[b]

Activity factor (AF)		Injury factor (IF)	
Confined to bed	1.2	Surgery	1.1–1.2
Ambulatory	1.3	Infection	1.2–1.6
		Trauma	1.1–1.8
		Sepsis	1.4–1.8

Estimated energy needs (EEN) = BEE × AF × IF

[a]Resting energy needs increase 13% for each degree Celsius, or 7.2% for each degree Fahrenheit.
[b]Wt = weight in kg; ht = height in cm; age = years.

ments and serum studies. Relevant measurements include current height, weight, and weight change over time; triceps skinfold thickness to evaluate fat reserves; and midarm circumference to assess somatic protein status. The patient's pre-illness weight is the best reference in evaluating weight changes [3]. Laboratory studies should include serum albumin, transferrin, and total protein. Serum albumin less than 2.5 gm/dl is associated with decreased bowel wall oncotic pressure and impaired gut function; albumin less than 2.0 gm/dl correlates with severe malnutrition and reduced survival [16]. Other studies, such as serum folate and cyanocobalamin levels, are directed by the clinical features of the case.

A patient's basal caloric requirements can be calculated using the basal energy expenditure (BEE) equation multiplied by an appropriate injury and activity factor [17, 18] (Table 5-2). Optimally, one wishes to provide 150 calories per gram nitrogen; protein needs can thus be estimated by

$$PN = EEN \times \frac{gm\ nitrogen}{150} \times \frac{6.25\ gm\ protein}{gm\ nitrogen}$$

where PN = protein needs and EEN = estimated energy needs [19].

Management

General Issues in Nutritional Support

The goals of nutritional support are preservation of lean body mass and provision of adequate protein, calories, and other nutrients in a formulation that minimizes side effects, especially malabsorption. Currently, there is no clinically proven superior oral, enteral, or parenteral diet for patients with symptomatic HIV disease, and, therefore, nutrition management must be individualized. Nutritional support is indicated if a patient has sustained a 20-lb or 10 percent weight loss in 6 months or is unable to meet 100 percent of his/her nutritional needs [7]. Early intervention may prevent the complications of malnutrition and maintain or improve quality of life.

In the patient with a functioning gut, oral delivery of nutrients maintains the structural and functional integrity of the gastrointestinal mucosa, minimizes costs, and decreases the risk of infection. A high-calorie, high-protein diet with a multivitamin supplement is recommended; modification of fat and lactose content is often necessary, especially in the patient with diarrhea. An enteral formula, administered orally or transnasally (and rarely per gastric tube), may supplement or replace the oral diet and should be selected with reference to fat content ($<5\%$ or as tolerated), viscosity, cost, osmolality, caloric density, patient acceptance, feasibility for home use, protein-calorie ratio, and lactose content. Patients with weight loss may be far more receptive to the initiation of enteral feedings as a choice in an outpatient setting than when such an intervention is presented during a hospitalization for acute illness. Enteral preparations include nutritionally complete elemental or polymeric formulas and modular formulas; many such commercial products have been used successfully in patients with HIV-associated syndromes [7]. If a patient with AIDS develops diarrhea while utilizing an enteral product, one must consider the myriad of potential causes other than the product itself, including hypoalbuminemia, antibiotic therapy, bacterial contamination, or a new infection. Formula-related problems include improper rate or strength of administration, specific content (fat, lactose), and temperature of feedings.

Parenteral nutrition can be used effectively to reestablish nutritional homeostasis in malnourished HIV-infected patients, but is generally reserved for those in whom oral and enteral methods have failed or cannot be used, or for those who have a clinical indication for rapid correction of nutritional deficiencies, such as impending surgery. Many causes of gut dysfunction in AIDS, with the notable exception of severe diarrhea due to cryptosporidiosis or HIV-induced enteropathy, or both, respond well to directed therapy. In some patients, parenteral nutrition may be required for only brief periods while specific therapy arrests or reverses gut dysfunction. A decision to implement chronic parenteral nutritional support should be made only after careful assessment of its likely effect on quality and duration of life.

Specific Nutrition Management Strategies

Anorexia is nearly universal at some point in the course of AIDS. Small frequent feedings; a high-calorie, high-protein diet; and an enteral supplementation are recommended. If oral intake is inadequate, transnasal tube feedings may be required. There is increasing experience with megestrol acetate, which has been shown to be effective in promoting improved appetite and weight gain among cachectic AIDS patients [20, 21]. Depressed patients may respond to tricyclic antidepressant therapy, with improvements in mood, appetite, and oral intake, although there are no published data demonstrating reversal of weight loss with these agents. Cyproheptadine may also enhance appetite but at the expense of sedation. In addition, nonsteroidal antiinflammatory drugs, fish oils (N-3 fatty acids), or more specific cytokine blockers may inhibit components of the anorexia and weight loss associated with HIV infection [9].

In patients with disorders of the oral cavity and esophagus, modifications in the acidity, temperature, texture, consistency, and seasoning of food may improve tolerance. If a patient's intake is compromised for more than 3 inpatient days, tube feedings should be considered. When esophageal ulcers preclude the use of nasogastric tube feedings, short-term (7–10 days) parenteral nutrition may be considered. Thrush, hairy leukoplakia, and herpetic infection occasionally pose barriers to oral intake, but generally respond to appropriate therapy. Symptomatic relief from painful mucosal lesions may be obtained with warm saline rinses, a mixture of Kaopectate and diphenhydramine oral suspension, viscous lidocaine, or sucralfate in suspension. Instruction and encouragement in good oral hygiene may pay dividends in retarding the development of accelerated caries and periodontal disease. With long-term dysfunction of the upper digestive tract, placement of a gastrostomy or jejunostomy feeding tube is an option. Nausea and vomiting can be managed through the use of antiemetics and postprandial timing of drug therapy. A low-fat, soft, bland diet with an enteral supplement is best tolerated. Patients should maintain an upright or semi-upright posture for such feedings. Tube feedings, especially nasojejunostomy feedings, may be indicated for refractory nausea and vomiting; one should always consider the possibility of a central nervous system lesion as the cause of such symptoms. Early satiety from HIV gastroparesis may respond to metoclopramide; mechanical obstruction from bulky abdominal or retroperitoneal tumors or adenopathy may be relieved with chemotherapy. It is also important to recognize that emotional stress and psychosocial issues may contribute to nausea and early satiety. Relaxation exercises before meals and institution of a regimen of small frequent feedings may be extremely helpful in this regard.

Diarrhea is the most common gastrointestinal manifestation of AIDS and often the most problematic to treat. The pattern of diarrhea may be enteropathic (frequent, large-volume, nonbloody stools without tenesmus), resulting in electrolyte abnormalities and profound wasting, colitic (painful bowel movements, with small-volume mucoid and/or bloody stools, abdominal pain, and often fever), or a combination. Patients with AIDS who have diarrhea manifest greater weight loss, lower CD4 lymphocyte counts, and a higher incidence of extraintestinal opportunistic infections than those without diarrhea. In the majority of such patients, enteric pathogens can be identified and treated successfully [22]. Diarrhea and other bowel problems arising from pathogenic bacteria, CMV, herpes simplex virus, and most protozoan and helminthic infestations generally respond to antimicrobial therapy. Unfortunately, the most severe diarrhea often occurs in the setting of cryptosporidiosis, for which there is, to date, no effective therapy. The possibility of iatrogenic diarrhea, such as Clostridium difficile–associated colitis, should always be considered.

Sometimes investigation does not reveal a specific cause of diarrhea in HIV-infected patients, and the syndrome is attributed to the enteropathogenic effects of HIV. A somatostatin analogue, octreotide, has shown promise in several case reports of severe secretory diarrhea in patients with AIDS, with or without cryptosporidial colonization [23, 24].

Several nutrition regimens have been espoused for use in the HIV-infected individual with diarrhea predicated on pattern of gut dysfunction and independent of the specific cause [6, 25, 26]. In the setting of severe small bowel disease and profound malabsorption, nutrition can only be effectively delivered parenterally. If the underlying cause of severe small bowel dysfunction can be ameliorated, an elemental enteral diet may promote gut function. With less profound small bowel dysfunction, frequent small feedings with low fat, low lactose, low fiber, low residue, and no caffeine should be administered. A similar diet in those with large bowel disease may be effective in reducing the frequency of bowel movements. Nonspecific mild enteropathy may respond to the addition of a bulking agent [26]. Most patients with AIDS and moderate or severe diarrhea require adjunctive therapy with an antidiarrheal agent. Institution of a "BRAT" (bananas, rice, apples, and tea or toast) diet may also be helpful in gaining control of diarrhea, but is nutritionally incomplete and inappropriate for extended use [6]. One should add an isotonic supplement, multivitamins, and appropriate fluids to the BRAT diet after a patient has followed it successfully for several days.

Weight loss and malnutrition are concomitant, in the absence of diarrhea, with systemic infections and malignancies associated with HIV infection. Antimicrobial therapy may readily control the fever and weight loss associated with Salmonella or Shigella bacteremia, Mycobacterium tuberculosis infection, or systemic fungal infection. Body mass repletion has also been accomplished with ganciclovir treatment of CMV infection [15]. The most common disseminated infection resulting in weight loss and fever in patients with AIDS is MAC; symptomatic improvement may occur with multidrug antimycobacterial regimens. Antineoplastic therapy for non-Hodgkin's lymphoma or Kaposi's sarcoma may reverse the fever and wasting that accompany these malignancies.

Conclusion

Involuntary weight loss occurs in virtually all patients with AIDS and is seen frequently in earlier stages of HIV infection. Most patients exhibit protein-calorie malnutrition with profound body cell mass depletion. There are numerous potential causes of weight loss in patients with HIV infection, many of which respond to specific therapy. Therefore, a complete nutritional assessment should be carried out in any patient who has lost 20 lb or 10 percent of usual weight. Nutritional management is individualized, with the goals of preservation of lean body mass and the provision of adequate protein, calories, and nutrients. While there is no clear evidence that nutritional support alters the course of HIV infection, such therapy is an accepted part of management.

References

1. O'Sullivan P, Linke RA, Dalton S. Evaluation of body weight and nutritional status among AIDS patients. *J Am Diet Assoc* 85:1483–1484, 1985.
2. Kotler DP, Wang J, Pierson RN. Body composition studies in patients with the acquired immunodeficiency syndrome. *Am J Clin Nutr* 42:1255–1265, 1985.
3. Garcia ME, Collins CL, Mansell PWA. The acquired immune deficiency syndrome: Nutritional complications and assessment of body weight status. *Nutr Clin Prac* 2:108–111, 1987.
4. Tindall B, Barker S, Donovan B, et al. Characterization of the acute clinical illness associated with human immunodeficiency virus infection. *Arch Intern Med* 148:945–949, 1988.
5. Centers for Disease Control. Revision of the CDC surveillance case definition for acquired immunodeficiency syndrome. *MMWR* 36 (suppl):3–15, 1987.
6. Ysseldyke LL. Nutritional complications and incidence of malnutrition among AIDS patients. *J Am Diet Assoc* 91:217–218, 1991.
7. Hickey MS, Weaver KE. Nutritional management of patients with ARC or AIDS. *Gastroenterol Clin North Am* 17:545–561, 1988.
8. Lahdevirta J, Maury CPJ, Teppo A-M, Repo H. Elevated levels of circulating cachectin/tumor necrosis factor in patients with acquired immunodeficiency syndrome. *Am J Med* 85:289–291, 1988.

9. Hellerstein MK, Kahn J, Mudie H, Viteri F. Current approach to the treatment of human immunodeficiency virus–associated weight loss: Pathophysiologic considerations and emerging management strategies. *Semin Oncol* 17 (suppl 9):17–33, 1990.
10. Greene JB. Clinical approach to weight loss in the patient with HIV infection. *Gastroenterol Clin North Am* 17:573–586, 1988.
11. Kotler DP. Intestinal and hepatic manifestations of AIDS. *Adv Intern Med* 34:43–72, 1989.
12. Resler SS. Nutrition care of AIDS patients. *J Am Diet Assoc* 88:828–832, 1988.
13. Serwadda D, Sewankambo NK, Carswell JW, et al. Slim disease: A new disease in Uganda and its association with HTLV-III infection. *Lancet* 2:849–852, 1985.
14. Greenson JK, Belitsos PC, Yardley JH, Bartlett JG. AIDS enteropathy: Occult enteric infections and duodenal mucosal alterations in chronic diarrhea. *Ann Intern Med* 114:366–372, 1991.
15. Kotler DP, Tierney AR, Altilio D, et al. Body mass repletion during gancyclovir treatment of cytomegalovirus infections in patients with acquired immunodeficiency syndrome. *Arch Intern Med* 149:901–905, 1989.
16. Justice AC, Feinstein AR, Wells CK. A new prognostic staging system for the acquired immunodeficiency syndrome. *N Engl J Med* 320:1388–1393, 1989.
17. Harris JA, Benedict FG. A biometric study of basal metabolism in man. Washington, DC: Carnegie Institution of Washington, 2:227, 1919.
18. Jan J, Van Lanschot B, Feenstra B, et al. Calculation versus measurement of total energy expenditure. *Crit Care Med* 14:982, 1986.
19. Krause MV, Mahan LK. *Food, Nutrition and Diet Therapy.* Philadelphia: Saunders, 1979.
20. Von Roenn JH, Murphy RL, Weber KM, et al. Megestrol acetate for treatment of cachexia associated with human immunodeficiency virus (HIV) infection. *Ann Intern Med* 109:840–841, 1988.
21. Von Roenn JH, Murphy RL, Wegener N. Megestrol acetate for treatment of anorexia and cachexia associated with human immunodeficiency virus infection. *Semin Oncol* 17 (suppl 9):13–16, 1990.
22. Smith PD, Lane HC, Gill VJ, et al. Intestinal infections in patients with the acquired immunodeficiency syndrome (AIDS). *Ann Intern Med* 108:328–333, 1988.
23. Cook DJ, Kelton JG, Andrzej MS, Collins SM. Somatostatin treatment for cryptosporidial diarrhea in a patient with the acquired immunodeficiency syndrome (AIDS). *Ann Intern Med* 108:708–709, 1988.
24. Robinson EN, Fogel R. SMS 201–995, a somatostatin analogue, and diarrhea in the acquired immunodeficiency syndrome (AIDS). *Ann Intern Med* 108:680–681, 1988.
25. O'Neill L. Acquired immune deficiency syndrome and nutrition. *Dietitians Nutr Support* 13:13–16, 1988.
26. Task Force on Nutrition Support in AIDS. Guidelines for nutrition support in AIDS. *Nutrition* 5:39–46, 1989.

6/Oral Manifestations

David L. Battinelli, Edward S. Peters

Oral lesions are often an early manifestation of HIV disease. They can be identified in 40 percent of all HIV-infected patients and in over 90 percent of AIDS patients [1–3]. While many different types of lesions have been described, a small number predominate [4]. Most HIV-related oral lesions are fungal, bacterial, viral, or neoplastic [5] (Table 6-1). Even though many are not specific to HIV disease, their presentation, natural history, and response to therapy are affected by the patient's degree of immunodeficiency [6]. Their course is also dependent on the presence of systemic disease and the individual's state of oral hygiene. Diagnosis of HIV-related oral disease is based primarily on clinical presentation in conjunction with routine smears and cultures; biopsy is rarely indicated.

Fungal Diseases

Oral Candidiasis

Candidiasis is the most common oral manifestation of HIV infection and often represents the initial symptom of HIV disease. In one study, 59 percent of patients with high-risk behaviors who had oral candidiasis developed AIDS, and over 90 percent of patients with AIDS experienced oral candidiasis sometime during their course [7]. Oral candidiasis is seen with advancing immunodeficiency, generally first occurring when the CD4 cell count falls below 400/mm^3 [5]. *Candida albicans,* part of the normal oral flora, is the most frequent pathogen, but other species have also been identified [8].

The clinical variants of oral candidiasis include pseudomembranous (thrush), hyperplastic, and atrophic forms, and angular cheilitis [8]. Oral candidiasis may be asymptomatic or associated with pain, burning, or irritation of the mouth [8]. The presence of odynophagia or retrosternal pain with swallowing suggests esophageal involvement. Pseudomembranous candidiasis, the most common variant, is characterized by white or cream-colored plaques, which, when scraped by a tongue blade, reveal reddened or bleeding mucosa (Plate 1). Multiple lesions may involve the buccal mucosa, dorsal tongue, gingiva, and hard and soft palates. Hyperplastic candidiasis, most often found on the buccal

Table 6-1 Oral manifestations of HIV infection

Fungal diseases
  Candidiasis
Viral diseases
  Herpes simplex virus
  Varicella-zoster virus
  Hairy leukoplakia
  Human papillomavirus
  Cytomegalovirus
Neoplastic diseases
  Kaposi's sarcoma
  Lymphoma
  Squamous cell carcinoma
Bacterial diseases
  Gingivitis
  Periodontitis
  Syphilis
  Gram-negative infection
  Mycobacterium avium complex infection
Miscellaneous conditions
  Aphthous ulcerations
  Idiopathic thrombocytopenic purpura
  Xerostomia
  Salivary gland enlargement

mucosa, manifests as white plaques (leukoplakia) that cannot be removed by scraping. Atrophic candidiasis is characterized by erythematous macular lesions of the buccal mucosa, hard palate, and dorsal surface of the tongue. Angular cheilitis presents as erythema, cracking, fissuring, and ulceration of the corners of the mouth.

Initial diagnosis of oral candidiasis is based on the clinical features and demonstration of budding yeast and pseudohyphae on smears examined with Gram's stain or potassium hydroxide. Diagnosis of recurrent episodes can be made clinically and by response to empiric therapy.

Oral candidiasis responds well to topical or systemic antifungal agents. Topical preparations include clotrimazole oral troches, 10 mg, dissolved slowly three to five times a day, and nystatin vaginal tablets 100,000 units, or oral pastilles, 200,000 units, one to two dissolved slowly three to five times a day. Nystatin suspension, 10 to 20 ml, swished and swallowed three to five times a day, is also effective but generally less well tolerated. Ketoconazole, an oral imidazole, 200 mg once or twice a day with food, is generally reserved for patients with refractory thrush or esophageal involvement; fluconazole, 50 to 100 mg orally once a day, is also effective but considerably more expensive [9]. Topical clotrimazole cream can be used to treat angular cheilitis.

Oral candidiasis generally improves within a few days of initiation of treatment. Reduced doses of topical or systemic agents are effective as maintenance therapy to prevent disease recurrence, which is common as immunosuppression progresses. Antimicrobial resistance may emerge in patients treated with chronic antifungal therapy [10].

Other Fungi

Other fungal diseases that less frequently cause oral lesions in HIV-infected patients include histoplasmosis, cryptococcosis, and geotrichosis [4, 11]. They generally manifest as persistent ulcerations, and their diagnosis is made by biopsy and culture.

Viral Infections

Herpesvirus infections are especially prevalent in HIV disease. Herpes simplex virus (HSV), varicella-zoster virus (VZV), Epstein-Barr virus (EBV), and, less commonly, cytomegalovirus (CMV) have been associated with a variety of acute and chronic oral lesions.

Herpes Simplex Virus

Herpes simplex virus produces painful ulcerations involving the oral mucosa (gingivostomatitis) or lips (herpes labialis), or both (Plate 2). Lesions appear abruptly as solitary or multiple small vesicles on an erythematous base that rupture to form ulcerations [12]. Herpes simplex virus infection frequently affects the hard and soft palate but may also involve the gingiva, floor of the mouth, and tongue. Labial lesions typically form large ulcerations that extend onto the facial skin. HIV-infected patients may have lesions that are atypical in appearance, aggressive, and persistent. Mucocutaneous HSV disease that lasts longer than 4 weeks in this population meets the Centers for Disease Control criteria for AIDS.

Diagnosis of HSV infection is made presumptively on clinical grounds and confirmed by culture or Tzanck smear, which shows multinucleated giant cells and viral inclusion bodies. Management consists of oral acyclovir, 200 to 800 mg five times a day; topical acyclovir is ineffective. Lesions generally clear within several days of initiation of therapy [12]. If response to oral therapy is inadequate, intravenous acyclovir, 5 to 10 mg/kg every 8 hours for one week, is indicated. Maintenance therapy at lower doses can be given in an effort to reduce the frequency of recurrent disease. Herpes simplex virus resistance to acyclovir has been described, and topical trifluridine or systemic foscarnet may be effective in this setting [9, 13].

Varicella-Zoster Virus

When VZV, the cause of shingles, involves the second (maxillary) or third (mandibular) branches of the trigeminal nerve, the oral mucosa may be affected. VZV infection of the mouth produces unilateral pain and a vesicular eruption that leads to mucosal ulceration [12, 14]. Diagnosis of VZV infection is made clinically. Oral acyclovir, 800 mg five times a day, is used to expedite healing and prevent dissemination. While recurrent VZV infection has been described in HIV-infected patients, maintenance therapy is generally not recommended.

Hairy Leukoplakia

Hairy leukoplakia (HL), which is caused by EBV, was originally thought to be unique to HIV infection in that it had not been described before the AIDS epidemic [15, 16]. However, there have since been case reports of HL in immunosuppressed heart, kidney, and bone marrow transplant recipients [17].

Hairy leukoplakia typically manifests as leukoplakia involving the lateral borders of the tongue that is corrugated or folded in appearance (Plate 3). The folds run vertically and have hair-like or "hairy" projections, which are best appreciated when the tongue is protruded and stretched to one side [18]. In severe HL, the entire dorsal surface of the tongue may be involved, and lesions are sometimes located on the buccal or labial mucosa. Hairy leukoplakia has negative prognostic implications; in over 50 percent of patients diagnosed with the condition, AIDS develops within 30 months of presentation [19].

Presumptive diagnosis of HL is based on its clinical appearance, and biopsy is generally not necessary. On histologic examination, hyperparakeratosis, acanthosis, and vacuolation of epithelial cells with minimal subepithelial inflammation are seen. A number of other white lesions can appear on the tongue in HIV-infected patients. Differential diagnosis includes candidiasis, tobacco-associated leukoplakia, lichen planus, traumatic mucositis, restorative dental material (galvanic lesion), and geographic tongue.

Hairy leukoplakia is asymptomatic and benign, and, therefore, generally requires no specific treatment. Temporary regression of HL has been observed in patients receiving antiviral therapy, including acyclovir, ganciclovir, and zidovudine [20–22]. Clinical improvement may be related to immunologic or antiviral effects [23]. An experimental analogue of acyclovir, given orally, has also caused regression of HL [24].

Human Papillomavirus

Human papillomavirus is the agent responsible for skin and mucosal warts, which may be more frequent and less responsive to treatment in HIV-infected patients [25–27]. Lesions are often multiple and located throughout the oral cavity. Diagnosis is made by recognition of the typical sessile-appearing or "cauliflower" papular lesions [8]. Some oral warts are well circumscribed and have a flat surface, and may disappear completely with stretching of the mucosa [28]. Treatment is by surgical excision, cryosurgery, or laser therapy, but recurrence is common.

Cytomegalovirus

Cytomegalovirus infection is most often associated with retinitis, and mucosal involvement is uncommon. Intraoral CMV infection may manifest as nonspecific mucositis, large well-demarcated shallow ulcerations, or salivary gland enlargement and xerostomia. Severe oral disease generally occurs in the context of systemic CMV infection. Diagnosis of oral CMV disease is made by biopsy. Treatment consists of systemic ganciclovir or foscarnet [14].

Neoplastic Diseases

Kaposi's Sarcoma

Kaposi's sarcoma (KS) is the most common neoplasm in AIDS, and more than 50 percent of patients with KS have oral involvement [29]. Intraoral lesions may occur alone or in conjunction with skin, visceral, and lymph node disease. In 10 percent of patients with KS, mouth lesions may be the only finding [20]. Oral KS presents as red or purple, nonblanching macules, papules, or nodules. Lesions are especially common on the hard palate and gingival margins, and are frequently asymptomatic [17]. Early oral KS may be only minimally different in color from normal mucosa, but, as lesions progress, they often ulcerate and bleed. Kaposi's sarcoma of the gingiva produces diffuse swelling and may be mistaken for gingivitis or periodontitis [17] (Plate 4). Diagnosis of oral KS is by biopsy. Therapy is with surgical excision, laser or radiation therapy, or systemic chemotherapy, depending on the number and size of the lesions and the presence of systemic disease. Lesions may recur following treatment.

Non-Hodgkin's Lymphoma

Occasionally HIV-related non-Hodgkin's lymphoma involves the oral mucosa, presenting as a firm, painless swelling, with or without ulceration, anywhere in the mouth but especially on the gingiva or palate [28, 30]. Any oral nodule and mass should be biopsied to rule out lymphoma. Non-Hodgkin's lymphoma is a systemic disease that requires chemotherapy.

Carcinoma

Squamous cell carcinoma, usually on the lateral and undersurface of the tongue, has also been described in HIV-infected patients [3]. Treatment consists of local excision and radiation therapy.

Bacterial Diseases

Gingivitis and Periodontal Disease

Human immunodeficiency virus infection is associated with severe gingival and periodontal disease that differs from that seen in normal hosts in its atypical appearance and rapid progression [31, 32]. While HIV-related gingivitis (HIV-G) and periodontitis (HIV-P) often involve the entire mouth, they can also present as discrete lesions adjacent to areas of healthy tissue.

HIV-G is a disease of the gingival margin, gingiva, and, occasionally, the alveolar mucosa that occurs in approximately 20 percent of HIV-infected patients [33]. It is characterized by marked erythema of the gingiva that may extend several millimeters away from the margin, and spontaneous or easy bleeding, ulceration, or necrosis of the interdental gingiva may be observed [32]. HIV-G often responds poorly to conventional therapy and may progress to HIV-P.

HIV-related periodontitis presents with gingival erythema and ulceration, soft-tissue necrosis, and rapid destruction of the periodontal attachment (Plate 5). Deep pain, bleeding, and exposure of the underlying bone may also be observed, with loss of more than 90 percent of the alveolar bone occurring within a few weeks. Significant tooth mobility is a common finding. HIV-P is usually seen as a localized lesion surrounded by areas of gingivitis. Untreated HIV-P is rapidly progressive and results in tooth loss [15, 29].

The management of HIV-G and HIV-P consists of removal of plaque and calculus by scaling and root planing and debridement of necrotic tissue. Povidone-iodine solution and chlorhexidine may be useful adjunctively, as may antibiotic therapy with penicillin, metronidazole, or clindamycin. Extraction of involved teeth is often necessary [29].

Other Bacteria

There have been a few case reports of oral lesions caused by gram-negative organisms, including *Klebsiella pneumoniae* and *Enterobacter cloacae* [2]. In addition, *Mycobacterium avium* complex infection presenting as mouth ulcerations has also been described [34]. Both of these diseases are managed with systemic antimicrobial therapy.

Miscellaneous Oral Conditions

Aphthous Ulcerations

Recurrent aphthous ulcerations are frequently associated with HIV infection [3]. While their etiology is unclear, trauma, systemic illness, and viruses have been implicated as contributing factors. Small, painful, shallow ulcers on an erythematous base with a raised white, glistening margin are observed, and these may enlarge and become necrotic over time (Plate 6). Symptomatic ulcers that do not heal spontaneously should be treated with topical steroids. Fluocinonide ointment 0.05% mixed with equal quantities of Orabase applied three to six times a day is effective [35]. Severe ulcers that do not respond to topical therapy can be treated with a short course of oral prednisone [35]. Recently, thalidomide, 100 mg per day orally, has also been reported to be useful in this setting [26]. Differential diagnosis of mouth ulcers includes HSV infection, CMV infection, syphilis, and lymphoma. They have also been associated with dideoxycytidine (ddC) therapy. Lesions that do not respond to empiric therapy should be biopsied.

Idiopathic Thrombocytopenic Purpura

Idiopathic thrombocytopenic purpura can manifest as gingival bleeding, oral petechia, mucosal ecchymosis, or hemorrhagic bullae. Lesions are occasionally mistaken for KS.

Xerostomia

Xerostomia, or dry mouth, has been described with or without parotid gland enlargement in the context of HIV infection. The syndrome is characterized by failure to express saliva from Wharton's or Stensen's ducts. Viral and autoimmune causes appear responsible for some cases, but the syndrome may also result from drug toxicity (e.g., tricyclic antidepressants). The presence of parotid enlargement may necessitate salivary gland biopsy to rule out lymphoma, Sjögren's syndrome, or sarcoidosis [3, 36].

References

1. Murray HW, Hillman JK, Rubin BY, et al. Patients at risk for AIDS-related opportunistic infections. *N Engl J Med* 313:1504, 1985.
2. Klein RS, Harris CA, Small CR, et al. Oral candidiasis in high-risk patients as the initial manifestations of the acquired immunodeficiency syndrome. *N Engl J Med* 311:354–358, 1984.
3. Silverman S, Migliorati CA, Lozada-Nur F, et al. Oral findings in people with or at high risk for AIDS: A study of 375 homosexual males. *J Am Dent Assoc* 112:187, 1986.
4. Phelan JA, Saltzman BR, Friedland GH, Klein RS. Oral findings in patients with acquired immunodeficiency syndrome. *Oral Surg* 64:50–56, 1987.
5. Barr C, Lopez M, Rau-Dobles A, et al. HIV-associated oral lesions; immunologic, virologic and salivary parameters. *J Oral Pathol Med* 21:295–298, 1992.
6. Orofacial manifestations of HIV infection (editorial). *Lancet* 1:976–977, 1988.
7. Greenspan JS, Greenspan D, Winkler JR. Diagnosis and management of the oral manifestations of HIV infections and AIDS. *Infect Dis Clin North Am* 2:373–383, 1988.
8. Reichart PA, et al. AIDS and the oral cavity. HIV infection: Virology, etiology, origin, immunology, precautions and clinical observations in 110 patients. *Int J Oral Maxillofac Surg* 16:129–153, 1987.
9. Scully C, McCarthy G. Management of oral health in persons with HIV infection. *Oral Surg Oral Med Oral Pathol* 73:215–225, 1992.
10. Leen CLS, Brettle RP, Willocks LJ, Milne LJR. Fluconazole-resistant candidiasis in patients with AIDS. Seventh International Conference on AIDS, Florence, Italy, June 1991.
11. Lynch DP, Naftolin LZ. Oral *Cryptococcus neoformans* infection in AIDS. *Oral Surg* 64:449, 1987.
12. Quinnan GV, Masur H, Rook AH, et al. Herpes virus infections in the acquired immunodeficiency syndrome. *JAMA* 252:72, 1984.
13. Kessler H, et al. ACTG 172: Treatment of acyclovir-resistant (ACV-R) mucocutaneous herpes simplex virus (HSV) infection in patients with AIDS: Open label pilot study of topical trifluridine (TFT). Eighth International Conference on AIDS, Amsterdam, July 1992.
14. Eversole L. Viral infections of the head and neck among HIV-seropositive patients. *Oral Surg Oral Med Oral Pathol* 73:155–163, 1992.
15. Winkler JR, Grassi M, Murray PA. Clinical Description and Etiology of

HIV-Associated Periodontal Diseases. In PB Robertson, JS Greenspan (eds), *Perspectives on Oral Manifestations of AIDS*. Littleton, MA: PSG Publishing, 1988. Pp 49–70.

16. Greenspan JS, Greenspan D, Lennette ET, et al. Replication of Epstein-Barr virus within the epithelial cells of oral "hairy" leukoplakia, an AIDS-associated lesion. *N Engl J Med* 313:1564–1571, 1985.

17. Greenspan D, Greenspan J. Significance of oral hairy leukoplakia. *Oral Surg Oral Med Oral Pathol* 73:151–154, 1992.

18. Schiodt M, Greenspan D, Daniels TE, et al. Clinical and histologic spectrum of oral hairy leukoplakia. *Oral Surg* 64:716–720, 1987.

19. Greenspan D, Greenspan JS, Hearst N, et al. Relation of oral hairy leukoplakia to infection with the human immunodeficiency virus and the risk of developing AIDS. *J Infect Dis* 155:475, 1987.

20. Lozada F, Silverman S, Migliorati CA, et al. Oral manifestations of tumor and opportunistic infections in the acquired immunodeficiency syndrome (AIDS): findings in 53 homosexual men with Kaposi's sarcoma. *Oral Surg* 56:491, 1983.

21. Newman C, Polk BF. Resolution of oral hairy leukoplakia during therapy with 9-(1,3-dihydroxy-2-propoxymethyl) guanine (DHPG). *Ann Intern Med* 107:348–350, 1987.

22. Resnick L, Herbst JS, Ablashi DV, et al. Regression of oral hairy leukoplakia after orally administered acyclovir therapy. *JAMA* 259:384–388, 1988.

23. Kessler HA, Benson CA, Urbanski P. Regression of oral hairy leukoplakia during zidovudine therapy. *Arch Intern Med* 148:2496–2497, 1988.

24. Greenspan D, Greenspan JS, Chapman S, et al. Efficacy of BWA515U in treatment of EBV infection in hairy leukoplakia. Third International Conference on AIDS, Washington, DC, June 1987.

25. Scully C, Laskaris G, Pindborg J, et al. Oral manifestations of HIV infection and their management: I. More common lesions. *Oral Surg Oral Med Oral Pathol* 71:158–166, 1991.

26. Owen WF. Sexually transmitted disease and traumatic problems in homosexual men. *Ann Intern Med* 92:805, 1980.

27. Scully C, Prime S, Maitland N. Papillomaviruses: Their possible role in oral disease. *Oral Surg* 60:166, 1985.

28. Greenspan D. Oral Manifestations of HIV Infection. In PB Robertson, JS Greenspan (eds), *Perspectives on Oral Manifestations of AIDS*. Littleton, MA: PSG Publishing, 1988. Pp 38–48.

29. Winkler JR, Robertson P. Periodontal disease associated with HIV infection. *Oral Surg Oral Med Oral Pathol* 73:145–150, 1992.

30. Ziegler JL, Miner RC, Rosenbaum E, et al. Outbreak of Burkitt's-like lymphoma in homosexual men. *Lancet* 2:261, 1982.

31. Winkler JR, Murray PA. AIDS update: Periodontal disease. *J Calif Dent Assoc* 15:20–24, 1987.

32. Winkler JR, Murray PA. Periodontal disease: A potential intraoral expression of AIDS may be rapidly progressive periodontitis. *J Calif Dent Assoc* 12:20, 1987.

33. Laskaris G, Potouridou I, Laskaris M, Stratigos J. Gingival lesions of HIV

infection in 178 Greek patients. *Oral Surg Oral Med Oral Pathol* 74:168–171, 1992.

34. Volpe F, Schimmer A, Barr C. Oral manifestations of disseminated *Mycobacterium avium-intracellulare* in a patient with AIDS. *Oral Surg* 60:567, 1985.

35. Silverman S, Jr, Lozada-Nur F, Migliorati C. Clinical efficacy of prednisone in the treatment of patients with oral inflammatory ulcerative diseases: A study of fifty-five patients. *Oral Surg* 59:360–363, 1987.

36. Ulirsch RC, Jaffe ES. Sjögren's syndrome–like illness associated with the acquired immunodeficiency syndrome–related complex. *Hum Pathol* 18:1063–1068, 1987.

7 / Ocular Manifestations

David L. Battinelli, Mariel Brittis

Nowhere is the importance of a multidisciplinary approach to the care of HIV-infected patients more evident than in the management of eye disease. Careful evaluation of ocular symptoms by the primary care provider and referral for ophthalmologic examination are essential for early diagnosis and treatment. This chapter reviews the common ocular manifestations of HIV infection (Table 7-1). Comprehensive reviews of the subject are also available [1–4].

Noninfectious Etiologies

Conjunctivitis and Keratitis

Nonspecific conjunctivitis, keratitis, and keratoconjunctivitis sicca have been reported in up to 10 percent of AIDS patients. The patient should be asked about conjunctival and corneal irritation, as well as symptoms related to dry eyes. Examination reveals inflammation of the affected part of the eye without pain or change in visual acuity. Treatment of conjunctivitis and keratitis consists of topical antibiotics; artificial tears are used in the management of keratoconjunctivitis sicca [1].

Ocular Hemorrhages

Multiple subconjunctival, scleral, and retinal hemorrhages may indicate the presence of thrombocytopenia related to idiopathic thrombocytopenic purpura or drug toxicity.

Cotton-Wool Spots

Cotton-wool spots (CWS) are the most common ocular abnormality in HIV disease, occurring in up to 50 percent of patients [3]. Cotton-wool spots are asymptomatic, white, fluffy, superficial retinal lesions with feathered edges generally distributed near the large vessels of the posterior retinal vascular arcade adjacent to the optic nerve [4] (Plate 7). Histologically they represent infarction of the nerve fiber layer of the retina. HIV-related CWS can be distinguished from those occurring with

Table 7-1 Ocular manifestations of HIV infection

Noninfectious	Infectious
Nonspecific conjunctivitis	Conjunctivitis
Nonspecific keratitis	Keratitis
Keratoconjunctivitis sicca	Iridocyclitis
Hemorrhages	Uveitis
Cotton-wool spots	Vitreitis
Papilledema	Retinitis
Kaposi's sarcoma	Multifocal choroiditis
Lymphoma	
Ocular palsies	

diabetes mellitus and hypertension by the absence of associated vascular retinopathy.

Diagnosis of CWS is made by their typical appearance on ophthalmoscopic examination. Differential diagnosis includes early retinitis caused by cytomegalovirus (CMV) and, less commonly, other opportunistic pathogens. Unlike retinitis, CWS regress spontaneously in about 2 months, are rarely associated with hemorrhage, and do not produce visual impairment. No specific treatment is indicated.

Cotton-wool spots, retinal hemorrhages, and other microvascular anomalies are collectively referred to as HIV retinopathy, the etiology of which is uncertain [5]. It has been suggested that CMV enters the retina at CWS, but evidence supporting this hypothesis is inconclusive [6, 7]. One report described isolation of Pneumocystis carinii from CWS [8]. Others have suggested that CWS result directly from HIV infection of the retina with immune complex deposition [9]. Increased serum viscosity secondary to high fibrinogen levels with resultant "sludging" and retinal infarction has also been proposed as the pathogenesis [5].

Papilledema

Papilledema occurs secondary to increased intracranial pressure. In HIV-infected patients, this is often an indication of an expanding infectious or neoplastic mass lesion of the central nervous system. Toxoplasmosis and lymphoma are the two most frequent causes.

Kaposi's Sarcoma

Ocular Kaposi's sarcoma (KS) occurs in up to 20 percent of AIDS patients who have systemic KS and is rarely the initial site of involvement [1]. Presenting signs include proptosis, ptosis, eyelid edema, conjunctival infection, and diplopia resulting from ocular nerve palsies. The characteristic deep-red or violaceous lesion is most often found along the eyelid margins or bulbar conjunctivae and can be easily confused with a conjunctival hemorrhage [2]. Diagnosis is made by biopsy of an associated mucocutaneous lesion.

Lymphoma

Aggressive non-Hodgkin's lymphoma is commonly associated with HIV infection and may involve ocular structures. Symptoms and signs, similar to those of KS, are related primarily to local infiltration of the tumor. Computed tomography and magnetic resonance imaging (MRI) scans together with biopsy are used to diagnose retroorbital mass lesions; vitrectomy permits cytologic sampling for intraocular involvement.

Ocular Palsies

Abnormalities of extraocular movements may be an early manifestation of retroorbital and intracranial mass lesions, described above.

Infectious Etiologies

A variety of bacterial, fungal, viral, and parasitic organisms are responsible for many of the ocular complications of HIV disease.

Conjunctivitis and Keratitis

Herpes simplex virus (HSV) keratitis in HIV-infected patients tends to be difficult to treat and prone to relapse [1]. Symptoms include eye pain and blurred vision. Diagnosis is by clinical examination, scrapings, and culture. Treatment is with topical trifluridine; prognosis is variable [10]. Varicella-zoster virus (VZV) ophthalmicus may be the initial manifestation of HIV infection. It presents as severe eye pain associated with keratitis, anterior uveitis, and cutaneous vesicles in a dermatomal distribution. Diagnosis is made clinically, and treatment consists of systemic acyclovir [1]. In addition to keratoconjunctivitis, both HSV and VZV are rare causes of necrotizing retinitis, which is discussed later in this section.

Iridocyclitis and Anterior Uveitis

Symptoms of iridocyclitis and anterior uveitis include pain and photophobia, and the eyes may appear grossly inflamed. Slit-lamp examination is necessary for diagnosis. Syphilis is an important consideration in the differential diagnosis of eye disease in HIV-infected patients. It may present atypically, be more aggressive, and relapse more frequently than in immunocompetent hosts [11–13]. While relatively uncommon, secondary syphilis may manifest as ocular disease, including iridocyclitis, anterior uveitis, retinitis, and vitreitis. Serologically false-negative cases of syphilis have been reported in HIV disease but are probably unusual [14]. HIV-infected patients with ocular syphilis should be treated with an antibiotic regimen appropriate for neurosyphilis, and close clinical and serologic follow-up study is essential [15].

Vitreitis

Inflammation of the vitreous occurs in many retinal infections. Symptoms include "floaters" and blurred vision, and, with marked inflammation, the vitreous appears cloudy on funduscopic examination.

Retinitis

Cytomegalovirus

The most common cause of retinitis and visual loss associated with HIV disease is CMV infection [2, 3, 16]. The incidence of CMV retinitis ranges from 15 to 46 percent, the vast majority of cases occurring when the CD4 cell count is below 100/mm^3 [2, 3, 17]. Approximately 40 percent of patients lose central vision in both eyes by the time of death despite antiviral treatment [6, 18, 19]. Cytomegalovirus retinitis is probably the result of hematogenous spread of the virus to the retina after reactivation of latent infection [18]. Cytomegalovirus spreads along the retinal nerve fiber layer at a rate of 250 μm per week, with proliferating virus found in the leading edge and spreading in a "brush fire" manner [20].

Symptoms of CMV infection depend on its location in the retina [16, 20]. The disease generally starts in one eye, with the onset gradual over a period of weeks. If retinitis does not involve the macula or optic nerve, the patient may have no symptoms, or the only symptoms may be floaters or peripheral field loss. If the lesion lies closer to the posterior retina near the macula or optic nerve, a corresponding scotoma or defect in the visual field may occur [16]. Ocular pain, photophobia, and erythema of the eye are unusual [1, 2, 21].

Untreated unilateral CMV infection becomes bilateral in up to 80 percent of cases. Visual loss results from retinal necrosis, edema, and detachment. Involvement of the optic nerve results in visual loss regardless of disease in the surrounding retina [18]. With resolution of edema and necrosis, the retina is left as an atrophic, thin tissue susceptible to breaks or tears [1]. Sudden onset of multiple floaters, flashing lights, visual field defects, and decreased vision portend retinal detachment.

Ophthalmologic examination is somewhat variable [3,19]. Early CMV retinitis is often subtle and characterized by one or two small white granular lesions, similar to CWS, often without hemorrhage. Early lesions are more commonly seen in the anterior or peripheral retina (Plate 8). More advanced CMV retinitis is characterized by perivascular, fluffy, yellow-white infiltrates accompanied by hemorrhage ("scrambled eggs and ketchup" or "pizza pie" pattern). Late lesions are often found in the posterior retina near the major vascular arcade, macula, and optic nerve.

Diagnosis of CMV retinitis is based on findings on funduscopic examination [16]. Serology and blood and urine cultures are nondiagnostic, and vitreal aspiration is not specific. Retinal biopsy, although possible, is impractical and should be reserved for progressive retinitis of uncertain etiology [1]. Lesions that are suspicious for but not diagnostic of CMV infection should be followed closely by serial funduscopic examinations and retinal photographs.

Two antiviral agents, ganciclovir and foscarnet, offer effective treatment but not cure for CMV retinitis. Ganciclovir is a nucleotide analogue of acyclovir that is 10 to 100 times more effective against CMV. Approximately 85 percent of patients respond to a 2-week course of ganciclovir given at the dose of 5 mg/kg intravenously every 12 hours [21, 22]. Maintenance therapy with ganciclovir at 5 mg/kg/day intravenously five to seven times per week is required to prevent relapse [20]. Eventually, progressive retinitis may occur in up to 50 percent of patients despite institution of therapy [1]. Neutropenia is the major toxicity of ganciclovir, occurring in up to 40 percent of patients and often requiring a dose reduction, the addition of granulocyte colony stimulating factor, or substitution of foscarnet. The concurrent use of ganciclovir and zidovudine is generally not recommended [23]. Intravitreal ganciclovir injection and implants used to avoid systemic toxicity are currently under investigation [24].

Foscarnet also has antiviral activity against CMV, and response and relapse rates are similar to those of ganciclovir [25–27]. Primary therapy consists of 60 mg/kg intravenously every 8 hours for 2 to 3 weeks. Renai dysfunction and metabolic abnormalities, including hypocalcemia and hypomagnesemia, are common [28]. Maintenance therapy with 90 to 120 mg/kg/day intravenously is necessary to prevent relapse. A recent trial comparing foscarnet and ganciclovir showed that they were equally effective in the treatment of CMV retinitis, but that patients who received foscarnet lived a median of 4 months longer [29]. This survival advantage has been postulated to be due to inherent antiretroviral activity of foscarnet.

The combination of ganciclovir and foscarnet has recently been proposed for primary therapy of CMV infection, with the use of alternating agents for maintenance therapy [30]. While this regimen appears to be effective and well tolerated, it has not yet been compared to conventional therapies.

Toxoplasma gondii
Toxoplasma gondii is the second most common cause of retinitis in AIDS [31, 32]. It may occur during the course of primary infection or from relapse of latent extraocular infection with dissemination of organisms to the retina. Ten percent of patients with toxoplasmic encephalitis have retinitis, and over 50 percent of those with retinitis are diagnosed with encephalitis [31]. Symptoms include photophobia, floaters, and decreased vision; physical findings consist of anterior uveitis, vitreitis, and necrotizing retinitis [32]. Although toxoplasmic retinitis may be confused with CMV disease, it is seldom associated with hemorrhage and frequently causes a marked vitreitis or anterior uveitis [32, 33]. Diagnosis is clinical; central nervous system involvement should be ruled out by computed tomography or MRI scanning. Serologic tests are not clinically useful. Treatment with pyrimethamine/sulfadiazine is effective, with regression of lesions occurring in 2 to 3 weeks [31, 32]. Maintenance therapy is required to prevent relapse.

Herpes Simplex and Varicella-Zoster Viruses
Although retinitis caused by these viruses has been reported with HIV infection, it is much less frequent than CMV disease [1]. Symptoms are ocular and periocular, with photophobia, floaters, and decreased vision. Diagnosis is based on the presence of cutaneous or corneal involvement. Acyclovir may accelerate healing, but untreated cases usually resolve spontaneously within 6 weeks. Visual loss as the result of retinal necrosis and detachment occurs in over 50 percent of cases.

Candida albicans
Fungal retinitis is unusual in AIDS [1-3]. Candidal involvement produces one or more fluffy, yellow-white, deep retinal lesions, which may be associated with significant vitreitis but not hemorrhage. Positive blood cultures may assist in the diagnosis. Treatment consists of systemic and sometimes intravitreal amphotericin B and removal of the source of primary infection (e.g., intravascular catheter).

Bacteria
Bacterial retinitis and endophthalmitis are also uncommon but should be considered, especially if the patient uses injection drugs or has con-

comitant endocarditis. Diagnosis is made by blood or vitreous cultures, or both. Treatment consists of systemic antibiotics.

Other Pathogens

Pneumocystis carinii, Mycobacterium avium complex, *Cryptococcus neoformans, Histoplasma capsulatum*, and other opportunistic organisms can cause ocular disease in HIV-infected patients, presenting as a multifocal choroiditis, although less commonly than CMV and toxoplasmosis. Vitrectomy with culture establishes the specific diagnosis.

References

1. Freeman, WR, Gross JG. Management of ocular disease in AIDS patients. *Ophthalmol Clin North Am* 1:91–100, 1988.
2. Freeman WR, Lerner CW, Mines JA, et al. A prospective study of the ophthalmologic findings in the acquired immune deficiency syndrome. *Am J Ophthalmol* 97:133–142, 1984.
3. Holland GN, Pepose JS, Pettit TH, et al. Acquired immune deficiency syndrome: Ocular manifestations. *Ophthalmology* 90:859–873, 1983.
4. Mansour AM, Jampol IM, Logani S, Reed J. Cotton wool spots in acquired immunodeficiency syndrome compared with diabetes mellitus, systemic hypertension, and central retinal vein occlusion. *Arch Ophthalmol* 106:1074–1077, 1988.
5. Engstrom RE, Holland GN, Hardy WD, Meiselman HJ. Hemorrheologic abnormalities in patients with human immunodeficiency virus infection and ophthalmic microvasculopathy. *Am J Ophthalmol* 109:153–161, 1990.
6. Mill J, Jacobson MA, O'Donnell JJ, et al. Treatment of cytomegalovirus retinitis in patients with AIDS. *Rev Infect Dis* 10 (suppl 3):5522–5531, 1988.
7. Newsome DA, Green RW, Miller ED, et al. Microvascular aspects of acquired immune deficiency syndrome retinopathy. *Am J Ophthalmol* 98:590–601, 1984.
8. Kwok S, O'Donnell JJ, Wood I. Retinal cotton wool spots in a patient with *Pneumocystis carinii* infection. *N Engl J Med* 307:184–185, 1982.
9. Pomerantz RJ, Kuritzkes DR, de la Monte SM, et al. Infection of the retina by human immunodeficiency virus type I. *N Engl J Med* 317:1643–1647, 1987.
10. Young TL, Robin JB, Holland GN, et al. Herpes simplex keratitis in patients with acquired immune deficiency syndrome. *Ophthalmology* 96:1476–1479, 1989.
11. Tramont EC. Syphilis in the AIDS era. *N Engl J Med* 316:1600–1601, 1987.
12. Johns DR, Tierney M, Felsenstein D. Alteration in the natural history of neurosyphilis by concurrent infection with the human immunodeficiency virus. *N Engl J Med* 316:1569–1572, 1987.
13. Passo MS, Rosenbaum JT. Ocular syphilis in patients with human immunodeficiency virus infection. *Am J Ophthalmol* 106:1–6, 1988.

14. Hicks CB, Benson PM, Lupton GP, et al. Seronegative secondary syphilis in a patient with the human immunodeficiency virus (HIV) with Kaposi sarcoma. *Ann Intern Med* 107:492–495, 1987.
15. Berry CD, Hooten TM, Collier AC, Lukehart SA. Neurologic relapse after benzathine penicillin therapy for secondary syphilis in a patient with HIV infection. *N Engl J Med* 316:1587–1589, 1987.
16. Bloom JN, Palestine AG. The diagnosis of cytomegalovirus retinitis. *Ann Intern Med* 109:963–969, 1988.
17. Henderly DE, Freeman WR, Smith RE, et al. Cytomegalovirus as the initial manifestation of the acquired immune deficiency syndrome. *Am J Ophthalmol* 103:316–320, 1987.
18. Grossniklaus HE, Frank KE, Tomsak RL. Cytomegalovirus retinitis optic neuritis in acquired immune deficiency syndrome. *Ophthalmology* 94:1601–1604, 1987.
19. Pepose JS, Holland GN, Nestor MS, et al. Acquired immune deficiency syndrome. Pathogenic mechanisms of ocular disease. *Ophthalmology* 92:472–484, 1985.
20. Henderly DE, Freeman WR, Causey DM, Rao NA. Cytomegalovirus retinitis and response to therapy with ganciclovir. *Ophthalmology* 94:425–434, 1987.
21. Collaborative DHPG Study Group. Treatment of serious cytomegalovirus infections with 9-(1,3-dihydroxy-2-propoxymethyl) guanine in patients with AIDS and other immunodeficiencies. *N Engl J Med* 314:801–805, 1986.
22. Culbertson WW. Discussion of DE Henderly, WR Freeman, DM Casey, NA Rao. Cytomegalovirus retinitis and response to therapy with ganciclovir. *Ophthalmology* 94:432–434, 1987.
23. Hochster H, Dieterich D, Bozzette S, et al. Toxicity of combined ganciclovir and zidovudine for cytomegalovirus disease associated with AIDS. *Ann Intern Med* 113:111–117, 1990.
24. Ussery F, Gibson S, Conklin R, et al. Intravitreal ganciclovir in the treatment of AIDS associated with cytomegalovirus retinitis. *Ophthalmology* 95:640–648, 1988.
25. Farthing CF, Dalgleish AG, Clark A, et al. Phosphonoformate (foscarnet): A pilot study in AIDS and AIDS-related complex. *AIDS* 1:21–25, 1987.
26. Walmsley S, Chew E, Fanning MM, et al. Treatment of cytomegalovirus retinitis with trisodium phosphonoformate hexahydrate (foscarnet). *J Infect Dis* 157:569–572, 1988.
27. Palestine AG, Polis MA, DeSmet MD, et al. A randomized, controlled trial of foscarnet in the treatment of cytomegalovirus retinitis in patients with AIDS. *Ann Intern Med* 115:665–673, 1991.
28. Foscarnet. *Med Lett Drugs Ther* 34:3–4, 1992.
29. Studies of Ocular Complications of AIDS Research Group in collaboration with the AIDS Clinical Trials Group. Mortality in patients with the acquired immunodeficiency syndrome treated with either foscarnet or ganciclovir for cytomegalovirus retinitis. *N Engl J Med* 23:213–220, 1992.
30. Malte P, Bergmann F, Grunewald T, et al. Safety and efficacy of combined and alternating ganciclovir and foscarnet in acute and maintenance ther-

apy for CMV infection in HIV positive patients. Eighth International Conference on AIDS, Amsterdam, July 1992.

31. Holland, GN, Engstrom RE, Glasgow BJ, et al. Ocular toxoplasmosis in patients with the acquired immunodeficiency syndrome. *Am J Ophthalmol* 106:653–667, 1988.
32. Weiss A, Margo CE, Ledford DK, et al. Toxoplasmic retinochoroiditis as an initial manifestation of the acquired immune deficiency syndrome. *Am J Ophthalmol* 101:248–249, 1986.
33. Parke DW, Font RL. Diffuse toxoplasmic retinochoroiditis in a patient with AIDS. *Arch Ophthalmol* 104:571–575, 1986.

8/Dermatologic Manifestations

Howard K. Koh, Bret E. Davis

Dermatologic disorders may be the first or most prominent signs of HIV infection (Table 8-1). In this chapter, we present an overview of the assessment and management of these conditions. The reader is also referred to additional references for further discussion [1–4].

Approach to the Patient

One should consider HIV infection when encountering patients with skin disease that is severe, atypical, or does not respond to routine treatment. In addition to performing an HIV risk assessment, the physician should ask about local skin symptoms (such as burning, pain, or itch), the length of time a lesion has been present, its distribution, and its initial appearance. Dermatologic examination should be an organized regional survey, which includes inspection and palpation.

Viral Infections

HIV Exanthem

Approximately 75 percent of patients with primary HIV infection will have an exanthem in addition to fever, lethargy, malaise, and adenopathy [5].

Clinical Manifestations
The exanthem appears much like that seen in other acute viral infections. Asymptomatic, oval, erythematous macules or urticarial plaques, usually 0.5 to 2.0 cm in diameter, may be generalized, involving the palms and soles, or affect the trunk and upper body only. The lesions may be centrally hemorrhagic, and desquamation may occur. Frequently, patients will also have an oral enanthem, with superficial ulcerations of the soft palate extending into the esophagus.

Laboratory Data
Patients may have leukopenia, lymphopenia with reversed CD4:CD8 lymphocyte ratio, or thrombocytopenia, and p24 antigenemia is often

Table 8-1 *Dermatologic manifestations of HIV infection*

Disease	Clinical manifestations	Diagnosis	Treatment
		Viral infections	
Acute HIV exanthem (primary HIV infection)*	Fever, myalgias, urticaria Truncal maculopapular eruption	HIV antibodies usually within 12 wk of infection Low white blood cell count, thrombocytopenia, hypergammaglobulinemia	Symptomatic treatment
Herpes simplex*	May be widely disseminated, persistent erosions and perirectal ulcers (see Plate 9)	HSV culture Tzanck smear for multinucleated giant cells	Acyclovir, 200–800 mg po five times/day Foscarnet for acyclovir-resistant strains
Varicella-zoster*	May be severe, persistent, dermatomal (see Plate 10), disseminated, or deeply scarring Intractable herpetic pain	Herpes virus culture Tzanck smear for multinucleated giant cells	Acyclovir, 800 mg po five times/day for dermatomal Acyclovir, 10–12 mg/kg IV q8h for disseminated
Molluscum contagiosum*	Clusters of white umbilicated papules (see Plate 11)	Biopsy or KOH preparations of soft central material show large viral inclusions	Cryosurgery Topical tretinoin Curettage
Oral hairy leukoplakia*	Whitish, nonremovable verrucous plaques on sides of tongue	Biopsy	Topical tretinoin Oral acyclovir Antiretroviral therapy
Warts (human papillomavirus)	Increased number, size of verrucous lesions	Biopsy or clinical appearance Cryosurgery	Topical agents Blunt dissection

Fungal infections

Candida albicans*	Oral mucosal white plaques, sore throat, dysphagia, deep tongue erosions Intractable vaginal infection Nail infection	Culture KOH slide preparation	Topical: nystatin suspension, clotrimazole troche Systemic: oral ketoconazole, fluconazole or IV amphotericin B
Tinea versicolor	Thick, scaly hypopigmented or light-brown plaques on trunk	KOH slide shows numerous short hyphae and spores Wood's light accentuates lesions	Topical: selenium sulfide, miconazole, clotrimazole, sodium thiosulfate Oral: ketoconazole
Dermatophytes (tinea corporis, pedis, cruris)	Extensive involvement, especially groin and feet	KOH slide preparation shows branched, septated hyphae	Topical: miconazole, naftifine Oral: griseofulvin, ketoconazole

Bacterial infections

Staphylococcal*	Superficial and subcutaneous infections Impetigo (see Plate 12)	Culture	Dicloxacillin First-generation cephalosporin
Syphilis*	Painless chancre (primary, see Fig. 21-1) Generalized plaques and papulosquamous lesions (secondary, see Plate 13) Incubation period for neurosyphilis may be very short (mo)	VDRL or RPR *and* FTA-abs or MHA-TP Skin biopsy	Standard recommended treatment may not be sufficient to prevent central nervous system disease
Bacillary angiomatosis*	Dome-shaped or pedunculated solitary or multiple papules and nodules (4 mm–2 cm) Visceral angiomatosis	Biopsy	Erythromycin, 250–500 mg orally q6h × 2 wk to one mo or longer

Table 8-1 (continued)

Disease	Clinical manifestations	Diagnosis	Treatment
Arthropod infestation			
Scabies	Generalized crusted papules and eczematous lesions	KOH or oil preparations show mites	Lindane Pyrethrin Permethrin
Miscellaneous disorders			
Seborrheic dermatitis*	Red scaling plaques (see Plate 14) with yellow greasy scales and distinct margins, on the face and scalp	Biopsy KOH to rule out tinea	Ketoconazole cream Oral ketoconazole, 200–400 mg/day Low-potency topical steroids
Psoriasis	Activation of previous disease or no previous history	Biopsy	Treatment-resistant cases may respond to etretinate or zidovudine
Xeroderma	Severe dry skin, possible erythroderma	Clinical presentation	Lactic acid emollients Lac-Hydrin
Papular eruption	2–5 mm skin-colored papules on head, neck, upper trunk Pruritic, chronic	Biopsy shows lymphocytic perivascular infiltrate	Low-potency topical steroids Antipruritic lotions Antihistamines
Eosinophilic pustular (EPF) and bacterial folliculitis*	Groups of small vesicles and pustules that can become confluent EPF: Polycyclic plaques with central hypopigmentation Severe, intractable pruritus	Biopsy Negative culture for atypical organisms	Ultraviolet B phototherapy for EPF Topical/systemic antibiotics for bacterial folliculitis

Thrombocytopenic purpura	Petechiae	Complete blood count	Antiretroviral therapy
Yellow nails	Yellow discoloration of nail plate May be associated with *Pneumocystis carinii* pneumonia	Clinical examination	None
Darkened nailbeds	Dark blue appearance at bases of fingernails	Recent history of zidovudine treatment	None
Premature hair graying, long eyelashes	Usually follow other AIDS signs and symptoms	Physical examination	None
Drug reactions	Most commonly sulfonamides, ampicillin Widespread maculopapular eruption	Clinical examination	Alternative drugs
Neoplastic disorders			
Kaposi's sarcoma*	Pale to deep violaceous, oval plaques (see Plate 15) and papules (see Plate 16) Oral lesions (usually palate) Visceral lesions	Biopsy	Individual lesions: radiation, cryotherapy, intralesional chemotherapy Multiple lesions: chemotherapy, interferon

*Discussed in text.
Source: Modified from TP Habif, *Clinical Dermatology: A Color Guide to Diagnosis and Therapy.* (2nd ed). St. Louis: Mosby, 1990; some data also from *Med Lett Drugs Ther* 33:95–102, 1991.

present. The HIV antibody test, initially negative, usually becomes positive within 3 months.

Differential Diagnosis
Viral infections (including mononucleosis and aseptic meningitis), *Mycoplasma* and bacterial infections, toxoplasmosis, and strongyloidiasis must be distinguished from primary HIV infection. Secondary syphilis is another important diagnostic consideration, especially when lesions involve the palms and soles.

Evaluation
The clinical impression should be confirmed by HIV seroconversion or demonstration of p24 antigenemia. Skin biopsy findings are nonspecific, showing a lymphocytic perivascular infiltrate in the papillary dermis.

Management
The exanthem and symptoms usually resolve with supportive care over a period of several weeks.

Herpesviruses

Chronic herpes simplex virus (HSV) and varicella-zoster virus (VZV) lesions may be early indicators of HIV disease. These infections usually reflect reactivation of latent disease. Herpesvirus infections in HIV-infected patients can cause severe morbidity, and genital ulcerations may increase the risk of transmitting and acquiring HIV infection.

Clinical Manifestations
Classic HSV type 1 and 2 infections present as self-limited, grouped vesicles, often with an erythematous base, affecting the lips or genitalia. However, in patients with advanced HIV disease, nonhealing HSV erosions may enlarge into severe, painful ulcers that can reach up to 20 cm in diameter (Plate 9). Any ulcerative lesion in an HIV-infected patient should be considered herpetic until proven otherwise. Herpes simplex virus infection may occasionally affect the oropharynx and esophagus, with resultant dysphagia and odynophagia.

Varicella-zoster virus infection occurs seven times more frequently in HIV-infected persons than in the general population. Typically, zoster appears as a painful, unidermatomal vesicular eruption on an erythematous base (Plate 10). However, in the context of HIV infection, it is sometimes multidermatomal or disseminated, with hemorrhagic and necrotic lesions. Painful, hyperkeratotic nodules may persist for months.

Serious eye complications, including visual loss, may follow zoster ophthalmicus.

Laboratory Data
For rapid diagnosis, Tzanck stain of scrapings from the base of a lesion may show multinucleated giant cells. Viral culture of vesicular fluid can also be performed. Skin biopsy is rarely necessary.

Differential Diagnosis
In most cases, grouped vesicles for HSV or dermatomal vesicles for VZV will lead to an accurate diagnosis. On occasion, contact dermatitis can be confused with herpetic infection, as can chancroid, cellulitis, and mycobacterial or fungal disease.

Evaluation
Cutaneous HSV and VZV infections are usually diagnosed clinically.

Management
For HSV, the treatment is oral acyclovir, 200 to 800 mg five times a day, or, if necessary, intravenously 5 to 10 mg/kg (adjusted for renal function) every 8 hours until lesions heal. Maintenance therapy may be necessary in patients with advanced HIV disease. Ulcerative HSV lesions that fail to respond to acyclovir may indicate resistant virus, and foscarnet is indicated in such instances. For VZV infection, the treatment is oral acyclovir, 800 mg five times a day, or, if necessary, 10 to 12 mg/kg intravenously every 8 hours for 7 days. Topical soaks (Domeboro's Solution) can be used to help dry wet lesions.

Molluscum Contagiosum

Approximately 20 percent of symptomatic HIV-infected patients develop these pox virus–associated lesions.

Clinical Manifestations
Classic lesions are pearly, dome-shaped, 2- to 4-mm papules with central umbilication (Plate 11). In immunocompetent adults, papules typically appear on the thigh or genital regions after intimate contact. However, in HIV-infected patients, lesions may disseminate widely and are especially common on the face. Individual lesions can enlarge to one centimeter or more.

Laboratory Data
Pathognomonic "molluscum bodies" (large viral inclusion formations) can be demonstrated by both potassium hydroxide touch preparations and skin biopsy.

Differential Diagnosis
The most common differential diagnosis is warts caused by human papillomavirus. Disseminated fungal disease, such as cryptococcosis, histoplasmosis, or coccidioidomycosis, may mimic molluscum, but tends to have a more acute onset. Large lesions, especially of the face and head, may be confused with basal cell carcinoma or keratoacanthoma.

Evaluation
The diagnosis of molluscum contagiosum is usually made clinically. However, the presence of atypical lesions in the patient with fever, headache, confusion, or pulmonary infiltrate requires biopsy to rule out systemic fungal infection. Biopsy may also be necessary to exclude malignancy.

Management
Liquid nitrogen applications every 1 to 2 weeks may be helpful. Alternatives include the application of cantharidin to nongenital lesions for 4 to 6 hours followed by curettage. Patients can prevent spread of mollusca by discontinuing blade shaving. Nightly use of topical tretinoin has also been used with some success. Electrodesiccation, while effective, is painful, potentially scarring, and has raised concerns about potential aerosolization of HIV.

Fungal Infections

Candidiasis

Mucocutaneous candidal infection is common in HIV-infected patients. Vaginitis and cutaneous infection are typically seen with early disease, whereas thrush and esophageal disease are associated with more advanced immunodeficiency.

Clinical Manifestations
In cutaneous disease, *Candida* species have a predilection for warm, moist, intertriginous regions, such as the groin, axillae, and inframammary areas. Most commonly, candidal infection presents as a tender, erythematous patch with satellite pustules. In severely immunocompromised patients, candidal balanitis, distal urethritis, or paronychia may occur.

Laboratory Data
Potassium hydroxide preparations of smears from affected areas show diagnostic pseudohyphae and budding yeast.

Differential Diagnosis
Dermatophyte infections and intertrigo occur in similar locations but do not have satellite lesions. Thrush must be distinguished from oral hairy leukoplakia.

Evaluation
Clinical appearance and smear are diagnostic. Biopsy is generally unnecessary.

Management
Management includes topical antifungal cream, such as clotrimazole, and local preventive measures to maintain a dry surface, effective both for treatment and prevention of recurrence. Drying macerated skin with twice-daily soaks may also decrease pain.

Bacterial Infections

Staphylococcal Disease

Staphylococcus aureus is a common cutaneous pathogen in HIV-infected patients. There is increased risk for *Staph. aureus* infection from disruptions of the skin barrier (dermatoses, intravenous catheters), qualitative and quantitative neutrophil defects (neutropenia, ineffective cytotoxic and chemotactic responses), and increased nasal carriage.

Clinical Manifestations
Cutaneous presentations of *Staph. aureus* infection include folliculitis, impetigo (Plate 12), ecthyma, furuncles, carbuncles, cellulitis, pyomyositis, and toxic shock syndrome. *Staphylococcus aureus* may secondarily infect other skin lesions, such as those caused by herpesvirus infections and eczema.

Folliculitis (hair-centered inflammation) is the most common manifestation of staphylococcal skin infection. Follicular pustules may affect the trunk, face, or groin, and usually heal without scarring. Other types of folliculitis include *Pityrosporum* disease (a fungal process confirmed by potassium hydroxide [KOH] scraping) and eosinophilic pustular folliculitis (EPF), which is culture negative and of unknown etiology. EPF is generally an acneiform, pruritic, papular, or pustular eruption. EPF lesions may coalesce to form keratotic, lichenified, or indurated plaques that are bordered by active papular, vesicular areas. Severe pruritus is a cause of significant morbidity in many patients with EPF.

With warmer weather, the blisters or erosions of bullous impetigo frequently involve the axilla or groin. Ecthyma, a pyoderma formed of "punched out" firm ulcerations with a purulent base, is sometimes seen in HIV-infected injection drug users. Staphylococcal abscesses at sites of needle entry are also common in this population.

Laboratory Data
Leukocytosis may be present. Cultures in bacterial folliculitis generally grow *Staph. aureus*, *Streptococcus pneumoniae*, and, less commonly, diphtheroids or gram-negative organisms. Bacterial cultures in EPF yield no growth; histologic findings on skin biopsy include diagnostic follicular destruction with striking eosinophilic infiltration.

Differential Diagnosis
Follicular inflammation is ordinarily seen with acne, local shaving, and topical steroid withdrawal. In the setting of HIV infection, acneiform papules may occur with histoplasmosis, cryptococcosis, and mycobacterial infection. Differential diagnosis also includes dermatophytosis, pustular psoriasis, superficial pemphigus, *Demodex* or scabies infestations, and dermatitis herpetiformis. Candidal folliculitis usually appears with characteristic satellite lesions. Ecthyma gangrenosum presents with a distinctive dark discoloration.

Evaluation
Gram's stain and culture of swab or biopsy specimens, or both, comprise the initial evaluation of suspected staphylococcal skin infection. EPF is diagnosed by skin biopsy.

Management
Treatment of folliculitis may prevent progression to furuncles, carbuncles, abscess, or cellulitis. Uncomplicated folliculitis is treated with topical antibacterial agents such as clindamycin or mupirocin and antibacterial soap (chlorhexidine). For more advanced lesions, any areas of enclosed infection should be incised and drained. Oral antistaphylococcal penicillins (e.g., dicloxacillin) and first-generation cephalosporins are useful. Some authors recommend the addition of rifampin or topical mupirocin in an attempt to clear staphylococcal nasal carriage and augment clinical response. Occasionally, HIV-infected patients require chronic low-dose oral antibiotics, but most staphylococcal pyodermas are curable. In EPF, remissions have occurred with the use of ultraviolet B light treatments (290–320 nm) [6]. Progressively increasing doses three times per week has been associated with significant relief of pruritus.

Syphilis

The incidence of syphilis rose in the late 1970s and early 1980s, concomitant with onset of the HIV epidemic. Persons with primary syphilis have disruption of normal skin integrity and are at increased risk for HIV transmission. Any patient diagnosed with syphilis is a candidate for HIV counseling and testing, and all patients with HIV disease should be routinely screened for syphilis. HIV-infected patients with *Treponema pallidum* infection may have false-negative serologic tests, severe or atypical clinical presentations, poor response or early relapse with antibiotic therapy, and accelerated progression to meningovascular syphilis.

Clinical Manifestations
Most HIV-infected patients with syphilis have typical skin lesions. These include the painless chancre of primary syphilis and the diffuse copper-colored papulosquamous eruption of secondary syphilis, which has predilection to palms, soles, and mucocutaneous surfaces (Plate 13). However, atypical presentations, such as painful ulcers and slowly growing isolated papules or nodules, are also common.

Laboratory Data
Serologic tests are generally positive in primary and secondary syphilis. Skin biopsy shows typical findings of perivascular lymphocytic and plasma cell infiltrates. Multinucleated giant cells and vascular degenerative changes are seen with more chronic lesions. Warthin-Starry silver stains and immunofluorescent staining may demonstrate the pathogenic spirochete.

Differential Diagnosis
The differential diagnosis of primary syphilis includes chancroid, HSV infection, and trauma. Secondary syphilis should be considered in the differential diagnosis of generalized maculopapular eruptions.

Evaluation
Serologic tests are used to confirm the clinical diagnosis. Nontreponemal tests (RPR, VDRL) are used both to screen for the disease and to follow response to treatment. Treponemal tests (FTA-abs, MHA-TP) are employed to confirm positive nontreponemal tests. Nontreponemal tests may be falsely negative in secondary syphilis because of the prozone effect, in which extreme titers yield such antibody excess that the cross-linking necessary for agglutination is absent. Testing of progressively diluted samples eliminates this problem. Both nontreponemal and treponemal serologies may be falsely negative in primary syphilis.

Management

Penicillin continues to be the drug of choice for patients with primary and secondary syphilis. Treatment consists of 2.4 to 4.8 million units of intramuscular benzathine penicillin G with clinical and serologic monitoring of response. Controversy exists as to whether HIV-infected patients with early syphilis require lumbar puncture as part of their evaluation. This and other issues pertaining to diagnosis and management of syphilis are discussed in Chap. 21.

Bacillary Angiomatosis

Bacillary angiomatosis (BA) is a vascular proliferative disorder of the skin, lymph nodes, and viscera [7–9]. Associated organisms include the rickettsia-like species, *Rochalimaea quintana*, the cause of body louse–transmitted trench fever, and *R. henselae* [10]. While the cutaneous lesion is asymptomatic, hematogenous or lymphatic spread may result in weight loss, nausea, vomiting, and hepatosplenomegaly; untreated BA can be fatal. Environmental sources for the bacillus remain unclear, although some patients report cat scratch or tick bite a short time before the illness.

Clinical Manifestations

Moderately firm lesions (approximately 1 cm in diameter) are most often red to purple, dome-shaped, friable papules. Scale and erythematous border may be present. Superficial lesions, which may be single or number 100 or more, may ulcerate and crust. Distribution frequently includes face, trunk, and extremities but usually spares palms, soles, and mouth. Other manifestations include subcutaneous lesions, and plaques or masses with erythema resembling cellulitis. Atypical presentations with generalized or zosteriform patterns may also occur.

Laboratory Data

Skin biopsy shows increased endothelial-lined vascular spaces in the dermis, with large cuboidal cells containing gram-negative rods. The fastidious, motile, curved organisms stain by the Warthin-Starry method and can be grown in culture with blood cell lysis technique.

Differential Diagnosis

Kaposi's sarcoma (KS) is the lesion most difficult to distinguish from BA both clinically and histologically. Less frequently, dermatofibroma, cherry angioma, or pyogenic granuloma (PG) appears similar to BA. Because superficial thinning and ulceration are often present in BA, shave biopsy may suggest PG, but full-thickness biopsy should distinguish between the two conditions. BA may occasionally be confused with angiosarcoma.

Evaluation
Full-thickness biopsy is the diagnostic method of choice. Lesions bleed profusely after sharp instrumentation.

Management
Oral erythromycin is the treatment of choice. Recommended doses range from 250 to 500 mg every 6 hours until lesions resolve (generally 2 weeks to one month). Less consistent success has been obtained with trimethoprim-sulfamethoxazole, isoniazid, rifampin, or doxycycline. Chronic suppressive therapy may be necessary to prevent relapse.

Miscellaneous Disorders

Seborrheic Dermatitis
Seborrheic dermatitis (SD), a common skin disease of the face and scalp, may occur as a severe variant in HIV-infected patients, afflicting 50 to 80 percent of this population [11]. The etiology of SD is unknown, although *Pityrosporum* is thought by some authorities to have a causative role.

Clinical Manifestations
In normal hosts, SD typically appears as a mildly erythematous scaly eruption involving the scalp, forehead, eyebrows, cheeks, and nose. In HIV-infected patients, there is often sudden production of markedly erythematous, inflammatory, papular, or even psoriasiform lesions (Plate 14). Lesions may have adherent yellow scales with a greasy appearance, crusts, and distinct margins. Distribution is often symmetric and may include posterior auricular, neck, and back areas; less frequently the trunk, groin, and extremities are involved. With chronic disease, there may be central atrophy, with hypopigmentation and loss of skin lines.

Laboratory Data
Biopsy of HIV-related SD may reveal unusual histologic features, including plasma cells, leukocytoclasis, focal obliteration of the dermoepidermal interface by lymphoid clusters, psoriasiform hyperplasia of the epidermis, widespread nuclear retention in the outer epidermal layers, overproduction of keratin, and dilated, thick-walled vessels of the upper dermis. *Pityrosporum* may be present.

Differential Diagnosis

More severe SD cases resemble psoriasis, but do not exhibit extensor surface extremity or gluteal cleft involvement. Also, the yellow scale and associated crusting are distinct from the usual silvery psoriatic scale. Other considerations in differential diagnosis include contact or exfoliative dermatitis, parapsoriasis, drug eruption, ichthyosis, and tinea faciale.

Evaluation

Diagnosis is generally made by clinical appearance. Potassium hydroxide preparation of scrapings should be done to rule out tinea infection. Skin biopsy is generally not necessary.

Management

Low-potency topical steroids result in improvement of mild SD. For resistant cases, topical ketoconazole cream or oral ketoconazole in doses of 200 to 400 mg per day can be used.

Kaposi's Sarcoma

Kaposi's sarcoma is a multifocal endothelial cell–derived tumor that primarily affects the skin but may involve other tissues as well [12, 13]. Classic KS is a rare tumor involving the lower extremities of men from well-defined ethnic groups, including Central European Jews, Poles, Russians, and Italians, in their sixth and seventh decades. HIV-infected patients have a 20,000-fold increased rate of KS.

Clinical Manifestations

In the early (patch or macular) stage, cutaneous lesions are irregular, reddish-blue, or purple to violaceous macules. Some have a bruise-like or "contusiform" appearance. Macules may become papular or nodular, or coalesce to form enlarging patches, plaques, and fusiform and oval tumors (Plates 15 and 16). Individual lesions are usually asymptomatic, although pain, itching, and burning are occasionally noted. Lymphadenopathy, both reactive and neoplastic, is common, as is oral and mucous membrane involvement. Gastrointestinal tract lesions, while generally asymptomatic, may cause abdominal pain, bowel obstruction, or bleeding. The lungs, liver, abdominal lymph nodes, spleen, adrenal glands, and heart are less often involved. AIDS-related KS lesions differ from those of classic KS by their smaller size (commonly <1 cm in diameter), their tendency to follow the lines of cutaneous cleavage, and their generalized distribution.

Laboratory Data

In early KS, histopathologic differentiation from granulation tissue may be difficult. Biopsy of these lesions shows the upper half of the dermis to contain irregular, thin-walled vascular channels with jagged and dilated lumina lined by flattened to slightly plump endothelial cells. As lesions evolve, capillary-sized vascular channels and spindle-shaped cell components proliferate. Intertwining fascicles and aggregates of spindle-shaped cells lining erythrocyte-filled vascular slits allow a definitive histologic diagnosis of KS.

The histogenesis of KS has been debated for years, but recent studies involving factor VIII–related antigen and *Ulex europaeus* agglutinin suggest an endothelial cell of origin. Whether these endothelial cells are of lymphocytic or blood vessel derivation, or both, is unclear.

Differential Diagnosis

Although cutaneous lesions of KS usually have distinctive coloration, differential diagnosis includes other vascular lesions, such as pyogenic granuloma, BA, hemangioma, or glomus tumor; granulomatous diseases, such as sarcoidosis; and cancers, such as malignant melanoma and lymphoma. Parasitic and fungal infections should also be considered when ulcerated lesions are present.

Management

Initiation of antiretroviral therapy is the first step in management. Localized disease can be treated with radiation therapy. Destructive modalities, including cryotherapy, and intralesional agents, such as vinblastine sulfate or alpha-interferon, are also of value. Treatment options for more widespread disease are addressed in Chap. 26.

References

1. James W, Thiers BH (eds). AIDS: A ten-year perspective. *Dermatol Clin* 9:465–501, 1991.
2. Habif TP. *Clinical Dermatology: A Color Guide to Diagnosis and Therapy* (2nd ed). St. Louis: Mosby, 1990.
3. Friedman-Kien AE. *Color Atlas of AIDS*. Philadelphia: Saunders, 1989.
4. Dover JS, Johnson RA. Cutaneous manifestations of human immunodeficiency virus infection. *Arch Dermatol* 127:1383–1391 and 1549–1558, 1991.
5. Hulsebosch HJ, Claessen FAP, van Ginkel CJW, et al. Human immunodeficiency virus exanthem. *J Am Acad Dermatol* 23:483–486, 1990.
6. Buchness MR, Lim HW, Hatcher VA, et al. Eosinophilic pustular folliculitis

in the acquired immunodeficiency syndrome: Treatment with ultraviolet B phototherapy. *N Engl J Med* 318:1183–1186, 1988.

7. Relman DA, Loutit JS, Schmidt TM, et al. The agent of bacillary angiomatosis: An approach to the identification of uncultured pathogens. *N Engl J Med* 323:1573–1580, 1990.

8. Slater LN, Welch DF, Hensel D, et al. A newly recognized fastidious gram-negative pathogen as a cause of fever and bacteremia. *N Engl J Med* 323:1587–1593, 1990.

9. Cockerell CJ, LeBoit PE. Bacillary angiomatosis: A newly characterized, pseudoneoplastic, infectious, cutaneous vascular disorder. *J Am Acad Dermatol* 22:501–512, 1990.

10. Koehler JE, Quinn FD, Berger TG, et al. Isolation of *Rochalimaea* species from cutaneous and osseous lesions of bacillary angiomatosis. *N Engl J Med* 327:1625–1631, 1992.

11. Soeprono FF, Schinella RA, Cockerell CJ, et al. Seborrheic-like dermatitis of acquired immunodeficiency syndrome. *J Am Acad Dermatol* 14:242–248, 1986.

12. Rutherford GW, Schwarcz SK, Lemp GF, et al. The epidemiology of AIDS-related Kaposi's sarcoma in San Francisco. *J Infect Dis* 159:3:569–571, 1989.

13. Chachoua A, Krigel R, Lafleur F, et al. Prognostic factors and staging classification of patients with epidemic Kaposi's sarcoma. *J Clin Oncol* 7:774–780, 1989.

9/Cardiac Manifestations

Sheilah A. Bernard

The epidemic of HIV infection has resulted in a low but significant cardiac morbidity (6–7%) and mortality (1–6%) based on reports from the United States and Europe [1]. Cardiac disease may occur at any stage of HIV infection, but important manifestations are more frequent with advanced immunodeficiency.

The first reports documenting cardiac involvement in AIDS were published in 1983. In their review of pathologic findings in 10 patients with AIDS, Reichert and associates [2] reported one case of Kaposi's sarcoma (KS) adjacent to the right coronary artery. The following year, Welch and colleagues [3] described cardiac involvement at autopsy in 11 of 36 AIDS patients; findings included myocardial infiltrates and necrosis, KS of the epicardium and myocardium, and cytomegalovirus (CMV) infection of the myocardium. In 1989, Lewis [4] identified cardiac disease in 59 of 115 postmortem examinations, including pericardial effusion, secondary right ventricular hypertrophy, KS of the pericardium and myocardium, nonbacterial thrombotic endocarditis, myocardial infiltrates, congestive cardiomyopathy, and focal abscess.

Human immunodeficiency virus infection can affect all parts of the heart, including the pericardium, myocardium, and endocardium (Table 9-1).

Pericardial Disease

Clinical Manifestations

Significant pericardial effusion has been identified in up to 46 percent of AIDS patients by echocardiography or autopsy [5]. While generally an incidental finding not associated with symptoms, it can sometimes present as or progress to cardiac tamponade, especially in the setting of advanced HIV disease. Acute pericarditis can be silent or present with fever, cough, dyspnea, and chest pain. Patients with a prior history of pericarditis may develop chronic pericarditis with recurrent pericardial effusion.

Physical findings of pericardial disease include tachypnea, friction rub, and Ewart's sign (dullness to percussion with tubular breath sounds

Table 9-1 Cardiac manifestations of HIV infection

Pericardial disease
   Viral infection: cytomegalovirus, herpes simplex virus
   Bacterial infection: tuberculosis, *Mycobacterium avium* complex
   Disseminated fungal infection
   Neoplasia: Kaposi's sarcoma, lymphoma
Myocardial disease
   HIV myocarditis/cardiomyopathy
   Disseminated opportunistic infections
   Neoplasia: Kaposi's sarcoma, lymphoma
   Medications: pentamidine, alpha-interferon, antiretroviral therapy
Endocardial disease
   Bacterial endocarditis
   Nonbacterial thrombotic endocarditis
   Disseminated fungal infection

between the left scapula and spine associated with large effusions). The manifestations of tamponade include tachypnea, hypotension with pulsus paradoxus, elevated jugular venous pressure with absent "y descent," and remote heart sounds. Of note is the phenomenon of "low-pressure tamponade," which is sometimes observed in HIV-infected patients. Severe volume depletion or cachexia may cause reduced right ventricular filling pressures, and minimal pericardial effusion may increase intrapericardial pressures sufficiently to exceed right atrial pressure at low levels. In this setting, jugular venous pressure or pulsus paradoxus may be absent despite hemodynamic tamponade.

Laboratory Data

Routine chest x-ray may be nondiagnostic with small pericardial effusions (<200 cc). As the effusion increases, the cardiac silhouette develops a classic "water bottle" appearance. Cardiomegaly with a straightened left heart border and absence of pulmonary vascular redistribution should also raise the question of pericardial effusion. Electrocardiography (ECG) may demonstrate ST-T wave changes of pericarditis. With large effusions, loss of QRS voltage and electrical alternans may appear.

Differential Diagnosis

Most pericardial effusions are idiopathic. Once non–HIV-related conditions, such as renal failure, trauma, radiation effect, drug toxicity, and hypothyroidism, are excluded, differential diagnosis includes viral, bacterial, fungal, and neoplastic etiologies.

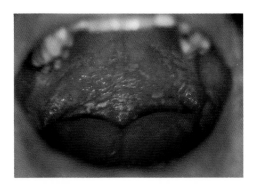

Plate 1. *Pseudomembranous candidiasis of the palate. (Courtesy of Dr. ES Peters.)*

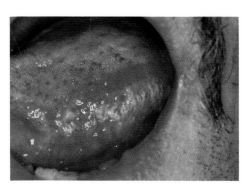

Plate 2. *Herpes simplex virus infection of the lip. (Courtesy of Dr. SB Woo.)*

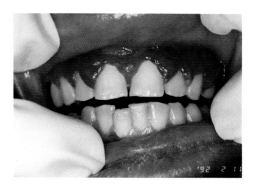

Plate 3. *Hairy leukoplakia. (Courtesy of Dr. ES Peters.)*

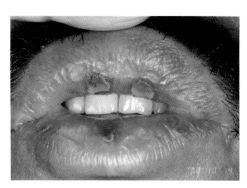

Plate 4. *Kaposi's sarcoma of the gingiva. (Courtesy of Dr. SB Woo.)*

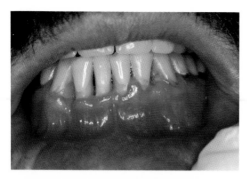

Plate 5. HIV-related periodontitis. (Courtesy of Dr. ES Peters.)

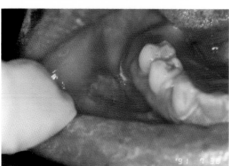

Plate 6. Aphthous ulceration of the buccal mucosa. (Courtesy of Dr. SB Woo.)

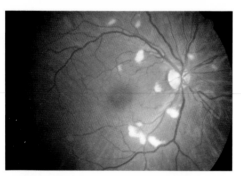

Plate 7. Cotton-wool spots.

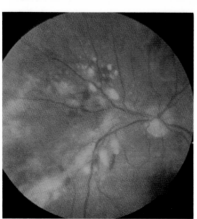

Plate 8. Cytomegalovirus retinitis. (Reprinted with permission from JN Bloom, AG Palestine, The diagnosis of cytomegalovirus retinitis. Ann Intern Med 109:963-969, 1988.)

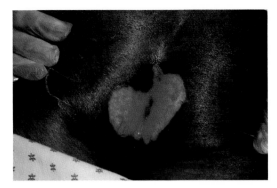

Plate 9. Perianal ulcerative herpes simplex infection.

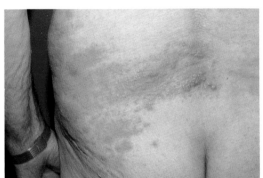

Plate 10. Varicella-zoster infection (shingles).

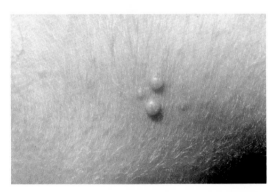

Plate 11. Molluscum contagiosum.

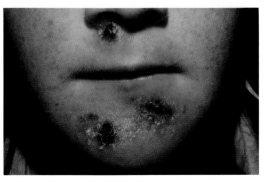

Plate 12. Impetigo. (Reprinted with permission from JJ O'Connell, J Groth (eds), The Manual of Common Communicable Diseases. Boston: Boston Health Care for the Homeless Program, 1991.)

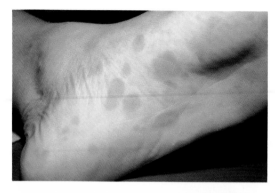

Plate 13. Secondary syphilis.
(Reprinted with permission from
JJ O'Connell, J Groth (eds),
The Manual of Common
Communicable Diseases. Boston:
Boston Health Care for the Homeless
Program, 1991.)

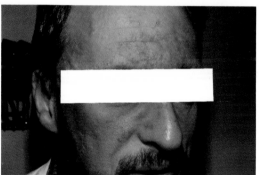

Plate 14. Seborrheic dermatitis.

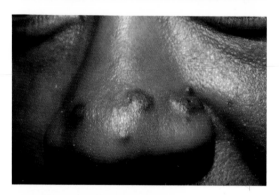

Plate 15. Kaposi's sarcoma (plaque-like lesions).

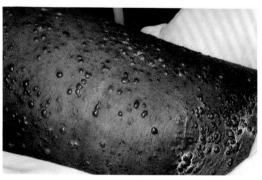

Plate 16. Kaposi's sarcoma (papular lesions).

Cytomegalovirus has been reported to cause cardiac tamponade in a patient with cryptococcal meningitis [6]. While pericardial fluid analysis was not diagnostic, the pericardium revealed characteristic intranuclear inclusion bodies. Herpes simplex virus pericarditis has also been reported in AIDS patients [7, 8]. It remains unclear whether HIV can independently cause pericarditis. Both *Mycobacterium tuberculosis* and *Mycobacterium avium* complex (MAC) have been identified in pericardial fluid or tissue of HIV-infected patients with disseminated infection [9, 10]. *Nocardia asteroides* has been cultured from pericardial fluid in two patients with AIDS [11]. *Staphylococcus aureus* pericarditis has been reported in AIDS-related complex [12]. Disseminated fungal infections may involve the pericardium. *Cryptococcus neoformans* pericarditis has been diagnosed by pericardial fluid stain and culture, and elevation of antigen titer [13]. Aspergillus pericarditis with mycotic plaques has been described in an immunocompromised patient [14].

Kaposi's sarcoma can involve the pericardium as well as the epicardium [15] (Fig. 9-1). Silver and associates [16] reported 5 of 18 AIDS necropsies with cutaneous and subepicardial KS. Kaposi's sarcoma of the pericardium has caused sanguineous pericarditis and tamponade [17]. Isolated cardiac KS has been described in one patient [18]. Cardiac involvement with AIDS-related lymphoma has been described in several cases, with evidence of pericardial effusion or fibrinous pericarditis [19–21].

Evaluation

The evaluation of pericardial disease in the HIV-infected patient is directed at diagnosis of the underlying pathology. A CD4 lymphocyte count and skin testing for tuberculosis should be performed. As pericardial disease is sometimes associated with bacteremia, blood cultures should be obtained in all patients.

Echocardiography is highly sensitive and specific for detecting pericardial effusion and cardiac tamponade. An echo-free space with or without fibrinous strands is diagnostic of pericardial effusion. Right ventricular compression or prolonged right atrial collapse indicates cardiac tamponade. In this setting, Doppler study demonstrates inspiratory augmentation of right-sided flow with simultaneous reduction of left-sided flow, representing the pulsus paradoxus of tamponade physiology. Tamponade physiology may be confirmed by Swan-Ganz monitoring, which reveals elevation and equalization of right atrial, right ventricular, and pulmonary artery end-diastolic pressures. Intrapericardial pressure at the time of pericardiocentesis is elevated and equal to right atrial pressure. Pericardial thickening associated with KS can be identified echo-

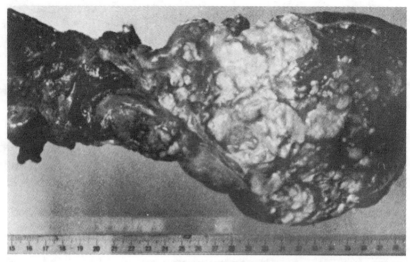

A

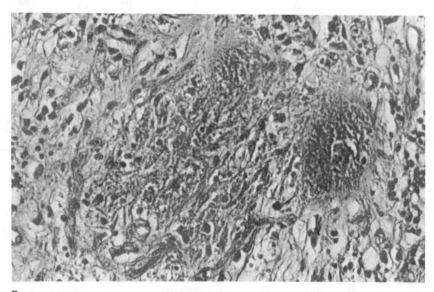

B

Figure 9-1. Kaposi's sarcoma in AIDS patient. A. Nodular neoplastic infiltration of anterior surface of heart. B. Hemorrhagic necrosis typical of Kaposi's sarcoma. (Reprinted with permission from the American College of Cardiology. G Baroldi, S Corallo, M Moroni, et al., Focal lymphocytic myocarditis in acquired immunodeficiency syndrome (AIDS): A correlative morphologic and clinical study in 26 consecutive total cases. J Am Coll Cardiol 12:463–469, 1988.)

cardiographically, but computed tomography and magnetic resonance imaging may provide more accurate assessment of neoplastic cardiac disease.

Management

Small asymptomatic pericardial effusions that require only serial evaluation and no specific therapy occur in up to 10 percent of HIV-infected patients. Nonsteroidal antiinflammatory agents have been used with success in larger asymptomatic effusions [22]. Corticosteroid therapy is generally avoided. The diagnostic utility of aspirating an asymptomatic pericardial effusion is low. Febrile patients often have an etiology identified from blood cultures or biopsy of other involved organs; pericardiocentesis is performed only when presumed infectious pericarditis fails to respond to appropriate antibiotics.

Pericardiocentesis can be used as a therapeutic procedure. In cases of tamponade, it offers immediate resolution of hemodynamic compromise. Pericardial fluid should be stained and cultured for bacteria, mycobacteria, and fungi. Draining pericardiotomy/pericardiectomy may be appropriate for recurring effusion or when pericardial tissue is necessary to diagnose KS or tuberculous pericarditis.

The prognosis of pericardial involvement in AIDS depends on the etiology. Multiple opportunistic infections bode a poor prognosis. It appears that tuberculous pericarditis is less likely to respond to therapy than extracardiac tuberculosis [23].

Myocardial Disease

Clinical Manifestations

Myocardial disease in the context of HIV infection takes three forms. The first is myocarditis, with pathologic specimens revealing opportunistic pathogens, lymphocytic myocarditis (with or without myocardial fiber necrosis), and noninflammatory myocardial necrosis [24]. The second form, dilated cardiomyopathy, reflects severe cardiac dysfunction, which may be either primary or secondary to systemic disease. Finally, the myocardium can be replaced or infiltrated with neoplastic disease.

Myocarditis is a biopsy or postmortem finding that is generally clinically silent. Cardiac symptoms may be obscured by underlying opportunistic infection or neoplasm. Baroldi and associates [15] found lymphocytic infiltrates in 20 of 26 hearts in AIDS patients without cardiac symptoms ([25], Fig. 9-2). Reilly and colleagues [26] noted that 6 of 26 AIDS patients with myocarditis had symptoms of congestive heart fail-

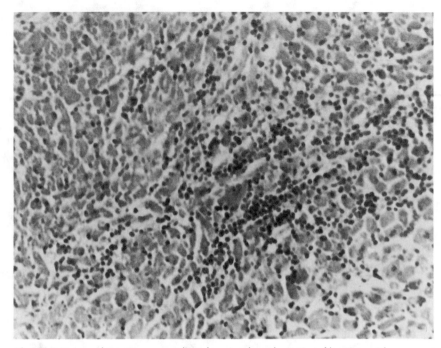

Figure 9-2. *Lymphocytic myocarditis showing lymphocytic infiltration with myocardial degeneration. (Reprinted with permission from M Klima, SM Escudier, Pathologic findings in the hearts of patients with acquired immunodeficiency syndrome. Tex Heart Inst J 18:116–121, 1991.)*

ure. Neoplastic involvement may present as heart failure, chest pain, or dysrhythmia [27]. Patients with symptomatic myocarditis/cardiomyopathy complain of dyspnea and fatigue, and biventricular dysfunction may result in peripheral edema and ascites. Symptoms of dysrhythmia, a manifestation of end-stage cardiac disease, include palpitations, dizziness, and syncope.

Vital signs may show relative hypotension, tachypnea, tachycardia, and ectopy. Physical examination may reveal elevated neck veins, diminished pulses, and rales on auscultation of the lungs. The cardiac examination may show a displaced point of maximal impulse. The S1 and S2 may be quiet, and an S3 gallop may be present. Mitral and tricuspid regurgitant murmurs secondary to biventricular dilatation may be heard. Hepatomegaly with hepatojugular reflex, ascites, and peripheral edema may be present.

Laboratory Data

Chest x-ray commonly shows cardiomegaly, with left atrial and ventricular dilatation and pulmonary vascular redistribution. Electrocardiography may reveal dysrhythmias, including premature ventricular contractions or atrioventricular block. A pseudoinfarct pattern may occur if focal patches of infiltrates or neoplasm are present. Left ventricular hypertrophy or nonspecific ST-T wave changes may be associated with ventricular dilatation.

Differential Diagnosis

Non–HIV-related etiologies for myocarditis/cardiomyopathy must be excluded. These include hypertension, diabetes mellitus, ischemia, and alcoholic or valvular heart disease. In injection drug users (IDUs), consideration should also be given to hypersensitivity reactions. Cocaine has been shown to produce a myocarditis as well as a myopathy due to coronary spasm and ischemia [28].

Multiple pathogens have been found in the myocardium at postmortem or biopsy. Cytomegalovirus has been identified in the myocardium, both with and without inflammatory infiltrate [26]. Neidt and Schinella [29] reported that 43 of 56 AIDS postmortem examinations had evidence of CMV infection, but only four patients had myocarditis with clinical heart failure, dysrhythmia, or ECG changes. *Toxoplasma gondii* is an uncommon cause of myocarditis, but the *Toxoplasma* cyst has been identified in myocardium [30]. *Mycobacterium tuberculosis*, MAC, *C. neoformans* (Fig. 9-3), *Candida albicans*, *Aspergillus fumigatus*, *Histoplasma capsulatum*, and *Pneumocystis carinii* have all been associated with myocarditis in the presence of underlying systemic disease [4, 15, 31, 32]. Homosexual patients have myocarditis associated with protozoal and fungal pathogens, KS, and mycobacteria, while IDUs have fungal, viral, and protozoal causes [15, 32].

Not all myocarditis associated with AIDS is the result of opportunistic infections. Anderson and associates [32] reported myocarditis in 37 of 71 (52%) necropsies of AIDS patients; in only seven cases was there an identified etiologic agent. The Dallas criterion for the diagnosis of myocarditis—inflammatory infiltrate with focal myocyte damage or necrosis—may not be appropriate in HIV-infected patients [33]. The AIDS virus may cause myocytic degeneration without inflammation [34]. RNA probes have identified HIV nucleic acid sequences in the myocardium at autopsy in 6 of 22 AIDS patients who did not have cardiac symptoms [35]. Possible immune-mediated mechanisms of myocarditis include anti-HIV antibodies cross-reacting with myocardium, autoantibodies directed against damaged myocardium, cytotoxic T lymphocytes lysing HIV-infected myocytes that express viral antigen on their surface, and natural killer cells lysing uninfected myocytes. Nutritional deficiencies and malnutrition are probably not as important contributing factors as was originally thought [36].

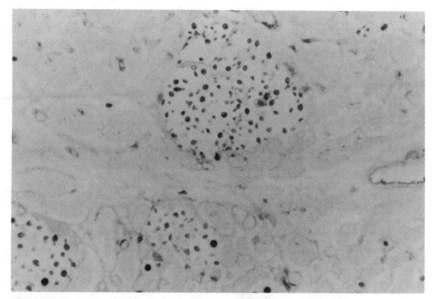

Figure 9-3. Cryptococcus myocarditis showing intact myocytes with foci of necrosis and clumps of periodic acid–Schiff positive capsules. An inflammatory reaction is notably absent. (Reprinted with permission from the American College of Cardiology. C Cammarosano, W Lewis, Cardiac lesions in acquired immune deficiency syndrome (AIDS). J Am Coll Cardiol 5:703–706, 1985.)

Evaluation

Echocardiography remains the single best noninvasive procedure to assess chamber size and left ventricular function. Infiltration of myocardium by lymphoma or subepicardial KS may also be seen echocardiographically. Right ventricular hypertrophy and pulmonary hypertension are commonly identified in patients with concomitant pulmonary disease [24]. Holter monitoring is valuable in detecting dysrhythmias, such as bradycardias or ventricular ectopy, caused by patchy infiltration of the conduction system. Signal-averaged ECGs, which reveal late potentials in patients prone to ventricular tachycardia, may be abnormal in HIV-infected patients [37]. Computed tomography or magnetic resonance imaging is helpful in the detection of cardiac tumors. Gallium scanning is nonspecific but may be useful in selected cases [38, 39]. Elevated serum immunoglobulin levels and cardiac antibodies may be associated with myocarditis [40]. Endomyocardial biopsy is of limited utility because blood contamination of specimens may give spurious immunocytochemistry results. Biopsy underestimates the prevalence of myocarditis, found to be 50 percent on postmortem studies, because of sampling error due to focal inflammation [41]. Rarely, it may prove useful in diagnosing unusual cases such as isolated cardiac lymphoma [42].

Management

Infectious myocarditis is treated with appropriate antibiotic therapy. Steroids are not recommended as therapy for myocarditis. One patient with HIV-associated lymphocytic myocarditis was successfully treated with zidovudine (ZDV), as documented by serial biopsies [43]. Recent data also suggest fewer cardiac abnormalities by noninvasive testing in ZDV-treated subjects [37]. Conventional treatment of congestive heart failure with bed rest, inotropic agents, vasodilators, diuretics, and, where indicated, antidysrhythmics and anticoagulants should be implemented, although it is not clear that this regimen improves survival. Although spontaneous regression of dilated cardiomyopathy may occur rarely, the prognosis of this condition is generally poor [44].

While lymphomatous cardiac involvement is rare and usually fatal, a case report has been published of complete remission of a large cell lymphoma in an HIV-infected patient following combination chemotherapy with cyclophosphamide, doxorubicin, vincristine, and prednisone [27]. Kaposi's sarcoma of the heart is generally a pathologic diagnosis, and there is no evidence that chemotherapy, interferon, or radiotherapy is beneficial.

Of concern recently is the appearance of cardiac disease as a result of HIV-related therapies. Pentamidine, both intravenous and intramuscular, has been associated with torsade de pointes, with or without potassium, calcium, and magnesium deficiency [45]. This is treated by drug termination and repletion of electrolytes, with a possible role for type IB antidysrhythmics, overdrive atrial or ventricular pacing, or isoproterenol administration. Alpha-interferon, used in the treatment of KS, may act synergistically with HIV to produce a reversible cardiomyopathy [46]. There have been case reports of cardiomyopathy associated with ZDV and didanosine (ddI), and ZDV has been implicated in the exacerbation of preexisting cardiac disease [47]. Amphotericin B may cause dysrhythmias, hypertension, and cardiac arrest.

Endocardial Disease

Clinical Manifestations

Endocardial disease in HIV-infected patients takes the form of bacterial endocarditis and marantic (nonbacterial thrombotic) endocarditis. It is curious that endocarditis in AIDS has been relatively infrequent, despite

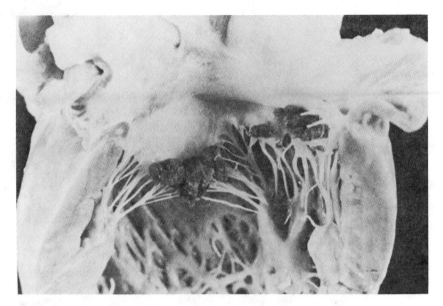

Figure 9-4. Nonbacterial thrombotic endocarditis showing large, friable vegetations on the atrial surface of both mitral valve leaflets. No organisms are demonstrated histologically. (Reprinted with permission from the American College of Cardiology. C Cammarosano, W Lewis, Cardiac lesions in acquired immune deficiency syndrome (AIDS). J Am Coll Cardiol 5:703–706, 1985.)

the fact that IDUs account for the second largest patient population with HIV infection. It is possible that HIV-infected IDUs with endocarditis die from bacterial infection before they become significantly immunocompromised or that they succumb prematurely to other diseases related to substance abuse.

Clinical features of bacterial endocarditis include the acute or insidious onset of fever, malaise, anorexia, and weight loss. In IDUs, right-sided valvular lesions may present with chest pain, cough, and dyspnea. Left-sided involvement may be evident from peripheral embolization or symptoms of heart failure due to aortic or mitral regurgitation.

Marantic endocarditis, associated with severe wasting diseases, has been infrequently reported in AIDS (Fig. 9-4). It is characterized by large, friable vegetations that may embolize or become secondarily infected. Marantic endocarditis may cause systemic embolization and disseminated intravascular coagulation [48–50].

Physical examination may reveal fever; peripheral stigmata of endocarditis, such as petechiae, splinter hemorrhages, Osler's nodes, or Janeway lesions; splenomegaly; and an abnormal cardiac examination. Although up to 15 percent of patients with subacute bacterial endocarditis may not have a murmur when they are initially examined, in the majority evidence of mitral, tricuspid, or aortic regurgitation will develop [51]. Signs of congestive heart failure are most often present with left-sided involvement.

Laboratory Data

Anemia is a common laboratory finding in infective endocarditis, but the white blood cell count may not be elevated in HIV disease. The urinary sediment may show hematuria or proteinuria, or both. Bacteremia is present in 90 percent of cases; recent exposure to antibiotics may cause negative culture results. Fungal and other nonbacterial pathogens are infrequently identified. Chest x-ray may reveal pulmonary infiltrates from right-sided septic emboli, pulmonary venous congestion, and/or vascular redistribution with overt heart failure. Electrocardiography may show progressive heart block from ring abscess formation involving the conduction system.

Differential Diagnosis

Endocarditis in the immunocompromised host may be more virulent than in the normal host. Bacterial endocarditis in the HIV-infected IDU is most commonly caused by *Staph. aureus* (over 75% of cases), *Streptococcus pneumoniae*, and *Haemophilus influenzae* [52]. Fungal endocarditis is often the result of systemic spread from an extracardiac source; pathogens include *Aspergillus* and *Candida* species and *C. neoformans* [24, 31, 53].

Evaluation

Although endocarditis is often a clinical diagnosis, echocardiography remains an important diagnostic test. The sensitivity of transthoracic echocardiography in the detection of vegetations is approximately 75 percent, and that of transesophageal echocardiography is 96 percent [54]. Transesophageal technique is superior to transthoracic in the detection of ring abscesses (sensitivity 84 vs. 19%) [55]. Echocardiography and Doppler studies can also provide information on ventricular function and degree of valvular insufficiency. Computed tomography is useful in the evaluation of cerebral embolic events. Cardiac catheterization, which can be performed safely during active endocarditis, is recommended for patients over the age of 40 who are anticipating valvular surgery [56].

Management

Bacterial endocarditis should be presumed in the HIV-infected IDU with fever and a new regurgitant murmur or peripheral stigmata. After blood cultures are obtained, empiric antibiotic therapy directed against the most likely pathogens should be initiated. Once the etiologic agent has been identified, treatment can be made specific. Duration of intravenous therapy is generally 4 weeks. Peak and trough levels of antibiotics should be monitored. Measurement of serum bactericidal titer may be helpful clinically when the organism or antibiotic regimen is unusual or when treatment appears to be failing.

There is evidence that patients with advanced HIV disease in whom endocarditis develops have a poor prognosis. In one study, endocarditis patients with advanced HIV disease had a 40 percent mortality, compared to 10 percent in asymptomatic HIV-infected individuals [52]. It appears that most HIV-infected patients can undergo successful valve replacement, but those with continued bacteremia at the time of surgery do poorly [57]. Patients should agree to substance abuse treatment before undergoing valvular surgery. Persons with advanced symptomatic HIV disease are generally not good surgical candidates.

References

1. Anderson DW, Virmani R. Emerging patterns of heart disease in human immunodeficiency virus infection. *Hum Pathol* 21:253–259, 1990.
2. Reichert CM, O'Leary TJ, Levens DL, et al. Autopsy pathology in the acquired immune deficiency syndrome. *Am J Pathol* 112:357–382, 1983.
3. Welch K, Finkbeiner W, Alpers CE, et al. Autopsy findings in the acquired immunodeficiency syndrome. *JAMA* 252:1152–1159, 1984.
4. Lewis W. AIDS: Cardiac findings from 115 autopsies. *Prog Cardiovasc Dis* 32:207–215, 1989.
5. Fink L, Reichek N, St John Sutton M. Cardiac abnormalities in acquired immune deficiency syndrome. *Am J Cardiol* 54:1161–1163, 1984.
6. Nathan PE, Arsura EL, Zappi M. Pericarditis with tamponade due to cytomegalovirus in the acquired immunodeficiency syndrome. *Chest* 99:765–766, 1991.
7. Freedberg RS, Gindea AJ, Dietrich DT, et al. Herpes simplex pericarditis in AIDS. *NY State J Med* 87:304–306, 1987.
8. Toma E, Poisson M, Claessens MR, et al. Herpes simplex type 2 pericarditis and bilateral facial palsy in a patient with AIDS (letter). *J Infect Dis* 160:553–554, 1989.
9. Dalli E, Quesada A, Juan A, et al. Tuberculous pericarditis as the first manifestation of acquired immunodeficiency syndrome. *Am Heart J* 114:905–906, 1987.
10. Woods GL, Goldsmith JC. Fatal pericarditis due to *Mycobacterium avium-*

intracellulare in acquired immunodeficiency syndrome. *Chest* 95:1355–1357, 1989.

11. Holtz HA, Lavery DP, Kapila R. Actinomycetales infection in the acquired immunodeficiency syndrome. *Ann Intern Med* 102:203–205, 1985.

12. Stechel RP, Cooper DJ, Greenspan J, et al. Staphylococcal pericarditis in a homosexual patient with AIDS-related complex. *NY State J Med* 86:592–593, 1986.

13. Schuster M, Valentine F, Holtzman R. Cryptococcal pericarditis in an IVDA. *J Infect Dis* 152:842, 1985.

14. Schwartz DA. Aspergillus pancarditis following bone marrow transplantation for chronic myelogenous leukemia. *Chest* 95:1338–1339, 1989.

15. Baroldi G, Corallo S, Moroni M, et al. Focal lymphocytic myocarditis in acquired immunodeficiency syndrome (AIDS): A correlative morphologic and clinical study in 26 consecutive fatal cases. *J Am Coll Cardiol* 12:463–469, 1988.

16. Silver MA, Macher AM, Reichert CM, et al. Cardiac involvement by Kaposi's sarcoma in acquired immune deficiency syndrome (AIDS). *Am J Cardiol* 53:983–985, 1984.

17. Stotka JL, Good CB, Downer WR, et al. Pericardial effusion and tamponade due to Kaposi's sarcoma in acquired immunodeficiency syndrome. *Chest* 95:1359–1361, 1989.

18. Autran B, Gorin I, Leibowitch M, et al. AIDS in a Haitian woman with cardiac Kaposi's sarcoma and Whipple's disease. *Lancet* 1:767–768, 1983.

19. Gill PS, Chandraratna AN, Meyer PR, et al. Malignant lymphoma: A clinicopathologic study. *Cancer* 49:944–951, 1982.

20. Ioachim HL, Cooper MC, Hillman GC. Lymphoma in men at high risk for acquired immune deficiency syndrome (AIDS). *Cancer* 56:2831–2842, 1985.

21. Balasubramanyam A, Waxman M, Kazal HL, et al. Malignant lymphoma of the heart in acquired immune deficiency syndrome. *Chest* 90:243–246, 1986.

22. Himelman RB, Chung WS, Chernoff DN, et al. Cardiac manifestations of human immunodeficiency virus infection: A two dimensional echocardiographic study. *J Am Coll Cardiol* 13:1030–1036, 1989.

23. Kinney EL, Monsuez JJ, Kitzis M, et al. Treatment of AIDS-associated heart disease. *Angiology* 40:970–976, 1989.

24. Acierno LJ. Cardiac complications in acquired immunodeficiency syndrome (AIDS): A review. *J Am Coll Cardiol* 13:1144–1154, 1989.

25. Klima M, Escudier SM. Pathologic findings in the hearts of patients with acquired immunodeficiency syndrome. *Tex Heart Inst J* 18:116–121, 1991.

26. Reilly JM, Cunnion RE, Anderson DW, et al. Frequency of myocarditis, left ventricular dysfunction and ventricular tachycardia in the acquired immune deficiency syndrome. *Am J Cardiol* 62:289–293, 1988.

27. Kelsey RC, Saker A, Morgan M. Cardiac lymphoma in a patient with AIDS. *Ann Intern Med* 115:370–371, 1991.

28. Isner JM, Chokski SK. Cardiovascular complications of cocaine. *Curr Prob Cardiol* 16:95–123, 1991.

29. Neidt GW, Schinella RA. Acquired immunodeficiency syndrome: Clinicopathologic study of 56 autopsies. *Arch Pathol Lab Med* 109:727–734, 1985.
30. Klatt EC, Meyer PR. Pathology of the heart in acquired immunodeficiency syndrome (AIDS). *Arch Pathol Lab Med* 112:114, 1988.
31. Cox JN, diDio F, Pizzolato GP, et al. Aspergillus endocarditis and myocarditis in a patient with the acquired immunodeficiency syndrome (AIDS): A review of the literature. *Virchows Arch* 417:255–259, 1990.
32. Anderson DW, Virmani R, Reilly JM, et al. Prevalent myocarditis at necropsy in the acquired immunodeficiency syndrome. *J Am Coll Cardiol* 11:792–799, 1988.
33. Aretz HT, Billingham ME, Edwards WD, et al. Myocarditis: A histopathologic definition and classification. *Am J Cardiovasc Pathol* 1:1–14, 1986.
34. Calabrese LH, Proffitt MR, Yen-Lieberman B, et al. Congestive cardiomyopathy and illness related to the acquired immunodeficiency syndrome (AIDS) associated with isolation of retrovirus from myocardium. *Ann Intern Med* 107:691–692, 1987.
35. Grody WW, Cheng L, Lewis W. Infection of the heart by the human immunodeficiency virus. *Am J Cardiol* 66:203–206, 1990.
36. Fisher LL, Fisher EA. Myocarditis associated with human immunodeficiency virus infection. *Primary Cardiol* 16:49–60, 1990.
37. Hsia J, Adams S, Ross AM. Natural history of human immunodeficiency virus (HIV) associated heart disease. *Circulation* 84:II-3 (abstract), 1991.
38. Cregler LL, Sosa I, Ducey S, et al. Myopericarditis in acquired immunodeficiency syndrome diagnosed by gallium scintigraphy. *J Natl Med Assoc* 82:511–513, 1990.
39. Constantino A, West TE, Gupta M, et al. Primary cardiac lymphoma in a patient with acquired immune deficiency syndrome. *Cancer* 60:2801–2805, 1987.
40. Hershowitz A, de Oliveria M, Willoughby S, et al. Cardiomyopathy: An initial presentation of human immunodeficiency virus (HIV) infection. *Circulation* 82:III-118 (abstract), 1990.
41. Dittrich H, Chow L, Denaro F, et al. Human immunodeficiency virus, coxsackievirus, and cardiomyopathy. *Ann Intern Med* 108:308–309, 1988.
42. Andress JD, Polish LB, Clark DM, et al. Transvenous biopsy diagnosis of cardiac lymphoma in an AIDS patient. *Am Heart J* 118:421–423, 1989.
43. Wilkins CE, Sexton DJ, McAllister HA. HIV-associated myocarditis treated with zidovudine (AZT). *Tex Heart Inst J* 16:44–45, 1989.
44. Hakas JF, Jr, Generalovich T. Spontaneous regression of cardiomyopathy in a patient with the acquired immunodeficiency syndrome. *Chest* 99:770–772, 1991.
45. Grogin H, Liem LB. Pentamidine-induced torsades de pointes. *Cardiology* 2:114–115, 1991.
46. Deyton LR, Walker RE, Kovacs JA, et al. Reversible cardiac dysfunction associated with interferon alpha therapy in AIDS patients with Kaposi's sarcoma. *N Engl J Med* 321:1246–1249, 1989.
47. Herskowitz A, et al. Cardiomyopathy associated with antiretroviral ther-

apy in patients with HIV infection: A report of six cases. *Ann Intern Med* 116:311–313, 1992.

48. Cammarosano C, Lewis W. Cardiac lesions in acquired immune deficiency syndrome (AIDS). *J Am Coll Cardiol* 5:703–706, 1985.

49. Guarda LA, Luna MA, Smith LJ, et al. Acquired immune deficiency syndrome: Postmortem findings. *Am J Clin Pathol* 81:549–557, 1984.

50. Kaul S, Fishbein MC, Siegel RJ. Cardiac manifestations of acquired immune deficiency syndrome: A 1991 update. *Am Heart J* 122(2):535–544, 1991.

51. Durack DT. Endocarditis. In JW Hurst (ed), *The Heart, Arteries and Veins* [7th ed]. New York: McGraw-Hill, 1990. Pp 1230–1255.

52. Nahass RG, Weinstein MP, Bartels J, et al. Infective endocarditis in intravenous drug users: A comparison of human immunodeficiency virus type 1–negative and –positive patients. *J Infect Dis* 162:967–970, 1990.

53. Francis CK. Cardiac involvement in AIDS. *Curr Probl Cardiol* 15:572–639, 1990.

54. Mugge A, Daniel WG, Frank G, et al. Echocardiography in infective endocarditis: Reassessment of prognostic implications of vegetation size determined by the transthoracic and the transesophageal approach. *J Am Coll Cardiol* 14:631–638, 1989.

55. Daniel WG, Mugge A, Martin RP, et al. Improvement in the diagnosis of abscesses associated with endocarditis by transesophageal echocardiography. *N Engl J Med* 324:795–800, 1991.

56. Welton DE, Young JB, Raizner AE, et al. Value and safety of cardiac catheterization during active infective endocarditis. *Am J Cardiol* 44:1306–1310, 1977.

57. Frater RWM, Sisto D, Condit D. Cardiac surgery in human immunodeficiency virus (HIV) carriers. *Eur J Cardio-Thorac Surg* 3:146–151, 1989.

10/Pulmonary Manifestations

Randall P. Wagner, Harrison W. Farber

The spectrum of pulmonary diseases associated with HIV infection continues to broaden (Table 10-1). More than 80 percent of patients with AIDS have pulmonary disorders, of which 90 percent are infectious in origin [1–4]. In addition, the prevalence of noninfectious pulmonary disorders is increasing, perhaps as a result of improved survival.

Infectious Pulmonary Disorders

Infections involving the respiratory tract are the result of a failure of one or more components of the immune system to protect against a nearly continuous assault of infectious agents. In early HIV disease, when the CD4 lymphocyte count is relatively preserved, patients have an increased incidence of the same pulmonary infections that afflict the general population [5]. When the CD4 cell count falls below $200/mm^3$, or 20 percent of total lymphocytes, the patient becomes at risk for opportunistic infections [6]. Although *Pneumocystis carinii* is still the most frequently recognized opportunistic pathogen, other protozoans, fungi, nontuberculous mycobacterial species, viruses, and unusual bacteria can also cause illness in patients with advanced HIV disease. The probability of infection with specific pathogens depends on the patient's residence, travel history, past medical history, and, to some extent, socioeconomic status.

Bacterial Infections

Community-acquired pneumonia may be the most frequent pulmonary manifestation of HIV infection, with the annual incidence of pneumococcal pneumonia as high as five times that of the general population [7]. Pneumonias caused by *Haemophilus influenzae*, *Mycobacterium tuberculosis*, *Staphylococcus aureus*, *Legionella* species, and *Klebsiella* species are also more common. Bacterial pneumonias in HIV-infected patients are often associated with bacteremia and may recur after appropriate antibiotic therapy.

Table 10-1 Common etiologies of pulmonary disease in the HIV-infected patient

Infectious diseases
    Bacterial: *Streptococcus pneumoniae, Haemophilus influenzae,* tuberculosis,
        Mycobacterium avium complex*
    Protozoal: *Pneumocystis carinii**
    Viral: Cytomegalovirus*
    Fungal: Cryptococcosis,* histoplasmosis, coccidioidomycosis
Neoplastic diseases
    Kaposi's sarcoma
    Non-Hodgkin's lymphoma*
Miscellaneous
    Lymphoid interstitial pneumonitis

*Conditions generally associated with advanced HIV disease.

Nocardia asteroides infection has become increasingly common in patients with advanced HIV disease. Patients usually present with fever, cough, dyspnea, and chest pain. The chest x-ray (CXR) typically shows an upper-lobe process with cavitation, consolidation, or interstitial infiltrate; pleural effusions or hilar adenopathy, or both, also occur [8]. Diagnosis is made by demonstrating branching, beaded, filamentous, gram-positive, weakly acid-fast organisms in respiratory secretions, on transbronchial biopsy or biopsy of skin lesions or lymph nodes. Treatment with sulfonamides or ampicillin for at least 6 months is necessary; the choice of antibiotics should be guided by culture and sensitivity results since resistant organisms have been identified [9]. Because CXR findings often mimic those of reactivation tuberculosis, bronchoscopy should be performed if expectorated sputum fails to yield a diagnosis.

Rhodococcus equi infection generally develops in HIV-infected patients who have been exposed to farm animals or to soil where such animals have been kept. Pneumonia usually occurs in patients with advanced immunosuppression, presenting as fever, cough, fatigue, pleuritic chest pain, and progressive dyspnea evolving over 2 to 3 weeks [10]. The CXR usually shows dense consolidation with cavitation; pleural effusions are common. Although cultures of sputum and blood are often diagnostic, bronchoscopy, biopsy, and/or thoracentesis may be required. Therapy is individualized based on culture and sensitivity results; surgical resection of abscess is occasionally required [11]. The optimal duration of treatment is unknown, but lifelong suppressive therapy may be necessary.

Nosocomial pneumonia is common in HIV-infected patients. Frequent hospitalization and impaired local and systemic immune function magnify the risk of pulmonary infection with *Staph. aureus, Pseudomonas aeruginosa,* and enteric gram-negative organisms.

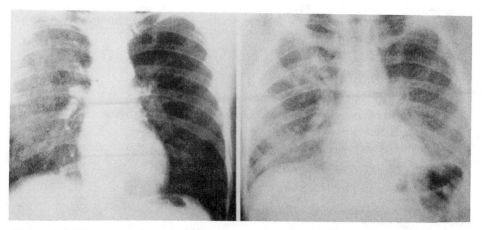

Figure 10-1. Chest x-ray showing the development of Pneumocystis carinii pneumonia. (Reprinted with permission of J. Golden, Pneumocystis lung disease in homosexual men. West J Med 137:400–407, 1982.)

Pneumocystis carinii

Pneumocystis carinii pneumonia (PCP) is the most commonly diagnosed AIDS-related infection in the United States [1, 12]. It occurs at least once in approximately 70 percent of HIV-infected patients, and, despite early recognition and aggressive therapy, still carries a 10 to 20 percent mortality per episode [13]. Because the clinical and roentgenographic features of PCP are nonspecific, diagnosis requires a high index of suspicion. Symptoms often develop more gradually than in other immunosuppressed patients but may present abruptly. Usual symptoms include fever, dyspnea, malaise, and a nonproductive cough, but chills, chest pain, and sputum production may also occur. Physical examination is notable for fever and tachypnea; auscultation of the lungs may be normal.

The CXR typically shows diffuse, bilateral interstitial infiltrates, although cavitary lesions, focal infiltrates, and nodular densities have also been described (Fig. 10-1). Apical infiltrates and pneumothorax have become more common in recent years, probably as the result of aerosol pentamidine (AP) prophylaxis. The CXR is normal in a minority of cases [1, 12]. Enlarged hilar or mediastinal lymph nodes and pleural effusions are unusual and suggest another diagnosis or a copathogen [14].

Arterial blood gas (ABG) determination usually reveals hypoxemia and an abnormal alveolar-arterial oxygen gradient, but may be normal in mild or early cases. Exercise-induced oxygen desaturation is common and often occurs with normal or near-normal ABGs. Pulmonary function testing usually demonstrates a diminished diffusing capacity for carbon monoxide; gallium scintigraphy reveals diffuse parenchymal uptake [15]. Several investigators have noted elevation of serum lactic dehydrogenase (LDH) at the time of diagnosis, the level of which correlates with disease severity [16, 17].

Diagnosis of PCP has depended traditionally on the identification of the organism on methenamine-silver or Giemsa staining of lung tissue or respiratory secretions. The recent development of fluorescent antibody staining (sensitivity 60–80%) has made sputum induction the initial diagnostic test of choice [18, 19]. In facilities that lack the capacity to perform induced sputum analysis or in patients with a negative induced sputum and a high clinical suspicion of PCP, fiberoptic bronchoscopy with bronchoalveolar lavage (BAL) remains the diagnostic mainstay. Although the sensitivity of BAL is approximately 90 percent, it is somewhat less in the first episode of PCP in patients receiving AP prophylaxis; transbronchial biopsy improves the yield in this population [20].

Empiric therapy can be initiated without affecting the ability to establish a definitive diagnosis. Trimethoprim-sulfamethoxazole (TMP-SMZ) in a 1 mg : 5 mg ratio (dose based on the trimethoprim content) is the drug of choice, with therapeutic serum levels attainable with 15 to 20 mg/kg/day given in four divided doses for 21 days. Although TMP-SMZ is available in both intravenous and oral preparations, there is no advantage to IV administration for patients with normal gastrointestinal function, since absorption is complete and equivalent serum drug levels are achievable [21]. HIV-infected patients treated with TMP-SMZ have an unusually high incidence of adverse effects, including fever, rash, leukopenia, thrombocytopenia, and renal dysfunction. If the patient has no clinical response after 5 to 7 days or if drug toxicity develops, pentamidine is used as an alternative agent.

Pentamidine isethionate is given in a dose of 3 to 4 mg/kg/day intravenously. Intramuscular administration should be avoided because injections are painful and sterile abscesses are common. Intravenous pentamidine may cause severe hypotension if the drug is administered too rapidly. Neutropenia, renal impairment, and hepatic dysfunction are frequent complications. Hypoglycemia is common, and glucose intolerance or frank diabetes mellitus may occur following completion of therapy [22]. Combination therapy with TMP-SMZ and pentamidine offers no additional benefit and should be avoided because of cumulative toxicity [1, 12].

The combination of dapsone and trimethoprim has also been shown to be highly effective for treatment of mild to moderate PCP. Both components are given orally, dapsone, 100 mg, once a day and trimethoprim, 15 to 20 mg/kg/day in four divided doses; glucose 6-phosphate dehydrogenase (G6PD) deficiency is a contraindication to the use of this regimen [23]. Side effects have been milder than with TMP-SMZ but are of a similar nature. Methemoglobinemia has been detected but is rarely of clinical significance [24]. Initial success of aerosol pentamidine (AP) prophylaxis has led to its use as treatment of mild to moderate PCP. Although systemic side effects are minimal, AP is not as effective as TMP-SMZ, and early relapses are common. Given these limitations and the cost of this regimen, AP should be reserved for patients with mild disease who are intolerant to other forms of therapy [25, 26].

Several other alternative regimens have been evaluated as rescue therapy for patients who fail to improve with, or who are intolerant to, conventional treatment. In these settings, intravenous clindamycin (600 mg four times a day) and oral primaquine (15 mg base po daily) has resulted in a response rate of approximately 90 percent [27]. Trimetrexate, an analogue of methotrexate, has been effective in approximately 70 percent of patients [28]. The lack of an oral trimetrexate preparation, the expense of the required adjuvant therapy with folinic acid, and high early relapse rates have limited its use. A recently approved hydroxynaphthoquinone, atovaquone, has also been tried as rescue therapy with encouraging results [29].

Sufficient data now exist to support the use of systemic corticosteroids in some patients with PCP [30, 31]. Prednisone, 40 mg, or its equivalent, twice daily for 5 days, followed by 40 mg daily for 5 days, and 20 mg daily for an additional 11 days is now recommended for patients with moderate to severe PCP (room air PaO_2 < 70 torr, or A-a gradient of >35) [32]. Currently, no data are available to justify the use of steroids in mild PCP, in children, or as rescue therapy.

Clinical response of PCP to antimicrobial therapy usually becomes evident between the second and sixth day of treatment [33]. If no improvement is noted by the seventh day, the diagnosis of PCP should be confirmed (if therapy was empiric) or a second diagnosis should be considered. Patients treated initially with TMP-SMZ have a survival rate of greater than 80 percent. Patients who are begun on TMP-SMZ but switched to pentamidine have lower survival rates: 70 percent if pentamidine is used because of TMP-SMZ toxicity and 30 percent in patients who have no clinical response to TMP-SMZ [1, 12]. Subsequent episodes of PCP and the need for assisted mechanical ventilation are associated with a poorer prognosis [1–4, 12, 34, 35] (Table 10-2).

Because of the high incidence of relapse, numerous regimens of PCP chemoprophylaxis have been devised, including TMP-SMZ, intravenous or aerosol pentamidine, dapsone, and Fansidar (see Chap. 17). The Centers for Disease Control has recently published updated recommendations for PCP prophylaxis [36].

Table 10-2 *Predictors of poor outcome in* Pneumocystis carinii *pneumonia*

Prolonged history of dyspnea/dry cough ($>$ 4 wk)

Admission respiratory rate $>$ 30/min

Recurrent *Pneumocystis carinii* pneumonia

Copathogens on BAL

Poor oxygenation on admission (PaO_2 $<$ 53 mm Hg or alveolar-arterial oxygen gradient $>$ 30 mm Hg)

Low serum albumin on admission ($<$ 3.5 mg%)

Severe radiographic abnormalities (diffuse bilateral interstitial infiltrates with or without alveolar consolidation)

Elevated white blood cell count on admission ($>$ 10,900/mm^3)

Increased serum lactate dehydrogenase activity ($>$ 300 IU/liter)

Severe interstitial edema in transbronchial biopsy specimens

Source: Adapted from RF Miller and DM Mitchell, Management of respiratory failure in the acquired immune deficiency syndrome and *Pneumocystis* pneumonia. *Thorax* 45:140–146, 1990.

Mycobacterial Infections

Tuberculosis

The rise in the incidence of tuberculosis (TB) in the US, which began in 1986, is largely due to cases occurring in the HIV-infected population [37–40]. Presenting symptoms include cough, fever, weight loss, and night sweats. Extrapulmonary disease is common, and symptoms resulting from liver, bone marrow, central nervous system, or lymphatic involvement may predominate [41–43]. Chest x-rays frequently do not reveal cavities, apical scarring, or pleural effusions and may be normal in up to 10 percent of patients [42–45]. The most common abnormalities are diffuse or miliary infiltrates, focal infiltrates, and mediastinal or hilar adenopathy (Fig. 10-2). The wide variety of clinical and roentgenographic findings makes the diagnosis of TB problematic in the AIDS population [46].

All HIV-infected patients with suspected mycobacterial disease should receive a treatment regimen effective against *M. tuberculosis,* as untreated TB is both fatal and transmissible [38]. Pending culture results, initial therapy should consist of isoniazid (INH; 300 mg/day) and rifampin (600 mg/day); pyrazinamide (25 mg/kg/day) should be added for the first 2 months, and ethambutol (15 mg/kg/day) added if there is suspicion of INH resistance or evidence of central nervous system involvement or disseminated disease [38, 47–49]. Therapy should be adjusted once culture results are available and continued for 9 to 12 months for INH-sensitive organisms and 18 months for INH-resistant

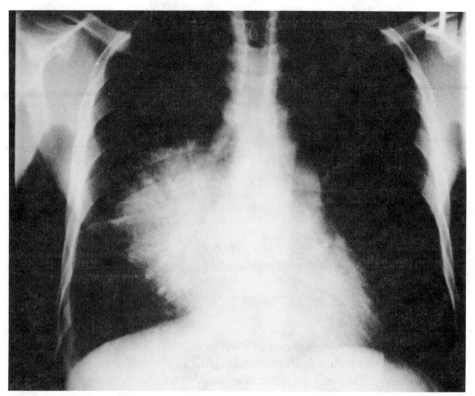

Figure 10-2. *Pulmonary tuberculosis presenting as localized right middle lobe infiltrate in HIV-infected patient.*

organisms. Recently, outbreaks of multidrug-resistant tuberculosis (MDR-TB) have been reported in health care facilities in Miami and New York City [50, 51]. MDR-TB has primarily affected patients with advanced HIV disease, and, despite the use of multidrug regimens, it has been uniformly fatal in this population.

Tuberculosis is a largely preventable disease, and chemoprophylaxis should be considered for all patients with documented HIV infection. All HIV-infected patients with induration greater than or equal to 5 mm on an intermediate-strength (5TU) PPD should receive prophylaxis, regardless of age, once active disease has been excluded [38, 52]. Patients who are anergic on skin testing but at high risk for TB ($>$10% prevalence), such as drug users, alcoholics, the homeless, past or current prison inmates, and patients from an endemic area, should also receive prophylaxis [38, 52]. In addition, patients with a history of a positive PPD who have never received treatment, patients with CXR abnormalities suggestive of previous untreated TB, and close contacts of patients with active TB should receive preventive therapy [38, 48, 52]. Prophylaxis consists of INH or rifampin (in patients in whom INH resistance is suspected) for a minimum of 12 months [38].

Mycobacterium avium *Complex*

Mycobacterium avium complex (MAC) infection occurs most often in patients with advanced HIV disease. MAC is typically cultured from blood or bone marrow, but lymph nodes, spleen, bone marrow, liver, stool, and sputum may also yield the organism. MAC infection is generally disseminated even in its early stages, and, because the lungs are frequently involved, they may be the initial site from which the organism is identified [53]. Most of the clinical manifestations are extrapulmonary, and pulmonary involvement does not seem to alter prognosis. In some studies the yield of MAC by bronchoscopy is approximately 50 percent but increases to 80 percent with the addition of transbronchial biopsy [1]. Combination therapy with ethambutol, rifampin, clofazimine, and ciprofloxacin, with or without amikacin, is often associated with symptomatic improvement, but clinical response may be modest, drug toxicity is common, bacteriologic cure is unusual, and the overall prognosis is poor [54–56]. Recently, newer macrolide antibiotics, such as clarithromycin and azithromycin, have been used with success as part of a multidrug regimen for the treatment of MAC [57]. Rifabutin has been demonstrated to be effective in preventing MAC bacteremia in HIV-infected patients with CD4 cell counts of $200/mm^3$ or lower [58]. It may also have a role in combination with other agents in the treatment of MAC infection.

Viral Infections

Disseminated cytomegalovirus (CMV) infection occurs commonly in patients with advanced HIV disease. Clinical manifestations include chorioretinitis, encephalitis, esophagitis, hepatitis, colitis, adrenalitis, and pneumonitis [59]. Pulmonary symptoms and signs, as well as CXR findings of a diffuse interstitial infiltrate, are nonspecific. Definitive diagnosis requires demonstration of characteristic intranuclear inclusions on histologic examination of lung parenchyma obtained by fiberoptic bronchoscopy with transbronchial biopsy [60]. Cytomegalovirus pneumonitis is often associated with other pulmonary infections such as PCP. There appears to be no relationship between pulmonary CMV and survival in patients with a first episode of PCP [61]. Evidence of pulmonary involvement should prompt a careful ophthalmologic examination, since therapy for CMV chorioretinitis has been shown to prevent blindness [62]. Therapy for pulmonary CMV infection with ganciclovir is probably ineffective [63].

Herpesvirus infections are an infrequent cause of pneumonia in patients with HIV disease. Because oral herpes simplex infection is common, isolation of the virus from respiratory tract specimens is not unusual. Herpes simplex pneumonitis should only be considered when there is histologic evidence of pulmonary infection and no other pathogen is isolated [5]. The diagnosis of varicella-zoster pneumonia is generally less difficult; patients present with diffuse, bilateral infiltrates on CXR in the setting of widely disseminated varicella infection [64]. Acyclovir is the drug of choice for both herpes simplex and varicella-zoster pneumonitis; foscarnet can be used to treat resistant organisms [65].

Fungal Infections

Cryptococcal infection usually presents as meningitis, with evidence of coexisting pneumonitis in 10 to 30 percent of cases [66]. The CXR usually demonstrates a focal or diffuse interstitial infiltrate, but cavitary lesions, adenopathy, and/or pleural effusions may also be seen. Identification of this organism in sputum or BAL specimens should prompt a lumbar puncture to rule out meningeal involvement. Cryptococcal pneumonitis, like meningitis, is treated with either fluconazole or amphotericin B followed by lifelong suppressive therapy [67].

Disseminated histoplasmosis has emerged as a common diagnosis in HIV-infected patients from endemic areas, such as the Ohio and Mississippi River Valleys, Haiti, Puerto Rico, and South and Central America [68]. Cases in patients who have not visited endemic areas for many years likely represent reactivation of latent infection. Chest x-rays generally show bilateral nodular infiltrates with or without adenopathy; evident pulmonary involvement is not required for dissemination. In the presence of infiltrates, the diagnostic yield of bronchoscopy is approximately 80 percent; for disseminated disease, bone marrow biopsy or blood culture has a sensitivity of approximately 90 percent [69, 70]. Amphotericin B is the drug of choice, but, even with therapy, the initial episode has a mortality of 20 to 50 percent; relapse is common and lifelong suppressive therapy is required [69]. Itraconazole has also been successfully used for the treatment and suppression of histoplasmosis.

Coccidioidomycosis with dissemination is a relatively frequent diagnosis in AIDS patients living in endemic areas [71]. The CXR is abnormal in approximately 70 percent of cases, with diffuse reticulonodular infiltrates or focal infiltrates with hilar adenopathy and pleural effusions [72, 73]. The organism may be isolated from lymph nodes, blood, urine, and skin, in addition to pulmonary specimens. Despite severe immunosuppression, tube precipitins or complement-fixing antibodies are present in greater than 90 percent of cases. Patients with a diffuse nodular pattern on CXR have a poor prognosis, with 50 percent dying within one month of diagnosis despite aggressive therapy with amphotericin B [74]. Ketoconazole and fluconazole may be useful for treatment as well as prophylaxis.

Pulmonary aspergillosis has only recently been recognized as a complication of HIV infection [74, 75]. Pulmonary infection with aspergillus occurs as an invasive parenchymal process or as obstructing bronchial disease. The majority of patients have had significant periods of neutropenia, and almost all have had a prior AIDS-defining disorder. The clinical picture consists of cough and fever; many patients also have chest pain. In patients with invasive aspergillosis, the CXR demonstrates unilateral or bilateral reticulonodular infiltrates with cavities or pleural-based lesions. Diffuse interstitial infiltrates may be seen in patients with obstructing bronchial disease, as well as in those with invasive aspergillosis [74, 75]. Despite aggressive therapy with amphotericin B, median survival has been approximately 3 months. Itraconazole may be useful in patients who cannot tolerate amphotericin.

Although cultures obtained at bronchoscopy frequently grow *Candida* species, the diagnosis of pulmonary candidiasis rests on the demonstration of fungal forms invading the lung parenchyma. Pulmonary candidiasis is exceedingly uncommon and rarely occurs except in gravely ill patients in the setting of disseminated disease. Patients may respond to treatment with amphotericin B, ketoconazole, or fluconazole, but mortality remains high [73].

Protozoal Infections

Toxoplasmosis occurs in only 1 to 3 percent of AIDS patients in the US but is more common in patients from Spain, Haiti, and other endemic areas. It usually presents as a necrotizing encephalitis with multiple ring-enhancing lesions on CT scan [76]. Pneumonitis may occur alone or as a complication of central nervous system disease. The CXR generally shows a nodular infiltrate or irregular consolidation. The demonstration of the parasite on Wright or Giemsa stain of biopsy material is required for diagnosis [73]. Treatment with sulfadiazine and pyrimethamine is generally effective, but lifelong suppressive therapy is required.

The intestinal parasites *Strongyloides* and *Cryptosporidium* may cause pulmonary symptoms in patients with gastrointestinal infestation. Identification of *Strongyloides* in the sputum denotes pulmonary infection [77]. Patients with respiratory cryptosporidiosis complain of unremitting cough. Examination of tissue specimens usually demonstrates localization of the organism to bronchial epithelial cells; identification of the pathogen in alveoli is rare, and invasion of the lung parenchyma has not been reported [78, 79]. Isolated pulmonary cryptosporidial disease does not appear to alter survival [80]. In contrast to *Strongyloides* infection, there is no effective therapy for disseminated cryptosporidiosis, and patients usually succumb to overwhelming gastrointestinal infestation.

Noninfectious Pulmonary Disorders

Kaposi's Sarcoma

Kaposi's sarcoma (KS) in the setting of AIDS usually presents as a multicentric disease involving the skin and oral mucosa. Internal organ involvement, particularly of the lymphatic system and gastrointestinal tract, occurs in 50 percent of patients with cutaneous KS [81, 82]. Thirty percent of patients with KS have symptomatic lung involvement, which accounts for 8 to 12 percent of the pulmonary complications of AIDS [83]. Pulmonary KS most often occurs in the context of disseminated disease, although isolated pulmonary involvement has been reported [1, 84, 85]. While nonspecific systemic symptoms such as fever and weight loss are most common, patients may complain of wheezing, hemoptysis, pleuritic chest pain, or stridor [86]. Physical examination is usually not revealing, although stridor suggests bulky lesions of the upper airway [87]. Chest x-ray findings include bilateral interstitial or alveolar infiltrates, or both, often with poorly defined nodularity and accompanying pleural effusions [86] (Fig. 10-3).

Definitive diagnosis of pulmonary KS usually requires open lung biopsy. However, visualization of the typical macular or plaque-like cherry-red lesions of KS in the trachea or endobronchial tree during bronchoscopy is considered adequate in patients with established disease. Endobronchial biopsy, transbronchial biopsy, or bronchial brushing with cytology is generally not diagnostic [1, 14, 83, 84]. Pleural biopsy occasionally provides useful specimens. Therapy for pulmonary KS is palliative and consists of radiation, combination chemotherapy, and/or alpha-interferon.

Lymphoma

Unlike non-Hodgkin's lymphoma in the seronegative population, HIV-associated lymphoma is likely to be comprised of multiple clones with highly malignant histology, and is usually disseminated and extranodal at the time of presentation [88]. The central nervous system, gastrointestinal tract, and liver are most commonly involved; the lungs are not usually the initial site of symptomatic disease. In patients with thoracic involvement, CXR reveals mediastinal nodes, interstitial and nodular infiltrates, solitary parenchymal nodules, or pleural thickening with effu-

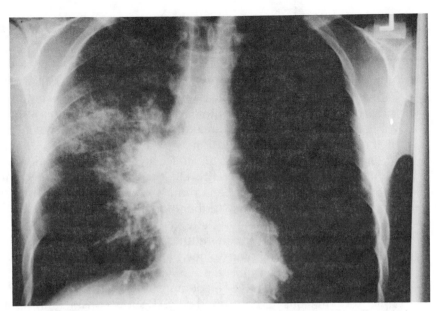

Figure 10-3. *Pulmonary Kaposi's sarcoma. Radiologic findings generally include nodular parenchymal infiltrates.*

sions [86]. Transbronchial biopsy is rarely diagnostic, and open lung biopsy is generally required.

Hodgkin's lymphoma is also more frequent in HIV-infected patients, but thoracic involvement is less common than in non-Hodgkin's lymphoma. Similar to non-Hodgkin's lymphoma, advanced disease at the time of presentation is common, and open lung biopsy is required for diagnosis. In the few cases of HIV-related pulmonary Hodgkin's lymphoma that have been reported, the CXRs demonstrated either mediastinal involvement or bilateral infiltrates [89, 90]. In general, therapy does not produce lasting control of HIV-related lymphoma.

Lymphoid Interstitial Pneumonitis

Lymphoid interstitial pneumonitis (LIP) is an immunologic disorder of unknown etiology; it typically occurs in pediatric AIDS patients but is also described in adults [86]. The characteristic lymphocytic and plasma cell infiltration of the alveolar interstitium suggests a response to chronic antigenic stimulation. Although the antigen has not been defined, direct infection of the pulmonary parenchyma with HIV or Epstein-Barr virus has been suggested [91, 92].

Patients typically present with slowly progressive dyspnea and nonproductive cough; fever and weight loss may also be present. Physical examination often reveals adenopathy, hepatosplenomegaly, uveitis, and/or parotid gland enlargement. Although examination of the chest may be normal, crackles at the bases are frequently noted on auscultation [93]. The CXR demonstrates bilateral lower-lobe interstitial or reticulonodular infiltrates with occasional areas of alveolar filling defects, similar to the pattern seen with PCP [94]. Pleural effusions are rare in LIP, and hilar adenopathy is uncommon in adults [93]. Hypergammaglobulinemia and lymphocytosis may occur [93, 94].

Diagnosis of LIP in adults is difficult. The clinical presentation is nonspecific, and, because of its rarity, LIP is usually not considered early in the evaluation of dyspnea. Recurrent bacterial pneumonia is strongly associated with LIP and may further hinder diagnosis. Patients with LIP may respond to treatment of pathogens recovered from sputum, and CXRs may improve but rarely return to normal. Histology from transbronchial or open lung biopsy shows alveolar and interstitial infiltration of lymphocytes and plasma cells [95].

Therapeutic benefit has been demonstrated with corticosteroid therapy. Abnormalities demonstrated on CXR show considerable improvement, and oxygenation may return to normal or near normal. In many cases, no recurrence of symptoms occurs after discontinuation of corticosteroid treatment [93]. However, in some patients, clinical and radiologic deterioration follows within days of stopping therapy, and steroids must be continued long term [96].

Nonspecific Interstitial Pneumonitis

Nonspecific interstitial pneumonitis is a histologic entity characterized on biopsy by a mild mononuclear cell infiltrate, with varying degrees of interstitial edema, fibrin deposition, alveolar cell hyperplasia, septal thickening, and fibrosis [4, 97]. Patients usually have nonspecific respiratory symptoms but may also be asymptomatic [98]. Diagnosis relies on demonstration of typical histologic abnormalities and the exclusion of another underlying process. The clinical course usually stabilizes or improves without specific therapy. Steroids may be useful in symptomatic patients [4, 97].

Pneumothorax

The insidious onset of PCP allows significant pulmonary parenchymal destruction, leading to the development of cysts, cavities, bullae, and pneumothorax [99, 100]. The risk of pneumothorax is increased in patients with recurrent PCP and in those receiving AP prophylaxis [101]. Treatment of pneumothorax with chest tube suction is adequate in fewer than 50 percent of patients; air leaks are slow to resolve and sclerotherapy or thoracotomy, or both, are frequently required [101, 102]. Treatment of PCP in AIDS patients with pneumothorax should be considered because of the common association of these two conditions.

Lymphadenopathy

Persistent generalized lymphadenopathy is a common finding in patients with HIV disease. Hilar and mediastinal adenopathy are not, however, a part of this syndrome [103, 104]. Consequently, patients with radiographic evidence of thoracic adenopathy should be evaluated carefully for infectious or neoplastic diseases. Extrathoracic lymph node biopsy will often identify the cause, but, if it is nondiagnostic, open biopsy of the chest should be considered.

Diagnostic Approach for Respiratory Symptoms

A physician caring for an HIV-infected patient with respiratory symptoms faces a lengthy differential diagnosis that requires a rational management plan. In 1984, the National Heart, Lung and Blood Institute, in a report of its workshop on pulmonary complications of AIDS, presented a series of algorithms designed to facilitate the diagnosis of pulmonary problems [3]. The following diagnostic approach, modified by more recent information, is recommended.

1. Patients with fever, cough, dyspnea, or weight loss should have chest roentgenography performed. Differential diagnosis and evaluation of commonly observed CXR patterns are presented in Table 10-3 and Fig. 10-4.
2. If the CXR is normal, one should measure the alveolar-arterial oxygen gradient, the diffusing capacity for carbon monoxide (DLCO), and/or perform gallium scanning of the lungs. If all three studies are unremarkable, pulmonary disease is highly unlikely.
3. If the CXR reveals a focal abnormality, an attempt should be made to identify a "routine" infection. Staining and culturing of sputum for conventional bacteria and acid-fast bacilli (AFB) should be included in this evaluation. If the CXR shows diffuse infiltrates, an empiric trial of therapy for PCP is reasonable in patients previously diagnosed with AIDS who have only mild to moderate gas exchange abnormalities.
4. A firm diagnosis should be pursued for those patients who lack an AIDS-defining illness. Induced sputum studies for PCP, AFB, and other pathogens should be the first step in such an evaluation. In institutions that lack the capacity to perform this procedure, flexible fiber-

Table 10-3 *Differential diagnosis of chest x-ray patterns in the HIV-infected patient*

CXR pattern	Differential diagnosis
Diffuse reticulonodular infiltrate	*Pneumocystis carinii* pneumonia Tuberculosis Disseminated histoplasmosis Disseminated coccidioidomycosis Lymphoid interstitial pneumonitis
Focal air space consolidation	Bacterial pneumonia Kaposi's sarcoma Cryptococcosis
Normal	*Pneumocystis carinii* pneumonia Disseminated MAC infection Disseminated histoplasmosis
Lymphadenopathy	Tuberculosis Kaposi's sarcoma Disseminated MAC infection Non-Hodgkin's lymphoma
Pleural effusion	Kaposi's sarcoma Tuberculosis Non-Hodgkin's lymphoma Pyogenic empyema

Source: Adapted from JF Murray, J Mills, Pulmonary infectious complications of human immunodeficiency virus infection (part 1). *Am Rev Respir Dis* 141:1356–1372, 1990.

optic bronchoscopy with BAL is appropriate. A similar approach is warranted in patients whose CXR abnormalities are focal, mild, or otherwise atypical of PCP after a "routine" pneumonia has been excluded.

5. If examination of induced sputum or initial fiberoptic bronchoscopy with BAL is nondiagnostic, fiberoptic bronchoscopy with BAL, bronchial brushing, and multiple transbronchial biopsies should be performed. The biopsy and lavage specimens should be processed with appropriate stains or cultures, or both, for bacterial pathogens, including *Legionella, P. carinii,* AFB, fungi, and CMV. Specimens should also undergo routine cytologic and histologic analysis.

6. If fiberoptic bronchoscopy with transbronchial biopsy is nondiagnostic and the patient's clinical condition is deteriorating, either repeat bronchoscopy with transbronchial biopsy or open lung biopsy should be performed.

7. If fiberoptic bronchoscopy with transbronchial biopsy is nondiagnostic and the patient's clinical condition is stable, diffusing capacity and alveolar-arterial oxygen gradient should be measured, and/or gallium scanning performed. If the results of these tests show that the patient's condition is stable or improving, clinical observation is

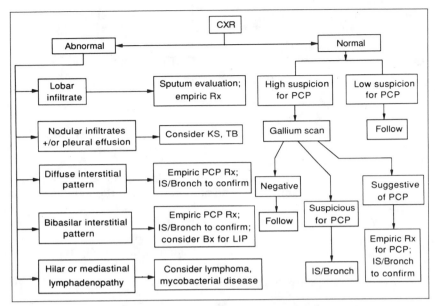

Figure 10-4. Algorithm for evaluation of pulmonary disease associated with HIV infection, based on chest x-ray appearance. (IS/Bronch = induced sputum/bronchoscopy; Bx = biopsy; LIP = lymphoid interstitial pneumonitis.) (Courtesy of Dr. Jon Fuller, Boston City Hospital.)

appropriate; if the results show a worsening condition, either repeat bronchoscopy or open lung biopsy should be considered.

References

1. White DA, Stover DE. Pulmonary effects of AIDS. *Clin Chest Med* 9:363–535, 1988.
2. Hopewell PC, Luce JM. Pulmonary involvement in the acquired immunodeficiency syndrome. *Chest* 87:104–112, 1985.
3. Murray JF, Felton CP, Garay SM, et al. Pulmonary complications of the acquired immunodeficiency syndrome: Report of a National Heart, Lung and Blood Institute workshop. *N Engl J Med* 310:1682–1688, 1984.
4. Stover DE, White DA, Roman PA, et al. Spectrum of pulmonary diseases associated with the acquired immune deficiency syndrome. *Am J Med* 78:429–437, 1985.
5. Murray JF, Mills J. Pulmonary infectious complications of human immunodeficiency virus infection (part 1). *Am Rev Respir Dis* 141:1356–1372, 1990.
6. Masur H, Ognibene FP, Yarchoan R, et al. CD4 counts as predictors of opportunistic pneumonias in human immunodeficiency virus (HIV) infection. *Ann Intern Med* 111:223–231, 1989.

7. Polsky B, Gold JWM, Whimbey E, et al. Bacterial pneumonia in patients with the acquired immunodeficiency syndrome. *Ann Intern Med* 104:38–41, 1986.
8. Kramer MR, Uttamchandani RB. The radiographic appearance of pulmonary nocardiosis associated with AIDS. *Chest* 98:382–385, 1990.
9. Joshi N, Hamory BH. Drug resistant *Nocardia asteroides* infection in a patient with acquired immunodeficiency syndrome. *South Med J* 84:1155–1156, 1991.
10. Harvey RL, Suntrum JC. *Rhodococcus equi* infection in patients with and without human immunodeficiency virus infection. *Rev Infect Dis* 13:139–145, 1991.
11. Emmons W, Reichwein B, Winslow DL. *Rhodococcus equi* infection in the patient with AIDS: Literature review and report of an unusual case. *Rev Infect Dis* 13:91–96, 1991.
12. Catterall JR, Potasman I, Remington JS. *Pneumocystis carinii* pneumonia in the patient with AIDS. *Chest* 88:758–762, 1985.
13. Freedberg KA, Tosteson ANA, Cohen CJ, Cotton DJ. Primary prophylaxis for *Pneumocystis carinii* pneumonia in HIV-infected people with CD4 counts below 200/mm^3: A cost-effectiveness analysis. *J AIDS* 4:521–531, 1991.
14. Weissler JC, Mootz AR. Southwestern internal medicine conference: pulmonary disease in AIDS patients. *Am J Med Sci* 300:330–343, 1990.
15. Stover D, Greeno R, Gagliardi A. The use of a simple exercise test for the diagnosis of *Pneumocystis carinii* pneumonia in patients with AIDS. *Am Rev Respir Dis* 139:1343–1346, 1989.
16. Garay SM, Green J. Prognostic indicators in the initial presentation of *Pneumocystis carinii* pneumonia. *Chest* 95:769–772, 1989.
17. Zaman MK, White DA. Serum lactate dehydrogenase levels and *Pneumocystis carinii* pneumonia: Diagnostic and prognostic significance. *Am Rev Respir Dis* 137:796–800, 1988.
18. Kovacs JA, Ng VL, Masur H, et al. Diagnosis of *Pneumocystis carinii* pneumonia: improved detection in sputum with use of monoclonal antibodies. *N Engl J Med* 318:589–593, 1988.
19. Pitchenik AE, Ganjei P, Torres A, et al. Sputum examination for the diagnosis of *Pneumocystis carinii* pneumonia in the acquired immunodeficiency syndrome. *Am Rev Respir Dis* 133:226–229, 1986.
20. Jules-Elysee K, Stover D, Zaman M, et al. Aerosolized pentamidine: Effect on diagnosis and presentation of *Pneumocystis carinii* pneumonia. *Ann Intern Med* 112:750–757, 1990.
21. Sattler FR, Cowan R, Nielsen DM, Ruskin J. Trimethoprim-sulfamethoxazole compared with pentamidine for treatment of *Pneumocystis carinii* pneumonia in the acquired immunodeficiency syndrome: A prospective, noncrossover study. *Ann Intern Med* 109:280–287, 1988.
22. Sands M, Kron MA, Brown RB. Pentamidine: A review. *Rev Infect Dis* 7:625–637, 1985.
23. Leoung G, Mills J, Hopewell P, et al. Dapsone-trimethoprim for *Pneumocystis carinii* pneumonia in the acquired immunodeficiency syndrome. *Ann Intern Med* 105:45–48, 1986.

24. Gallant JE, Hoehn-Saric E, Smith MD. Respiratory insufficiency from dapsone induced methemoglobinemia. *AIDS* 5:1392–1393, 1991.
25. Montgomery AB, Debs R, Luce J, et al. Aerosolized pentamidine as sole therapy for *Pneumocystis carinii* pneumonia in patients with acquired immunodeficiency syndrome. *Lancet* 2:480–483, 1987.
26. Conte J, Hollander H, Golden J, et al. Selective delivery of pentamidine to the lung by aerosol. *Am Rev Respir Dis* 137:477–478, 1988.
27. Toma E, Fournier S, Poisson M, et al. Clindamycin with primaquine for *Pneumocystis carinii* pneumonia. *Lancet* 1:1046–1048, 1989.
28. Allegra CJ, Chabner BA, Tuazon CU, et al. Trimetrexate for the treatment of *Pneumocystis carinii* pneumonia in patients with acquired immunodeficiency syndrome. *N Engl J Med* 317:978–985, 1987.
29. Fallon J, Kovacs J, Hughes W, et al. The preliminary evaluation of 566C80 for the treatment of *Pneumocystis* pneumonia in patients with the acquired immunodeficiency syndrome. *N Engl J Med* 325:1534–1538, 1991.
30. Gagnon S, Booth AM, Fischl MA, et al. Corticosteroids as adjunctive therapy for severe *Pneumocystis carinii* pneumonia in the acquired immunodeficiency syndrome. *N Engl J Med* 323:1444–1450, 1990.
31. Bozzette SA, Sattler FR, Chui J, et al. A controlled trial of early adjunctive treatment for *Pneumocystis carinii* pneumonia in the acquired immunodeficiency syndrome. *N Engl J Med* 323:1451–1457, 1990.
32. NIH-UC expert panel for corticosteroids as adjunctive therapy for *Pneumocystis* pneumonia. Consensus statement for use of corticosteroids as adjunctive therapy for *Pneumocystis* pneumonia in AIDS. *N Engl J Med* 323:1500–1504, 1990.
33. Mitchell DM, Johnson MA. Treatment of lung disease in patients with the acquired immune deficiency syndrome. *Thorax* 45:219–224, 1990.
34. Miller RF, Mitchell DM. Management of respiratory failure in the acquired immune deficiency syndrome and *Pneumocystis* pneumonia. *Thorax* 45:140–146, 1990.
35. Wachter RM, Luce JM, Turner J, et al. Intensive care of patients with the acquired immunodeficiency syndrome: Outcome and changing patterns of utilization. *Am Rev Respir Dis* 134:891–896, 1986.
36. Centers for Disease Control. Recommendations for prophylaxis against *Pneumocystis carinii* pneumonia for adults and adolescents infected with human immunodeficiency virus. *MMWR* 41(RR-4):1–11, 1992.
37. Centers for Disease Control. Update: Tuberculosis elimination—United States. *MMWR* 39:153–156, 1990.
38. Centers for Disease Control. Tuberculosis and human immunodeficiency virus infection: Recommendations of the advisory committee for the elimination of tuberculosis (ACET). *MMWR* 38:236–250, 1989.
39. Rieder HL, Cauthen GM, Bloch AB, et al. Tuberculosis and acquired immunodeficiency syndrome—Florida. *Arch Intern Med* 149:1268–1273, 1989.
40. Chaisson RE, Slutkin G. Tuberculosis and human immunodeficiency virus infection. *J Infect Dis* 159:96–99, 1989.
41. Chaisson RE, Schecter GF, Theuer CP, et al. Tuberculosis in patients with

the acquired immunodeficiency syndrome: Clinical features, response to therapy, and survival. *Am Rev Respir Dis* 136:570–574, 1987.

42. Theuer CP, Hopewell PC, Elias D, et al. Human immunodeficiency virus infection in tuberculosis patients. *J Infect Dis* 162:8–12, 1990.

43. Pitchenik AE, Cole C, Russell BW, et al. Tuberculosis, atypical mycobacteriosis, and the acquired immunodeficiency syndrome among Haitian and non-Haitian patients in south Florida. *Ann Intern Med* 101:610–615, 1984.

44. Pitchenik AE, Rubinson A. The radiographic appearance of tuberculosis in patients with the acquired immune deficiency syndrome (AIDS) and pre-AIDS. *Am Rev Respir Dis* 131:393–396, 1985.

45. Colebunders RE, Ryder RW, Nzilambi N, et al. HIV infection in patients with tuberculosis in Kinshasa, Zaire. *Am Rev Respir Dis* 139:1082–1085, 1989.

46. Kramer F, Modilevsky T, Waliany AR, et al. Delayed diagnosis of tuberculosis in patients with human immunodeficiency virus infection. *Am J Med* 89:451–456, 1990.

47. Davidson PT. Treating tuberculosis; what drugs, for how long? *Ann Intern Med* 112:393–395, 1990.

48. American Thoracic Society. Treatment of tuberculosis and tuberculosis infection in adults and children. *Am Rev Respir Dis* 134:355–363, 1986.

49. American Thoracic Society. Mycobacterioses and the acquired immunodeficiency syndrome. *Am Rev Respir Dis* 136:492–496, 1987.

50. Fischl M, Uttamchandani R, Daikos G, et al. Outbreak of multiple drug resistant tuberculosis (MDR-TB) among patients with HIV infection. Eighth International Conference on AIDS, Amsterdam, July 1992.

51. Edlin BR, et al. An outbreak of multidrug-resistant tuberculosis among hospitalized patients with the acquired immunodeficiency syndrome. *N Engl J Med* 326:1514–1521, 1992.

52. Centers for Disease Control. Screening for tuberculosis and tuberculosis infection in high-risk populations and the use of preventive therapy for tuberculosis infection in the United States: Recommendations of the Advisory Committee for Elimination of Tuberculosis. *MMWR* 39:1–12, 1990.

53. Hawkins C, Gold J, Whimbey E, et al. *Mycobacterium avium* complex in patients with acquired immunodeficiency syndrome. *Ann Intern Med* 105:184–188, 1986.

54. Hoy J, Mitch A, Sandland M, et al. Quadruple drug therapy for *Mycobacterium avium-intracellulare* bacteremia in AIDS patients. *J Infect Dis* 161:801–805, 1990.

55. Chiu J, Nussbaum J, Bozzette S, et al. Treatment of disseminated *Mycobacterium avium* complex infection in AIDS with amikacin, ethambutol, rifampin and ciprofloxacin. *Ann Intern Med* 113:358–361, 1990.

56. Agins BC, Berman DS, Spicehandler D, et al. Effect of combined therapy with ansamycin, clofazamine, ethambutol and isoniazid for *Mycobacterium avium* infection in patients with AIDS. *J Infect Dis* 159:784–787, 1989.

57. Chaisson RE, Benson CA, Dube M, et al. Clarithromycin for disseminated *Mycobacterium avium* complex in AIDS patients. Eighth International Conference on AIDS, Amsterdam, July 1992.

58. Cameron W, Sparti P, Pietroski N, et al. Rifabutin therapy for the prevention of MAC bacteremia in patients with AIDS and CD4 $\leq$ 200. Eighth International Conference on AIDS, Amsterdam, July 1992.

59. Wallace JM, Hannah J. Cytomegalovirus pneumonitis in patients with AIDS: Findings in a autopsy series. *Chest* 92:198–203, 1987.

60. Jacobson MA, Mills J. Cytomegalovirus infection. *Clin Chest Med* 9:443–448, 1988.

61. Jacobson MA, Mills J, Rush J, et al. Morbidity and mortality of patients with AIDS and first-episode *Pneumocystis carinii* pneumonia unaffected by concomitant pulmonary cytomegalovirus infection. *Am Rev Respir Dis* 144:6–9, 1991.

62. Jacobson MA, Mills J. Serious cytomegalovirus disease in the acquired immunodeficiency syndrome (AIDS). *Ann Intern Med* 108:585–594, 1988.

63. Collaborative DHPG Treatment Study Group. Treatment of serious cytomegalovirus infection with 9-(1,3-dihydroxy-2-propoxymethyl) guanine in patients with AIDS and other immunodeficiencies. *N Engl J Med* 314:801–805, 1986.

64. Cohen PR, Belltrani VP, Grossman ME, Disseminated herpes-zoster in patients with human immunodeficiency virus infection. *Am J Med* 84:1076–1080, 1988.

65. Erlich K, Jacobson, Loehler J, et al. Foscarnet therapy for severe acyclovir resistant herpes simplex virus infections in patients with acquired immunodeficiency syndrome. *Ann Intern Med* 109:710–713, 1989.

66. Cameron ML, Bartlett JA, Gallos HA, Waskin HA. Manifestations of pulmonary cryptococcosis in patients with acquired immunodeficiency syndrome. *Rev Infect Dis* 13:64–67, 1991.

67. Saag MA, Powderly WG, Cloud GA, et al. Comparison of amphotericin B with fluconazole in the treatment of acute AIDS-associated cryptococcal meningitis. *N Engl J Med* 326:83–89, 1992.

68. Mandell W, Goldberg DM, Neu HC. Histoplasmosis in patients with the acquired immune deficiency syndrome. *Am J Med* 81:974–978, 1986.

69. Wheat LJ, Connolly-Stringfield PA, Baker RL, et al. Disseminated histoplasmosis in the acquired immune deficiency syndrome: Clinical findings, diagnosis and treatment, and review of the literature. *Medicine* 69:361–374, 1990.

70. Prechter GC, Prakash UBS. Bronchoscopy in the diagnosis of pulmonary histoplasmosis. *Chest* 95:1033–1036, 1989.

71. Sobonya RE, Barbee RA, Wiens J, Trego D. Detection of fungi and other pathogens in immunocompromised patients by bronchoalveolar lavage in an area endemic for coccidioidomycosis. *Chest* 97:1349–1355, 1990.

72. Fish DG, Ampel NM, Galgiani JN, et al. Coccidioidomycosis during human immunodeficiency virus infection: A review of 77 patients. *Medicine* 69:384–391, 1990.

73. Murray JF, Mills J. Pulmonary infectious complications of human immunodeficiency virus infection (part 2). *Am Rev Respir Dis* 141:1582–1598, 1990.

74. Denning DW, Follansbee SE, Scolaro M, et al. Pulmonary aspergillosis in the acquired immunodeficiency syndrome. *N Engl J Med* 324:654–662, 1991.

75. Klapholz A, Salomon N, Perlman DC, Talavera W. Aspergillosis in the acquired immunodeficiency syndrome. *Chest* 100:1614–1618, 1991.

76. McCabe RE, Remington JS. *Toxoplasma gondii*. In GL Mandell, RG Douglas, JE Bennett (eds), *Principles and Practices of Infectious Diseases* (3rd ed). New York: Churchill Livingstone, 1989. Pp 2093–2094.

77. Armignacco O, Capecchi A, DeMori P. *Strongyloides stercoralis* hyperinfection and the acquired immunodeficiency syndrome. *Am J Med* 86:258, 1989.

78. Brady EM, Margolis ML, Korzeniowski OM. Pulmonary cryptosporidiosis in acquired immune deficiency syndrome. *JAMA* 252:89–90, 1984.

79. Ma P, Villanueva TG, Kaufman D, Gillooley JF. Respiratory cryptosporidiosis in the acquired immune deficiency syndrome. *JAMA* 252:1298–1301, 1984.

80. Hojlyng N, Jensen BN. Respiratory cryptosporidiosis in HIV-positive patients. *Lancet* 1:590–591, 1988.

81. Safai B, Johnson KG, Myskowski PL, et al. The natural history of Kaposi's sarcoma in the acquired immunodeficiency syndrome. *Ann Intern Med* 102:471–475, 1985.

82. Friedman, SL, Wright TL, Altman DF. Gastrointestinal Kaposi's sarcoma in patients with the acquired immune deficiency syndrome. Endoscopic and autopsy findings. *Gastroenterology* 890:102–108, 1985.

83. Garay S, Belenko M, Fazzini E, Schinella R. Pulmonary manifestations of Kaposi's sarcoma. *Chest* 91:39–43, 1987.

84. Meduri GU, Stover DE, Lee M, et al. Pulmonary Kaposi's sarcoma in the acquired immune deficiency syndrome. *Am J Med* 81:11–18, 1986.

85. Zibrak JD, Silvestri RC, Costello P, et al. Bronchoscopic and radiologic features of Kaposi's sarcoma involving the respiratory system. *Chest* 90:476, 1986.

86. White DA, Matthay RA. Noninfectious complications of infection with the human immunodeficiency virus. *Am Rev Respir Dis* 140:1763–1787, 1989.

87. Malabonga VM, Smith PR. Upper airway obstruction due to Kaposi's sarcoma in the acquired immunodeficiency syndrome. *NY State J Med* 90:613–614, 1990.

88. Kaplan LD, Abrams DI, Feigal E, et al. AIDS-associated non-Hodgkin's lymphoma in San Francisco. *JAMA* 261:719–724, 1989.

89. Knowles, LD, Chamulak GA, Subar M, et al. Lymphoid neoplasia associated with the acquired immunodeficiency syndrome (AIDS). *Ann Intern Med* 108:744–753, 1988.

90. Scheib RG, Seigal RS. Atypical Hodgkin's disease and the acquired immunodeficiency syndrome. *Ann Intern Med* 102:554, 1985.

91. Resnick L, Pitchenik AE, Fisher E, Croney R. Detection of HTLV-III/LAV-

specific IgG and antigen in bronchoalveolar lavage fluid from two patients with lymphocytic interstitial pneumonitis associated with AIDS-related complex. *Am J Med* 82:553–556, 1987.

92. Lin RY, Gruber PJ, Saunders R, Perla EN. Lymphocytic interstitial pneumonitis in adult HIV infection. *NY State J Med* 88:273–276, 1988.

93. Oldham SAA, Castillo M, Jacobson FL, et al. HIV associated lymphocytic interstitial pneumonia: radiologic manifestations and pathologic correlation. *Radiology* 170:83–87, 1989.

94. Rubinstein A, Morecki R, Silverman B, et al. Pulmonary disease in children with the acquired immunodeficiency syndrome and AIDS-related complex. *J Pediatr* 108:498–503, 1986.

95. Barrio JL, Harcup C, Baier HJ, Pitchenik AE. Value of repeat fiberoptic bronchoscopies and significance of nondiagnostic bronchoscopy results in patients with the acquired immunodeficiency syndrome. *Am Rev Respir Dis* 135:422–425, 1987.

96. Morris JC, Rosen MJ, Marchevsky A, Tierstein AS. Lymphocytic interstitial pneumonitis in patients at risk for the acquired immunodeficiency syndrome. *Chest* 91:63–67, 1987.

97. Suffredini AF, Ognibene FP, Lack EE, et al. Nonspecific interstitial pneumonitis: A common cause of pulmonary disease in the acquired immunodeficiency syndrome. *Ann Intern Med* 107:7–13, 1987.

98. Ognibene FP, Masur H, Rogers P, et al. Nonspecific interstitial pneumonitis without evidence of *Pneumocystis carinii* in asymptomatic patients with human immunodeficiency virus (HIV). *Ann Intern Med* 109:874–879, 1988.

99. Joe L, Gordin F, Parker RH. Spontaneous pneumothorax with *Pneumocystis carinii* infection. *Arch Intern Med* 146:1816–1817, 1986.

100. Feurerstein IM, Archer A, Pluda JM, et al. Thin walled cavities, cysts, and pneumothorax in *Pneumocystis carinii* pneumonia: Further observations with histopathologic correlation. *Radiology* 177:697–702, 1990.

101. Sepkowitz KA, Telzak EE, Gold JWM, et al. Pneumothorax in AIDS. *Ann Intern Med* 114:455–459, 1991.

102. Fleisher AG, McElvaney G, Lawson L, et al. Surgical management of spontaneous pneumothorax in patients with acquired immunodeficiency syndrome. *Ann Thorac Surg* 45:21–23, 1988.

103. Stern RG, Gamsu G, Golden JA, et al. Intrathoracic adenopathy: Differential features of AIDS and diffuse lymphadenopathy syndrome. *Am J Radiol* 142:689–692, 1984.

104. Suster B, Akerman M, Orenstein M, Wax MR. Pulmonary manifestations of AIDS; review of 106 episodes. *Radiology* 161:87–93, 1986.

11 / Gastrointestinal Manifestations

Nezam H. Afdhal

Gastrointestinal (GI) involvement in AIDS is almost universal, and clinically significant disease occurs in 50 to 90 percent of patients [1, 2]. Common and opportunistic infections, malignancies, and specific HIV-related syndromes all affect the GI tract. Symptoms include diarrhea with associated weight loss and wasting, odynophagia, and abdominal pain. Hepatobiliary disease, although commonly associated with HIV infection, is often asymptomatic. Prompt diagnosis and treatment of HIV-related GI disorders are necessary to prevent significant morbidity from weight loss and malnutrition.

Diarrhea

Diarrhea is experienced by nearly all patients with HIV infection at some time during their disease. It is considered significant when the stool output is greater than 500 gm per day. Over 70 percent of cases of diarrhea are caused by infection [3]. The diarrhea may be mild and intermittent, or severe and disabling; spontaneous exacerbations and remissions are common. The history can prove useful in localizing the site of diarrhea to the small or large bowel. Large-volume diarrhea, frequently pale and bulky, is generally associated with small bowel disease such as that seen with cryptosporidiosis. Frequent small-volume stools associated with tenesmus, hematochezia, or rectal discharge may suggest perianal disease, such as herpes simplex proctitis, or an invasive viral or bacterial colitis. Epidemiologic factors may be useful in differential diagnosis. For example, patients from the Caribbean are at increased risk for infection with parasites such as *Isospora belli* and *Strongyloides stercoralis*.

The initial evaluation of diarrhea is the same as that performed in an immunocompetent patient. Examination of the stool is essential and should include (1) wet prep of fresh stool for leukocytes and motile trophozoites; (2) test for occult blood; (3) bacterial culture for common pathogens, such as *Salmonella, Campylobacter,* and *Shigella;* and (4) three stool samples for ova and parasites. In patients with advanced

Table 11-1 Differential diagnosis of diarrhea in the HIV-infected patient

Infections
  Bacterial
    Mycobacterium avium complex
    Salmonella species
    Shigella species
    Campylobacter species
    Clostridium difficile
  Viral
    Cytomegalovirus
    Rotavirus
    Norwalk agent
  Fungal
    Candida species
    Histoplasmosis
  Parasitic
    Cryptosporidium
    Isospora belli
    Microsporidia
    Giardia lamblia
    Entamoeba histolytica
Neoplasms
  Lymphoma
  Kaposi's sarcoma
HIV enteropathy
Drug toxicity

HIV disease (CD4 cell count $< 200/mm^3$), an acid-fast or Kinyoun stain for *Mycobacterium avium* complex (MAC) and modified acid-fast stains for cryptosporidial and *I. belli* oocysts should also be included. Patients receiving antimicrobial therapy should have their stool assayed for *Clostridium difficile* cytotoxin.

If results of these studies are negative and significant diarrhea persists, further investigations should include upper-GI endoscopy with biopsy and duodenal juice aspiration, and flexible sigmoidoscopy. Small bowel biopsy and aspirate can be useful in excluding parasites that are intermittently shed in stool. Villous atrophy is characteristic of HIV enteropathy but may also be associated with MAC-laden macrophages. Sigmoidoscopy may reveal evidence of colitis or proctitis. Tissue obtained at endoscopy should be sent for histopathologic examination, as well as viral, fungal, and mycobacterial cultures.

The differential diagnosis for HIV-associated diarrhea is presented in Table 11-1. Gastroenteritis may result from bacterial, viral, and parasitic infections. Diarrhea may also be the result of neoplasms, HIV enteropathy, or drug toxicity.

Bacterial Infections

Salmonella *Species*

HIV-infected patients have a 20-fold increased risk of salmonellosis, usually nontyphoidal, which is associated with bacteremia in 50 to 80 percent of cases [4, 5]. Bacteremia may occur in the presence of negative stool cultures. Recurrent *Salmonella* infection may be an early manifestation of AIDS and has also been described with HIV-2 infection. *Salmonella* species are resistant to ampicillin in 50 percent of cases, and trimethoprim-sulfamethoxazole (TMP-SMZ) or a quinolone (ciprofloxacin or ofloxacin) is recommended [6]. Parenteral therapy is necessary for patients with evidence of sepsis. In cases of chronic relapsing disease, long-term suppressive therapy with a quinolone antibiotic may be necessary.

Shigella *Species*

Shigella flexnerii is the usual pathogen, and bacteremia is uncommon. Blood and leukocytes are frequently identified in the stool. A quinolone antibiotic is the treatment of choice.

Campylobacter *Species*

Infection may present with diarrhea, cholecystitis, or a Crohn's-disease–like terminal ileitis. Treatment is with erythromycin, 500 mg orally four times a day, or a quinolone antibiotic in resistant cases.

Viral Infections

Cytomegalovirus

Disseminated cytomegalovirus (CMV) infection is associated with advanced HIV disease and can affect any part of the GI tract [7]. Frequent bloody bowel movements are common [8]. The disease is characterized endoscopically by a patchy colitis with vasculitis and histologically by typical intranuclear inclusions. Enteritis manifested by abdominal pain may also occur, and fistula formation with perforation is not unusual. Inflammatory masses that mimic tumors— "CMVoma's"—have been described in the cecum, colon, and small bowel. Treatment with ganciclovir (10 mg/kg/day intravenously in two divided doses for 14 days) results in clinical improvement in a majority of cases. Maintenance therapy is generally necessary, and CMV colitis is associated with a poor long-term prognosis.

Herpes Simplex Virus

Herpes simplex virus (HSV) (usually type II) proctitis is common in patients who practice receptive anal intercourse and manifests as diarrhea, rectal pain, and discharge. Diagnosis is based on flexible sigmoidoscopic biopsy and culture. Oral acyclovir (200–800 mg five times/day) is the treatment of choice; intravenous administration is reserved for severe cases.

Parasitic Infections

Cryptosporidium
Cryptosporidiosis in the severely immunocompromised host is characterized by chronic, voluminous small bowel diarrhea (up to 20 liters per day) associated with cramping abdominal pain and weight loss [9]. In HIV-infected patients with earlier disease, its course may be self-limited [10]. Diagnosis is made by identification of the oocyst in stool (Fig. 11-1A). Spiramycin, erythromycin, and clindamycin have proven ineffective, but immune bovine dialyzable leukocyte extract may be useful in some patients [11, 12].

Isospora belli
This sporozoan is frequently seen in patients from the Caribbean and causes a clinical syndrome similar to cryptosporidiosis [13] (Fig. 11-1B). Treatment with TMP-SMZ (double-strength tablet four times a day for 10 days, then twice a day for 3 weeks) is effective, but relapse rates as high as 50 percent are seen following initial therapy. Pyrimethamine plus folinic acid is an alternative regimen for patients who cannot tolerate TMP-SMZ.

Strongyloides stercoralis
This nematode helminth is endemic to the tropics and can be transmitted sexually. Latent infection has been reported to last for as long as 30 years. Diarrhea is watery with few leukocytes. A hyperinfection syndrome with larvae invading the bowel wall has been reported in AIDS, presenting as respiratory symptoms, meningitis, and polymicrobial sepsis [14]. Stool and duodenal juice aspirates are frequently required for diagnosis. Thiabendazole, 25 mg/kg orally twice a day for 5 to 10 days, is the treatment of choice.

Entamoeba histolytica
Cyst carriage is seen in 5 percent of the United States population and in 20 to 30 percent of homosexuals. Active infection is indicated by bloody stools containing the trophozoites with ingested red cells (hemophagocytosis). Treatment is with metronidazole, 750 mg orally three times a day, for 10 days, followed by iodoquinol, 650 mg orally three times a day for 20 days.

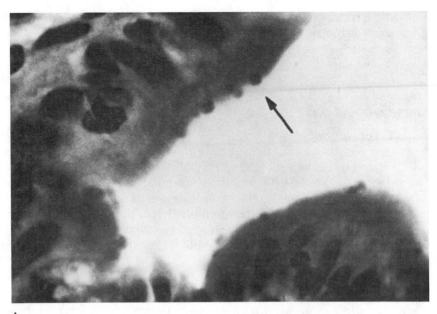

A

B

Figure 11-1. A. Cryptosporidial cysts in small bowel biopsy. (Courtesy of Dr. Jonathan W. M. Gold, Cornell University Medical College, and Centers for Disease Control, Atlanta, GA.) B. Isospora belli cyst in stool. (From JA DeHovitz, et al., Clinical manifestations and therapy of Isospora belli infection in patients with AIDS. N Engl J Med 315:87–90, 1986. Reprinted by permission of the New England Journal of Medicine.)

Giardia lamblia

This flagellated protozoan is a common cause of traveler's diarrhea, and 3 to 7 percent of the US population are asymptomatic cyst carriers. Giardiasis can cause diarrhea, flatulence, abdominal cramps, and bloating; the illness appears to be no more severe in HIV-infected patients than in the immunocompetent host. The syndrome may be acute or chronic, and diagnosis depends on demonstration of trophozoites in stool or duodenal fluid. Metronidazole, 250 mg orally three times a day for 10 days, is the treatment of choice.

Microsporidia

This unicellular protozoan, which can cause nonbloody diarrhea, has been shown in the small bowel of AIDS patients by Giemsa stain and electron microscopy [15]. No effective therapy has been described to date.

HIV Enteropathy

In 20 to 30 percent of HIV-infected patients with diarrhea, no specific pathogen can be isolated [16]. There is evidence of malabsorption, and small bowel biopsy generally demonstrates partial villous atrophy, with evidence of tissue injury and increased intraepithelial lymphocytes (Fig. 11-2). The etiology of this syndrome is unclear, but may include a direct enterocytopathic effect of HIV or other viral pathogens. Immunologic injury induced by these agents is also a possibility. Treatment is supportive, and there may be some benefit from octreotide administration (see section on general management of diarrhea).

Gay Bowel Syndrome

A syndrome of perianal pain with diarrhea and rectal discharge has been described in homosexual men [17, 18]. It appears most commonly to be caused by sexually transmitted diseases, including syphilis, gonorrhea, chlamydia, and HSV. Rectal Kaposi's sarcoma (KS) and squamous cell carcinoma of the anus may produce a similar syndrome. In addition to stool examination and sigmoidoscopy, a high rectal swab and culture should be performed.

General Management of Diarrhea

Diarrhea in HIV-infected patients can be associated with severe dehydration and weight loss; appropriate fluid and electrolyte management is vital. For patients who do not require hospitalization, oral rehydration therapy with fluids containing electrolytes and glucose (juice, soda,

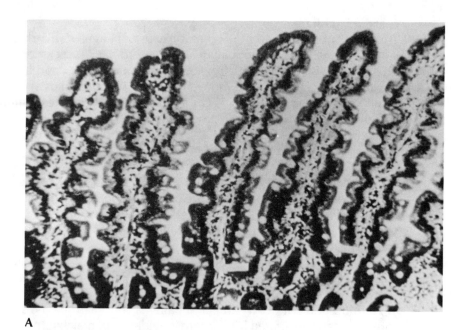

A

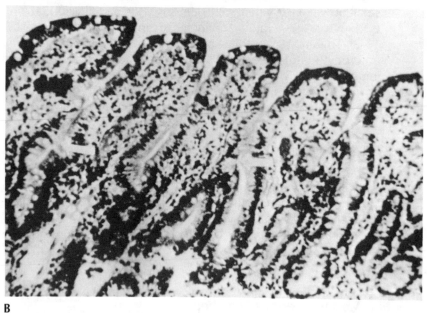

B

Figure 11-2. A. Normal small intestinal villi. B. Abnormal villi in HIV enteropathy. (Reprinted with permission of DP Kottler, HP Gaetz, M Lange, et al., Enteropathy associated with the acquired immunodeficiency syndrome. Ann Intern Med 101:421–428, 1984.)

soup) may be sufficient. In the absence of *Salmonella* infection or antibiotic-associated colitis, antidiarrheal agents, such as diphenoxylate hydrochloride (Lomotil), loperamide hydrochloride (Imodium), or deodorized tincture of opium (DTO), can be safely given and are often effective. In resistant cases in which no treatable pathogen is identified, therapy with a somatostatin analogue, octreotide (doses of 50–500 μg three times a day subcutaneously), has proven useful [19, 20]. Nutritional support in patients with chronic diarrhea is important since severe weight loss may exacerbate the degree of immunodeficiency. Enteral or parenteral nutrition may be required in severe cases.

Odynophagia

Odynophagia, or pain on swallowing, a manifestation of esophageal disease, is described in up to 90 percent of patients with AIDS. Infective esophagitis, either fungal or viral, is the usual cause. Esophageal candidiasis, which can occur in the absence of oral involvement, is characterized by white plaque-like lesions with associated erythema and ulceration [21]. Viral infections, such as CMV or HSV, usually manifest as discrete or giant ulcers of the esophagus; esophageal perforation or severe GI bleeding may ensue [22, 23]. In about 10 percent of cases, multiple pathogens can be identified. Definitive diagnosis requires endoscopy with biopsy and brushings for histology, as well as viral and fungal culture [24]. Unusual causes of odynophagia include tumors, such as lymphoma or KS, and MAC infection. When endoscopy is negative, computed tomography of the thorax may identify disease in the submucosa or mediastinum.

Treatment of odynophagia is initially empiric. A trial of ketoconazole, 200 to 400 mg orally daily, can be given, but if improvement is not seen within one week, endoscopy with biopsy and cultures should be performed. Esophageal candidiasis may become resistant to ketoconazole, but such cases generally respond well to fluconazole. Cytomegalovirus and HSV infections are managed with ganciclovir or foscarnet, and acyclovir, respectively. Isolated giant esophageal ulcers not caused by a known pathogen have been treated with submucosal injection of steroids with encouraging results.

Abdominal Pain

HIV-infected patients are susceptible to common causes of abdominal pain seen in the immunocompetent host, such as appendicitis and cholecystitis. These should be excluded by careful clinical evaluation and appropriate diagnostic tests. Opportunistic diseases may also cause abdominal pain. Cytomegalovirus and MAC enterocolitis may result in deep ulcers, fistulas, and bowel perforation. Nodal involvement by MAC and lymphoma can give rise to severe postprandial pain secondary to mesenteric compression. Pancreatitis may be related to drug therapy (pentamidine, sulfa drugs) or opportunistic diseases; CMV, toxoplasmosis, candidiasis, lymphoma, and KS have all been implicated. Typhlitis, a clinical syndrome described in patients receiving chemotherapy for hematologic malignancy, has also been associated with HIV infection [25]. It presents as fever and right lower quadrant pain and is characterized by cecal wall thickening on CT scan. Treatment consists of bowel rest and intravenous antibiotics.

Hepatic Disease

The clinical and histologic spectrum of hepatobiliary disease in HIV infection is extremely diverse and is outlined in Table 11-2 [26, 27].

Viral Hepatitis

Evidence of past or present hepatitis is seen in 90 percent of HIV-infected patients [28, 29]. Careful serologic and biochemical evaluation is necessary to determine its significance.

Hepatitis B
Serologic evidence of previous hepatitis B infection (anti-HBc) is seen in 90 percent of patients. Only 10 percent have detectable hepatitis B surface antigen (HBsAg) and markers of active viral replication (HBeAg, HBV DNA). The immunosuppression associated with HIV infection results in active viral replication of HBV without significant evidence of biochemical or histologic injury. Serum transaminases are frequently normal, and progression to either severe chronic active hepatitis or fulminant liver failure is unusual, although paradoxically it may occur in response to antiretroviral therapy.

Hepatitis C
Hepatitis C virus (HCV) is a common cause of hepatitis in injection drug users and appears to be directly hepatotoxic. In HIV-infected patients, HCV-induced hepatic injury may be accelerated, with a rapid progression from chronic active hepatitis to cirrhosis. Alpha-interferon has been used successfully in HIV-infected patients for the treatment of chronic active hepatitis secondary to HCV [30].

Table 11-2 Hepatobiliary disease in HIV infection

Hepatic parenchymal disease

Viral pathogens
    Hepatitis B
    Hepatitis C
    Hepatitis D (delta)
    Cytomegalovirus
    Herpes simplex virus

Mycobacterial pathogens
    Mycobacterium avium complex
    Tuberculosis

Fungal pathogens
    Cryptococcosis
    Candida species
    Histoplasmosis

Neoplastic
    Lymphoma
    Kaposi's sarcoma

Drug-related
    Sulfonamides
    Ketoconazole
    Isoniazid
    Rifampicin
    Zidovudine
    Didanosine
    Pentamidine

Biliary tract disease

Acalculous cholecystitis
Papillary stenosis
Sclerosing cholangitis
Vanishing bile duct syndrome

Opportunistic Infections

The liver is susceptible to the many opportunistic infections seen in AIDS. Patients may present with a variety of symptoms, including fever, abdominal pain, and hepatomegaly. If noninvasive diagnostic testing is unhelpful, liver biopsy for histology and culture may be necessary.

Mycobacteria

Tuberculosis and MAC are the most common bacterial liver infections in AIDS patients [31]. Hepatic involvement is often associated with widely disseminated disease. Liver function test abnormalities include a mixed picture of both hepatitis and cholestasis (elevated transaminases and alkaline phosphatase). Hepatic imaging is not useful, and definitive diagnosis can only be made by liver biopsy. Patients with a positive acid-fast stain on liver biopsy should be placed on antituberculous therapy pending culture results.

Cytomegalovirus
CMV hepatitis is associated with disseminated infection in advanced HIV disease. Treatment consists of ganciclovir or foscarnet.

Fungal Infections
Candidiasis, cryptococcosis, and histoplasmosis can all affect the liver. Each of these fungi is associated with granuloma formation. Definitive diagnosis requires liver biopsy.

Peliosis Hepatitis

Peliosis is a histologic diagnosis characterized by multiple small blood-filled cysts throughout the liver. Similar lesions are seen in the lymph nodes, spleen, and bones. A bacilliform organism has been isolated from the liver of patients with HIV infection [32]. These bacilli resemble *Bartonella bacilliformis* and may release an angiogenesis factor. Treatment with erythromycin has resulted in resolution of the histologic abnormality.

Drug-Induced Liver Injury

Many of the common therapeutic drugs used in HIV-infected patients are potentially hepatotoxic. If significantly abnormal liver function or clinical hepatitis develops, hepatotoxic agents should be discontinued and the patient's clinical course observed. Drugs frequently associated with hepatotoxicity include isoniazid, rifampin, sulfa agents, and ketoconazole.

Role of Liver Biopsy

Liver biopsy seldom influences therapy or survival in patients with AIDS. However, it should be considered in the following clinical situations: (1) fever, hepatomegaly, and/or abnormal liver function tests of undetermined cause; (2) suspected drug-induced hepatotoxicity where discontinuation of the agent may be harmful; and (3) chronic cholestasis with a negative ultrasound and endoscopic retrograde cholangiopancreatography (ERCP). Anecdotal cases suggest a higher morbidity and mortality associated with liver biopsy in patients with AIDS.

Biliary Tract Disease

Disorders of the intrahepatic and extrahepatic ducts and gallbladder have been reported in AIDS. Biliary tract disease is manifested by right upper quadrant pain with or without fever and/or jaundice.

Acute Cholecystitis

Acute acalculous cholecystitis has been reported in AIDS patients, sometimes with systemic toxicity [33]. Etiologic agents include CMV, *Candida* species, and *Cryptosporidium*. Diagnosis is by HIDA scan. Urgent cholecystectomy may be necessary to prevent rupture of the gallbladder and peritonitis.

Papillary Stenosis

Papillary stenosis is a syndrome characterized by recurrent episodes of right upper quadrant pain accompanied by transient liver function test abnormalities with or without common bile duct (CBD) dilatation on ultrasonography [34]. Diagnosis is confirmed by ERCP, which reveals an edematous and swollen ampulla; biopsy may reveal CMV or cryptosporidiosis. Sphincterotomy may relieve the pain and fever and provide adequate biliary drainage.

Sclerosing Cholangitis

Sclerosing cholangitis can involve either the CBD alone, CBD and ampulla, CBD and intrahepatic ducts, or intrahepatic ducts alone [35, 36]. Patients generally present with right upper quadrant pain and an elevated alkaline phosphatase. Diagnosis is made by ERCP, and any significant strictures can be bypassed with an endoprosthesis at the time of the procedure. Cytomegalovirus and cryptosporidiosis may be detected on biopsy. Intrahepatic disease appears to progress rapidly and is relatively inaccessible to interventional therapy. Recently, we have achieved both symptom relief and biochemical improvement of cholestasis with the synthetic bile salt ursodeoxycholic acid at 15 mg/kg/day in three divided doses (unpublished observation).

Vanishing Bile Duct Syndrome

Chronic progressive cholestasis with normal extrahepatic ducts has been described in HIV-infected patients. Liver biopsy reveals a paucity of intrahepatic ducts similar to that seen in primary biliary cirrhosis or liver allograft rejection. Treatment with ursodeoxycholic acid may be effective in slowing progression of this disease to end-stage biliary cirrhosis.

References

1. Dworkin B, et al. Gastrointestinal manifestations of the acquired immunodeficiency syndrome. *Am J Gastroenterol* 80:774, 1985.
2. Malenbranche R, et al. AIDS with severe gastrointestinal manifestations in Haiti. *Lancet* 2:873, 1983.
3. Smith PD, et al. Intestinal infections in patients with the acquired immunodeficiency syndrome. *Ann Intern Med* 108:328, 1988.
4. Glaser JB, et al. Recurrent *Salmonella typhimurium* bacteremia associated with the acquired immunodeficiency syndrome. *Ann Intern Med* 102:189, 1985.
5. Jacobs JL, et al. *Salmonella* infections in patients with AIDS. *Ann Intern Med* 102:186, 1985.
6. Rolston KVI, et al. Antimicrobial therapy for *Salmonella* infections in the acquired immunodeficiency syndrome. *Ann Intern Med* 108:309, 1988.
7. Jacobsen MA, et al. Serious cytomegalovirus infection in AIDS. *Ann Intern Med* 108:585, 1988.
8. Meiselman MS, et al. Cytomegalovirus colitis: Report of the clinical, endoscopic and pathological findings in 2 patients with the acquired immunodeficiency syndrome. *Gastroenterology* 88:171, 1984.
9. Soave R, et al. *Cryptosporidium* and *Isospora belli* infections. *J Infect Dis* 157:225, 1988.
10. Flanigan T, et al. *Cryptosporidium* infection and CD4 counts. *Ann Intern Med* 116:840–842, 1992.
11. Portnoy D, et al. Treatment of intestinal cryptosporidiosis with spiramycin. *Ann Intern Med* 101:202, 1984.
12. MeMeeking, et al. A controlled trial of bovine dialyzable leukocyte extract for cryptosporidiosis in patients with AIDS. *J Infect Dis* 161:108, 1990.
13. DeHovitz JA, et al. Clinical manifestations and therapy of *Isospora belli* infection in patients with AIDS. *N Engl J Med* 315:87, 1986.
14. Maayan S, et al. *Strongyloides stercoralis* hyperinfection in a patient with the acquired immunodeficiency syndrome. *Am J Med* 83:945, 1987.
15. Modigliani R, et al. Diarrhea and malabsorption in acquired immunodeficiency syndrome. *Gut* 26:179, 1985.
16. Ullrich R, et al. Small intestinal structure and function in patients infected with HIV: Evidence for HIV induced enteropathy. *Ann Intern Med* 111:15, 1989.
17. Weller IVD. The gay bowel. *Gut* 26:869, 1985.
18. Laughon BE, et al. Prevalence of enteric pathogens in homosexual men with and without AIDS. *Gastroenterology* 94:984, 1988.

19. Robinson EW, et al. SMS 201-995 a somatostatin analogue and diarrhea in AIDS. *Ann Intern Med* 111:15, 1989.
20. Cello JP, et al. Effect of octreotide on refractory AIDS-associated diarrhea. *Ann Intern Med* 115:705–710, 1991.
21. Tavitian A, et al. Oral candidiasis as a marker for esophageal candidiasis in AIDS. *Ann Intern Med* 104:54, 1986.
22. Balthazar EJ, et al. Cytomegalovirus esophagitis in AIDS; radiographic features in 16 patients. *Am J Radiol* 149:919, 1987.
23. Agha FP, et al. Herpetic esophagitis: A diagnostic challenge in immunocompromised patients. *Am J Gastroenterol* 81:246, 1986.
24. McBane RD, et al. Herpes esophagitis: Clinical syndrome, endoscopic appearance and diagnosis in 23 patients. *Gastrointest Endosc* 37:600, 1991.
25. Till M, et al. Typhilitis in patients with HIV infection. *Ann Intern Med* 116:998–1000, 1992.
26. Lebovics E, et al. The liver in AIDS: A clinical and histological study. *Hepatology* 5:293, 1985.
27. Schneiderman DJ, et al. Hepatic disease in patients with AIDS. *Hepatology* 7:925, 1987.
28. Rustgi VK, et al. Hepatitis B virus infection in AIDS. *Ann Intern Med* 101:795, 1984.
29. Ravenholt RT. Role of hepatitis B virus in AIDS. *Lancet* 2:885, 1983.
30. Boyer N, et al. Recombinant interferon-alpha for chronic hepatitis C in patients positive for antibody to human immunodeficiency virus. *J Infect Dis* 165:723–726, 1992.
31. Hawkins CC, et al. *Mycobacterium avium* complex infection in patients with AIDS. *Ann Intern Med* 105:184, 1986.
32. Perkocha LA, et al. Clinical and pathological features of bacillary peliosis hepatis in association with HIV infection. *N Engl J Med* 23:1581, 1990.
33. Blumberg RS, et al. Cytomegalovirus and cryptosporidium associated acalculous gangrenous cholecystitis. *Am J Med* 76:1118, 1984.
34. Schneiderman DJ, et al. Papillary stenosis and sclerosing cholangitis in AIDS. *Ann Intern Med* 106:546, 1987.
35. Margulis SJ, et al. Biliary tract obstruction in AIDS. *Ann Intern Med* 105:207, 1986.
36. Cello JP. Acquired immunodeficiency syndrome cholangiopathy; spectrum of disease. *Am J Med* 86:539, 1989.

12/Hematologic Manifestations

Paul E. Berard

The hematologic consequences of HIV infection are dominated by peripheral blood cytopenias. These have become more common with the advent of antiretroviral therapy and treatments for HIV-associated infections and malignancies [1]. Anemia occurs in approximately 60 to 70 percent, granulocytopenia in 50 percent, and thrombocytopenia in 40 percent of AIDS patients [2]. Current research efforts are focused on better understanding the pathophysiology and treatment of these hematologic complications.

In general, the incidence and severity of low cell counts increases with advancing HIV disease. An exception is thrombocytopenia, which may be the presenting manifestation of HIV infection, occurring in 3 to 12 percent of asymptomatic patients [3]. Whereas thrombocytopenia is most often the result of immune-mediated peripheral destruction, present data suggest that the anemia and neutropenia of HIV infection reflect an abnormally maturing, hypoproliferative bone marrow. Myelo-suppressive therapies or marrow-infiltrating opportunistic diseases may further contribute to the development of cytopenia.

Bone Marrow Findings in HIV Infection

Bone marrow cellularity in the presence of HIV infection is decreased in 5 to 20 percent of patients [3–5]. A dry tap or difficult aspiration is observed in up to 40 percent of cases; however, this does not correlate with the presence of increased marrow reticulin [4]. Increased plasma cells are frequently seen and, together with a polyclonal gammopathy, may reflect an immune response to unusual antigenic stimulation or dysregulation of B-lymphocyte activity [2]. Increased eosinophils may also be present, as well as a slight increase in reticulin, the latter often associated with granulomas or lymphoid aggregates [3, 5]. Megakary-ocytes are normal or increased in most cases [3, 5, 6]. Mild to moderate megaloblastoid erythrocytic changes are commonly present, reflecting abnormal erythroid maturation [6]. Dysplasia of the megakaryocytic and myeloid cell lines is also observed and appears to correlate with the presence of peripheral blood cytopenias, or concurrent infection or drug therapy [3, 6]. Granulomas due to acid-fast organisms or fungi, or infiltration by aggressive-histology B-cell lymphoma, are sometimes seen. Kaposi's sarcoma rarely involves the bone marrow [7].

Pathophysiology of Hematologic Complications

Multiple defects in hematopoiesis have been reported consistent with the described changes in bone marrow morphology. These include (1) decreased numbers of bone marrow progenitors, (2) HIV infection of bone marrow progenitors with resulting abnormal maturation/proliferation, (3) deficient production of hematopoietic growth factors by bone marrow accessory cells, and (4) HIV-induced factors that inhibit normal hematopoiesis.

Several investigators have reported decreased erythrocyte and granulocyte/monocyte colony formation in vitro using bone marrow progenitor cells from HIV-infected individuals [8]. However, other researchers using sera from subjects without HIV infection and growth factors from different sources have demonstrated no differences in colony formation [9, 10]. Interpretation of these results is clouded by variability in culture media and cell culture techniques.

Human immunodeficiency virus infection of hematopoietic progenitor cells both in vitro and in vivo has been described using techniques such as in situ hybridization and immunohistochemistry [11–13]. Interpretation of these results is difficult due to the potential contamination in vitro of myeloid colonies by differentiated HIV-infected monocytes [2]. A recent study using the sensitive polymerase chain reaction technique was unable to demonstrate HIV DNA within colonies derived from hematopoietic progenitor cells of HIV-infected individuals [10].

Within the bone marrow environment, T lymphocytes, monocytes/macrophages, and stromal cells produce growth factors that stimulate proliferation and differentiation of normal hematopoietic tissue. T cells and macrophages are infected in vivo with HIV, and this may result in a perturbation in their ability to produce these factors. Sera from individuals with certain hematologic disorders characterized by peripheral cytopenias, such as aplastic anemia, are able to support colony growth of normal bone marrow progenitor cells, even in the absence of exogenous stimulating factors. Sera from patients with advanced HIV disease with cytopenia do not promote colony formation, raising the possibility of deficient growth factor production [9]. This view is supported by the apparent ability of progenitor cells from HIV-infected patients to respond normally in vitro to exogenous growth factors [10].

Additionally, there is evidence to suggest that HIV may induce factors that inhibit normal hematopoietic activity. Stella and associates [8] demonstrated that depleting the bone marrow of T cells before culture resulted in increased colony growth. Molina observed inhibition of colony formation by sera from HIV-infected patients [10]. As this inhibitor activity was isolated to the antibody fraction, it was thought to be immune mediated. Leiderman and colleagues [14] described a unique glycoprotein of 84 kilodaltons isolated from bone marrow cultures of AIDS patients that specifically inhibited granulopoiesis. This glycoprotein did not react with HIV antibodies and was believed to represent an induced, rather than direct, product of HIV infection. In addition, the increased production of cytokines, such as tumor necrosis factor (TNF) and interleukin-1 (IL-1), by HIV-infected monocytes may be a potential source of inhibition of hematopoiesis [2].

Anemia

Anemia is a common manifestation of AIDS, occurring in 65 to 80 percent of patients [3, 15]. The anemia is consistent with a chronic disease state and is typically normochromic and normocytic. Microcytosis is uncommon and has been found to correlate poorly with bone marrow iron stores [16]. Macrocytosis is rarely seen in patients who have not received zidovudine (ZDV).

Anti–red blood cell antibodies cause a positive Coombs' test in approximately 20 percent of HIV-infected patients with hypergammaglobulinemia [17]. These antibodies appear to behave as polyagglutinins and may be induced by infections associated with HIV disease. McGinniss and associates [18] observed autoantibodies of anti-u and anti-i specificity in most of the AIDS patients in their study, but in none of their seronegative control subjects. Despite this high incidence of positive Coombs' tests, immunohemolysis in nonbacteremic patients is rare [19].

Burkes and associates [20] have reported that 20 percent of HIV-infected patients have low vitamin B_{12} levels. However, these patients all had normal folate levels and mean corpuscular volumes and neutrophil lobe counts, and bone marrow biopsies did not show megaloblastic changes. Furthermore, no patients had clinical manifestations of B_{12} deficiency, and parenterally administered B_{12} did not lead to hematologic improvement. Other studies have shown an abnormal Schilling test in up to 75 percent of AIDS patients, but clinically significant B_{12} deficiency appears to be rare [21].

When evaluating the HIV-infected patient with anemia, special consideration should be given to the possibility of gastrointestinal bleeding, hypersplenism, liver disease, and bone marrow infiltration. Drug-related hemolysis, such as that caused by dapsone in glucose 6-phosphate dehydrogenase (G6PD)–deficient patients, may also occur.

Perhaps of greatest significance is the progressive anemia that often accompanies ZDV therapy. Richman and associates [22] reported that 31 percent of ZDV-treated patients had reduction in hemoglobin level to less than 7.5 gm/dl compared to only 2.7 percent of those given placebo. These patients required red blood cell transfusions, and approximately 20 percent became transfusion dependent. Despite the current use of lower ZDV doses, anemia remains a significant clinical problem [23].

In the past, management of ZDV-induced anemia included discontinuation of the agent or chronic transfusion therapy. Presently, multiple therapeutic options are available, including (1) substitution of a nonmyelosuppressive drug such as didanosine (ddI), (2) addition of a nonmyelosuppressive drug to a reduced-dose ZDV regimen, and (3) treatment with recombinant erythropoietin (r-EPO) [24–26].

Many HIV-infected patients with anemia have low levels of erythropoietin [27]. In a randomized, double-blind controlled trial of recombinant erythropoietin, 63 patients treated with ZDV were randomized to either placebo or r-EPO [26]. Patients received r-EPO at a dose of 100 IU/kg intravenously three times a week, and a statistically significant decrease in the number of patients requiring transfusion was observed in the r-EPO–treated group. Retrospective analysis showed that an entry serum erythropoietin level of less than 500 IU/L was predictive of a response to r-EPO. Responding patients also typically had a macrocytosis.

Thus, the majority of patients who are intolerant of ZDV because of anemia and not candidates for other antiretroviral agents may be managed effectively with r-EPO [26, 28]. A starting dose of 50 IU/kg is given subcutaneously three times a week. If no reticulocyte response is seen after 2 weeks of therapy, the dose can be increased to 100 IU/kg and then 150 IU/kg after an additional 2 weeks if the patient still has no response.

Neutropenia

In addition to the evidence for abnormal granulopoiesis, antigranulocyte antibodies have been described in 30 to 67 percent of HIV-infected patients [29, 30]. The significance of this finding is unclear, but some investigators believe that it contributes to neutropenia in some patients [29]. Qualitative defects in neutrophil function have also been described in HIV disease, and these may predispose to bacterial infection [31]. Similar to the anemia of HIV infection, the major clinical significance of the HIV-induced neutropenia is that it often precludes therapy with ZDV and other drugs used for the treatment of opportunistic diseases.

Granulocyte macrophage colony stimulating factor (GM-CSF) is a cytokine produced by T cells that is known to stimulate the proliferation and function of myeloid cells. It has been produced in bacteria, yeast, and human cells by recombinant technology. Baldwin and associates [31] have shown that GM-CSF may reverse the neutrophil phagocytic and killing defects in patients with HIV infection.

The first clinical study of GM-CSF, in 1987, included 16 neutropenic AIDS patients and demonstrated a rapid increase in granulocytes and monocytes [32]. However, several in vitro studies have demonstrated stimulation of HIV replication in peripheral blood monocytes/macrophages [33, 34]. Other clinical trials have shown little or no effect on HIV expression by GM-CSF, although a recent trial conducted at the National Cancer Institute found a statistically significant increase in HIV p24 antigen when GM-CSF was used as a single agent [32, 35–37]. In vitro studies combining GM-CSF and ZDV have shown an increased inhibition of certain monocytotrophic HIV strains and human macrophages/monocytes. This has been ascribed to the increase in monocyte cellular thymidine kinase activity induced by GM-CSF, resulting in increased intracellular levels of the nucleoside triphosphate [34]. Presently, it is anticipated that the beneficial myeloproliferative effects of GM-CSF will more than offset any viral-enhancing effect [38]. Granulocyte colony stimulating factor (G-CSF), another cytokine, does not stimulate monocyte proliferation/differentiation and has not been shown to have a stimulatory effect on HIV replication in macrophages [33].

GM-CSF has had more extensive clinical testing than G-CSF to date. It has potential benefits in HIV-infected patients in whom neutropenia develops secondary to therapy with ZDV, ganciclovir, alpha-interferon, m-BACOD, and CHOP chemotherapy [39–44]. Phase I–II trials are addressing the role of GM-CSF in adriamycin-based regimens for Kaposi's sarcoma, as well as its optimal dose and timing of delivery. The major toxicities of GM-CSF have been pain or erythema at the injection site, fever, bone pain, and myalgias. When combined with alpha-interferon, it may potentiate the typical "flu-like" symptoms described with that agent [45].

G-CSF has also shown potential in ameliorating neutropenia resulting from ZDV therapy [46]. Within the population studied, all who required concurrent ganciclovir therapy were able to receive it without dose modification, and little toxicity was experienced. G-CSF may eventually prove more clinically useful than GM-CSF, given its low toxicity and lack of stimulatory effect on HIV activity.

Thrombocytopenia

Thrombocytopenia in heroin users was described at Boston City Hospital in 1978 [47]. At that time, it was ascribed to the type of heroin that was used, although a viral cause could not be excluded. In retrospect, this may have represented the first report of idiopathic thrombocytopenic purpura (ITP) in HIV-infected individuals. Thrombocytopenia is also sometimes the result of drug therapy with agents such as ZDV or trimethoprim-sulfamethoxazole. Transient thrombocytopenia has been described in primary HIV infection [48]. Thrombotic thrombocytopenic purpura has also been reported in HIV-infected patients [49].

The most common cause of HIV-related thrombocytopenia is immune-mediated peripheral destruction. The peripheral blood smear shows decreased numbers of platelets that are increased in size. As in classic ITP, the spleen is not enlarged, and the bone marrow biopsy reveals normal to increased numbers of megakaryocytes. Initially, it was thought that asymptomatic HIV-infected men with thrombocytopenia were more likely to advance to AIDS; this has not been borne out in other studies [50]. Hemorrhagic complications were first described as unusual, although more recently a high incidence of clinically significant bleeding with severe thrombocytopenia has been reported [51–53].

Much controversy exists regarding the pathogenesis of HIV-associated ITP. There is evidence to support both autoantibody-mediated and antigen-containing immune complex mechanisms [54]. Immune complexes containing HIV antibody have been demonstrated on the platelet surfaces of homosexual men and drug users [55]. An autoantibody that binds to a membrane glycoprotein of 25 kilodaltons (gp25) in seropositive thrombocytopenic homosexual men has also been identified [56]. This antibody was not detected in sera from hemophiliacs, drug users, or patients with transfusion-acquired HIV infection who had ITP. These discrepancies may be explained by different mechanisms of ITP in sexually acquired versus parenterally acquired HIV infection. Alternatively, an immune complex consisting of an autoantibody and a second anti-F(ab)$_2$ antibody might be involved [57].

The optimal management of HIV-associated ITP has not been clearly defined (Table 12-1). Zidovudine has an established role in managing ITP, although its mechanism is poorly understood [58, 59]. Most patients respond with a long-term remission. Prednisone produces an initial response in approximately 50 percent of patients, but its effect is

Table 12-1 Management of HIV-related ITP

Modality	Initial response (%)	Durable response (%)
Prednisone	40–60	10–20
Splenectomy	70–100	40–60
Intravenous immunoglobulin	70–90	< 10
Anti-Rh (D)	64	< 10
Zidovudine	30–90	Unknown

Source: Data compiled from [58–66].

often short lived [52, 60]. The risks of corticosteroid therapy in HIV-infected patients include further immunosuppression and progression of Kaposi's sarcoma [61]. Intravenous immunoglobulin is effective initially in 70 to 90 percent of patients, although the response is durable in fewer than 10 percent [62, 63]. Likewise, anti-Rh immunoglobulin therapy results in few long-term responses [64]. Splenectomy is generally effective, and in approximately 50 percent of patients the response is maintained [65, 66]. Low-dose splenic irradiation has been used successfully in some patients as an alternative to surgery [67]. Before splenectomy, all patients should have cultures performed for *Mycobacterium avium* complex (MAC), as the clinical course of patients with disseminated MAC following splenectomy is uniformly poor [68].

In general, ZDV should be considered the drug of choice for significant thrombocytopenia. If ZDV therapy fails, splenectomy should be performed. Intravenous immunoglobulin should be reserved for the management of acute hemorrhagic episodes or just prior to a surgical procedure.

References

1. Pluda JM, Mitsuya H, Yarchoan R. Hematologic effects of AIDS therapies. *Hematol Oncol Clin North Am* 5:229–248, 1991.
2. Scadden DT, Zon LI, Groopman JE. Pathophysiology and management of HIV-associated hematologic disorders. *Blood* 74:1455–1463, 1989.
3. Zon LI, Arkin C, Groopman JE. Haematologic manifestations of the human immune deficiency virus (HIV). *Br J Haemotol* 66:251–256, 1987.
4. Treacy M, Lai L, Costello D, Clark A. Peripheral blood and bone marrow abnormalities in patients with HIV related disease. *Br J Haemotol* 65:289–294, 1987.
5. Castella A, Croxson TS, Mildvan D, et al. The bone marrow in AIDS: A histologic, hematologic and microbiologic study. *Am J Clin Pathol* 84:425–431, 1985.

6. Schneider DR, Picker LJ. Myelodysplasia in the acquired immune deficiency syndrome. *Am J Clin Pathol* 84:144–152, 1984.
7. Little BJ, Spivak JL, Quin TC, et al. Case report: Kaposi's sarcoma with marrow involvement–occurrence in a patient with AIDS. *Am J Med Sci* 292:44–46, 1986.
8. Stella CC, Ganser A, Hoelzer D. Defective in vitro growth of the hemopoietic progenitor cells in the acquired immunodeficiency syndrome. *J Clin Invest* 80:286–293, 1987.
9. Donahue RE, Johnson MM, Zon LI, et al. Suppression of *in vitro* haematopoiesis following human immunodeficiency virus infection. *Nature* 326:200–203, 1987.
10. Molina J-M, Scadden DT, Sakaguchi M, et al. Lack of evidence for infection of or effect on growth of hematopoietic progenitor cells after *in vivo* or *in vitro* exposure to human immunodeficiency virus. *Blood* 76:2476–2482, 1990.
11. Busch M, Beckstead J, Gantz D, et al. Detection of human immunodeficiency virus infection of myeloid precursors in bone marrow samples from AIDS patients (abstract). *Blood* 68:122a, 1986.
12. Zucker-Franklin D, Cao Y. Megakaryocytes of human immunodeficiency virus–infected individuals express viral RNA. *Proc Natl Acad Sci USA* 86:5595, 1989.
13. Folks TM, Kessler SW, Orenstein JM, et al. Infection and replication of HIV-1 in purified progenitor cells of normal human bone marrow. *Science* 242:919–922, 1988.
14. Leiderman IZ, Greenberg ML, Adelsberg BR, et al. A glycoprotein inhibitor of *in vitro* granulopoiesis associated with AIDS. *Blood* 70:1267–1272, 1987.
15. Spivak JL, Bender BS, Quinn TC. Hematologic abnormalities in the acquired immune deficiency syndrome. *Am J Med* 77:224–228, 1984.
16. Osborne BM, Guarda LA, Butler JJ. Bone marrow biopsies in patients with AIDS. *Hum Pathol* 15:1048, 1984.
17. Aboulafia D, Mitsuyasu R. Hematologic abnormalities in AIDS. *Hematol Oncol Clin North Am* 5:195–214, 1992.
18. McGinniss MH, Macher AM, Rook AH, et al. Red cell autoantibodies in patients with acquired immune deficiency syndrome. *Transfusion* 26:405–409, 1986.
19. Perkocha LA, Rodgers GM. Hematologic aspects of human immunodeficiency virus infection: Laboratory and clinical considerations. *Am J Hematol* 29:94, 1988.
20. Burkes RL, Colten H, Krailo M, et al. Low serum cobalamin levels occur frequently in the acquired immunodeficiency syndrome and related disorders. *Eur J Haematol* 38:141, 1987.
21. Harriman GR, Smith PD, Horne MK, et al. Vitamin B12 malabsorption in patients with acquired immunodeficiency syndrome. *Arch Intern Med* 149:2039, 1989.
22. Richman DD, Fischl MA, Grieco MH, et al. The toxicity of azidothymidine (AZT) in the treatment of patients with AIDS and AIDS-related complex. *N Engl J Med* 317:192, 1987.

23. Fischl MA, Parker CD, Pettinelli C, et al. A randomized controlled trial of a reduced daily dose of zidovudine in patients with the acquired immunodeficiency syndrome. *N Engl J Med* 323:1009, 1990.
24. Cooley TP, Kunches LM, Saunders CA, et al. Once daily administration of 2'3'-dideoxyinosine (ddI) in patients with the acquired immunodeficiency syndrome or AIDS-related complex. *N Engl J Med* 322:1340, 1990.
25. Meng TC, et al. Combination therapy with zidovudine and dideoxycytidine in patients with advanced human immunodeficiency virus infection. *Ann Intern Med* 116:13–20, 1992.
26. Erythropoietin (EPO) Study Group, Rodnick SA. Human recombinant erythropoietin (r-HuEPO): A double blind, placebo controlled study in acquired immunodeficiency syndrome (AIDS) patients with anemia induced by disease and AZT. *Proc Am Soc Clin Oncol* 8:2, 1989.
27. Spivak JL, Barnes DC, Fuchs E, et al. Serum immunoreactive erythropoietin in HIV-infected patients. *JAMA* 261:3104, 1989.
28. Henry DH, et al. Recombinant human erythropoietin in the treatment of anemia associated with human immunodeficiency virus infection and zidovudine therapy. *Ann Intern Med* 117:739–748, 1992.
29. Murphy MF, Metcalfe P, Waters AH, et al. Incidence and mechanism of neutropenia and thrombocytopenia in patients with human immunodeficiency virus infection. *Br J Haematol* 66:337–340, 1987.
30. van der Lelie J, Lange JMA, Vos JJE, et al. Autoimmunity against blood cells in human immunodeficiency virus (HIV) infection. *Br J Haematol* 67:109–114, 1987.
31. Baldwin GC, Gasson JC, Quan SG, et al. Granulocyte-macrophage colony-stimulating factor enhances neutrophil function in acquired immunodeficiency syndrome patients. *Proc Natl Acad Sci USA* 85:2763–2766, 1988.
32. Groopman JE, Mitsuyasu RT, DeLeo MS, et al. Effect of recombinant human granulocyte-macrophage colony stimulating factor on myelopoiesis in the acquired immunodeficiency syndrome. *N Engl J Med* 317:593, 1987.
33. Koyangi Y, O'Brien WA, Zhao JQ, et al. Cytokines alter production of HIV-1 from primary mononuclear phagocytes. *Science* 241:1673, 1988.
34. Perno C-F, Yarchoan R, Cooney DA, et al. Replication of human immunodeficiency virus in monocytes: Granulocyte/macrophage colony stimulating factor (GM-CSF) potentiates viral production yet enhances the antiviral effect mediated by AZT and other dideoxynucleoside consumers of thymidine. *J Exp Med* 169:933, 1988.
35. Mitsuyasu R, Levine J, Miles SA, et al. Effect of long term subcutaneous (SC) administration of recombinant granulocyte-macrophage colony stimulating factor (GM-CSF) in patients with HIV-related leukopenia (abstract) *Blood* 72:357, 1988.
36. Krown SE, O'Boyle K, Gold JWM, et al. Recombinant human granulocyte-macrophage colony stimulating factor: A phase I trial in neutropenic AIDS patients. Fifth International Conference on AIDS, Montreal, June 1989.
37. Pluda JM, Yarchoan R, Smith PD, et al. Subcutaneous recombinant granulocyte-macrophage colony-stimulating factor used as a single agent and

in an alternating regimen with azidothymidine in leukopenic patients with severe human immunodeficiency virus infection. *Blood* 76:463–472, 1990.

38. Folks TM. Human immunodeficiency virus in bone marrow: Still more questions than answers. *Blood* 77:1625–1626, 1991.
39. Levine SD, Allan JD, Tesitore SH, et al. Granulocyte-macrophage colony stimulating factor ameliorates the neutropenia induced by azidothymidine in AIDS/ARC patients (abstract). *Proc Am Soc Clin Oncol* 8:1, 1989.
40. Hardy D, Spector S, Polsky B, et al. Safety and efficacy of combined ganciclovir (GCV) and granulocyte-macrophage colony stimulating factor (GM-CSF) vs ganciclovir alone for CMV retinitis in AIDS (ACTG 073): A preliminary report. Sixth International Conference on AIDS, San Francisco, June 1990.
41. Grossberg HS, Bonnem EM, Buhles WC. GM-CSF with ganciclovir for the treatment of CMV retinitis in AIDS (letter). *N Engl J Med* 320:1560, 1989.
42. Scadden D, Bering H, Levine J, et al. Combined AZT and interferon-alpha/GM-CSF for AIDS-associated Kaposi's sarcoma (KS) (abstract). *Blood* 74:127, 1989.
43. Walsh C, Werna J, Laubenstein L, et al. Phase I study of m-BACOD and GM-CSF in AIDS associated non-Hodgkin's lymphoma (NHL): Preliminary results (abstract). *Blood* 74:1260, 1989.
44. Kaplan LD, Kahn JO, Grossberg H, et al. Chemotherapy with or without rGM-CSF in patients with AIDS-associated non-Hodgkin's lymphoma (NHL). Fifth International Conference on AIDS. Montreal, June 1989.
45. Davey RT, Jr, Davey V, Zurlo J, et al. A phase I/II trial of zidovudine, interferon-alpha, and granulocyte-macrophage colony stimulating factor in treatment of HIV infection. Sixth International Conference on AIDS, San Francisco, June 1990.
46. Miles SA, Mitsuyasu R, Fink N, et al. Recombinant G-CSF and recombinant erythropoietin may abrogate the neutropenia and anemia of AIDS and may allow resumption of AZT. Fifth International Conference on AIDS, Montreal, June 1989.
47. Adams WH, Rufo RA, Talarico L, et al. Thrombocytopenia and intravenous heroin use. *Ann Intern Med* 84:2207–2211, 1978.
48. Goldman R, Lang W, Lyman D. Acute AIDS viral infection. *Am J Med* 81:1122, 1986.
49. Nair, JMG, Bellevue R, Bertrant M, et al. Thrombotic thrombocytopenic purpura in patients with the acquired immunodeficiency syndrome (AIDS)-related complex. *Ann Intern Med* 109:204–212, 1988.
50. Holzman RS, Walsh CM, Karputkin S. Risk for acquired immunodeficiency syndrome among thrombocytopenic and non-thrombocytopenic homosexual men seropositive for the human immunodeficiency virus. *Ann Intern Med* 106:383, 1987.
51. Goldsweig HG, Grossman R, Williams D. Thrombocytopenia in homosexual men. *Am J Hematol* 21:243–247, 1986.
52. Landmio G, Galli M, Nosari A, et al. HIV-related severe thrombocytopenia in intravenous drug users: Prevalence, response to therapy in a medium-term follow up and pathogenic evaluation. *AIDS* 4:24–34, 1990.

53. Brusamolino E, Malfitano A, Pagnullo O, et al. HIV-related thrombocy-topenic purpura: A study of 24 cases. *Haematologica* 74:51–56, 1989.
54. Karpatkin S. Immunologic thrombocytopenic purpura in HIV-seroposi-tive homosexuals, narcotic addicts and hemophiliacs. *Semin Hematol* 25:219–224, 1988.
55. Karpatkin S, Nardi M, Lannette ET, et al. Anti human immunodeficiency virus type I antibody complexes on platelets of seropositive thrombocy-topenic homosexuals and narcotic addicts. *Proc Natl Acad Sci USA* 85:9763–9767, 1988.
56. Stricker RB, Abrams DI, Corash L, et al. Target platelet antigen in homo-sexual men with immune thrombocytopenia. *N Engl J Med* 313:1375–1380, 1985.
57. Stricker RB. Hemostatic abnormalities in HIV disease. *Hematol Oncol Clin North Am* 5:249–266, 1991.
58. Hynes KB, Green JB, Karpatkin S. The effect of azidothymidine in HIV-related thrombocytopenia. *N Engl J Med* 318:516–517, 1988.
59. Oksenhendler E, Bierling P, Brossard Y, et al. Zidovudine for thrombo-cytopenic purpura related to human immunodeficiency virus (HIV) infec-tion. *Ann Intern Med* 110:365–368, 1989.
60. Rosenfelt FP, Rosenbloom BE, Weinstein IH. Immune thrombocytopenia in homosexual men. *Ann Intern Med* 104:583, 1989.
61. Gill PS, Loureiro C, Bernstein-Singer M, Rarick MU, et al. Clinical effect of glucocorticoids on Kaposi sarcoma related to the acquired immunodefi-ciency syndrome (AIDS). *Ann Intern Med* 110:937–940, 1989.
62. Bussel JB, Haimi JS. Isolated thrombocytopenia in patients infected with HIV: Treatment with intravenous gammaglobulin. *Am J Hematol* 28:79–84, 1988.
63. Pollack AT, Janinis J, Green D. Successful intravenous immune globulin therapy for human immunodeficiency virus–associated thrombocytope-nia. *Arch Intern Med* 148:695–697, 1988.
64. Oksenhendler E, Bierling P, Brossard Y, et al. Anti-Rh immunoglobulin therapy for human immunodeficiency virus–related immune thrombo-cytopenic purpura. *Blood* 71:1499–1502, 1988.
65. Landorio G, Nosari AM, Barbavno L, et al. Splenectomy for severe HIV-related thrombocytopenia in heroin abusers. *Br J Haematol* 69:290, 1988.
66. Ravikumar TS, Allen JD, Bothe A, Jr, et al. Splenectomy: The treatment of choice for human immunodeficiency virus–related immune thrombocy-topenia. *Arch Surg* 124:625–628, 1989.
67. Needleman SW, et al. Low-dose splenic irradiation in the treatment of autoimmune thrombocytopenia in HIV-infected patients. *Ann Intern Med* 116:310–311, 1992.
68. Mathew A, Raviglione MC, Niranjan U, et al. Splenectomy in patients with AIDS. *Am J Hematol* 32:184–189, 1989.

13/Renal Manifestations

Steven C. Borkan

Epidemiology

HIV-associated nephropathy (HIVAN) is characterized by the onset of nephrotic syndrome and rapidly progressive renal dysfunction associated with focal, segmental glomerulosclerosis (FSGS) [1–5]. Distinguishing HIVAN from other treatable causes of renal dysfunction is important [1, 4, 6, 7].

The disease now recognized as HIVAN was first described in patients with AIDS in 1984 [8, 9]. The absence of confirmatory studies initially supported speculation that HIVAN was either unrelated to HIV infection or resulted from host-specific factors such as injection drug use (IDU) or race [2]. Further confusing the issue were early reports that homosexual men with AIDS had no discernible renal pathology, and the existence of common epidemiologic and pathologic features delayed the distinction of HIVAN from heroin-associated nephropathy (HAN) [10]. The hypothesis that HIV is associated with a distinct nephropathy is now widely accepted [1, 4, 7].

The prevalence of HIVAN in HIV-infected patients is estimated to be 10 percent; men comprise 80 to 90 percent of cases [1, 2, 7, 11]. Approximately 50 percent of patients with HIVAN have a history of drug use, and the remainder are either homosexual or originate from regions where HIV infection is endemic [1, 2, 7, 11, 12]. In approximately 10 percent of patients, no specific risk factor for HIV can be identified [11]. African-American men appear to be at increased risk for development of HIVAN, but they also have a two- to fivefold increased risk for renal dysfunction associated with other systemic diseases, as well as for idiopathic focal, segmental glomerulosclerosis [2, 13, 14].

HIVAN is recognized throughout the spectrum of HIV disease, although, in one study, 57 percent of patients with HIVAN fulfilled Centers for Disease Control criteria for AIDS [7, 15]. HIVAN can be the first manifestation of HIV infection or even precede detection of HIV antibodies [1, 16]. HIVAN has also been reported as the presenting feature of HIV infection in infants born to seropositive mothers [17].

Clinical Manifestations

The onset of HIVAN is heralded by the appearance of heavy protein-uria, often with renal insufficiency. Azotemia, proteinuria, or both were the presenting features in over 90 percent of HIV-infected patients reported by inpatient renal consultation services [15, 18] (Table 13-1). Gross or microscopic hematuria and electrolyte abnormalities com-prised the other abnormalities. Most patients (89%) excreted 1 gm or more protein per day [15].

Some of the clinical and epidemiologic features of HIVAN overlap with HAN, leading to diagnostic confusion [19] (Table 13-2). Fortu-nately, several clinical features permit the distinction of HIVAN from HAN (Table 13-3). Features consistent with the diagnosis of HIVAN include the absence of hypertension, a characteristic urine sediment, normal or large kidneys, hypoalbuminemia disproportionate to the degree of proteinuria, and rapidly progressive renal insufficiency. The absence of hypertension in patients with HIVAN is striking and unex-plained, given the high prevalence of essential hypertension in black men and the presence of advanced renal failure with reduced salt and water clearance. Examination of the urine sediment in HIVAN often reveals evidence of severe proteinuria with oval fat bodies and frank lip-iduria. Large numbers of broad (giant) waxy casts (Fig. 13-1A) have also been observed in patients whose renal biopsies showed HIVAN (E Alex-ander, Boston City Hospital, personal communication).

Renal ultrasound in patients with HIVAN typically shows a normal or enlarged renal silhouette with increased echogenicity, even with advanced renal failure. In one series of patients with HIVAN, renal size averaged 12.3 cm [20]. Renal enlargement may be the result of (1) insuf-ficient time for global sclerosis and fibrosis given the rapid progression of renal disease; (2) marked dilatation of the tubules with numerous microcysts, in contrast to the tubular collapse frequently seen in other forms of chronic renal injury; and (3) interstitial edema [2, 4, 21]. The

Table 13-1 Clinical presentation of HIVAN

Presentation	% of patients
Azotemia	63
Proteinuria	19
Azotemia and protein	9
Electrolyte imbalances	6
Gross hematuria	3

Source: Adapted from JJ Bourgoignie, R Meneses, C Ortiz, et al., The clinical spectrum of renal disease associated with the acquired immunodeficiency syndrome. *Am J Kidney Dis* 12:131–137, 1988.

Table 13-2 Similar features of HAN and HIVAN

Age at presentation, 20–40 yr
Gender, > 90% men
IDU, 100% (HAN) vs. 40–50% (HIVAN)
Race at risk, 90% black
Renal insufficiency
Proteinuria ($\geq$ 3 gm) in most patients

Source: Adapted from [2] and [19].

dramatic decline observed in serum albumin concentration (to $\leq$1 gm/dl) with moderate albuminuria (<10 gm/day) may be caused by malnutrition or a defect in hepatic albumin synthesis, or both. HIVAN is a rapidly progressive form of renal failure; in one series of 55 patients, progression to end-stage disease occurred in an average of 10.9 weeks from the onset of mild azotemia [21].

Pathology

HIVAN is predominantly a glomerular disease with focal, segmental glomerulosclerosis. *FSGS* is a term that describes a pattern of renal response to a variety of insults and is not specific for HIVAN [2]. Autopsy data demonstrate that 90 percent of patients with the clinical diagnosis of HIVAN have focal and segmental glomerulosclerosis [4, 7]. Of 160 renal biopsies in patients with HIV infection reviewed by Rao

Table 13-3 Features that distinguish HAN from HIVAN

Feature	HAN	HIVAN
Clinical		
Hypertension	Usual	< 7%
Broad waxy casts	No	Yes
Renal size (late)	Small	Large (12.3 cm)
Severe hypoalbuminemia*	Unusual	Yes
Rate progression to ESRD	2–4 yr	4–16 wk
Histologic		
Light microscopy	Normal tubules	Microcystic tubules
Electron microscopy	No inclusions	No inclusions
Tissue HIV	No	Yes
Prognosis	Good	Poor

ESRD = end-stage renal disease.
*Disproportionate to the degree of proteinuria.
Source: Adapted from [2], [19], and [21].

and Friedman [2], 90 percent showed either FSGS or mesangial hyperplasia, a probable precursor lesion to FSGS.

Renal biopsy can confirm the clinical diagnosis of HIVAN. The light microscopic features include FSGS (Fig.13-1B, 1C) or mesangial hyperplasia with (1) severe epithelial cell injury; (2) interstitial infiltration by lymphocytes or monocytes; (3) dilated, degenerating proximal tubules filled with eosinophilic material, possibly representing cast formation in situ (Fig. 13-1D); (4) marked tubular microcyst accumulation (Fig. 13-1D); and (5) mesangial hyperplasia [2, 18, 22]. The presence of numerous tubuloreticular inclusions (TRI) within endothelial cells (Fig. 13-1E) is another important finding in HIVAN [16, 23]. TRI do not represent particles of HIV, since other diseases such as lupus nephritis are associated with similar findings, and exposure of cultured cells to exogenous interferon may result in the appearance of identical inclusions [24]. Rather, TRI may be a component of interferon or reflect a cellular response to interferon. Although renal tissue may stain for immunoglobulin M (IgM), C_{1q}, C_3, and kappa or lambda light chains in areas of focal sclerosis, immunologic mechanisms are probably not central to the genesis of HIVAN [22]. Both immunoglobulins and complement can be trapped nonspecifically by sclerosing glomeruli. In addition, similar glomerular deposits of immunoglobulins and complement occur in the majority of HIV-infected patients without nephropathy, and serum complement levels are normal in patients with HIVAN [25].

Pathogenesis

Human immunodeficiency virus appears to be trophic for specific cell types, including lymphocytes (T cells) and epithelial cells of the colon, central nervous system, and kidney. The basis of this tropism is complex and is not simply related to the presence of a surface CD4 receptor on susceptible cells [26, 27]. Regardless of the mechanism of viral entry, proliferation of HIV is generally associated with cytotoxicity. Within the kidney, tubular epithelial and glomerular epithelial cells undergo the

-->

Figure 13-1. Renal histopathology in HIVAN. A. Giant waxy cast with the characteristic rectangular shape, "squared-off" ends, and twists (rectangular indentations) along the longitudinal axis. Note the broad width of the cast compared to the diameter of the degenerating cell (polarized light at 400× magnification; kindly donated by Dr. Edward A. Alexander, Boston City Hospital). B. Renal biopsy specimen demonstrating regions of focal, segmental glomerulosclerosis (FSGS) in six glomeruli with partial collapse and expansion of Bowman's space. Markedly dilated tubules are noted, many containing eosinophilic material. The interstitium is moderately expanded by edema and cellular infiltrates (200× magnification).

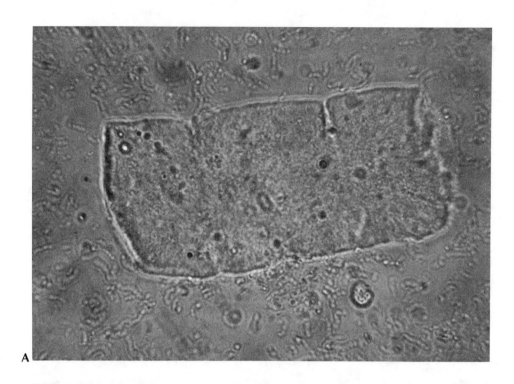

A

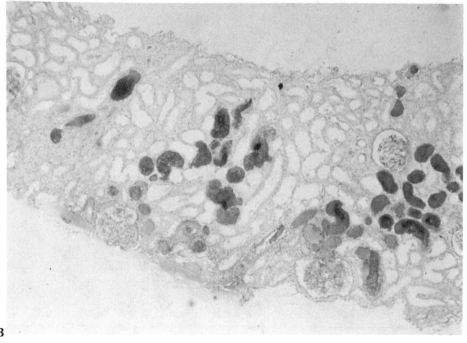

B

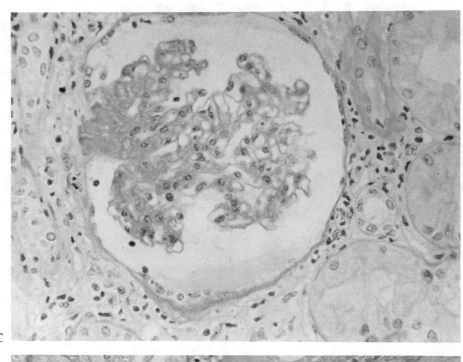

C

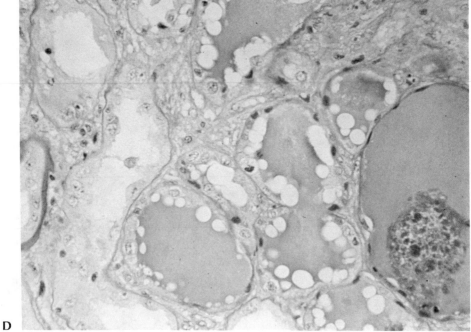

D

Figure 13-1 (continued)

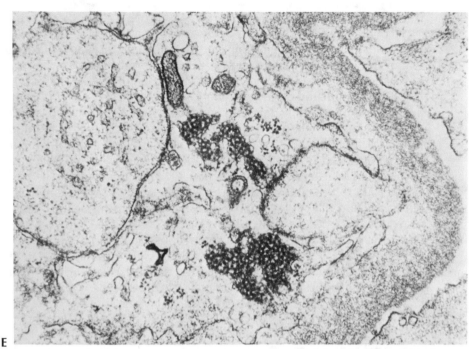

E

Figure 13-1 (continued). *Renal histopathology in HIVAN. C. Renal biopsy specimen showing segmental glomerulosclerosis, partial collapse of the glomerular tuft, and expansion of Bowman's space (400× magnification). D. Renal biopsy specimen illustrating microcystic dilatation of proximal tubules with severe degeneration of tubular epithelial cells. Tubular lumina are filled with eosinophilic staining material. Moderate interstitial infiltration with mononuclear cells is apparent (400× magnification). E. Electron micrograph of an endothelial cell with the characteristic intracellular accumulation of electron-dense tubuloreticular structures (TRI). (The micrographs of the renal biopsy tissue were donated by Dr. Helmut Renke.)*

most severe injury. Damage to renal epithelial cells probably accounts for leakage of filtered protein (nephrotic syndrome) and renal failure.

Although a causal link between human immunodeficiency virus and HIVAN has yet to be established, several lines of indirect evidence support a strong association. Viral DNA and protein markers specific for HIV have been localized within tubular and glomerular epithelial cells in renal biopsies from HIV-infected patients with nephrotic syndrome [28, 29]. A study using the transgenic murine model of HIV infection suggests a critical role of HIV in the pathogenesis of HIVAN; severe proteinuria, renal failure, and specific expression of HIV markers within the kidney were associated with FSGS in the offspring of parents in whom an HIV provirus had been introduced [30].

One of the most striking features of HIVAN is the prolonged period of dormancy between the detection of antiretroviral antibodies and the onset of renal disease. Since proliferation of HIV appears to be the major determinant of cytotoxicity, factors that precipitate viral replication within the kidney could explain the sudden onset of disease. Several mechanisms for rapid HIV proliferation have been suggested. HIV proliferation is regulated by at least two genes, *nef* and *vif,* with opposing actions. Minor diversification (mutation) in either of these could lead to rapid viral reproduction and death of the host cell. Concomitant infection with hepatitis, syphilis, or cytomegalovirus (CMV), all common in the HIV-infected population, could induce HIV replication. Recent in vitro studies have shown that susceptibility to HIV infection can be conferred to fibroblasts by a CMV-induced F_c receptor [31]. Cytomegalovirus infection may also promote viral proliferation through a mechanism that is dependent on tumor necrosis factor (TNF) [32]. Lastly, concomitant viral infection might remove inhibition to HIV replication by depleting CD4 lymphocytes, further depressing the immune system. The susceptibility of blacks, men, and IDUs suggests that both genetic and environmental factors may modulate the development of HIV-associated renal disease.

Prognosis and Management

HIVAN rapidly evolves from mild renal insufficiency to end-stage renal disease (ESRD) and is associated with shortened survival [6, 11, 13, 21, 33]. AIDS patients with HIVAN have increased mortality compared to AIDS patients without nephropathy (50% survival at 10 vs. 15 months) [33]. In a series of patients with HIVAN who were receiving maintenance hemodialysis, death occurred in 75 percent within 3 months, and 100 percent died within 9 months of the onset of ESRD [6]. Two subsequent reports have confirmed the poor prognosis for HIVAN patients on maintenance hemodialysis [13, 21]. Unrelenting cachexia, progressive neurologic deterioration, and opportunistic infections were the most common causes of death. In a study of patients with HIVAN who were undergoing dialysis, asymptomatic HIV-infected patients lived longer than those with symptomatic disease, and patients with AIDS had the shortest survival [13].

Treatment of early HIVAN to reverse or retard progression of renal insufficiency and proteinuria is based on anecdotal information. Oral prednisone decreased proteinuria in a patient with mesangial hyperplasia and intense, diffuse IgM deposition [34]. In a second case report, zidovudine (ZDV) restored renal function but did not decrease proteinuria in a patient with a clinical and histologic diagnosis of HIVAN [35].

Table 13-4 *Advantages of peritoneal dialysis for ESRD in HIVAN*

Reduced T-cell activation and cytokine release (mediators of HIV proliferation) attributed to hemodialysis membranes

Enhanced humoral immune function

Improved nitrogen balance from glucose absorption

Permits larger doses of antiretroviral agents in those patients with membrane-associated leukopenia

Higher average hematocrit

Lower risk of transmitting HIV infection

Source: Adapted from P Schoenfeld, NJ Feduska, Acquired immunodeficiency syndrome and renal disease: Report of the National Kidney Foundation–National Institutes of Health Task Force on AIDS and Kidney Disease. *Am J Kidney Dis* 16:14–25, 1990.

Whether antiretroviral drug therapy can avert ESRD in patients with early HIVAN or prolong survival once ESRD ensues remains to be determined.

The role of renal transplantation in patients with HIV infection is controversial. HIV infection shortens life expectancy, and the requirement for chronic immunosuppressive therapy to prevent allograft rejection may have detrimental effects on HIV proliferation. A National Institutes of Health task force concluded that HIV infection should not be a contraindication to transplantation given the paucity of data regarding the outcome of asymptomatic HIV carriers with renal allografts [11]. Rarely, seronegative organ and tissue donors have transmitted HIV infection [36]. In patients who have undergone renal transplantation for non–HIV-related renal disease and have identifiable risk factors for HIV infection, the diagnosis of AIDS should be considered when atypical opportunistic infections occur [37].

Patients with HIVAN and ESRD can be managed by either hemodialysis or peritoneal dialysis. Theoretically, peritoneal dialysis has several advantages compared to hemodialysis in patients who are equally suited for either modality (Table 13-4), but no controlled trials comparing the two types of dialysis have been reported [11].

Incidental HIV Infection in the ESRD Patient

Seronegative patients with ESRD are susceptible to HIV infection. Although unrelated to dialysis per se, the occurrence of AIDS from drug use or sexual contact in patients receiving chronic dialysis is associated with rapid demise from opportunistic infection [13]. Routine testing for

HIV is not recommended in the ESRD population when no risk factors are identified [11].

Other Renal and Electrolyte Abnormalities in the HIV-Infected Patient

The HIV-infected population is at increased risk for renal and electrolyte abnormalities apart from HIVAN. Conditions such as diarrhea, volume depletion, malnutrition, loss of muscle mass (leading to diminished generation of creatinine and overestimation of renal function), and opportunistic infections treated with potentially nephrotoxic agents all predispose to a spectrum of renal and electrolyte disorders. Non–HIV-related reversible causes of renal insufficiency associated with HIV infection include kidney infection, exposure to nephrotoxic antibiotics or radiologic contrast agents, endotoxemia, and hypoperfusion (Table 13-5). Although rare, progressive renal insufficiency may result from parenchymal infiltration with Kaposi's sarcoma or lymphoma.

Of the electrolyte abnormalities observed in HIV-infected patients, two—hyponatremia and hyperkalemia—have the most significance. Hyponatremia has been reported in 40 to 50 percent of hospital admissions in patients with symptomatic HIV infection or AIDS, and severe hyponatremia may be associated with decreased survival [4, 38]. Excess total body water was attributed either to hypovolemia with physiologic stimulation of antidiuretic hormone (ADH), administration of hypotonic fluids, or the syndrome of inappropriate ADH secretion (SIADH). SIADH in HIV-infected patients is usually associated with central nervous system or pulmonary disease. Hyperkalemia and mild metabolic acidosis may be the presenting features of adrenal insufficiency. In addition, hyporeninemic hypoaldosteronism with hyperkalemia has been reported in patients with AIDS [39]. Hypoadrenalism with hyperkalemia has been associated with ketoconazole therapy [40].

Drug Therapy in the HIV-Infected Patient with Renal Insufficiency

Dosage adjustment of agents that are nephrotoxic, undergo significant renal metabolism, or depend on glomerular filtration for their elimination is frequently necessary in the HIV-infected patient with renal insufficiency [41]. Potentially nephrotic agents commonly used in the management of HIV-infected patients include acyclovir, amikacin, amphotericin B, foscarnet, pentamidine, sulfadiazine, and trimethoprim-sulfamethoxazole (TMP-SMZ). When available, drug levels should

Table 13-5 Etiologies of acute renal failure in HIV-infected patients

Prerenal azotemia
  Volume depletion (diarrhea, bleeding, decreased intake)
  Early obstructive uropathy

Acute tubular necrosis
  Ischemia/hypoperfusion
  Sepsis/endotoxemia
  Nephrotoxic antibiotics
  Radiocontrast exposure

Infiltrative lesions
  Kaposi's sarcoma
  Renal cell carcinoma
  Lymphoma
  Amyloidosis

Allergic interstitial nephritis
  Nephrotoxic antibiotics
  Nonsteroidal agents

Systemic infections
  Mycobacterium species
  Candida species
  Cryptococcus
  Aspergillosis
  Cytomegalovirus
  Bacterial endocarditis
  Renal microabscess formation

Vasculitis
  Hemolytic-uremic syndrome
  Thrombotic thrombocytopenic purpura
  Renal cortical infarction

Miscellaneous
  Heroin (HAN)
  "Nephrosarca" (renal edema with severe hypoalbuminemia)
  Primary glomerulonephropathies
  Chemical interference with the creatinine assay
    Trimethoprim-sulfamethoxazole
    Cephalosporins
    Cimetidine

Source: Adapted from [1], [2], and [4].

be used to monitor treatment. TMP-SMZ and pentamidine cause acute renal insufficiency in 15 and 60 percent of cases, respectively [42]. Drug therapy can also produce relatively unusual renal complications. In one case report, sulfadiazine treatment for toxoplasmosis resulted in acute obstructive uropathy from renal stone formation [43]. Table 13-6 shows dose adjustments for commonly used agents at various levels of renal dysfunction.

Table 13-6 HIV drug dosage adjustments for renal insufficiency

Drug	Glomerular filtration rate (GFR)				HD	PD
	> 50 ml/min	25–50 ml/min	10–25 ml/min	< 10 ml/min		
Sulfadiazine	1.0–1.5 gm q6h	0.5–0.75 gm q6h or 1–1.5 gm q8–12h	0.5–0.75 gm q12h or 1–1.5 gm q24h	Avoid or use 1–1.5 gm q48–72 hr[a]	No Δ	No Δ
TMP-SMZ[b]						
TMP	5 mg/kg q6h	2.5 mg/kg q6h or 5 mg/kg q12h	1.7 mg/kg q6h or 5 mg/kg q18h	1.25 mg/kg q6h or 5 mg/kg q24h	No Δ	No Δ
SMZ	25 mg/kg q6h	12.5 mg/kg q6h or 25 mg/kg q12h	8 mg/kg q6h or 25 mg/kg q18h	6.25 mg/kg q6h or 25 mg/kg q24h	Add 6.25 mg/kg post-HD	No Δ
Acyclovir[c]	5–10 mg/kg q8h	5–10 mg/kg q12h	5–10 mg/kg q24h	2.5–5 mg/kg q24h	5–10 mg/kg post-HD q48h or 2.5–5 mg/kg q24h	2.5–5 mg/kg q24h
Ganciclovir	2.5 mg/kg q8h or 5 mg/kg q12h	3 mg/kg q12h	3 mg/kg q24h	1.5 mg/kg q24h	Add 1.25–2.5 mg/kg post-HD	U
Ethambutol	15–25 mg/kg/day	No Δ	15–25 mg/kg q24–36h or 7.5–15 mg/kg q24h	15–25 mg/kg q48h or 3–10 mg/kg q24h	No Δ	No Δ

Drug						
Fluconazole	50–400 mg/day	No Δ	25–200 mg/day	12.5–100 mg/day	FDD after each HD	50–100 mg/day
Foscarnet	60 mg/kg q8h (B) or 9–20 mg/kg (L) then 0.16–0.19 mg/kg/min (C)	Decrease dose for each ml/min loss of GFR (B): reduce by 3.5 mg/kg for each 0.1 ml/min/kg loss in GFR < 1.6 ml/min/kg (C): reduce dose by 0.02 mg/kg/min for each 20 μmole/liter[d] rise in serum Cr > 70 μmole/liter[e] Stop drug if GFR < 0.6 ml/min/kg or serum Cr > 250 μmole/liter[f]			Removed, check serum level[g]	U

HD = hemodialysis; PD = peritoneal dialysis; h = hours, d = days; no Δ = no change; (U) = unknown; (B) = bolus dose; (L) = loading dose; (C) = continuous infusion; Cr = creatinine; FDD = full daily dose.

[a]If essential.

[b]Can be given by oral or intravenous routes at equivalent dosage.

[c]Oral dose of acyclovir with renal insufficiency is 200 mg twice daily.

[d]20 μmole/liter creatinine = 0.2 mg%.

[e]70 μmole/liter creatinine = 0.8 mg%.

[f]250 μmole/liter creatinine = 2.8 mg%.

[g]Foscarnet clearance by HD estimated to be 80 ml/min.

Note: When available, drug levels should be followed, especially in patients with renal insufficiency. To convert serum creatinine in μmole/liter to mg/dL, divide by 88.40.

Source: Adapted from JS Berns, RM Cohen, RJ Stumacher, et al. Renal aspects of therapy for immunodeficiency virus and associated opportunistic infections. J Am Soc Nephrol 1:1061–1080, 1991.

Conclusion

Patients with HIV infection may develop a form of renal disease characterized by severe proteinuria, profound hypoalbuminemia, rapid deterioration of renal function, and focal, segmental glomerulosclerosis. HIVAN is found throughout the clinical spectrum of HIV disease. Renal disease may be the first manifestation of HIV infection, occasionally preceding the detection of HIV antibodies. HIVAN is most common in urban centers, with a prevalence of about 10 percent. Most patients with HIVAN in the United States are black, male, or use injection drugs. The prognosis for patients with HIVAN is poor and may depend on the clinical status of the HIV infection, the presence of end-stage renal disease, or both. Although FSGS represents a nonspecific pattern of renal injury, HIVAN is associated with characteristic histologic changes. Severe glomerular and tubular epithelial cell injury, markedly dilated tubules with microcysts, and moderate interstitial inflammation are observed on light microscopy. Electron microscopy reveals abundant tubuloreticular inclusions in glomerular and vascular endothelial cells. Clinical presentation and histopathologic findings can be used to distinguish HIVAN from HAN. Until the factors that precipitate HIVAN are identified and randomized drug trials performed, the therapy of HIVAN will remain empiric and be limited to suppression of viral proliferation.

References

1. Rao TKS. Clinical features of human immunodeficiency virus associated nephropathy. *Kidney Int* 40(suppl):13–18, 1991.
2. Rao TKS, Friedman EA. AIDS (HIV)-associated nephropathy; does it exist? *Am J Nephrol* 9:441–453, 1989.
3. Bourgoignie JJ, Pardo V. The nephropathology in human immunodeficiency virus (HIV-1) infection. *Kidney Int* 40:S19-S23, 1991.
4. Glassock RJ, Cohen AH, Danovitch G, Parsa P. Human immunodeficiency virus (HIV) infection and the kidney. *Ann Intern Med* 112: 35–49, 1990.
5. Langs C, Gallo GR, Schacht RG, et al. Rapid renal failure in AIDS-associated focal glomerulosclerosis. *Arch Int Med* 150:287–292, 1990.
6. Rao TKS, Friedman EA, Nicastri AD. The types of renal disease in the acquired immuno-deficiency syndrome. *N Engl J Med* 316:1062–1068, 1987.
7. Bourgoignie JJ, Jacques J. Renal complications of human immunodeficiency virus type I. *Kidney Int* 37:1571–1584, 1990.
8. Rao TKS, Fillippone EJ, et al. Associated focal and segmental glomerulosclerosis in AIDS. *N Engl J Med* 310:669–673, 1984.
9. Pardo V, Aldana M, Colton RM, et al. Glomerular lesions in AIDS. *Ann Intern Med* 101:429–434, 1984.

10. Mazbar S, Humphreys MH. AIDS-associated nephropathy is not seen at San Francisco General Hospital. *Kidney Int* 33:202, 1988.
11. Schoenfeld P, Feduska NJ. Acquired immunodeficiency syndrome and renal disease: Report of the National Kidney Foundation–National Institutes of Health Task Force on AIDS and Kidney Disease. *Am J Kidney Dis* 16:14–25, 1990.
12. Frasetto L, Schoenfeld PY, Humphreys MH. Increasing incidence of human immunodeficiency virus–associated nephropathy at San Francisco General Hospital. *Am J Kidney Dis* 18:655–659, 1991.
13. Ortiz C, Meneses R, Jaffe D, et al. Outcome of patients with immunodeficiency virus on maintenance hemodialysis. *Kidney Int* 34:248–253, 1988.
14. Cantor ES, Kimmel PL, Bosch JP. Effect of race on expression of acquired immunodeficiency syndrome–associated nephropathy. *Arch Intern Med* 151:125–128, 1991.
15. Bourgoignie JJ, Meneses R, Ortiz C, et al. The clinical spectrum of renal disease associated with the acquired immunodeficiency syndrome. *Am J Kidney Dis* 12:131–137, 1988.
16. Chander P, Agarwal A, Soni A, et al. Renal cytomembranous inclusions in idiopathic renal disease as predictive markers for the acquired immunodeficiency syndrome. *Hum Pathol* 19:1060–1064, 1988.
17. Pardo V, Meneses R, Ossa L, et al. AIDS-related glomerulopathy: Occurrence in specific risk groups. *Kidney Int* 31:1167–1173, 1987.
18. Gardenschwartz MH, Lerner CW, Seligson GR, et al. Renal disease in patients with AIDS: A clinicopathologic study. *Clin Nephrol* 21:197–204, 1984.
19. Cunningham EE, Brentjens JR, Zielenzy MA, et al. Heroin nephropathy: A clinical and epidemiologic study. *Am J Med* 68:47–53, 1980.
20. Schaffer RM, Schwartz GE, Becker JA, et al. Renal ultrasound in acquired immunodeficiency syndrome. *Radiology* 153:511–513, 1984.
21. Carbone L, D'Agati V, Cheng JT, Appel GB. Course and prognosis of human immunodeficiency virus–associated nephropathy. *Am J Med* 87:389–395, 1989.
22. D'Agati V, Suh JI, Carbone L, et al. Pathology of HIV-associated nephropathy: A detailed morphologic and comparative study. *Kidney Int* 35:1358–1370, 1989.
23. Alpers CE, Harawi S, Rennke HG. Focal glomerulosclerosis with tubuloreticular inclusions: Possible predictive value for acquired immunodeficiency syndrome (AIDS). *Am J Kidney Dis* 12:240–242, 1988.
24. Grimley PM, Kang Y-H, Frederick W, et al. Interferon-related leukocyte inclusions in acquired immunodeficiency syndrome: Localization in T-cells. *Am J Clin Pathol* 81:147–155, 1984.
25. Bourgoignie JJ, Meneses R, Pardo V. The nephropathy related to acquired immunodeficiency syndrome. *Adv Nephrol* 17:113–126, 1988.
26. Edelman AS, Zolla-Pazner S. AIDS: A syndrome of immune dysregulation, dysfunction and deficiency. *FASEB J* 3:22–30, 1989.
27. Camerini D, Seed B. A CD4 domain important for HIV-mediated syncytium formation lies outside the virus binding site. *Cell* 60:747–754, 1990.

28. Cohen AH, Sun NCJ, Shapshak P, et al. Demonstration of human immunodeficiency virus in renal epithelium in HIV-associated nephropathy. *Mod Pathol* 2:125–128, 1989.
29. Farkas-Szallasi T, Fereira-Centeno A, Abraham AA, et al. Viral DNA in biopsy material from HIV infected patients with nephrotic syndrome (abstract). *J Am Soc Nephrol* 2:306, 1991.
30. Dickie P, Felser J, Eckhaus M, et al. HIV-associated nephropathy in transgenic mice expressing HIV-1 genes. *Virology* 185:109–119, 1991.
31. McKeating JA, Griffiths PD, Weiss RA. HIV susceptibility conferred to human fibroblasts by cytomegalovirus-induced Fc receptor. *Nature* 343:659–661, 1990.
32. Peterson PK, Gekker G, Chao CC, et al. Human cytomegalovirus-stimulated peripheral blood mononuclear cells induce HIV-1 replication via a tumor necrosis factor-a–mediated mechanism. *J Clin Invest* 89:574–580, 1992.
33. Valeri A, Neusy AJ. Acute and chronic renal disease in hospitalized AIDS patients. *Clin Nephrol* 35:110–118, 1991.
34. Appel RG, Neill J. A steroid responsive nephrotic syndrome in a patient with human immunodeficiency virus (HIV) infection. *Ann Intern Med* 113:892–893, 1990.
35. Lam M, Park MC. HIV-associated nephropathy: Beneficial effect of zidovudine therapy. *N Engl J Med* 323:1775–1776, 1990.
36. Simonds RJ, Holmberg SD, Hurwitz RL, et al. Transmission of human immunodeficiency virus type I from a seronegative organ and tissue donor. *N Engl J Med* 326:726–732, 1992.
37. Carbone LG, Cohen DJ, Hardy MA, et al. Determination of acquired immunodeficiency syndrome (AIDS) after renal transplantation. *Am J Kidney Dis* 11:387–392, 1988.
38. Vitting KE, Gardenschwartz MH, Zabetakis PM, et al. Frequency of hyponatremia and nonosmolar vasopressin release in the acquired immunodeficiency syndrome. *JAMA* 263:973–978, 1990.
39. Kalin MF, Poretsky L, Seres DS, Zumoff B. Hyporeninemic hypoaldosteronism associated with acquired immune deficiency syndrome. *Am J Med* 82:1035–1038, 1987.
40. Best TR, Jenkins JK, Nicks SA, et al. Persistent adrenal insufficiency secondary to low-dose ketoconazole therapy. *Am J Med* 82:676–680, 1988.
41. Berns JS, Cohen RM, Stumacher RJ, et al. Renal aspects of therapy for immunodeficiency virus and associated opportunistic infections. *J Am Soc Nephrol* 1:1061–1080, 1991.
42. Sattler FR, Cowan R, Nielsen DM, Ruskin J. Trimethoprim-sulfamethoxazole compared with pentamidine for treatment of *Pneumocystis carinii* pneumonia in the acquired immunodeficiency syndrome. *Ann Intern Med* 109:280–287, 1988.
43. Carbone LG, Bendixen B, Appel GB. Sulfadiazine-associated obstructive uropathy in a patient with the acquired immunodeficiency syndrome. *Am J Kidney Dis* 2:72–75, 1988.

14/Rheumatologic Manifestations

Robert W. Simms

The spectrum of HIV disease includes a number of rheumatologic disorders, ranging from relatively benign arthralgia and fibromyalgia to potentially life-threatening conditions such as septic arthritis and systemic vasculitis [1–12] (Table 14-1). A variety of noninfectious articular syndromes, including Reiter's syndrome, psoriatic arthritis, and nonspecific oligoarthritis, have also been associated with HIV infection, as has the development of autoantibodies [13–17]. The precise relationship of these conditions to HIV itself remains to be determined.

Clinical Manifestations

Arthralgia

Arthralgia is the most common rheumatic manifestation of HIV infection, with a prevalence ranging from 10 to 35 percent of unselected patients [1, 18]. A particularly disabling, severe, painful articular syndrome has also been identified [1]. Transient arthralgias may occur at the time of HIV seroconversion or become part of a more chronic syndrome without the development of actual arthritis [1, 3]. Most often arthralgia is intermittent and involves large joints such as the shoulders and knees [1].

Fibromyalgia Syndrome

Two recent studies have identified fibromyalgia syndrome (FMS) in patients with HIV infection [2, 3]. FMS is a common cause of chronic musculoskeletal pain, manifested by widespread pain and characteristic sites of muscle tenderness ("trigger points"), as defined by recently published American College of Rheumatology (ACR) criteria [19]. The etiology of FMS is unknown, but it has been linked to depression and, possibly, chronic viral infection [20, 21]. The reported prevalence of FMS in the setting of HIV infection ranges between 10 and 20 percent [2, 3]. Patients with chronic musculoskeletal pain should be carefully

Table 14-1 *Rheumatologic manifestations of HIV infection*

Arthralgia
Fibromyalgia syndrome
Reiter's syndrome
Psoriatic arthritis
Infectious arthritis
Myositis
Sjögren's-like syndrome
Vasculitis
Autoantibody production

evaluated for FMS; symptoms are sometimes confused with other conditions, such as myositis or arthritis, for which the treatment is quite different. FMS in HIV-infected patients, similar to FMS occurring without HIV infection, is often associated with fatigue, sleep disturbance, and depressive symptoms [3].

Arthritis

Several arthritis syndromes have been described in the setting of HIV infection, including Reiter's syndrome, psoriatic arthritis, nonspecific oligoarthritis, and septic arthritis.

Reiter's Syndrome

Reiter's syndrome, one of the seronegative spondyloarthropathies, is classically described as a triad of arthritis, conjunctivitis, and urethritis [22]. Recently published ACR criteria do not require the presence of all three components of the triad simultaneously [22]. Reiter's syndrome in patients with and without HIV infection has been strongly associated with the presence of HLA-B27 [22, 31]. Both enteric and sexually transmitted infection are important risk factors for the development of this condition [22]. It has been estimated that approximately 20 percent of HLA-B27–positive individuals (5–8% of the adult white population) who experience bacterial gastroenteritis will subsequently develop Reiter's syndrome [23].

The relative risk of Reiter's syndrome in HIV-infected patients is 144- to 312-fold greater than that of the general population, and a particularly aggressive form of Reiter's syndrome has been described [1, 13]. The majority of patients report homosexuality as their risk behavior, and a specific infectious precipitant is often identified [13]. The arthritis is characteristically a large-joint, lower-extremity, asymmetric oligoarthritis, frequently associated with Achilles tendonitis and dactylitis or "sausage digits." Radiographic evidence of joint destruction is reported in approximately 50 percent of patients [13].

HIV-associated Reiter's syndrome may precede symptomatic HIV infection by up to 12 months, although most patients develop it along with manifestations of immunodeficiency. It is unclear whether Reiter's syndrome is actually caused by HIV, the result of an immune alteration secondary to HIV infection, or the consequence of known risk factors, such as enteric or sexually transmitted pathogens, which are highly prevalent in some populations with HIV infection. Two recent preliminary studies have found that among homosexual men the prevalence of Reiter's syndrome is the same with or without HIV infection [24, 25].

Psoriatic Arthritis

Arthritis occurs in approximately 7 percent of patients with psoriasis [26]. An asymmetric oligoarthritis is the most common finding on presentation; others include a symmetric polyarthritis similar to rheumatoid arthritis, classic distal interphalangeal joint (DIP) disease, arthritis mutilans, and spondyloarthropathy [26]. HLA-B27 is associated only with spondyloarthropathy [27].

A wide variety of psoriatic or psoriasiform skin lesions, including vulgaris, guttate, and erythrodermic varieties, have been described in HIV-infected patients [28]. Psoriatic arthritis has also been reported in a small number of individuals [1, 14, 29]. As in Reiter's syndrome, enthesopathy and dactylitis, especially of the foot, are common. Onychodystrophy is highly correlated with arthritis, particularly of the DIP joints [14]. Recently, HIV p24 antigen was detected in synoviocytes and lymphocytes in synovial biopsy material from patients with HIV-associated psoriatic arthritis [30]. Since psoriatic fibroblasts in vitro have an increased response to growth factor stimulation (including epidermal growth factor, transforming growth factor beta, and platelet-derived growth factor), similar proteins could be encoded by HIV genes, inducing direct stimulation of keratinocytes, fibroblasts, and vascular cells, and resulting in dermal, synovial, and blood vessel proliferation [31].

Nonspecific Oligoarthritis

A few patients with arthritis and HIV infection cannot be classified as having either Reiter's syndrome or psoriatic arthritis [1, 16]. Typically, they have lower-extremity oligoarthritis with pain out of proportion to the degree of inflammation [2, 16]. No association with HLA-B27 or other autoantibodies has been found. Synovial biopsy demonstrates mild chronic synovitis, and synovial fluid is characteristically noninflammatory [16].

Septic Arthritis

Joint infection due to a variety of pathogens, including *Staphylococcus aureus, Campylobacter* species, *Cryptococcus neoformans,* and *Sporothrix schenckii,* has been described in patients with HIV infection [10, 32, 33]. Although no studies have addressed the prevalence of joint infection in this population, it appears to be less frequent than might be expected given the profound state of immunodeficiency that may occur [18]. Septic arthritis caused by *Staph. aureus* in patients with HIV infection presents much the same way as in patients without HIV infection. Injection drug use is a common risk factor, and, although the presentation most often seen is large-joint, lower-extremity monoarthritis, unusual sites of articular infection, including the acromioclavicular joint, have been described [10]. Hemophiliacs with HIV infection may be particularly prone to joint sepsis due to the high frequency of hemarthrosis [34, 35]. The outcome of septic arthritis in HIV infection, as in the case of non-HIV–associated septic arthritis, is dependent on the duration of symptoms before diagnosis and institution of antimicrobial therapy.

Myositis

A variety of myopathies have been described in patients with HIV infection, including polymyositis, zidovudine (ZDV)-associated mitochondrial myopathy, and pyomyositis [8, 9, 36, 37]. Polymyositis in the setting of HIV infection presents with myalgias and proximal muscle weakness with elevated serum creatine phosphokinase (CPK) levels. In one report, polymyositis was the only clinical manifestation of HIV infection [8]. Immunohistochemical studies of muscle biopsies have shown that anti-HIV antibodies react with CD4 lymphocytes in the inflammatory infiltrate but not with muscle fibers, suggesting that HIV induces an autoimmune inflammatory response rather than a direct cytopathic effect [8]. Long-term ZDV therapy has been shown to produce a mitochondrial myopathy that may be clinically indistinguishable from that caused by HIV alone [37]. Muscle biopsy in this condition shows abundant "ragged red" fibers indicative of abnormal mitochondria with paracrystalline inclusions [37]. Interestingly, ZDV-associated myopathy, non-zidovudine–associated myopathy, and HIV-seronegative polymyositis all appear to be mediated by suppressor-cytotoxic (CD8) T cells and macrophages expressing class I major histocompatibility complex (MHC-1) antigens. This suggests the possibility of a common inflammatory mechanism [37].

Sjögren's-like Syndrome

Sjögren's syndrome is a chronic, inflammatory autoimmune disease characterized by diminished lacrimal and salivary secretions, resulting

Table 14-2 Comparison of Sjögren's syndrome and HIV diffuse lymphocytosis syndrome

Feature	Sjögren's syndrome	Diffuse lymphocytosis syndrome
Extraglandular manifestations	Infrequent	Prominent
Infiltrative lymphocytic phenotype	CD4	CD8
Autoantibodies	High frequency of RF, ANA, anti-SSA/Ro, anti-SSB/La	Low frequency of RF, absent ANA, absent anti-SSA/Ro, SSB/La
HLA association	B8, DR2, DR3, DR4	DR5

RF = rheumatoid factor; ANA = antinuclear antibody.
Source: Adapted from S Itescu, L Brancato, J Buxbaum, et al., A diffuse infiltrative CD8 lymphocytosis in human immunodeficiency virus (HIV) infection: A host immune response associated with HLA-DR5. *Ann Intern Med* 112:3–10, 1990.

in the keratoconjunctivitis sicca symptom complex [38]. Rarely, associated polymyositis, renal tubular acidosis, or vasculitis occurs. Ninety percent of patients with idiopathic Sjögren's syndrome are women. Salivary gland biopsy typically shows an inflammatory infiltrate consisting of predominantly CD4 cells, and there is a strong association with SSA/Ro and SSB/La autoantibodies [38, 39]. A secondary form of Sjögren's syndrome may be associated with rheumatoid arthritis, systemic lupus erythematosus, or scleroderma [38].

A Sjögren's-like syndrome, also known as diffuse lymphocytosis syndrome (DLS), has been reported in a number of patients with HIV infection [5, 6]. The majority have dry mouth but not dry eyes, and most have generalized lymphadenopathy [6]. Table 14-2 contrasts the features of this HIV syndrome with those of the primary or secondary forms of Sjögren's syndrome not associated with HIV infection. Of particular note is the prominence of extraglandular features in the HIV syndrome, typically lymphocytic interstitial pneumonitis (LIP), which was present in 10 of 17 patients in one series [6]. The severity of parotid involvement and LIP correlates directly with the peripheral circulating CD8 count [6]. It is of interest that the rate of progression to AIDS may be slowed in patients with DLS, although the reason for this is unclear [6].

Vasculitis

A small number of cases of necrotizing vasculitis have been associated with HIV infection (Table 14-3). Underlying infection has been a prominent feature, although four apparent cases of polyarteritis nodosa had negative hepatitis B serologies [12]. All of these patients had a periph-

Table 14-3 *Necrotizing vasculitis associated with HIV infection*

Vasculitis type	Number (n = 14)	Associated infection/malignancy
PAN	4	None
PA-CNS	2	1 disseminated varicella-zoster
LCV	1	CMV infection
AIL	6	3 non-Hodgkin's lymphoma 1 staphylococcal, cryptococcal infection
Overlap	1	Kaposi's sarcoma

PAN = polyarteritis nodosa; PA-CNS = primary angiitis of central nervous system; LCV = leukocytoclastic vasculitis; AIL = angiocentric lymphoproliferative disorder; CMV = cytomegalovirus.
Source: Adapted from J Marcef-Valeriano, L Ravichandran, LD Kerr, HIV-associated systemic necrotizing vasculitis. *J Rheumatol* 17:1091–1093, 1990.

eral sensory or sensorimotor neuropathy, and were found to have vasculitis on sural nerve biopsy [12]. Of particular interest are six cases of angiocentric lymphoproliferative disorder, also known as lymphomatoid granulomatosis; three were associated with non-Hodgkin's lymphoma [11]. On biopsy, an angiocentric lesion without HIV antigen was found, suggesting that HIV-induced immune dysregulation led to uncontrolled T-cell proliferation, which eventually resulted in lymphoma [11].

Laboratory Data

Serologic Studies

A wide variety of autoantibodies have been described in association with HIV infection (Table 14-4). Their significance is unknown, although the majority likely represent epiphenomena of polyclonal B-cell activation [17]. Anticardiolipin antibodies, for example, are found in up to 40 percent of patients with HIV infection, but are not associated with clinical thrombosis as in systemic lupus erythematosus [40]. The presence of lupus anticoagulant antibody tends to mirror the activity of opportunistic infections [41].

Creatine phosphokinase is the most sensitive marker of inflammatory muscle disease, although it is similarly elevated in HIV-associated polymyositis and ZDV-associated mitochondrial myopathy and, therefore, cannot be used to distinguish between these two disorders [37].

Table 14-4 *Autoantibodies associated with HIV infection*

Anticardiolipin antibodies
Rheumatoid factor
Circulatory immune complexes
Antilymphocyte antibodies
Antisperm antibodies
Antimyelin antibodies
Antiplatelet antibodies
Anti–red blood cell antibodies

Synovial Fluid and Synovial Biopsy

Synovial fluid white blood cell (WBC) count is elevated in Reiter's syndrome (approximately 11,000 WBC/mm³) and psoriatic arthritis (approximately 15,000 WBC/mm³), with a predominance of polymorphonuclear leukocytes [1]. Nonspecific HIV-associated oligoarthritis typically demonstrates noninflammatory synovial fluid, with the WBC count generally less than 2,000 cells/mm³; HIV is rarely isolated [16, 42]. In one patient with HIV-associated oligoarthritis, in situ HIV DNA was found in small numbers of synovial fluid lymphocytes and dendritic cells [43]. Synovial fluid findings in HIV-infected patients with septic arthritis generally show WBC counts exceeding 50,000 cells/mm³, low glucose levels, and organisms on Gram's stain and culture [10].

Few synovial biopsy studies have been done, and these have been primarily in patients with nonspecific oligoarthritis demonstrating only mild, chronic inflammatory changes [16]. Synovial biopsy may show noncaseating granulomas in patients with *S. schenckii* infection [33].

Muscle Studies

Electromyography

Electromyography (EMG) in patients with HIV-associated polymyositis shows nonspecific myopathic changes, such as low-amplitude EMG signals, increased insertional activity with fibrillation potentials, and F waves [8, 9].

Muscle Biopsy

Muscle biopsies of both ZDV-associated myopathy and HIV-associated polymyositis show perivascular or endomysial inflammation, varying degrees of necrotic muscle fibers, rod (nemaline) bodies, and cytoplasmic bodies in many fibers [37]. Only ZDV-associated myopathy, however, demonstrates the presence of "ragged red" fibers, indicative of abnormal mitochondria, with paracrystalline inclusions by electron microscopy [37].

Roentgenographic Studies

Roentgenographic studies of patients with Reiter's syndrome, psoriatic arthritis, and septic arthritis may show evidence of joint destruction, but are typically normal in patients with arthralgia, fibromyalgia syndrome, myositis, and vasculitis [44]. In patients with HIV-associated Sjögren's-like syndrome, the chest x-ray may show interstitial changes characteristic of LIP [6].

HLA Testing

HLA-B27 is found in approximately 80 percent of patients with Reiter's syndrome with or without HIV infection [13].

Clinical Evaluation

History and Physical Examination

Patients with rheumatic symptoms should undergo a careful history and physical examination. The history should focus on specific joint or muscle complaints, or both, including the presence or absence of joint swelling or muscle weakness. A detailed functional history is also critical; for example, eliciting a history of difficulty in combing the hair or rising from a seated position will provide important clues as to the presence of proximal myopathy. For patients with suspected Reiter's syndrome, a prior history of enteric or sexually transmitted infection and transient eye or urethral symptoms is important. Physical examination should focus on the joint and periarticular examination, including the presence of enthesopathy (Achilles tendonitis or plantar fasciitis) and nonarticular point tenderness. The presence of a joint effusion is almost always indicative of arthritis and should prompt further evaluation.

Laboratory Evaluation

Patients with fibromyalgia syndrome should have serum CPK and thyroid function assessed to rule out polymyositis and hypothyroidism. Patients with muscle weakness should have a CPK drawn and possibly further evaluation, including EMG and muscle biopsy. Patients with arthritis and joint effusion(s) should generally undergo arthrocentesis; this is mandatory in the case of suspected joint infection. Roentgenographic studies of involved joints are helpful if a destructive arthropathy is part of the differential diagnosis, and HLA-B27 testing should be considered in patients with suspected Reiter's syndrome. For patients with suspected vasculitis (e.g., palpable purpura, mononeuritis multiplex), biopsy of the involved organ should be considered before treatment is initiated.

Management

Arthralgia

Most arthralgias without arthritis can be managed with nonnarcotic analgesics, such as acetaminophen or nonsteroidal antiinflammatory drugs (NSAIDs). On occasion, short courses of narcotic analgesics may be required [1].

Fibromyalgia Syndrome

Most patients with FMS can be managed with the combination of low-dose tricyclic antidepressants and nonnarcotic analgesics. Severely depressed patients may require intensive antidepressant therapy and psychiatric referral.

Reiter's Syndrome, Psoriatic Arthritis, and Nonspecific Oligoarthritis

These disorders are generally treated with NSAIDs initially, although this therapy is not uniformly effective [13]. Sulfasalazine has been tried in several patients with Reiter's syndrome without substantial benefit [13]. Methotrexate should be used with caution, since rapid progression to AIDS was noted in two patients shortly after this agent was initiated in low doses for treatment of Reiter's syndrome [13].

Septic Arthritis

The management of septic arthritis in patients with HIV infection is similar to that in patients without HIV infection: systemic antibiotic therapy and adequate joint drainage. Most authorities recommend a minimum of four weeks of antibiotics for bacterial arthritis in this setting.

Zidovudine-Associated Myopathy and HIV-Associated Polymyositis

It is not known if ZDV-associated myopathy is dose related and whether the lower doses currently recommended will prove less myotoxic with long-term therapy. The management of these myopathies has been reviewed by Dalakas and associates [37]. An NSAID should be tried first, with or without dose reduction of ZDV. If this is not effective, ZDV should be discontinued, and the patient's level of strength followed (serum CPK may normalize without improvement in muscle strength). If the patient's strength increases, another antiretroviral agent should be started; if the patient's strength decreases or remains unchanged, ZDV therapy should be resumed with prednisone (40–60 mg daily).

Vasculitis

Once the possibility of infection as underlying cause has been eliminated, a cautious trial of prednisone and a cytotoxic drug should be considered, particularly in the patient with more serious organ involvement.

Sjögren's-like Syndrome

In one study, early corticosteroid or chlorambucil therapy appeared to prevent progression to interstitial fibrosis [6].

References

1. Berman A, Espinoza LR, Diaz JD, et al. Rheumatic manifestations of human immunodeficiency virus infection. *Am J Med* 85:59–64, 1988.
2. Buskila D, Gladman DD, Langevitz P, et al. Fibromyalgia in human immunodeficiency virus infection. *J Rheumatol* 17:1202–1206, 1990.
3. Simms RW, Zerbini CAF, Ferrante N, et al. Fibromyalgia syndrome in patients infected with the human immunodeficiency virus. *Am J Med* 92:368–374, 1992.
4. De Clerck LS, Couttenye MM, de Broe ME, Stevens WJ. Acquired immunodeficiency syndrome mimicking Sjogren's syndrome and systemic lupus erythematosus. *Arthritis Rheum* 31:272–275, 1988.
5. Ulirsch RC, Jaffe ES. Sjogren's syndrome-like illness associated with the acquired immunodeficiency syndrome-related complex. *Hum Pathol* 18:1063–1068, 1987.
6. Itescu S, Brancato L, Buxbaum J, et al. A diffuse infiltrative CD8 lymphocytosis in human immunodeficiency virus (HIV) infection: A host immune response associated with HLA-DR5. *Ann Intern Med* 112:3–10, 1990.
7. Dalakas MC, Pezeshkpour GH, Gravell M, Sever JL. Polymyositis associated with AIDS retrovirus. *JAMA* 256:2381–2383, 1986.
8. Nordstrom DM, Petroposis AA, Giorno R, et al. Inflammatory myopathy and acquired immunodeficiency syndrome. *Arthritis Rheum* 32:475–479, 1989.
9. Glickstein SL, Strickland SR, Rusin LH. Acute myositis in a patient with acquired immunodeficiency syndrome. *Arthritis Rheum* 33:298, 1990.

10. Zimmerman B, Erickson AD, Milkolich DJ. Septic acromio-clavicular arthritis and osteomyelitis in a patient with acquired immunodeficiency syndrome. *Arthritis Rheum* 32:1175–1178, 1989.
11. Calabrese LH, Estes M, Yen-Lieberman B, et al. Systemic vasculitis in association with human immunodeficiency virus infection. *Arthritis Rheum* 32:569–576, 1989.
12. Marcef-Valeriano J, Ravichandran L, Kerr LD. HIV-associated systemic necrotizing vasculitis. *J Rheumatol* 17:1091–1093, 1990.
13. Winchester R, Bernstein H, Fischer H, et al. The co-occurrence of Reiter's syndrome and acquired immunodeficiency. *Ann Intern Med* 106:19–26, 1987.
14. Duvic M, Johnson TM, Rapini RP, et al. Acquired immunodeficiency syndrome–associated psoriasis and Reiter's syndrome. *Arch Dermatol* 123:1622–1632, 1987.
15. Espinoza LR, Berman A, Vasey FB, et al. Psoriatic arthritis and acquired immunodeficiency syndrome. *Arthritis Rheum* 31:1034–1040, 1988.
16. Rynes RI, Goldenberg DL, di Giacomo R, et al. Acquired immunodeficiency syndrome–associated arthritis. *Am J Med* 84:810–816, 1988.
17. Calabrese LH. Autoimmune manifestations of human immunodeficiency virus (HIV) infection. *Clin Lab Med* 8:269–279, 1988.
18. Monteagndo I, Rivera J, Lopez-Lungo J, et al. AIDS and rheumatic manifestations in patients addicted to drugs. An analysis of 106 cases. *J Rheumatol* 18:1038–1041, 1991.
19. Wolfe F, Smythe HA, Yunus M, et al. The American College of Rheumatology 1990 criteria for the classification of fibromyalgia: Report of the multicenter criteria committee. *Arthritis Rheum* 33:160–172, 1990.
20. Hudson JI, Hudson MS, Pliner LF, et al. Fibromyalgia and psychopathology: Is fibromyalgia a form of "affective spectrum disorder?" *J Rheumatol* 16 (suppl):15–22, 1989.
21. Goldenberg DL. Fibromyalgia and other chronic fatigue syndromes: Is there evidence for chronic viral disease? *Semin Arthritis Rheum* 18:111–120, 1988.
22. Calin A. Reiter's Syndrome. In WN Kelly, E Harris, S Ruddy, C Sledge (eds), *Textbook of Rheumatology* (3rd ed). Philadelphia: Saunders, 1989. Pp 1038–1049.
23. Calin A, Fries JF. An "experimental" epidemic of Reiter's syndrome revisited: Follow-up evidence on genetic and environmental factors. *Ann Intern Med* 84:564, 1976.
24. Clark M, Kinsolving M, Chernoff D. The prevalence of arthritis in two HIV-infected cohorts (abstract). *Arthritis Rheum* 32:S85, 1989.
25. Hochberg MC, Fox R, Nelson KR. Reiter's syndrome is not associated with HIV infection (abstract). *Arthritis Rheum* 33:17S, 1989.
26. Kammer GM, Soter NA, Gibson DJ, Schur PH. Psoriatic arthritis: A clinical immunologic and HLA study of 100 patients. *Semin Arthritis Rheum* 9:75–97, 1979.
27. Bennett RM. Psoriatic Arthritis. In DJ McCarty, *Arthritis and Allied Conditions* (11th ed). Philadelphia: Lea & Febiger, 1989. Pp 954–971, 1989.

28. Kaplan MH, Sadick N, McNutt S, et al. Dermatologic findings and manifestations of acquired immunodeficiency syndrome (AIDS). *J Am Acad Dermatol* 16:485–506, 1987.
29. Reveille JD, Cewant MA, Duvic M. Human immunodeficiency virus–associated psoriasis, psoriatic arthritis, and Reiter's syndrome: A disease continuum? *Arthritis Rheum* 33:1574–1578, 1990.
30. Aguilar JL, Espinoza LR, Berman A, et al. HIV antigen demonstration in synovial membrane from patients with HIV-associated arthritis and HIV-associated psoriatic arthritis. *Arthritis Rheum* 32:587, 1989.
31. Aguilar JL, Espinoza LR. Psoriatic arthritis: A current perspective. *J Musculoskel Med* 6:11–28, 1989.
32. Ricciardi DD, Sepkowitz LB, Bienenstoch H, Maslow ML. Cryptococcal arthritis in a patient with acquired immune deficiency syndrome: A case report and review of the literature. *J Rheumatol* 13:455–458, 1986.
33. Lipstein-Kresch E, Isenberg HD, Singer C, et al. Disseminated *Sporothrix schenckii* infection with arthritis in a patient with acquired immunodeficiency syndrome. *J Rheumatol* 12:805–808, 1985.
34. Pappo AS, Buchanan GR, Johnson A. Septic arthritis in children with hemophilia. *Am J Dis Child* 143:1226–1228, 1989.
35. Rogni MV, Hanley EN. Septic arthritis in hemophiliac patients and infection with human immunodeficiency virus. *Ann Intern Med* 110:168–169, 1989.
36. Widrow CA, Kellie SM, Saltzman BR, Mathur-Wagh V. Pyomyositis in patients with the human immunodeficiency virus: An unusual form of disseminated bacterial infection. *Am J Med* 91:129–136, 1991.
37. Dalakas MC, Illa I, Pezeshkpour GH, et al. Mitochondrial myopathy caused by long-term zidovudine therapy. *N Engl J Med* 322:1098–1105, 1990.
38. Talal N. Sjogren's Syndrome and Connective Tissue Diseases Associated with other Immunologic Disorders. In DJ McCarty, *Arthritis and Allied Conditions* (11th ed). Philadelphia: Lea & Febiger, 1989. Pp 1197–1213.
39. Adamson TC, Fox RI, Frismen DM, et al. Immunohistochemical analysis of lymphoid filtrates in primary Sjogren's syndrome using monoclonal antibodies. *J Immunol* 130:203–208, 1983.
40. Canoso RT, Zow LI, Goopman JE. Anticardiolipin antibodies associated with HTLV-III infection. *Br J Haematol* 65:495–498, 1987.
41. Cohen A, Phillips TM, Kessler CM. Circulating coagulation inhibitors in the acquired immunodeficiency syndrome. *Ann Intern Med* 104:175–180, 1986.
42. Withrington RH, Cornes P, Harris JRW, et al. Isolation of human immunodeficiency virus from synovial fluid of a patient with reactive arthritis. *Br Med J* 294:484, 1987.
43. Espinoza LR, Aguilar JL, Espinoza CW, et al. HIV associated arthropathy: HIV antigen demonstration in the synovial membrane. *J Rheumatol* 17:1195–1201, 1990.
44. Rosenberg ZS, Norman A, Solomon G. Arthritis associated with HIV infection: Radiographic manifestations. *Radiology* 173:171–176, 1989.

15/Neurologic Manifestations

Nagagopal Venna

Manifestations of HIV infection involving the central, peripheral, and autonomic nervous systems are protean [1, 2] (Table 15-1). Disorders characteristic of primary HIV infection include acute aseptic meningitis and encephalitis, demyelinating polyneuropathy, and acute mononeuropathy; HIV encephalopathy, vacuolar myelopathy, distal symmetric polyneuropathy, and opportunistic infections and neoplasms generally occur with advanced HIV disease. Many neurologic disturbances in HIV-infected patients improve spontaneously or in response to therapeutic intervention.

HIV Meningoencephalitides

See Table 15-2 for a list of brain and meningeal disorders common to HIV infection.

Chronic Asymptomatic Meningitis

Human immunodeficiency virus penetrates the blood-brain barrier early, as demonstrated by the presence of increased cerebrospinal fluid (CSF) mononuclear cells and protein, oligoclonal immunoglobulins, and positive HIV culture. While meningeal inflammation persists throughout life, the critical factors that determine progression to neurologic injury are not known.

Acute Meningitis

Acute meningitis may appear during HIV seroconversion, presenting as fever, myalgias, headache, neck stiffness, and, rarely, transient Bell's palsy [3]. Cerebrospinal fluid (CSF) analysis shows lymphocytosis, moderately increased protein, normal glucose, and positive HIV culture. Clinical recovery generally occurs within 2 weeks, but the syndrome may recrudesce periodically.

Table 15-1 Neurologic manifestations of HIV disease

Brain and meninges
    HIV-related meningoencephalitides
    Opportunistic infections
    Neoplasms
    Stroke syndrome
    Seizure disorder

Spinal cord
    HIV-related vacuolar myelopathy
    Acute myelopathy due to opportunistic infections

Peripheral nerves
    Distal symmetric polyneuropathy
    Drug-induced symmetric neuropathy
    Bell's palsy
    Neuralgic amyotrophy
    Mononeuritis multiplex
    Lumbosacral polyradiculopathy
    Demyelinating polyneuropathies
    Autonomic neuropathy

Acute Encephalitis

Acute encephalitis is a rare presentation of HIV seroconversion that manifests as fever, malaise, confusion, lethargy, seizures, and focal neurologic signs evolving over a few days [4]. Cerebrospinal fluid analysis shows mild lymphocytosis, increased protein, and normal glucose; computed tomography (CT) scan of the brain is unremarkable. Patients recover spontaneously.

HIV Encephalopathy

This common and progressive complication of HIV infection usually affects patients with advanced disease but may present earlier [5, 6]. Pathologic abnormalities, identified in approximately 90 percent of patients dying from AIDS, include demyelination, accumulation of mononuclear cells, microglial nodules, and multinucleated cells in the subcortical gray and white matter. HIV antigens are demonstrable in macrophages, monocytes, microglia, oligodendrocytes, astrocytes, and capillary endothelial cells but not in neurons.

The syndrome begins with insidious alteration of behavior, intellect, and motor control. Behavioral changes are usually noted by family and friends as a decline in spontaneity and drive resembling depression. Cognitive changes lead to difficulty in tasks that demand sustained concentration and complex sequential steps. Later, memory becomes increasingly impaired. These changes are punctuated or sometimes

Table 15-2 *Brain and meningeal disorders in HIV infection*

HIV infection
  Chronic asymptomatic meningitis
  Acute meningitis
  Acute encephalitis
  HIV encephalopathy

Opportunistic infections
  Viral infections
    Cytomegalovirus encephalitis
    Varicella-zoster virus meningoencephalitis
    Herpes simplex virus encephalitis
    Progressive multifocal leukoencephalopathy
  Protozoal infections
    Toxoplasmic encephalitis
    Chagas' disease
    Amebic encephalitis
  Fungal infections
    Cryptococcosis
    Mucormycosis
    Aspergillosis
    Candidiasis
  Bacterial infections
    Nocardiosis
    Tuberculosis
    Syphilis
    Bacillary angiomatosis

Neoplastic diseases
  Lymphoma, primary and metastatic
  Kaposi's sarcoma

brought to light by dramatic psychosis [7]. Mania, acute schizophreni-form illness with bizarre behavior, suicidal ideation, and labile affect have all been described. The patient experiences gradual disintegration of motor skills: Hands become clumsy, gait is slowed and unsteady, and eye movements lose normal smoothness in pursuit.

In the early stages of HIV encephalopathy, neuropsychological tests may help detect subtle changes of memory, concentration, and frontal system involvement, such as speed of processing information and sequential complex tasks, but later dementia is apparent. The impairment of ocular pursuit, decrease in rapid fine finger movements, and other early signs of upper motor neuron system dysfunction provide supportive evidence of the diagnosis. Computed tomography and magnetic resonance imaging (MRI) scans show diffuse and progressive cerebral gyral atrophy, dilatation of ventricles, and patchy abnormal signals in subcortical white and gray matter (Fig. 15-1). Positron emission tomography (PET) and single photon emission computed tomography

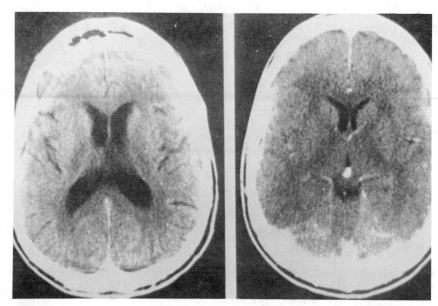

Figure 15-1. Computed tomographic scan of cerebral atrophy associated with HIV encephalopathy. (Reprinted with permission of DM Barnes, AIDS-related brain damage unexplained. Science 232:1091–1093, 1986.)

(SPECT) scans may indicate subcortical hypometabolism, and electro-encephalography (EEG) shows nonspecific slowing over the hemi-spheres. Cerebrospinal fluid analysis reveals mononuclear pleocytosis, modestly increased protein, and sometimes oligoclonal bands.

Although nonspecific, the clinical picture of dementia without decreased alertness is characteristic of HIV encephalopathy. Differen-tial diagnosis includes depression, infectious and neoplastic diseases of the central nervous system (CNS), and toxic and drug-induced enceph-alopathies. Zidovudine (ZDV) has produced modest clinical improve-ment in some patients as documented by brain metabolic mapping studies [8]. The efficacy of didanosine (ddI) and dideoxycytidine (ddC) is unknown. Careful use of tricyclic antidepressant drugs, methylphe-nidate (to treat apathy), and neuroleptics may be helpful in ameliorating symptoms.

Meningoencephalitides Caused by Opportunistic Infections

Cytomegalovirus Encephalitis

Cytomegalovirus encephalitis is a common pathologic finding in patients dying from AIDS [9]. Microglial nodules, some of which contain

CMV, are scattered in the subcortical gray and white matter, accompanied by multifocal parenchymal necrosis without inflammation. Cytomegalovirus encephalitis is not well characterized clinically because of its frequent coexistence with herpes simplex virus (HSV) infection and other systemic illnesses [10]. Brain CT and MRI scans are generally nonfocal, but may show periventricular enhancement due to ventriculitis and small multifocal subcortical lesions. The CSF reveals lymphocytosis, increased CMV antibody titers, and, occasionally, a positive CMV culture. While the antiviral agent ganciclovir, used in the treatment of CMV retinitis, penetrates the brain well, its role in the management of encephalitis has not been established.

Varicella-Zoster Virus Meningoencephalitis

Varicella-zoster virus (VZV) encephalitis is characterized pathologically by multifocal demyelination, necrosis, and thrombosis with viral antigens and inclusions in neurons and glia [11]. This rare illness manifests as the subacute onset of confusion, lethargy, memory impairment, upper motor neuron paresis, and ataxia [12]. Brain CT and MRI scans may be normal or show multifocal white and gray matter lesions. Cerebrospinal fluid abnormalities are nonspecific, and VZV antibodies are rarely present. Brain biopsy and culture are necessary for definitive diagnosis. Therapy with acyclovir may be beneficial but has not been demonstrated to be effective.

Herpes Simplex Virus Encephalitis

Herpes simplex virus may coinfect the CNS with CMV in patients with advanced HIV disease, but the focal, frontotemporal encephalitis characteristic of HSV infection in immunocompetent patients has not been documented.

Progressive Multifocal Leukoencephalopathy

Progressive multifocal leukoencephalopathy (PML) is caused by JC virus infection of oligodendroglia. This previously rare condition affects approximately 3 percent of AIDS patients, resulting in large patches of demyelination in the cerebral, brainstem, and cerebellar white matter without inflammation [13, 14]. Patients have hemiparesis, dysarthria, hemianopsia, cortical blindness, cerebellar ataxia, evidence of brainstem dysfunction, and dementia, but remain alert and without seizures. Computed tomographic scan shows hypodense, nonenhancing white matter lesions. MRI scan demonstrates distinctive abnormalities in the subcortical region, including sparing of the cortex, lack of mass effect,

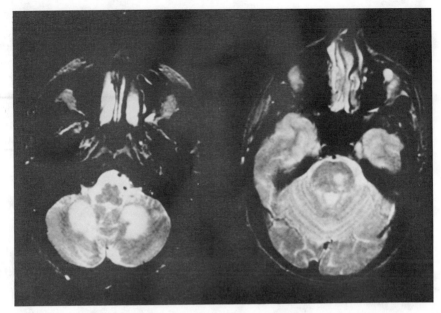

Figure 15-2. *Progressive multifocal leukoencephalopathy on T2-weighted MRI scan of brain. Image on left shows extensive area of abnormal high signal in the cerebellar peduncles; image on right shows high signal in the white matter of pons.*

predilection to periventricular areas, and lack of contrast enhancement (Fig. 15-2). Cerebrospinal fluid analysis is typically normal, and EEG often reveals delta wave slowing. Brain biopsy, necessary for definitive diagnosis, shows demyelination, axonal sparing with bizarre astrocytes, and viral particles in the oligodendrocytes. No treatment has been demonstrated to be effective. Patients generally experience a progressive downhill course over months, but extended survival and spontaneous clinical improvement have been reported in some cases [15, 16].

Toxoplasmic Encephalitis

Toxoplasmosis, which causes a multifocal necrotizing encephalitis, is the most common opportunistic infection of the brain in AIDS, affecting approximately 10 percent of patients [17]. Clinical manifestations include headache, confusion, lethargy, and, less commonly, focal abnormalities, such as seizures, hemiparesis, gait ataxia, hemiballismus, and evidence of brainstem dysfunction. Brain CT scan shows single or multiple, noncalcified mass lesions with contrast enhancement (Fig. 15-3); gadolinium-enhanced MRI scan appears to be even more sensitive. Most patients with cerebral toxoplasmosis have detectable serum *Toxo-*

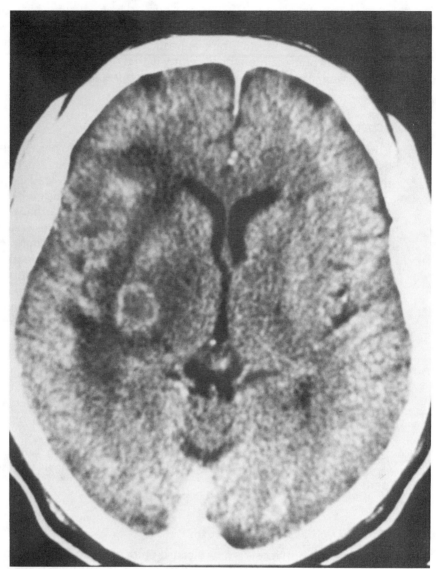

Figure 15-3. *Computed tomographic scan of cerebral toxoplasmosis.*

plasma antibodies; the role of CSF antibodies is uncertain. Brain biopsy, although necessary for definitive diagnosis, is generally reserved for patients who fail to respond to empiric therapy.

Empiric treatment with pyrimethamine/sulfadiazine is indicated when toxoplasmic encephalitis is suggested by clinical and radiologic findings. Improvement generally occurs within days to a couple of weeks of initiation of therapy. Dexamethasone should be administered only if clinically significant cerebral edema is present, although its indiscriminate use may obscure the diagnostic value of empiric antimicrobial therapy. Chronic maintenance therapy with reduced doses of the drugs used for initial management is necessary to prevent relapse.

Cryptococcal Meningitis

Cryptococcus neoformans causes a subacute or chronic basal meningitis, with occasional involvement of the lumbosacral, cervical, or thoracic meninges and nerve roots [18]. The basal meningitis may lead to hydrocephalus, intracranial hypertension, and cranial nerve palsies.

Cryptococcal meningitis is manifested by headache, lethargy, confusion, and numbness and weakness in the extremities; neck stiffness is frequently absent. Papilledema, blindness, and deafness may occur. Cerebral granulomas or cysts may cause progressive hemiparesis or other focal signs. Brain CT and MRI scans are generally normal, but granulomas are occasionally seen. Diagnosis is made by lumbar puncture with CSF analysis, which shows variable pleocytosis, increased protein, and/or decreased glucose. Cerebrospinal fluid cryptococcal antigen and India ink preparation are usually positive, and organisms can be readily cultured. In some patients, very high CSF pressure develops without hydrocephalus by an unknown mechanism.

Amphotericin B or fluconazole is used for primary treatment; fluconazole is the drug of choice for maintenance therapy. In patients with progressive obtundation and visual failure associated with high CSF pressure without hydrocephalus, large-volume spinal taps or lumboperitoneal shunt should be attempted [19]. Obstructive hydrocephalus is relieved by ventricular drainage with a CSF reservoir or ventriculoperitoneal shunt.

Cerebral Mucormycosis

Cerebral mucormycosis is a rare cause of focal necrotizing encephalitis that should be considered in HIV-infected patients who use injection drugs [20]. The clinical presentation is nonspecific, as are brain scans, which show focal mass lesions, and the CSF, from which organisms cannot generally be recovered. Unlike mucormycosis associated with diabetic ketoacidosis, paranasal sinusitis and orbital cellulitis are typically absent in HIV-infected patients. Diagnosis is by brain biopsy with silver methenamine stain, which shows nonseptate hyphae with right-angled branches. Treatment consists of amphotericin B.

Cerebral Aspergillosis

Cerebral aspergillosis is a focal encephalitis that is uncommon in AIDS, developing in the context of severe systemic illness and broad-spectrum antibiotic therapy [21]. Fulminant hemorrhagic infarction of the brain with prominent invasion of blood vessels by the fungus is characteristic. Diagnosis is generally by brain biopsy, although repeated CSF examinations, especially by cisternal tap, may sometimes reveal the pathogen. Therapy is with amphotericin B, but the prognosis is poor.

Candidal Encephalitis

Only a few cases of candidal abscesses of the CNS have been described in AIDS patients despite the high prevalence of candidiasis in HIV infection. The clinical picture is nonspecific, with brain imaging studies showing multiple small abscesses. Candida albicans is often cultured from the blood and CSF. Amphotericin B is the drug of choice.

Nocardial Encephalitis

Nocardial abscesses have been documented in AIDS but are unusual [22]. Clinical features and CSF analysis are nonspecific, and brain scans show focal ring-like abscesses. Diagnosis is made by biopsy of the brain or other involved sites. Antibiotic therapy with trimethoprim-sulfamethoxazole or sulfonamides is effective, but surgical excision may be necessary for large multiloculated lesions.

Mycobacterial Infection

Extrapulmonary infection with Mycobacterium tuberculosis is commonly associated with HIV infection [23]. Neurologic involvement is characterized by subacute basal meningitis complicated by cranial nerve palsies, hydrocephalus, and infectious arteritis leading to brain infarction. Brain tuberculomas and abscesses may occur with or without meningitis. Pulmonary disease may not be evident, and the tuberculosis skin test (purified protein derivative, or PPD) may be negative with advanced immunodeficiency.

Clinically, fever, headache, confusion, lethargy, and cranial nerve palsies steadily progress over days. Sudden stroke syndrome may be the presenting feature or punctuate the illness, and seizures are common with intracerebral tuberculomas. Brain CT and MRI scans often reveal basal meningeal enhancement, obstructive hydrocephalus, focal hypodensities due to brain infarction, granulomas with or without calcification, and, rarely, abscesses. Cerebrospinal fluid analysis shows progressive lymphocytic pleocytosis, increased protein, and decreased glucose. Acid-fast stains rarely reveal the organism, but CSF culture is generally positive.

Treatment should be started promptly based on the clinical presentation and CSF analysis pending definitive diagnosis. Combination antituberculous drug therapy with isoniazid, rifampin, ethambutol, and pyrazinamide is indicated pending culture and drug sensitivity testing results. Corticosteroids may have a role in the management of severe meningitis. Clinical and radiologic improvement generally occurs within a few weeks of initiation of therapy. Occasionally, brain biopsy may be necessary for diagnosis.

Syphilitic Meningoencephalitis

Central nervous system infection with *Treponema pallidum* in HIV-seropositive patients may present without symptoms or with acute meningitis, meningitis with cerebral vasculitis, or encephalitis [24]. In the meningovascular form, obliterative vasculitis of the small and the penetrating arteries causes small lacunar infarctions. In the rare encephalitic form, characterized by dementia, seizures, and myoclonus, there is diffuse infection of the brain. Some HIV-infected patients with syphilis may have atypical clinical manifestations, accelerated disease progression, and false-negative serologic studies, and inadequate therapeutic responses to conventional antibiotic regimens [24, 25].

Acute syphilitic meningitis causes fever, headache, neck stiffness, and, sometimes, cranial nerve palsies, especially of the second and eighth nerves; conjunctivitis, uveitis, and retinitis may accompany the neurologic syndrome. Cerebrospinal fluid examination shows lymphocytosis, increased protein, and decreased glucose, and the CSF VDRL is generally positive. Meningovascular syphilis is most often characterized by the abrupt onset of hemiplegia, but a variety of cerebral and brainstem syndromes have also been noted. Brain CT and MRI scans show focal infarctions, especially of the basis pontis and internal capsule.

Syphilis is part of the differential diagnosis of any neurologic problem in the HIV-infected patient, and serum and CSF serologies should always be obtained. Nervous system involvement may be associated with other manifestations of syphilis or occur in isolation. Conventional treatment of neurosyphilis consists of parenteral penicillin G, 12 to 16 million units per day for 10 days, followed by benzathine penicillin, 2.4 million units given intramuscularly for 3 consecutive weeks. Oral tetracycline or erythromycin should be used in those who are allergic to penicillin. Patients diagnosed with syphilis should be monitored clinically and serologically following completion of their treatment regimen.

Miscellaneous Infections

A case of focal encephalitis caused by the protozoan *Trypanosoma cruzi* was described in an AIDS patient who came from an endemic area [26]. Temporal lobe bacillary angiomatosis has been reported in a patient who had a characteristic skin lesion [27]. Biopsy of skin and brain lesions confirmed the presence of microvascular proliferation and pleomorphic bacilli, and the condition responded to erythromycin therapy. Focal hemorrhagic encephalitis due to ameba has also been described in the context of HIV infection [28].

Neoplastic Meningoencephalopathies

Primary CNS Lymphoma

Primary B-cell brain lymphoma occurs in approximately 5 to 10 percent of patients with AIDS, but is an otherwise rare tumor [29]. Highly malignant and multicentric, it has a predilection for the basal ganglia, thalami, and periventricular regions. The tumor presents with headache, lethargy, and confusion, sometimes accompanied by hemiparesis and cerebellar or brainstem dysfunction. The patient experiences steady clinical deterioration over a few weeks, with increasing obtundation secondary to infiltrating tumor or hydrocephalus, or both. Brain CT and MRI scans show single or multiple lesions with minimal mass effect (Fig. 15-4). With the administration of contrast, there is diffuse irregular enhancement of the mass and, sometimes, ventricular lining. In approximately 25 percent of cases, immunocytology of the CSF reveals monoclonal malignant cells. Definitive diagnosis requires brain biopsy, although, presumptive diagnosis is sometimes made on the basis of clinical and radiologic features. Dexamethasone combined with radiation treatment is used palliatively, but survival rarely exceeds 3 months.

Metastatic Lymphoma

Systemic lymphoma may spread to the brain and meninges. Meningeal lymphomatosis presents with multiple cranial and extremity nerve palsies and may be complicated by obstructive hydrocephalus. Cytologic examination of CSF reveals malignant cells. Intrathecal methotrexate or

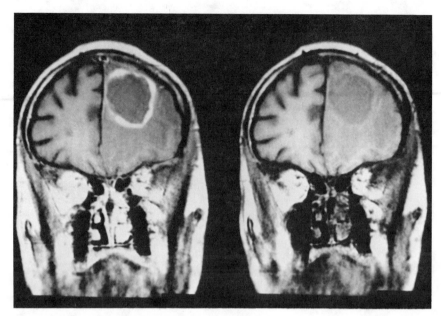

Figure 15-4. *Primary central nervous system lymphoma on MRI scan of brain. Image on left shows a large gadolinium-enhanced lesion of the frontal lobe with surrounding edema; image on right is without enhancement.*

cytosine arabinoside have been used therapeutically, but survival longer than 6 months is unusual.

Kaposi's Sarcoma

Central nervous system involvement by Kaposi's sarcoma is very rare, manifesting with the rapid onset of focal neurologic signs [30]. Brain CT scan shows multiple, hemorrhagic nodules with mass effect, but definitive diagnosis requires brain biopsy. There are no data available regarding the efficacy of therapy.

Stroke Syndrome

HIV-infected patients have a markedly increased incidence of stroke. Cerebral infarctions may be sequelae to infectious vasculitis of mycobacterial, treponemal, viral, or cryptococcal origin, or to embolism from endocarditis [31]. In some patients, cerebral infarction occurs without a specific identifiable etiology, ascribed to an "HIV arteriopathy." The CSF should be examined for evidence of infection in all HIV-infected patients who present with stroke.

Seizure Disorder

Seizure activity occurs frequently in HIV infection and may be a presenting symptom of neurologic disease [32]. In approximately 50 percent of patients, it indicates the presence of a focal meningoencephalitis. In about 25 percent of cases, it is a manifestation of HIV encephalopathy, and, in the remaining cases, no specific cause can be found. Although seizure activity generally responds well to conventional anticonvulsive agents, HIV-infected patients seem to have an unusually high incidence of hypersensitivity reactions to phenytoin. Carbamazepine and valproic acid should be used with caution in this population because of the frequent coexistence of bone marrow and liver dysfunction.

Diagnostic Approach to Meningoencephalitis

Because clinical manifestations are often nonspecific, all HIV-infected patients with evidence of significant CNS dysfunction should undergo brain CT or MRI scan, followed by lumbar puncture with CSF analysis (Table 15-3). Syphilis and *Toxoplasma* serologies should be performed, and a PPD with appropriate controls placed. Psychiatric examination or neuropsychological testing, or both, are also indicated if depression is part of the differential diagnosis. Injection drug and alcohol abuse histories should be reviewed, as both intoxication and withdrawal syndromes may result in altered mental status. Toxicity from prescription medications should also be a diagnostic consideration.

Opportunistic infections of the CNS are more common with advanced immunodeficiency (CD4 cell count $< 200/mm^3$), and patients with suspected toxoplasmosis or tuberculosis should be treated empirically. Brain biopsy is indicated if the diagnosis remains uncertain or clinical progression occurs despite empiric therapy. Stereotactic technique permits biopsy of even deep brain lesions with little morbidity and is quite safe in the absence of a bleeding diathesis. Specimens should be examined with fungal, acid-fast, and immunoperoxidase stains, by dark-field microscopy for spirochetes, and by electron microscopy for viral inclusions.

Spinal Cord Syndromes

The most common spinal cord syndrome associated with HIV infection is subacute vacuolar myelopathy. Rare cases of acute myelitis are

Table 15-3 *Evaluation of HIV-related meningoencephalitis*

History
    History of syphilis, tuberculosis
    Vegetative symptoms of depression
    Injection drug use
    Alcoholism
    Medication toxicity

Physical examination
    Alteration in mental status
    Focal neurologic findings

Laboratory evaluation
    CD4 cell count
    Syphilis serologies
    Toxoplasma serology
    PPD and controls
    Neuropsychological testing
    Brain CT or MRI scan
    Lumbar puncture with CSF analysis
        Cell count
        Glucose, protein
        Gram's, acid-fast, India ink stains
        Bacterial, mycobacterial, fungal cultures
        Cryptococcal antigen
        VDRL
    Brain biopsy*

*Indicated only if the diagnosis is uncertain based on less invasive tests or if clinical progression occurs despite empiric therapy.

caused by VZV, HSV, CMV, and *Toxoplasma gondii*, and as a complication of tuberculous and syphilitic meningitides.

Vacuolar Myelopathy

The striking pathologic picture seen with vacuolar myelopathy resembles subacute combined degeneration of the spinal cord of vitamin B_{12} deficiency, with vacuolation of the lateral and posterior columns, minimal inflammation, and no vascular changes [33]. HIV antigen has been identified in macrophages.

The myelopathy may be overshadowed clinically by HIV encephalopathy and peripheral neuropathy, but presents as a subacute spastic, ataxic paraparesis associated with upper motor neuron signs and impaired proprioception in the limbs. A mass lesion should be ruled out by MRI scan with gadolinium, and CSF analysis should be performed to exclude syphilis and tuberculosis. The role of antiretroviral therapy has not been examined systematically, although one case report suggested improvement with ZDV [34].

Acute Myelopathies

Although rare, acute myelopathies are important because some are potentially treatable [35–38]. Patients have rapidly developing paraparesis, bladder and bowel incontinence, and a transverse sensory level. VZV myelitis is suggested by its association with shingles. MRI scan of the spinal cord with gadolinium may reveal epidural abscess in the drug-using patient or focal swelling suggesting *Toxoplasma* or tuberculous myelitis. Cerebrospinal fluid examination should be performed to rule out syphilis, tuberculosis, or CMV infection as the cause.

Peripheral Neuropathies

A variety of peripheral nerve disorders have been reported in HIV infection [39].

Distal Symmetric Polyneuropathy

Distal symmetric polyneuropathy is a common neuropathy of unknown etiology that is characterized pathologically by diffuse axonal loss with variable lymphocytic infiltration and viral antigen in the axoplasm and mononuclear cells. It presents insidiously with prominent paresthesias and shooting pains in the lower extremities accompanied by contact hypersensitivity and disturbed sleep. Physical findings may be minimal early in the disease, with reduction in proprioception and diminished ankle reflexes, but later sensory impairment occurs in a stocking and glove distribution. Motor abnormalities are unusual. Nerve conduction velocities (NCV) and electromyography (EMG) demonstrate a symmetric, predominantly axonal neuropathy with decreased sensory action potentials. Cerebrospinal fluid analysis may show mild pleocytosis and increased protein, and sural nerve biopsy reveals nonspecific axonal degeneration. Other causes of neuropathy, such as alcoholism, and neurotoxic drugs, such as vincristine and ddI, should be considered in the differential diagnosis.

The neuropathy has an indolent course and may stabilize spontaneously. Some reports suggest that ZDV therapy may be beneficial [40]. Treatment of pain and dysesthesia is challenging. Tricyclic antidepressant drugs, such as amitriptyline, doxepin, and desipramine, given in modest doses are often helpful. Carbamazepine, clonazepam, baclofen, phenytoin, and acupuncture are used as alternative agents. In severe cases, narcotic analgesics may be necessary.

Drug-Induced Symmetric Polyneuropathy

This predominantly sensory polyneuropathy is a common toxicity of the antiretroviral agents ddI and ddC [41]. Significant symptoms may necessitate discontinuation of the drug but take weeks to months to abate. Vincristine, used in the treatment of Kaposi's sarcoma, is associated with a similar dose-dependent, reversible polyneuropathy. Isoniazid, lithium carbonate, and dapsone are other potential causes of polyneuropathy.

Bell's Palsy

Self-limited unilateral or bilateral Bell's palsy may develop during primary HIV infection, sometimes in association with aseptic meningitis.

Neuralgic Amyotrophy

A syndrome of self-limited unilateral or bilateral shoulder girdle neuropathy may also develop during HIV seroconversion. Intense pain in the shoulders is followed by rapid development of weakness and atrophy of the girdle muscles. Weakness of the serratus anterior, causing winging of the scapula, is particularly characteristic.

Mononeuritis Multiplex

In mononeuritis multiplex, an unusual variant of peripheral neuropathy, multiple cranial, limb, and truncal nerves are affected serially over days to weeks in a patchy, scattered pattern. Cerebrospinal fluid analysis is nonspecific; sural nerve biopsy may show mononuclear cell infiltration and, occasionally, necrotizing vasculitis. The condition may evolve into a symmetric diffuse, demyelinating polyneuropathy, stabilize, or improve spontaneously. Patients with progressive disease may respond to plasmapheresis, corticosteroids, and intravenous immunoglobulin therapy.

Lumbosacral Polyradiculopathy: Cauda Equina Syndrome

In lumbosacral polyradiculopathy, an unusual and potentially treatable neuropathy, the nerve roots of cauda equina are affected by a necrotizing vasculitis resulting from CMV infection [42]. Rapidly progressive weakness and numbness of the legs and the perianal area lead to sphincter paralysis. Physical examination shows bilateral asymmetric, areflexic paraparesis and anesthesia over the buttocks. CSF analysis is remarkable for polymorphonuclear pleocytosis, increased protein, decreased glucose, and the presence of CMV antibodies. Cytomegalovirus can be cultured from the cerebrospinal fluid, and sural nerve biopsy may reveal CMV inclusions in giant cells. Lumbar spine CT scan after intrathecal contrast and gadolinium-enhanced MRI show thickened lumbosacral nerve roots and enhancement of the lumbar thecal sac. Differential diagnosis includes syphilitic, tuberculous, cryptococcal, and lymphomatous meningoradiculopathies, and toxoplasmosis of the conus medullaris [43]. Empiric treatment with ganciclovir should be initiated based on characteristic clinical and cerebrospinal fluid findings.

Acute and Chronic Inflammatory Demyelinating Polyneuropathies

These conditions characteristically occur with primary HIV infection. The ascending quadriparesis usually begins in lower limbs and spreads to the upper extremities, bulbar and facial muscles, and, in severe cases, the respiratory muscles. The acute form (Guillain-Barré syndrome) evolves over 2 to 4 weeks, whereas the chronic variety develops over months with a tendency for a relapsing course. Cerebrospinal fluid analysis shows mononuclear pleocytosis. NCV testing reveals marked slowing in multiple peripheral nerves. Plasmapheresis accelerates neurologic recovery, and intravenous immunoglobulin therapy has been reported to ameliorate symptoms [44].

Autonomic Neuropathy

Evidence of autonomic dysfunction is being increasingly recognized in HIV-infected patients. Although usually asymptomatic, it may cause orthostatic hypotension, gastrointestinal dysfunction, urinary incontinence, impotence, and, rarely, cardiopulmonary arrest [45].

References

1. Snider WD, Simpson DM, Nielsen J. Neurological complications of acquired immunodeficiency syndrome: Analysis of 50 patients. *Ann Neurol* 14:403–418, 1983.
2. McArthur JC. Neurological manifestation of AIDS. *Medicine* 66:407–437, 1987.
3. Hollander H, Stringari S. Human immunodeficiency virus associated meningitis: Clinical course and correlations. *Am J Med* 83:813–815, 1987.
4. Carne CA, Smith A, Elkington SG, et al. Acute encephalopathy coincident with seroconversion for HTLV-III. *Lancet* 2:1206–1208, 1985.

5. Navia BA, Jordan BD, Price RW. The AIDS dementia complex: I. Clinical features. *Ann Neurol* 19:517–524, 1986.
6. Navia BA, Cho ES, Petito CK, et al. AIDS dementia complex: II. Neuropathology. *Ann Neurol* 19:525–535, 1986.
7. Perry SW. Organic mental disorders caused by human immunodeficiency virus: Update on early diagnosis and treatment. *Am J Psychiatry* 147:696–710, 1990.
8. Schmitt FA, Bigley JW, McKinnis R, et al. Neuropsychological outcome of zidovudine (AZT) in the treatment of patients with AIDS and AIDS-related complex. *N Engl J Med* 319:1573–1578, 1987.
9. Morgello S, Cho ES, Nielsen S, et al. Cytomegalovirus encephalitis in patients with acquired immunodeficiency syndrome: An autopsy study of 30 cases and a review of the literature. *Hum Pathol* 18:289–297, 1987.
10. Masdeu JC, Small CB, Weiss L, et al. Multifocal cytomegalic encephalitis in AIDS. *Ann Neurol* 23:97–99, 1988.
11. Morgello S, Block GA, Price RW, et al. Varicella-zoster leukoencephalitis and cerebral vasculopathy. *Arch Pathol Lab Med* 112:173–177, 1988.
12. Gilden DH, Murray RS, Wellish M, et al. Chronic progressive varicella-zoster encephalitis in an AIDS patient. *Neurology* 38:1150–1153, 1988.
13. Berger JR, Kaszovitz B, Donovan MJ, et al. Progressive multifocal leukoencephalopathy associated with human immunodeficiency virus infection: A review of the literature with a report of sixteen cases. *Ann Intern Med* 107:78–87, 1987.
14. Gillespie SM, et al. Progressive multifocal leukoencephalopathy in persons infected with human immunodeficiency virus, San Francisco, 1981–89. *Ann Neurol* 30:597–604, 1991.
15. Karahalios D, et al. Progressive multifocal leukoencephalopathy in patients with HIV infection: Lack of impact of early diagnosis of stereotactic brain biopsy. *J AIDS* 5:1030–1038, 1992.
16. Berger JR, Mucke L. Prolonged survival and partial recovery in AIDS associated progressive multifocal leukoencephalopathy. *Neurology* 38:1060–1065, 1988.
17. Luft BJ, Remington JS. Toxoplasmic encephalitis: AIDS commentary. *J Infect Dis* 157:1–6, 1987.
18. Dismukes WE. Cryptococcal meningitis in patients with AIDS: AIDS commentary. *J Infect Dis* 157:624–628,1988.
19. Denning D, Armstrong RW, Steven DA. Elevated cerebrospinal fluid pressure in patients with cryptococcal meningitis and acquired immunodeficiency syndrome. *Am J Med* 91:267–272, 1991.
20. Cuadrado LM, Guerrero A, Asenjo LG, et al. Cerebral mucormycosis in two cases of acquired immunodeficiency syndrome. *Arch Neurol* 45:109–111, 1988.
21. Woods GL, Goldsmith JC. Aspergillus infection of the central nervous system in patients with acquired immunodeficiency syndrome. *Arch Neurol* 47:181–184, 1990.
22. Adair JC, Beck AC, Apfelbaum RI, et al. Nocardial brain abscess in the acquired immunodeficiency syndrome. *Arch Neurol* 44:548–550, 1987.

23. Berenguer J, Moreno S, Laguna F, et al. Tuberculous meningitis in patients infected with the human immunodeficiency virus. *N Engl J Med* 326:668–672, 1992.
24. Katz DA, Berger JR. Neurosyphilis in acquired immunodeficiency syndrome. *Arch Neurol* 46:895–898, 1989.
25. Musher DM, Hanill RJ, Baughn RE. Effect of human immunodeficiency virus infection on the course of syphilis and on the response to treatment. *Ann Intern Med* 113:872–881, 1990.
26. Gluckstein D, Ciferri F, Ruskin J. Chagas' disease: Another cause of cerebral mass in the acquired immunodeficiency syndrome. *Am J Med* 92:429–432, 1992.
27. Spach DH, Panther LA, Thorning DR, et al. Intracerebral bacillary angiomatosis in a patient infected with human immunodeficiency virus. *Ann Intern Med* 116:740–742, 1992.
28. Gordner HAR, Martinez AJ, Visvesvara GS, et al. Granulomatous amebic encephalitis in an AIDS patient. *Neurology* 41:1993–1995, 1991.
29. Remick SC, Diamond C, Migliozzi JA, et al. Primary central nervous system lymphoma in patients with and without the acquired immunodeficiency syndrome. *Medicine* 69:345–360, 1990.
30. Gorin FA, Bale TF, Halks-Miller M, et al. Kaposi sarcoma metastatic to the CNS. *Arch Neurol* 42:162–165, 1985.
31. Engstrom JW, Lowenstein DH, Bredesen DE. Cerebral infarction and transient neurological deficits associated with acquired immunodeficiency syndrome. *Am J Med* 86:528–532, 1989.
32. Wong MC, Suite NDA, Labar DR. Seizures in human immunodeficiency virus infection. *Arch Neurol* 47:640–642, 1990.
33. Petito CK, Mavia BA, Cho ES, et al. Vacuolar myelopathy pathologically resembling subacute combined degeneration in patients with acquired immunodeficiency syndrome. *N Engl J Med* 312:874–879, 1985.
34. Oksenhendler E, Ferchal F, Cadranel J, et al. Zidovudine for HIV-related myelopathy. *Am J Med* 88:65N–66N, 1990.
35. Britton CB, Mesa-Tejada R, Fenoglio CM, et al. A new complication of AIDS: Thoracic myelitis caused by herpes simplex. *Neurology* 35:1071–1074, 1985.
36. Woolsey RM, Chambers TJ, Chung HD, et al. Mycobacterial meningomyelitis associated with human immunodeficiency virus infection. *Arch Neurol* 45:691–693, 1988.
37. Berger JR. Spinal cord syphilis associated with human immunodeficiency virus infection: A treatable myelopathy. *Am J Med* 922:101–103, 1992.
38. Herskovitz S, Siegel SE, Schneider AT, et al. Spinal cord toxoplasmosis in AIDS. *Neurology* 39:1552–1553, 1989.
39. Dalakas MC, Perzeshkpour GH. Neuromuscular disease associated with human immunodeficiency virus infection. *Ann Neurol* 23(suppl):38–48, 1988.
40. Dalakas MC, Harchoan MD, Spitzer R, et al. Treatment of human immunodeficiency virus-related polyneuropathy with 3-azido-2-3-dideoxythymidine. *Ann Neurol* 23 (suppl):92–94, 1988.

41. Schaumburg HH, Arezzo J, Berger A, et al. Dideoxycytidine (ddC) neuropathy in human immunodeficiency virus infections: A report of 52 patients. *Neurology* 40 (suppl):428, 1990.
42. Miller RG, Storey JR, Greco CM. Gancyclovir in the treatment of progressive AIDS-related polyradiculopathy. *Neurology* 40:569–574, 1990.
43. Lanska MJ, Lanska J, Schmidley JW. Syphilitic polyradiculopathy in an HIV-positive man. *Neurology* 38:1277–1301, 1988.
44. Malamut RI, Leopold N, Chester PA, et al. The treatment of HIV associated chronic inflammatory demyelinating polyneuropathy with intravenous immunoglobulin. *Neurology* 42 (suppl 3):355, 1992.
45. Cohen JA, Miller L, Polish L. Orthostatic hypotension in human immunodeficiency virus infection may be the result of generalized autonomic nervous system dysfunction. *J AIDS* 4:32, 1991.

16 / Psychological Manifestations

Alexandra Beckett, Marshall Forstein

Altered Mental Status in HIV Infection

HIV-infected patients with altered mental status require careful clinical assessment. Although psychological problems are common in this population, the assumption in such situations should always be that the etiology is central nervous system (CNS) dysfunction. Primary causes ensue directly from HIV infection, while secondary causes derive from opportunistic infections and malignancies, systemic derangements, and treatment complications (Table 16-1). Primary CNS dysfunction is often insidious in onset; a rapid or sudden change in mental state is more likely to represent a secondary disorder. Many causes of neurologic dysfunction are treatable or even reversible. These include anemia, hypoxia, electrolyte imbalance, drug toxicities (Table 16-2), and opportunistic infections and malignancies. Individuals with preexisting HIV encephalopathy, even of relatively minor clinical significance, may be particularly vulnerable to the superimposed psychological and neurologic challenges of acute medical illness. The evaluation of altered mental status in the HIV-infected patient is guided by clinical presentation and will often include head computed tomographic (CT) scan, lumbar puncture, electroencephalography (EEG), and neuropsychological testing.

HIV-Related Neurologic Disease

By 1982, clinicians noted a syndrome of depression, apathy, and social withdrawal that was often associated with AIDS. It was suspected that this syndrome, which was termed *subacute encephalitis* or *AIDS encephalopathy,* had an organic etiology. Evidence rapidly accumulated that CNS involvement led to the development of encephalopathy [1]. In 1987, in recognition of the prevalence and severity of HIV-related neurologic dysfunction, the Centers for Disease Control added dementia to its roster of AIDS-defining disorders [2]. HIV-related disease has been described at all levels of the central nervous system and represents a source of substantial morbidity.

219

Table 16-1 *Causes of altered mental status in the HIV-infected patient*

HIV-related syndromes
   Primary infection
   HIV encephalopathy
Infection
   Bacterial (tuberculosis, syphilis)
   Fungal (cryptococcoses, candidiasis)
   Parasitic (toxoplasmosis)
   Viral (herpes simplex, cytomegalovirus)
Neoplasms
   Primary or metastatic lymphoma
   Kaposi's sarcoma (rarely)
Cerebrovascular disease
Toxic/metabolic disorders
   Drug-related neurotoxicities
   Anemia
   Nutritional deficiencies
   Dehydration
   Hypoxia secondary to pulmonary disease
   Adrenal insufficiency
   Renal disease
   Hepatic encephalopathy
Psychiatric disorders
   Adjustment
   Major depression/bipolar disorders
   Psychosis
   Anxiety disorders
   Substance abuse disorders

HIV Encephalopathy

Pathogenesis

The precise mechanism by which HIV gains entry into the CNS has not been determined. It is conceivable that the virus penetrates directly from serum. Recent developments in neuroimmunology suggest that HIV-infected lymphocytes and macrophages enter the CNS circulation and then pass into the brain parenchyma through ruptured capillary endothelium [1]. Furthermore, it appears that HIV actively replicates in the cerebrospinal fluid (CSF) and sometimes in the brain itself. HIV has been recovered from brain tissue, CSF, spinal cord, and peripheral nerves of patients with neurologic dysfunction [3]. In a few cases, HIV has been isolated from the nervous system of patients in whom no virus was detected in peripheral blood [4]. Eighty to 90 percent of autopsied AIDS cases manifest histopathologic changes in the brain, with relative sparing of the cortex [5]. In white matter, there is diffuse gliosis and a

Table 16-2 Neuropsychiatric side effects of medications

Drug	Neuropsychiatric effects
Acyclovir	Visual hallucinations, depersonalization, tearfulness, confusion, hyperesthesia, hyperacusia, thought insertion, insomnia, agitation
Amphotericin B	Delirium, peripheral neuropathy, diplopia, weight loss, loss of appetite
Corticosteroids	Depression, euphoria, psychosis
Ganciclovir	Manic psychosis, agitation, delirium, irritability
Alpha-interferon	Depression, weakness
Isoniazid	Depression, agitation, hallucinations, paranoia, impaired memory
Methotrexate	Encephalopathy (high dose)
Pentamidine	Hypoglycemia, hypotension (leading to CNS dysfunction)
Procarbazine	Mania, loss of appetite, insomnia, nightmares, confusion, malaise
Trimethoprim-sulfamethoxazole	Depression, loss of appetite, insomnia, apathy, headache
Vinblastine	Depression, loss of appetite, headache
Vincristine	Hallucinations, headache, ataxia, sensory loss, depression, agitation
Zidovudine	Headache, restlessness, severe agitation, insomnia, mania, depression, irritability

loss of myelin and, less frequently, focal areas of demyelination. Gross atrophy derives from diffuse white matter disease.

Clinical Manifestations

HIV encephalopathy is a complex of cognitive, affective, behavioral, and motor abnormalities (Table 16-3). The clinical findings are often subtle and insidious in onset. Forgetfulness and loss of concentration are the most frequent early symptoms [6]. Patients may complain of difficulty with attention, confusion, and mental slowing. Attention lapses appear as an inability to read a book, follow a television program, or sustain a conversation. Patients may have trouble accomplishing complex tasks that were formerly automatic, and vegetative signs of depression, including loss of energy and appetite, sexual dysfunction, and sleep disturbance, are common. Some patients may become apathetic, socially withdrawn, or irritable. Agitation and anxiety may be troubling and at times incapacitating. Persons familiar with the patient may notice a "change in personality" characterized by heightened anxiety in

Table 16-3 Stages of HIV encephalopathy

Early
Cognitive: Short-term memory loss, impaired attention and concentration, comprehension difficulties, slowed information processing, mild frontal lobe dysfunction
Behavioral: Apathy, withdrawal, irritability
Motor: Slowing, unsteady gait, dysgraphia, dysarthria, hyperreflexia, weakness
Affective: Depression, psychotic features, hypomania
Late
Cognitive: Severe memory impairment, severe attention difficulties, marked frontal lobe dysfunction
Behavioral: Disinhibition, withdrawal
Motor: Slowing, spasticity, incontinence, ataxia
Affective: Depression, psychosis, hypomania/mania
End stage
Mutism, aphasia, incontinence, myoclonus, seizures

response to change and the development of a rigid, inflexible style [7]. The presentation of HIV encephalopathy is occasionally much more dramatic, with acute agitated psychosis, hallucinations, paranoid ideation, or frank mania [8]. In this setting, there is often evidence of cognitive dysfunction or focal neurologic deficits supporting the diagnosis of an organic mental disorder.

Nearly 50 percent of patients with HIV encephalopathy complain of motor dysfunction [9]. Motor impairment may include weakness, particularly of the lower extremities, and difficulty with fine motor coordination. There is often dysarthria, tremor, and physical slowing [7]. Patients may notice difficulty in walking or climbing stairs, deterioration in handwriting, or a slight slurring of speech. Some of these motor deficits may result from concomitant spinal cord disease (vacuolar myelopathy) and not solely from cerebral involvement.

The course of HIV encephalopathy is highly variable. There may be little or no progression of deficits, and affected individuals can often compensate for cognitive problems by keeping written records, using a pocket calendar, or making out a daily medication sheet. For some patients, the cognitive problems progress, rendering them dependent on others for help with daily tasks. Occasionally, the syndrome is characterized by a dramatic and catastrophic decline in mental function, resulting in severe dementia within weeks.

Neuroradiologic Imaging
The head CT scan in patients with HIV encephalopathy may be normal or demonstrate diffuse cerebral atrophy. In advanced HIV encephalop-

athy, the scan often shows a widening of the frontal horns or bilateral low-density changes of the adjacent white matter [1]. Magnetic resonance imaging (MRI) is more sensitive than CT because of its superior capacity to distinguish white matter disease [10]. MRI findings in HIV encephalopathy include cerebral atrophy and ventricular enlargement. Single photon emission computed tomography (SPECT) is a technique that visualizes blood perfusion in the brain. The imaging of individuals with HIV encephalopathy using 123-I-N-isopropyl-p-iodoamphetamine has identified focal uptake deficits [11].

Cerebrospinal Fluid Abnormalities
Cerebrospinal fluid abnormalities may occur in individuals with or without clinical findings of encephalopathy, although the prevalence of abnormal findings is greater in those who are symptomatic. Abnormalities include (1) white blood cell count greater than $5/mm^3$, (2) total protein greater than 40 mg/dl, (3) immunoglobulin G (IgG) greater than 6.1 mg/dl, (4) IgG index greater than 0.7, (5) oligoclonal bands greater than 2, (6) positive HIV culture, and (7) detectable HIV p24 antigen.

Neuropsychological Testing
There is a consensus among investigators that clinically significant cognitive impairment occurs in persons diagnosed with AIDS, although its prevalence is uncertain. Disagreement exists as to whether subtle neuropsychological dysfunction occurs in asymptomatic seropositive individuals [12]. In large numbers of subjects followed in the Multicenter AIDS Cohort Study neuropsychologically, no difference was detected between seronegative control subjects and asymptomatic seropositive individuals [13–15]. In another study, Grant and associates [16] found extremely high rates of neurologic impairment in all HIV-infected groups: asymptomatic seropositives, 44 percent; AIDS-related complex (ARC), 54 percent; and AIDS, 87 percent. Despite these conflicting findings, neuropsychological tests have been found to be useful in assessing the HIV-infected population. They measure attention and concentration, psychomotor speed, motor performance, short-term memory, abstraction, information processing, and complex tasks involving sequencing.

Psychiatric Syndromes

The most common psychiatric diagnoses in HIV-infected patients are adjustment disorder, major depression, substance abuse disorder, and anxiety [17, 18]. Because of the high incidence of organic brain disease in this population, a syndrome that manifests itself primarily as a psychiatric disorder merits careful medical evaluation [19]. Psychological symptoms may be part of an organic syndrome warranting medical intervention. For example, mania in an HIV-infected patient may signal an intracranial process, such as infection or tumor, or may represent an adverse drug effect (zidovudine [ZDV] or ganciclovir).

Symptoms of anxiety and depression are the most common findings in patients without clear organic pathology. Adjustment disorder with depressed or anxious mood, considered to be a reaction to the illness, is common, and may be severe enough to warrant psychotherapeutic or pharmacologic treatment. A clinical distinction can be made between the withdrawal, apathy, avoidance of complex tasks, and mental slowing associated with early HIV encephalopathy and the low self-esteem, irrational guilt, and other signs related to psychological depression. However, studies that suggest unusually high rates of mood disorders in people with and at risk for HIV infection make the distinction between organic disorders and psychological depression problematic [20, 21].

In addition to the CNS effects of HIV itself, the complications of systemic HIV-related disease and its treatments may alter brain function. More difficult to assess completely are the external (societal) and internal (intrapsychic) stressors associated with HIV infection. These can compound CNS dysfunction, making the accommodation to neuropsychiatric disturbances more difficult. These stressors may include (1) all of the psychological issues associated with a life-threatening illness, (2) stigmatization that threatens the patient's premorbid status in society, (3) uncertainty about the course of illness, (4) difficulty in obtaining adequate health care or financial resources, and (5) the loss of significant numbers of one's social support network to AIDS [22].

Suicidality

Assessment of suicidal risk in the HIV-infected population is important. The psychological use of suicidal ideation as a means of coping with difficult and intractable life circumstances is common. Neuropsychiatric disorders, such as delirium, dementia, or depression, may be contributing factors. Psychodynamically, suicidal ideation is used to cope with the fear of pain, death, or disfigurement. It may be a wish to have ultimate control over one's fate when all else seems to be slipping away. The onset of a new medical illness, a relapse of substance abuse, a precipitous drop in CD4 lymphocyte count, a loss of someone important, financial devastation, loss of living quarters, or rejection by others may engender suicidal thinking or behavior, or both.

Assurance from the provider that pain, depression, and cognitive impairment will be aggressively treated is comforting to patients and reduces the intrusive nature of self-destructive thoughts. Suicidal ideation may be the way that patients begin to talk about the fears and anxieties associated with dying and death. As patients become more impaired and face the inevitability of their own death, they may begin to withdraw emotionally from others around them, focusing more on themselves and the approaching end of life. Patients who perceive their provider as willing to talk about suicide, decisions concerning the rational termination of treatment, and anxiety about dying will be more likely to seek help before acting impulsively. The use of disinhibiting substances may contribute to impulsive self-destructive behavior.

Physicians must recognize that, in the presence of treatable organic illness or depression, suicide is not a rational choice. A newly diagnosed asymptomatic patient with early HIV disease who believes he or she is going to die soon cannot be considered to be acting rationally. Conversely, the decision by a patient to forgo further treatment or withhold life-sustaining medications when there is little more to be accomplished, as opposed to reversing an acute condition, must be differentiated from suicide.

Pain

HIV-infected patients often experience pain during the course of their illness. Since the severity of pain is impossible to measure objectively, providers are often faced with difficult management issues in affected patients, especially those with a history of drug abuse. Chronic, severe pain should be treated with a sufficient dose of a long-acting narcotic. Pain or the fear of pain may be a precipitant to suicidal ideation and behavior.

Sleep Disorders

Most patients with HIV infection complain of sleep disturbance at some time during the course of illness. Sleep may be disturbed as a consequence of acute anxiety or depression secondary to HIV infection or CNS disease, or a result of drug toxicity. Sleep deprivation may cause significant psychiatric morbidity and requires a careful evaluation and aggressive treatment.

Management

HIV Encephalopathy

Yarchoan and associates [23] reported improvement in clinical status, motor function, nerve conduction velocities, memory, general cognitive ability, and findings on neuroradiologic imaging in patients with HIV encephalopathy who received ZDV. Schmitt and colleagues [24] noted a significant improvement in neuropsychological performance in a double-blind, placebo-controlled trial of ZDV for persons with advanced symptomatic disease and AIDS. Measures of subjective distress were also lower in ZDV recipients.

Psychostimulants provide significant relief of symptoms for a number of patients. Fernandez and associates [25, 26] found improvement in most neuropsychological tests in cognitively impaired ARC and AIDS patients treated with psychostimulants. Pharmacotherapy with either methylphenidate or dextroamphetamine was "clinically effective" in 91 percent and moderately to markedly effective in 82 percent. Therapy with psychostimulants can be effective in bringing about qualitative and quantitative improvement in high cortical functions, self-esteem, and self-sufficiency. Few side effects have been seen.

Psychiatric Disorders

Recommendations on the use of antidepressants, antipsychotics, and benzodiazepines in HIV-infected patients are outlined below. General recommendations for prescribing psychoactive medications include: (1) start with low doses; (2) increase the dose slowly; (3) monitor closely for side effects; (4) prescribe small amounts in suicidal patients, but do not avoid using appropriate psychopharmacologic agents; and (5) distinguish the clinical indications for medications from the management issues related to patient personality or cognitive capacity.

Depression

For depression with marked slowing, apathy, and hypersomnia, treatment with desipramine should be considered. One should begin with a daily oral dose of 10 mg, increasing the daily dose by 10 mg po every 3 days with a maximal daily dose of 200 to 250 mg. For depression with difficulty in falling asleep or early-morning awakening, doxepin should be considered. One should begin with a daily oral dose of 10 mg and increase as above, with a maximum daily dose of 150 mg at bedtime. Trazodone, fluoxetine, and nortriptyline are other clinically useful antidepressants.

Psychosis

Antipsychotics are indicated for the treatment of agitation and hallucinations. Caution is warranted with respect to anticholinergic side effects and extrapyramidal symptoms. Haloperidol, 0.5 to 1.0 mg daily to twice a day orally or intramuscularly, should be used initially; agitated patients may require significantly higher doses. Adjunctive treatment with lorazepam may be helpful for anxiety. One should use perphenazine instead of haloperidol in patients with extrapyramidal symptoms or pre-existing movement disorders. Carbamazepine should be used cautiously (with hematologic parameters monitored) for bipolar disorder; valproic acid is an alternative. Lithium carbonate is indicated for manic episodes.

Anxiety

Benzodiazepines may exacerbate underlying cognitive problems. In general, they should be used sparingly. Short-acting benzodiazepines, such as triazolam (0.25–0.50 mg orally at bedtime) or temazepam (15–30 mg orally at bedtime), are useful for sleep disturbances. When rebound insomnia occurs after cessation of a short-acting benzodiazepine, one should switch to an every other day regimen or less frequent use of a longer-acting agent such as lorazepam or clonazepam.

Pain

When pain is neuropathic in origin, one should try carbamazepine, valproic acid, or amitriptyline in low doses, increasing as tolerated. Opiates should be used where necessary in sufficient dose to completely relieve rather than ameliorate severe pain. Acupuncture should be considered in the management of chronic pain.

CNS Drug Toxicities

Anticholinergic side effects of tricyclic antidepressant and antipsychotic agents may involve the central and peripheral nervous systems. CNS symptoms include confusion, delirium with disorientation, agitation, visual and auditory hallucinations, anxiety, and motor restlessness; peripheral nervous system manifestations include constipation, urinary retention, anhidrosis, mydriasis, dry mouth, flushing, and tachycardia. Extrapyramidal syndromes characteristic of antipsychotic agents include acute dystonic reactions (abnormal involuntary movements or oculogyric crisis), motor restlessness, Parkinson's syndrome (tremor, rigidity, akinesia or bradykinesia), and tardive dyskinesia (abnormal, involuntary choreoathetotic movements involving tongue, lips, jaw, face, extremities).

Psychotherapy

There is a significant body of literature demonstrating that primary care providers play an important role in the emotional life of their patients. The physician may be the most constant, stabilizing influence on the HIV-infected patient. It is important that the clinician conceptualize his or her role as having psychotherapeutic power, but not feel as if he or she has to carry that burden alone; the emotional needs of someone with AIDS can be exhausting to provider as well as patient. Thus, making use of other available resources, such as individual and group psychotherapy and peer-run support and psychoeducation groups, is essential. Many patients resist seeing a psychotherapist based on previous experience or cultural biases, or out of fear of losing control over their lives to someone else. Additionally, an unspoken fear may be that the therapist will identify cognitive impairment. Primary care providers can facilitate such a referral by taking time to talk with the patient about his or her fears and anxieties.

References

1. Levy JA. The Biology of the Human Immunodeficiency Virus and Its Role in Neurological Disease. In Rosenblum, Levy, Bredesen (eds), *AIDS and the Nervous System*. New York: Raven Press, 1988.
2. Centers for Disease Control. Revision of the CDC surveillance case definition for acquired immunodeficiency syndrome. *MMWR* 36 (suppl):1–16, 1987.
3. Ho DD, Sarngadgaran MG, Resnick L, et al. Primary human T-lymphotropic virus type III infection. *Ann Intern Med* 103:880–883, 1985.
4. Hollander H, Levy J. Neurological abnormalities and human immunodeficiency virus recovery from cerebrospinal fluid. *Ann Intern Med* 106:692–695, 1987.
5. Navia BA, Cho ES, Rosenblum ML. The AIDS dementia complex: II. Neuropathology. *Ann Neurol* 19:525–535, 1986.
6. Navia BA, Jordan BD, Price RW. The AIDS dementia complex: I. Clinical features. *Ann Neurol* 19:517–524, 1986.
7. Brew BJ, Sidtis JJ, Rosenblum M, et al. AIDS dementia complex. *J R Coll Physicians Lond* 3:140–144, 1988.
8. Beckett A, Summergrad P, Manshrek, et al. Symptomatic HIV infection of the CNS in a patient without clinical evidence of immune deficiency. *Am J Psychiatry* 144:1342–1344, 1987.
9. Gabuzda DH, Hirsch MS. Neurologic manifestations of infection with human immunodeficiency virus: Clinical features and pathogenesis. *Ann Intern Med* 107:383–391, 1987.
10. Post MJD, Sheldon JJ, Hensley GT, et al. Central nervous system disease in acquired immunodeficiency syndrome: Prospective correlation using CT, MR imaging, and pathologic studies. *Radiology* 158:141–148, 1986.
11. Pohl P, Vogle G, Heiko F, et al. Single photon emission computed tomography in AIDS dementia complex. *J Nucl Med* 29:1382–1386, 1988.
12. Perry SW. Organic mental disorders caused by HIV: Update on early diagnosis and treatment. *Am J Psychiatry* 147:696–710, 1990.
13. Neel JR. Predict no epidemic of dementing illness in HIV seropositives. *Clin Psychiat News* 1988;6.
14. McArthur JC, Cohen BA, Selnes OA. Low prevalence of neurological and

neuropsychiatric abnormalities in healthy HIV-1 infected individuals: Results from the Multicenter AIDS Cohort Study. *Ann Neurol* 26:5, 1989.

15. Goethke KE, Mitchell JE, Marshall DW, et al. Neuropsychological and neurological function of human immunodeficiency virus seropositive asymptomatic individuals. *Arch Neurol* 46:129–133, 1989.
16. Grant I, Atkinson JH, Hesselink JR. Evidence for early central nervous system involvement in the acquired immunodeficiency syndrome (AIDS) and other human immunodeficiency virus (HIV) infections. *Ann Intern Med* 107:828–836, 1987.
17. Holland JC, Tross S. The psychosocial and neuropsychiatric sequelae of the acquired immunodeficiency syndrome. *Ann Intern Med* 103:760–764, 1985.
18. Perry SW, Jacobsen P. Neuropsychiatric manifestations of AIDS spectrum disorders. *Hosp Community Psychiatry* 37:135–142, 1986.
19. Forstein M, Baer J. HIV Infection. In L Sederer (ed), *Inpatient Psychiatry: Diagnosis and Treatment.* Baltimore: Williams & Wilkins, 1991. Pp. 189–211.
20. Atkinson JH, Grant I, Kennedy J, et al. Prevalence of psychiatric disorders among men infected with human immunodeficiency virus. *Am J Psychiatry* 145:859–864, 1988.
21. Perry SW, Jacobsen LB, Fishman B, et al. Psychiatric diagnosis before serologic testing for the human immunodeficiency virus. *Am J Psychiatry* 147:89–93, 1990.
22. Dilley JW, Forstein M. Psychosocial aspects of the human immunodeficiency virus epidemic. In A Tasman, SM Goldfinger, CA Kaufmann (eds), *Review of Psychiatry.* Washington, DC: American Psychiatric Press, 1990.
23. Yarchoan R, Berg G, Brouwers P. Response of human-immunodeficiency virus-associated neurological disease to 3′-azido-3′-deoxythymidine. *Lancet* 1:132–135, 1987.
24. Schmitt FA, Bigley JW, McKinniss R, et al. Neuropsychological outcome of zidovudine (AZT) treatment of patients with AIDS and AIDS-related complex. *N Engl J Med* 319:1573–1578, 1988.
25. Fernandez F, Adams F, Levy JK, et al. Cognitive impairment due to AIDS-related complex and its response to psychostimulants. *Psychosomatics* 1:38–46, 1988.
26. Holmes VF, Fernandez F, Levy JK. Psychostimulant response in AIDS-related complex (ARC) patients. *J Clin Psychiatry* 50:5–8, 1989.

III/Opportunistic Diseases

17/Pneumocystis Pneumonia

Brant L. Viner

Epidemiology

Despite ultrastructural and genomic sequence data suggesting that *Pneumocystis carinii* may be a fungus, it has traditionally been classified as a protozoan [1, 2]. *Pneumocystis carinii* is a unicellular organism of global distribution that has been recovered from the lungs of many mammals including humans. Serologic evidence of infection with *P. carinii* develops in virtually all children before 4 years of age [3, 4]. Autopsy series of adults have demonstrated the organism in 4 to 8 percent of lung specimens, often without evidence of pneumonia [3, 5].

The first association of *P. carinii* with human disease was made after World War II, when outbreaks of interstitial plasma cell pneumonitis occurred in foundling homes that sheltered premature and debilitated infants. This epidemic form of disease has been seen subsequently in Korea, Iran, and Vietnam, and appears to represent primary infection in immunosuppressed hosts. Although evidence in humans is lacking, animal studies suggest the possibility of person-to-person respiratory transmission of the organism.

A totally distinct form of pneumocystosis emerged in the mid-1950s, manifesting as a diffuse alveolar pneumonitis that affected children and adults suffering from drug-induced, neoplastic, or congenital immune deficiency. Although sporadic in distribution, this reactivation type of pneumocystosis was the most common variety seen in developed countries before the AIDS epidemic. Extrapulmonary and disseminated disease was rare, almost always appearing in conjunction with pneumonitis [6, 7].

Pneumocystis carinii pneumonia (PCP) was one of the first opportunistic diseases described in association with AIDS. Despite the fact that PCP is generally easy to diagnose and treat, it remains one of the most serious HIV-related infections. PCP represents the AIDS-defining diagnosis in approximately 60 percent of HIV-infected patients, and it develops in up to 85 percent sometime in the course of their disease [8–12].

Clinical Manifestations

HIV-related PCP is etiologically and pathologically similar to the sporadic form of the disease previously described. However, its clinical features are unique [13]. Patients with PCP associated with non-HIV immunodeficiencies experience the sudden onset of severe respiratory compromise. Although AIDS patients may present in a similar fashion, they typically describe a subacute process that lasts for weeks to months. The indolent nature of this illness frequently permits a remarkable degree of physiologic compensation. Constitutional symptoms, such as fever, anorexia, and lethargy, may overshadow localized pulmonary complaints (Table 17-1). Although cough is usual, it is seldom productive. Dyspnea is common but may go unnoticed in a sedentary patient, and chest pain is rare. The patient may have a low-grade fever, and the lungs are either clear or reveal dry bibasilar rales on auscultation.

Routine laboratory studies may not be helpful. Serum lactate dehydrogenase (LDH) levels are usually increased but nonspecific, and normal values do not rule out PCP. Resting arterial blood gases generally show an increased alveolar-arterial oxygen gradient. Chest radiography is often remarkable for a diffuse interstitial infiltrate but may be normal in early disease.

AIDS-related extrapulmonary *P. carinii* infection has proved both more common and varied than that seen in other populations [6, 7, 14]. To date, over 70 cases have been reported, approximately one third of which have presented as fulminant, disseminated disease in patients previously diagnosed with AIDS. The vast majority of cases were fatal, and 50 percent were associated with pneumonia. Other cases took the form of more indolent, focal disease without pneumonia. While extrapulmonary pneumocystosis usually presents nonspecifically, symptomatic infiltration of lymph nodes, liver, spleen, pleura, bone marrow, gastrointestinal tract, thyroid, ears/mastoid, eyes, and skin has also been described. Patients receiving aerosol pentamidine (AP) prophylaxis appear to be at greatest risk for the development of extrapulmonary disease.

Diagnosis

Chest radiography is an imprecise tool for the diagnosis of PCP. A nonspecific diffuse interstitial pattern is described in 75 to 85 percent of cases, and 5 to 10 percent are associated with a normal study [15–17] (see Table 17-1, Fig. 17-1). Typically, infiltrates are bilateral (95%) and involve both central and peripheral fields (84%); localized infiltrates

Table 17-1 *Clinical and laboratory features of Pneumocystis pneumonia*

History
    CD4 cell count $< 200/mm^3$ or prior history of PCP
    Subacute or chronic onset
    Constitutional and/or respiratory symptoms

Physical examination
    Fever
    Lungs are clear or show nonspecific findings

Laboratory evaluation
    Nonspecific findings
        Increased serum LDH
        Increased alveolar-arterial oxygen gradient
        Diffuse interstitial pattern on chest x-ray[a]
        Abnormal postexercise diffusing capacity (DLCO)
        Positive gallium scan
    Specific findings
        Positive induced sputum
        Positive bronchoalveolar lavage
        Positive transbronchial or open lung biopsy[b]

[a]Normal chest x-ray in 5–10% of patients; atypical radiologic presentations are more common in patients receiving AP prophylaxis.
[b]Rarely necessary for diagnosis.

generally affect the lower lobes. Thin-walled cystic lesions and infiltrates with spontaneous pneumothorax, although infrequent, are highly suggestive of PCP. While unilobar or unilateral disease, cavitation, nodularity, pleural effusion, and intrathoracic adenopathy should raise suspicion for a different disease process, all have been described with PCP. Conversely, radiographic patterns that are "classic" for PCP may be seen with cytomegalovirus pneumonia, pulmonary Kaposi's sarcoma, nonspecific interstitial pneumonitis, tuberculosis, and cryptococcosis. Up to 15 percent of AIDS patients with a diffuse interstitial pattern on chest x-ray do not have PCP [17].

The use of AP prophylaxis appears to alter the radiographic presentation of PCP, resulting in an increased incidence of cystic disease and spontaneous pneumothorax [18, 19]. Only 26 to 52 percent of those receiving AP present with a diffuse interstitial pattern on chest x-ray [18, 20–24]. Infiltrates are often limited to, or predominate in, the upper lung fields.

Pulmonary function tests (PFTs) are not useful in establishing the diagnosis of PCP but may be helpful in excluding it. Postexertional arterial blood gases and diffusing capacity (DLCO) are extremely sensitive (90–100%), but not specific [25–27]. Thus, the finding of normal PFTs makes the diagnosis of PCP very unlikely.

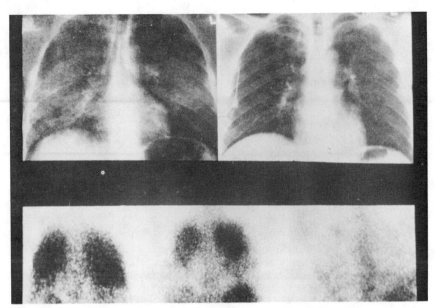

Figure 17-1. Pneumocystis carinii *pneumonia on chest x-ray and gallium scan. A. At time of diagnosis. B. Following treatment. (Reprinted with permission of JA Golden, et al.,* Pneumocystis carinii *pneumonia treated with α-difluoromethylornithine: A prospective study among patients with acquired immunodeficiency syndrome. West J Med 141:613–622, 1984.*

Nuclear lung scans suffer from the same limitations as PFTs. Gallium scans demonstrate high sensitivity (94–100%), but low specificity (20–74%) for PCP [28–31] (see Fig. 17-1). High-grade, diffuse gallium uptake in the lungs, classic for AIDS-related PCP, may be associated with other pulmonary processes, and atypical patterns have been reported in PCP patients receiving therapy [31]. Cases that "break through" AP prophylaxis may present with focal and/or decreased tracer uptake [18]. Thus, a negative gallium scan can only rule out PCP when clinical suspicion is low.

The definitive diagnosis of PCP requires direct visualization of *P. carinii* on sputum or tissue stains (Fig. 17-2). Experienced observers can readily identify sporozoites, trophozoites, and cysts with Giemsa, Wright, or methylene blue stains, but cysts are more easily seen with toluidine blue or methenamine silver stains [32].

In contrast to other immunocompromised hosts, in whom open lung biopsy is frequently required to demonstrate pneumocysts, fiberoptic bronchoscopy has proven a sensitive and reliable method of obtaining diagnostic specimens in HIV-infected patients. Transbronchial biopsy (TBB) provides the highest yield, with pneumocysts routinely detected

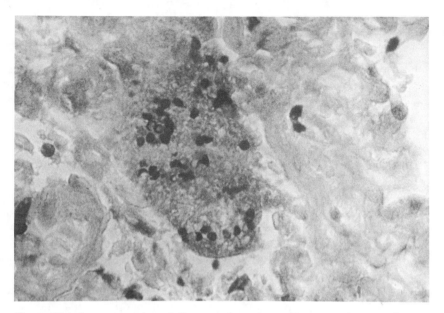

Figure 17-2. Pneumocystis carinii *cysts in lung tissue. (Courtesy of Centers for Disease Control, Atlanta, GA.)*

in 88 to 97 percent of PCP cases [11, 33–35]. However, pneumothorax occurs in 9 to 16 percent of patients who undergo this procedure, and, in those with a tenuous pulmonary and/or hematologic status, such risk may be prohibitive [33, 34, 36].

In most cases, bronchoalveolar lavage (BAL) is by itself only slightly less sensitive for the diagnosis of PCP than TBB [33, 35, 37]. It is a relatively benign procedure that is well tolerated by all except the most fragile patients. Because of its high sensitivity and low morbidity, BAL alone is generally satisfactory for the initial assessment of diffuse lung disease in the HIV-infected patient. In individuals receiving AP prophylaxis, BAL results must be interpreted cautiously, as there is evidence that its sensitivity may be reduced [18]. If BAL is negative or if there is accessible focal lung disease, repeat bronchoscopy with TBB may be useful. When TBB is combined with BAL, the sensitivity of flexible bronchoscopy approaches 100 percent, even in patients receiving AP [18, 33, 35]. Negative studies argue strongly for an alternative diagnosis [38].

At many institutions, examination of induced sputum is the diagnostic modality of choice, with bronchoscopy reserved for cases in which it is unrevealing. In experienced hands, stains of concentrated sputum obtained by induction with an ultrasonic saline nebulizer have achieved a sensitivity of 55 to 80 percent compared to fiberoptic bronchoscopy [39, 40–43]. Immunofluorescent staining techniques employing monoclonal antibodies specific for *P. carinii* appear to be even more promising. In small trials, direct and indirect fluorescent-antibody stains show a sensitivity of 85 to 92 percent when applied to induced, concentrated sputum, but the yield is reduced in persons receiving AP [22, 40, 44, 45].

Clinical Course

In non–HIV-infected populations, PCP typically responds rapidly to appropriate therapy, with clinical and radiologic improvement within several days; 2 weeks of treatment are sufficient for all but the exceptional case [13, 46]. In contrast, many AIDS patients demonstrate few, if any, objective signs of improvement during the first week of therapy. Improved oxygenation on arterial blood gases may be seen as soon as 2 or 3 days into treatment, but should not be expected for at least a week to 10 days. Patients may defervesce within a day or two but frequently this does not occur until the second week of therapy [9, 47].

Chest x-rays are also unreliable for evaluating clinical response. As many as 50 percent of patients who eventually improve have worsening radiographic studies early in therapy [12, 15]. Resolution of infiltrates may take as long as 2 weeks, and many survivors never clear them entirely [9, 13, 15, 47]. Extreme elevation of serum LDH and failure of serum LDH to fall with therapy have been associated with poor outcome [48–50]. Sequential PFTs have been shown to be of little value in the management of PCP [51].

Unless a patient is clearly deteriorating and the question of a second pulmonary process has been raised, repeat bronchoscopy is seldom useful. In contrast to other immunocompromised hosts, AIDS patients will continue to show *P. carinii* cysts in 38 to 90 percent of bronchoscopy specimens obtained after 2 to 3 weeks of therapy and in up to 25 percent of specimens obtained after more than 5 weeks of therapy [52–54]. Although one report has suggested that the failure to decrease *P. carinii* burden by at least 50 percent on BAL performed 21 days into therapy is predictive of early relapse, other investigators have found that neither the persistence nor the quantity of organisms recovered on follow-up bronchoscopy correlates with clinical status, outcome, or tendency to relapse [52, 55, 56].

Although the rate of clinical improvement is much slower, AIDS patients with a first episode of PCP otherwise respond much the same as other immunocompromised hosts [9, 13, 46, 57–59]. Ninety percent of patients in good clinical condition can be expected to improve on therapy, although, without prophylaxis, many would suffer recurrent PCP within months of the initial episode. Annual relapse rates of 25 to 85 percent have been reported in patients not receiving prophylactic therapy, with a median time of 6 to 10 months [57, 60, 61]. The survival rate of recurrent AIDS-related PCP is approximately 60 percent, significantly lower than that of the first episode [9, 13, 57, 59].

Early reports documented a survival rate of only 0 to 15 percent among AIDS patients who required intubation for respiratory distress [10, 13, 62]. Many died in the intensive care unit, and those who were successfully extubated often succumbed to other processes before they could leave the hospital. The grim prognosis of severe AIDS-related PCP has led some authors to question the value of intubation in this setting [10, 62]. However, using current standard management techniques, more recent studies describe a 40 to 53 percent immediate survival and 30 to 38 percent survival at 9 months in PCP patients who require intubation [48, 63].

Treatment

Despite scant scientific evidence, many clinicians believe that AIDS patients require a longer treatment course than other hosts with PCP. Three weeks of therapy is standard for uncomplicated cases. There are two widely accepted regimens for the treatment of PCP: pentamidine and trimethoprim-sulfamethoxazole (TMP-SMZ). Neither is fully satisfactory with respect to clinical outcome and toxicity. The average daily dose of TMP-SMZ costs a hospital pharmacy less than $10; pentamidine costs approximately $80 per day.

Pentamidine

Pentamidine is one of a family of guanidine analogues that were discovered to have antiprotozoal activity in the late 1930s. While its mechanism of action is not firmly established, it appears to function by inhibition of dihydrofolate reductase and interference with nucleic acid synthesis [64]. Pentamidine was first employed in the treatment of PCP in the late 1950s. When used early in the course of disease, pentamidine reduced the mortality of infantile plasma cell pneumonitis from 50 percent to as low as 3 percent and of alveolar disease in immunocompromised hosts from 100 percent to 25–32 percent [65].

Pentamidine must be administered parenterally. In the past, because of reports of severe hypotension following rapid intravenous administration, the intramuscular route was advised. Experience with AIDS patients suggests that this problem was rate-related rather than route-related. The Centers for Disease Control (CDC) has reviewed the first 108 AIDS cases in which pentamidine was employed; severe hypotension was documented only in patients treated intramuscularly [66]. When administered slowly over the course of at least one hour, intravenous pentamidine appears to be well tolerated. The recommended dosage of pentamidine isethionate is 4 mg/kg/day regardless of the route chosen.

The pharmacokinetics of pentamidine have not been fully defined. However, since it is in part cleared by the kidneys, dosage adjustment is required in the presence of renal failure. For a glomerular filtration rate (GFR) of 10 to 50 ml per minute, doses should be administered every 24 to 36 hours; if the rate is less than 10 ml per minute, doses should be given every 48 hours [67].

Toxicity

The major limitation of pentamidine is its toxicity. Although small series in patients with mild to moderate PCP suggest that a dose reduction to 3 mg/kg/day reduces the frequency and severity of side effects without lessening efficacy, most reports using the conventional dose confirm the pre-AIDS experience of a 40 to 50 percent risk of major adverse reactions [60, 64, 65, 68–71].The more important toxicities of pentamidine include renal failure, hypotension, hematologic disturbances, hypoglycemia, and hepatic dysfunction. Less common adverse reactions include sterile abscess formation at intramuscular injection sites, rash (including Stevens-Johnson syndrome), hypocalcemia, acute pancreatitis, ventricular tachycardia, Jarisch-Herxheimer reaction, fever, anorexia, nausea, and acute confusional states [64, 65, 69, 71].

Renal Failure (Approximately 25%).   Although pentamidine-induced nephrotoxicity usually presents with isolated elevation of serum creatinine, a clinical syndrome indistinguishable from type IV renal tubular acidosis has also been reported [72]. Occasional severe cases have required dialysis and/or treatment of hyperkalemia. Far more commonly, renal dysfunction has been mild and reversible with discontinuation of the agent. Preexisting renal failure is a relative contraindication to the use of pentamidine.

Hypotension (Approximately 10%).   This appears to be less common when pentamidine is given by slow intravenous infusion. If hypotension occurs during intravenous administration, the infusion should be stopped, and crystalloids and pressors should be used as needed. Once the patient's blood pressure has returned to baseline, there is no contraindication to restarting pentamidine at a slower infusion rate under close observation.

Hematologic Disturbances (Approximately 15%). Leukopenia is the most common problem but is usually mild. Severe neutropenia may require discontinuation of pentamidine in up to 7 percent of AIDS patients [73]. Thrombocytopenia has been described more rarely. Hematologic problems are almost always reversible.

Hypoglycemia (6–35%). Most pentamidine-induced hypoglycemia is subclinical, but severe hypoglycemia can occur within hours of the first dose and is seen more commonly late in the first week of therapy. Hypoglycemia can usually be controlled with glucose infusion and discontinuation of the drug, but diazoxide therapy may occasionally be required. Some patients who have suffered pentamidine-induced hypoglycemia have developed irreversible insulin-dependent diabetes mellitus within 6 to 150 days of initiation of the drug. Derangements of glucose metabolism are believed to be secondary to a streptozocin-like action of pentamidine on pancreatic beta cells [74].

Hepatic Dysfunction (Approximately 10%). Elevation of serum transaminase values is generally mild and reversible.

Trimethoprim-Sulfamethoxazole

Trimethoprim-sulfamethoxazole was first used for the treatment of pneumocystosis in the mid-1970s. Studies of immunocompromised children with alveolar PCP demonstrated equal efficacy for pentamidine, 4 mg/kg/day parenterally, and TMP, 20 mg/kg/day, plus SMZ, 100 mg/kg/day, orally. Adverse effects were seen far less often in patients treated with TMP-SMZ, and, for this reason, it came to be regarded as the drug of choice for PCP [58, 65].

Trimethoprim-sulfamethoxazole seems to derive its antiprotozoal activity from interference with folate metabolism. The drug is available in oral and parenteral preparations, and both have proved effective in the treatment of PCP. In the patient who is severely ill or who might not absorb a drug well from the gastrointestinal tract, parenteral therapy is indicated; for all others, there is no evidence to suggest it is superior to oral therapy.

Trimethoprim-sulfamethoxazole should be avoided in patients with sulfa allergy or glucose 6-phosphate dehydrogenase (G6PD) deficiency. Because TMP-SMZ must be given as a very dilute solution, it should be administered carefully in individuals with a low cardiac ejection fraction. Because TMP-SMZ is excreted primarily by the kidneys, dosage adjustment is required in the presence of renal failure. For a GFR greater than 50 ml per minute, TMP-SMZ should be given as 5 mg/kg TMP every 6 hours. For a GFR of 10 to 50 ml per minute, the same dose should be given every 8 hours, and, if the GFR is less than 10 ml per minute, every 12 hours [67].

The side effects of TMP-SMZ include drug fever, rash (including Stevens-Johnson syndrome), hepatitis, hepatic necrosis, serum sickness, acute hemolytic anemia, agranulocytosis, thrombocytopenia, and aplastic anemia. The concurrent administration of folate or folinic acid does not ameliorate the hematologic effects of the drug. AIDS patients experience a high rate of toxicity to TMP-SMZ, with a 38 to 65 percent incidence of major adverse reactions [9, 13, 57, 71, 75]. As many as 18 to 54 percent of patients require alteration of therapy, usually for drug fever, rash, leukopenia, thrombocytopenia, or increased serum transaminases. Classically, TMP-SMZ reactions occur 7 to 14 days into therapy and are almost invariably reversible with discontinuation of the drug. The use of diphenhydramine or epinephrine, or both may permit continued treatment with TMP-SMZ in the patient with a history of hypersensitivity [76]. Oral desensitization techniques have also been used successfully [77].

There is tenuous evidence in the pre-AIDS literature to suggest that successful clinical outcome correlates with achieving a peak TMP level of 3 to 8 μg/ml and a peak SMZ level of 100 to 150 μg/ml between 60 and 90 minutes after dosing [58, 78]. More recent data suggest that the frequency and severity of TMP-SMZ reactions can be reduced by maintaining serum levels in this same range [79]. Nevertheless, in most institutions, serum TMP-SMZ levels are not routinely monitored.

Initial Drug Therapy

There is considerable debate about whether to use pentamidine or TMP-SMZ as the first-line agent in the treatment of AIDS-related PCP (Table 17-2). This question is impossible to answer with certainty at this time because available data are derived largely from retrospective analysis of small samples of patients who were switched from one drug to the other according to variable definitions of "adverse drug reaction" and "therapeutic failure."

Trimethoprim-sulfamethoxazole has been studied far more extensively than pentamidine in AIDS patients. Of all patients with PCP, 58 to 86 percent have responded to TMP-SMZ therapy, with patients treated for an initial episode doing better than those with recurrent disease [13, 47, 57, 79]. Of patients started on TMP-SMZ, 42 to 85 percent have been switched to pentamidine because of therapeutic failure or adverse reactions [11, 13, 47, 57, 71, 75]. In general, survival rates are much higher for patients switched to pentamidine because of TMP-SMZ reactions (69–100%) than in those switched because of TMP-SMZ failure (11–36%) [11, 13, 47, 57, 75].

Table 17-2 Treatment of Pneumocystis pneumonia*

Drug therapy of choice

Trimethoprim-sulfamethoxazole: TMP, 20 mg/kg/day, and SMZ, 100 mg/kg/day, in four divided doses orally or intravenously, *or*

Pentamidine isethionate, 4 mg/kg/day intravenously, *and*
If $PaO_2 < 70$ or alveolar-arterial gradient > 35, *add*

Prednisone, 40 mg orally bid × 5 days, followed by 40 mg qd orally × 5 days, followed by 20 mg qd orally × 11 days

Alternative agents

Trimethoprim-dapsone
Primaquine-clindamycin
Atovaquone
Trimetrexate

*See text for drug toxicities and additional information.

Investigators have reported a response rate of 44 to 100 percent in PCP patients treated with pentamidine; there are no good data comparing response rates of initial compared to recurrent disease [13, 47, 57, 68, 70, 71, 79]. Of patients started on pentamidine, 22 to 92 percent were switched to TMP-SMZ because of therapeutic failure or adverse reactions [13, 71]. The only study to examine prognostic significance of change in regimen documented a fall in survival rate from 44 percent overall to 22 percent in crossover patients [13].

There have been only two prospective, randomized studies comparing TMP-SMZ to pentamidine in the treatment of AIDS-related PCP. Wharton and associates [71] found that patients started on pentamidine seemed to do better than those started on TMP-SMZ (95 vs. 75% survival). However, statistical significance was not achieved, and 60 percent of patients in both study groups crossed over because of therapeutic failure or adverse reactions. In a non-crossover study, Sattler and colleagues [79] found a significant difference in survival between patients treated with TMP-SMZ and those given pentamidine (86 vs. 61%).

Alternative and Adjunctive Therapies

TMP-SMZ and Pentamidine

Data on the simultaneous use of TMP-SMZ and pentamidine are scarce. Work with a rat model of PCP failed to demonstrate clinical benefit with this regimen, but human experience has been limited by concerns about combined toxicity [80]. In one study, 21 AIDS patients were incidentally discovered to have received 3 or more days of combination therapy after TMP-SMZ failure [57]. These patients fared slightly worse than others given pentamidine alone, but the difference was not significant.

TMP-Dapsone

In the rat model, dapsone and TMP-dapsone seem to be as effective as TMP-SMZ. Although dapsone monotherapy has not proved very successful in HIV-related PCP, TMP-dapsone appears more promising [81]. In an uncontrolled, nonblinded study, Leoung and associates [82] treated 15 AIDS patients suffering their first episode of mild to moderate PCP with TMP 20 mg/kg/day in four divided doses, plus dapsone, 100 mg per day, for 3 weeks. All patients survived, and only two were switched to alternative therapy because of adverse reactions. Medina and colleagues [83] randomized 60 AIDS patients with similar characteristics to receive either TMP-dapsone or a standard course of oral TMP-SMZ. Both groups had over a 90 percent survival rate, but significantly fewer of those treated with TMP-dapsone required a change in therapy because of adverse reactions (30 vs. 57%). Common side effects included rash, nausea and vomiting, methemoglobinemia, hematologic derangements, and hepatitis. Individuals who are candidates for dapsone therapy should be screened for G6PD deficiency.

Primaquine-Clindamycin

In the rat model, primaquine-clindamycin has demonstrated efficacy in the treatment and prophylaxis of PCP, and a growing body of evidence suggests that this combination may be useful in the treatment of HIV-related disease. In an ongoing study, Toma [84] has given primaquine, 15 mg orally once a day, and clindamycin, 300 to 450 mg every 6 hours orally, or 450 to 600 mg every 6 hours intravenously, for 3 weeks to a group of 109 patients, 36 percent of whom did not have firmly diagnosed PCP and 73 percent of whom had received prior treatment with standard agents; 73 percent were "cured" and another 19 percent "improved" with therapy. Black and associates [85] conducted a multicenter, nonrandomized, open-label, pilot study for mild to moderate AIDS-related PCP. Patients were treated with primaquine 30 mg orally once a day, and clindamycin, 1,800 to 2,700 mg per day in divided doses every 6 to 8 hours, for 21 days. The clinical response rate was 92 percent, with treatment-limiting toxicity seen in only 4 of 36 subjects. Ruf and colleagues [36] treated a study group of 19 patients with a first episode of mild to moderate PCP with primaquine, 30 mg orally each day, and clindamycin, 900 mg orally or intravenously four times a day, for 3 weeks. Comparing these subjects with a similar number of matched historical control subjects who had been treated with TMP-SMZ, no difference was found in response rate and no treatment-limiting toxicity was noted.

Side effects have been described in AIDS patients given primaquine-clindamycin, but they appear to be milder than those caused by TMP-SMZ or pentamidine and rarely require alteration of treatment [84–86]. Rash occurs in about 50 percent of cases but usually resolves in 3 to 5 days. Methemoglobinemia is common, but seldom causes symptoms that require intervention. Diarrhea, hepatitis, and leukopenia are seen infrequently.

Aerosol Pentamidine

With appropriate equipment and technique, pentamidine can be nebulized and delivered directly to the lung, with minimal systemic absorption of the drug [87]. Small, uncontrolled pilot studies suggested that AP is effective, nontoxic therapy for mild to moderate AIDS-related PCP, but subsequent trials have not confirmed these results. Soo Hoo and associates [70] randomized 30 patients with mild to moderate PCP to receive either pentamidine aerosol, 8 mg/kg/day, or intravenous pentamidine, 4 mg/kg/day, for 3 weeks. Although much less drug toxicity was seen in the group receiving AP, the clinical outcome was significantly worse (55% response rate vs. 100%). Conte and colleagues [68] obtained similar results when they randomized 45 patients with mild to moderate PCP to receive either pentamidine aerosol, 600 mg per day nebulized, or intravenous pentamidine, 3 mg/kg/day, for 2 to 3 weeks. Subjects who received intravenous treatment had a response rate of 81 percent with no deaths and no relapses, compared to a 53 percent response rate and 12 percent mortality in those receiving AP. Furthermore, 35 percent of the AP group recrudesced within 28 days of treatment and another 24 percent relapsed during a 3-month follow-up period. Given current regimens and delivery systems, AP does not appear particularly effective for the treatment of AIDS-related PCP.

Atovaquone

Atovaquone (formerly known as 566C80), a hydroxynaphthoquinone recently approved by the Food and Drug Administration, has been shown to be a potent and selective inhibitor of de novo pyrimidine synthesis in a number of protozoa. In a phase I study of 19 HIV-seropositive men, Hughes and associates [88] found that atovaquone was well tolerated up to a dose of 3 gm daily for 16 days. In a follow-up, open-label, dose-escalation phase I–II trial, Falloon and colleagues [89] studied the drug in a group of 34 HIV-infected patients with mild to moderate PCP, including 12 with recurrent disease. Overall, 79 percent were treated successfully. Side effects included fever, rash, hepatitis, neutropenia, and anemia, but only four patients (all receiving high-dose therapy) were withdrawn from the study for presumed drug toxicity. Although subjects were given PCP prophylaxis after completing therapy, in 26 percent of those successfully treated with atovaquone recurrent disease developed within 6 months.

Atovaquone appears to be an effective and fairly well-tolerated drug. However, the high PCP relapse rate seen in treated patients is worrisome. Until more data are available, it seems prudent to reserve atovaquone for patients with inadequate response or proven intolerance to traditional therapies. The recommended dose of atovaquone is 750 mg orally three times per day administered with food.

Trimetrexate

Trimetrexate, an antineoplastic agent related to methotrexate, is a potent inhibitor of dihydrofolate reductase. While potentially myelosuppressive, the simultaneous administration of folinic acid ameliorates its hematologic toxicity. In an uncontrolled pilot study performed by Allegra and associates [90], AIDS patients with PCP, including severely ill individuals and patients with recurrent disease, were given trimetrexate, 30 mg/m^2/day intravenously, and folinic acid, 20 mg/m^2 every 6 hours, for 21 days. Cure rates appeared comparable to those seen with standard agents, and the drug was well tolerated. In a subsequent phase I–II dose-escalation study, 54 patients with mild to moderate PCP were treated for 3 weeks, with an 85 percent survival rate [91]. Common side effects included fever, rash, anemia, neutropenia, thrombocytopenia, and hepatitis.

Trimetrexate in combination with folinic acid appears promising as salvage therapy in refractory PCP. The drug can be obtained from the National Institute of Allergy and Infectious Diseases (telephone: 1-800-537-9978) for patients with histologically confirmed PCP who have either failed or shown intolerance to both pentamidine and TMP-SMZ.

Corticosteroids

Data from prospective, randomized trials have demonstrated corticosteroid therapy to be useful adjunctively in the treatment of moderate to severe PCP. Although a study by Clement and associates [92] failed to show a clinical benefit of methylprednisolone for AIDS patients with PCP and room air PaO$_2$ of 50 mm Hg or less, most had not received the agent until after at least 2 days of antimicrobial therapy. In contrast, three groups have been able to demonstrate clinical benefit from early administration of corticosteroids.

Montaner and associates [93] studied patients with first-episode PCP and a room air oxygen saturation of 85% or greater. Although no difference in survival was noted, subjects given adjunctive prednisone within 48 hours were significantly less likely to suffer early clinical deterioration than those given placebo (6 vs. 42%). Gagnon and colleagues [94] studied nonintubated patients with PCP who had a resting respiratory rate of greater than 30 per minute, an alveolar-arterial oxygen gradient of greater than 30 mm Hg on room air, and a PaO_2 of less than 75 mm Hg on 35% oxygen but greater than 60 mm Hg on 100% oxygen. Subjects given adjunctive methylprednisolone within 72 hours were significantly less likely to suffer respiratory failure (25 vs. 82%) and more likely to survive until discharge (75 vs. 18%) than those given placebo. Bozzette and coworkers [95] studied patients with presumed or confirmed PCP who were not intubated and had a hypoxemia ratio (PaO_2:FIO_2) of 75 or greater. Subjects who received adjunctive prednisone or methylprednisolone within 36 hours were significantly less likely to develop respiratory failure (14 vs. 30%) and more likely to survive (86 vs. 70%) than those who did not. In subgroup analysis, clinical benefit could only be demonstrated for patients with moderate to severe disease.

Although there have been case reports of new and accelerated Kaposi's sarcoma in AIDS patients receiving corticosteroid therapy, relatively few complications have been noted with the use of adjunctive steroids for PCP [96, 97]. Gastrointestinal bleeding occurs rarely, and an increased incidence of thrush and localized herpes reactivation has also been described [95]. Thus far, however, there is no evidence that steroid therapy is associated with an increased risk of serious opportunistic infection or PCP relapse [98].

Despite considerable variation in study design, population examined, and steroid regimen employed, the aforementioned studies persuaded the National Institutes of Health (NIH) to issue a consensus statement on the use of corticosteroids as adjunctive therapy for AIDS-related PCP [99]. It recommends that steroids be given to all patients 13 years of age or older with HIV infection and documented or suspected PCP of at least moderate severity (defined as $PaO_2 < 70$ mm Hg or an alveolar-arterial gradient of > 35 mm Hg). It advises that adjunctive steroid therapy be initiated at the same time that antimicrobial agents are started, with a regimen of prednisone, 40 mg orally twice a day for 5 days, followed by 40 mg orally once a day for 5 days, followed by 20 mg orally once a day for 11 days. Intravenous methylprednisolone at 75 percent of the above dosages can be used instead if parenteral treatment is necessary. In the opinion of the NIH, insufficient data exist to allow useful conclusions about the benefit of corticosteroid therapy in patients in whom standard regimens fail or in patients with mild PCP.

Prophylaxis

The issue of PCP prophylaxis was first addressed in the pediatric literature. Success in the animal model of PCP led to large-scale trials of TMP-SMZ in children suffering from hematologic malignancies. In 1977, Hughes and colleagues [100] showed that an oral formulation of TMP, 150 mg/m^2/day, and SMZ, 750 mg/m^2/day, given as two divided doses provided virtually complete protection in a population known to have an attack rate of 20 percent. Ten years later, Hughes and associates [101] examined a similar population and showed that the same dose of TMP-SMZ given 3 consecutive days per week was just as effective for the prevention of PCP.

The high incidence of PCP in the HIV-infected population argues strongly for attempts at prophylaxis. Asymptomatic patients with an absolute CD4 lymphocyte count of fewer than 200 cells/mm^3 or a CD4:total lymphocyte ratio of less than 20 percent are at significant risk for PCP, as are individuals with a prior history of PCP [102, 103]. Patients with thrush or prolonged, unexplained fever may also be at increased risk for PCP despite a CD4 count of greater than 200 cells/mm^3 [103]. Several PCP prophylaxis regimens have been evaluated in HIV-infected patients, including TMP-SMZ, AP, dapsone, pyrimethamine-sulfadoxine, pyrimethamine-sulfadiazine, and zidovudine (ZDV).

Trimethoprim-Sulfamethoxazole

Fischl and associates [104] examined a group of 60 HIV-infected patients with biopsy-proven Kaposi's sarcoma and no history or evidence of opportunistic infection. Subjects were randomly assigned to receive either no therapy or an oral dose of 160 mg TMP and 800 mg SMZ twice a day, and were followed for up to 3 years. No patients receiving TMP-SMZ developed PCP, compared to 53 percent of the control group. Sixty percent of the patients randomized to TMP-SMZ died during the course of the study, compared to 93 percent of the control group.

Data concerning low-dose, intermittent TMP-SMZ prophylaxis of HIV-infected patients are beginning to become available. Wormser and associates [105] gave 160 mg TMP and 800 mg SMZ orally every other day to 67 HIV-seropositive patients with either a CD4 count of less than 200 cells/mm^3 or a history of proven or probable PCP. No episodes of PCP occurred among 32 subjects receiving primary prophylaxis over a mean of 7 months, and one case of recurrent PCP developed among 35 subjects receiving secondary prophylaxis over a mean of 11 months. Adverse reactions occurred in 40 percent of patients, usually leading to discontinuation of the drug. Ruskin and LaRiviere [106] evaluated the prophylactic use of TMP-SMZ, 160 mg/800 mg orally three times a week, in 116 HIV-infected patients. No cases of PCP were seen in primary prophylaxis patients over a mean of 24 months or in secondary prophylaxis patients over a mean of 19 months. Although adverse reactions occurred in 28 percent of individuals, they rarely necessitated discontinuation of the drug. Of note, none of the study subjects developed toxoplasmosis.

Aerosol Pentamidine

Although AP has been disappointing for the treatment of AIDS-related PCP, there is considerable evidence of its efficacy in both primary and secondary prophylaxis. In a prospective, randomized, double-blind, placebo-controlled trial evaluating primary prophylaxis, Hirschel and associates [107] studied 223 HIV-infected patients with CD4 counts of less than $200/mm^3$, advanced AIDS-related complex (ARC), or AIDS without prior PCP. Within a year, 23 cases of PCP had occurred in the placebo group compared to only 8 in the group receiving 300 mg pentamidine isethionate by Respirgard II nebulizer every 28 days. Only 4 percent of those given AP discontinued treatment because of drug toxicity. Montaner and colleagues [108] achieved equally impressive results in a similar trial of secondary prophylaxis. They studied 164 HIV-infected patients who had suffered one prior episode of PCP and no other AIDS-defining opportunistic infection. Over a mean follow-up period of 15.5 weeks, 27 of 32 (84%) PCP recurrences had occurred in the placebo group. Only one subject receiving pentamidine reported clinically significant side effects. Large dose-ranging studies by Leoung and coworkers [109] and Murphy and associates [24] confirm the efficacy and safety of both the Respirgard and Fisoneb AP prophylactic regimens [24,109].

Many patients treated with AP complain of metallic taste, but it usually resolves once treatment is completed and fluids are given. Drug-induced bronchospasm and coughing spells are common, especially in smokers and asthmatics. Inhaled bronchodilators given as needed or before treatment and cessation of smoking greatly ameliorate symptoms in most cases. Every effort must be made to rule out transmissible respiratory diseases such as tuberculosis before initiation of therapy. Since very little AP is absorbed from the lungs, systemic side effects are unusual. However, asymptomatic hypoglycemia and pancreatitis, including fatal episodes, have rarely been reported.

The failure of AP to achieve significant blood levels may not be altogether fortunate. Distribution of an aerosol drug is determined by ventilatory dynamics and the size of the particles generated by whatever delivery system is employed. Not all nebulizer systems are equally effective in delivering AP to the pulmonary alveoli [87]. Even under ideal circumstances, the upper lobes receive less drug than other regions. In patients who have preexisting lung damage or who are too debilitated to generate maximum inspiratory effort, drug distribution can be even more problematic. Breakthrough pneumocystosis may present atypically in patients receiving AP, displaying focal radiographic or gallium abnormalities, predominantly in the upper lung fields [18, 20–24]. Furthermore, approximately 50 percent of the cases of HIV-related extrapulmonary pneumocystosis reported to date have occurred in patients receiving AP prophylaxis [6, 7, 14].

Dapsone

Dapsone provides highly effective PCP prophylaxis in the rat model. Early studies by Metroka and coworkers [110, 111] suggested that patients given dapsone, 25 mg orally four times a day, received effective primary and secondary prophylaxis compared to untreated historical controls and to patients given oral TMP-SMZ, one double-strength tablet twice a day. Hughes and associates [112] gave dapsone—100, 200, or 300 mg weekly—to 61 AIDS patients as primary and secondary prophylaxis. Only one case of PCP developed over a time course in which 14 were expected based on historical controls. Lavelle and colleagues [113] are conducting a trial of dapsone, 200 mg once a week, with or without pyrimethamine, 25 mg once a week, for primary and secondary prophylaxis. Preliminary analysis of 45 patients over a median follow-up period of 40 weeks has documented only two cases of PCP, one in each group.

Studies suggest that 10 to 15 percent of patients treated with dapsone will experience side effects (described above), but they are seldom severe and almost always reversible with cessation of the drug. Dapsone can usually be employed safely in HIV-infected patients with a history of TMP-SMZ intolerance, including severe reactions [114].

Pyrimethamine-Sulfadoxine

Fansidar contains 25 mg pyrimethamine and 500 mg sulfadoxine. Two open, uncontrolled studies documented the efficacy of one tablet per week for the prophylaxis of AIDS-related PCP [115, 116]. However, Fischl and Dickinson [117] found pyrimethamine-sulfadoxine to be ineffective primary prophylaxis in a group of 30 HIV-seropositive patients with newly diagnosed Kaposi's sarcoma and no history or evidence of opportunistic infection.

Pyrimethamine-sulfadoxine possesses the same toxicity profile as other sulfa-containing compounds, but severe mucocutaneous reactions may be more common than with shorter-acting agents. One fatal and several nonfatal cases of Stevens-Johnson syndrome have been reported [118]. Thus, despite the obvious appeal of a simple, inexpensive, oral regimen, many clinicians are reluctant to use this agent routinely.

Pyrimethamine-Sulfadiazine

Pyrimethamine-sulfadiazine is commonly used in the treatment and prophylaxis of cerebral toxoplasmosis. In a large cohort study, Heald and associates [119] found that the incidence of PCP was substantially lower in patients receiving treatment for cerebral toxoplasmosis than in patients with other severe opportunistic infections and similar to that seen in individuals receiving AP prophylaxis. The most frequently used prophylactic regimens were 25 mg pyrimethamine with 3,000 mg sulfadiazine or 2,400 mg clindamycin daily. Only one of the six prophylaxis failures occurred in patients receiving pyrimethamine-sulfadiazine. There have been no prospective studies of pyrimethamine-sulfadiazine for PCP prophylaxis.

Zidovudine

Although ZDV has no intrinsic activity against *P. carinii*, it seems reasonable that an antiretroviral agent might have prophylactic value to the extent that it improves host immune function. In fact, several large, prospective, randomized trials found decreased PCP incidence and increased survival in ARC and AIDS patients receiving ZDV [109, 120, 121]. However, other studies have been less convincing. Recurrence rates equivalent to historical and untreated controls have been described in AIDS patients given ZDV after the first episode of PCP [122–124]. ARC and AIDS patients receiving ZDV alone suffer a significantly higher incidence of PCP than those also receiving specific prophylactic therapy [124, 125]. Furthermore, in patients receiving AP who have been followed prospectively, it has not been possible to demonstrate additional prophylactic benefit from ZDV therapy [20, 108].

Comparison of Regimens

In controlled trials, TMP-SMZ has been shown to be effective for primary PCP prophylaxis and AP effective for both primary and secondary prophylaxis [104, 107, 108]. However, it is only recently that data comparing these regimens have become available. A study performed by the AIDS Clinical Trials Group has convincingly demonstrated the superiority of TMP-SMZ over AP in secondary PCP prophylaxis [126]. In this study, 310 participants were randomized to receive either TMP-SMZ,

Table 17-3 Comparison of PCP prophylaxis regimens

Issue	TMP-SMZ	Dapsone	AP
Efficacy	High	?Moderate	Moderate
Toxicity	Moderate	Low	Low
Drug interaction	Zidovudine	Didanosine	None
Cost	Low	Low	High
Toxoplasmosis protection	Yes	?	No

one double-strength tablet daily, or AP, 300 mg every 4 weeks by means of a Respirgard II nebulizer for secondary prophylaxis. Interim analysis showed that in 4.5 percent of subjects receiving TMP-SMZ recurrent PCP developed within 12 months, compared to 18.5 percent of those receiving AP. Although side effect profiles were remarkably similar in the two groups, subjects initially treated with TMP-SMZ had to be crossed over more frequently than those who received AP (27 vs. 4%).

Another recent prospective study has shown TMP-SMZ to be superior to AP for primary PCP prophylaxis [127]. Subjects were randomized to receive AP, 300 mg once a month; TMP-SMZ, one single-strength tablet daily; or TMP-SMZ, one double-strength tablet daily. At 12 months follow-up, 8 percent of subjects receiving AP had a documented case of PCP, compared to none in both of the two TMP-SMZ groups. Of subjects who received TMP-SMZ, 25 percent experienced drug toxicity compared to 3 percent of those who received AP.

Management Recommendations

Prophylaxis with TMP-SMZ, AP, or dapsone reduces the incidence of PCP in patients with advanced HIV disease. Recent data indicate that the use of PCP prophylaxis is also associated with improved survival [128]. Table 17-3 compares key features of available PCP prophylaxis regimens. TMP-SMZ appears to be the most effective agent but has the greatest toxicity. Aerosol pentamidine and dapsone have been associated with breakthrough PCP infection, and extrapulmonary disease seems to be a significant problem with AP because it is not systemically absorbed. TMP-SMZ may be difficult to give to patients who are receiving other marrow suppressants such as ZDV; dapsone may interfere with the absorption of didanosine (ddI) if dosed at the same time. A potential benefit of AP therapy is the ability to monitor compliance. However, AP costs considerably more than either TMP-SMZ or dap-

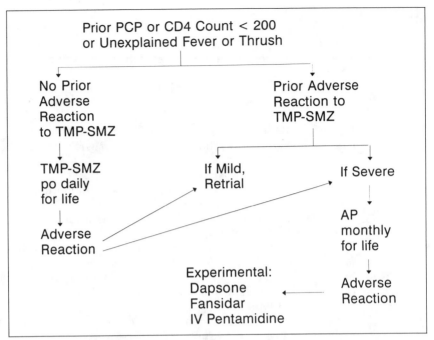

Figure 17-3. *Algorithm for prophylaxis of* Pneumocystis carinii *pneumonia. (Adapted from Centers for Disease Control, Recommendations for prophylaxis against* Pneumocystis carinii *pneumonia for adults and adolescents infected with human immunodeficiency virus. MMWR 41[RR-4]:1–11, 1992.)*

sone. TMP-SMZ appears to afford some protection against toxoplasmosis as well as PCP [129].

On the basis of available data, the United States Public Health Service has published guidelines for PCP prophylaxis [130] (Fig. 17-3). Current recommendations are that, unless contraindicated, lifetime PCP prophylaxis be initiated in HIV-infected adults who have a prior history of PCP, a CD4 count of less than 200 cells/mm^3, or constitutional symptoms such as thrush or unexplained fever greater than 100°F for 2 weeks or longer. Three prophylaxis regimens are endorsed: (1) 160 mg TMP and 800 mg SMZ orally once a day; (2) 300 mg AP once a month by means of a Respirgard II jet nebulizer; and (3) five 60-mg AP loading doses over a 2-week period, followed by a 60-mg dose every 2 weeks by means of a Fisoneb nebulizer. TMP-SMZ should be used initially. In patients who experience a mild reaction to TMP-SMZ, rechallenge is appropriate. In individuals with significant toxicity, AP should be given as alternative therapy. Dapsone may be used in patients who experience breakthrough PCP or toxicity on AP.

References

1. Edman JC, Kovacs JA, Masur H, et al. Ribosomal RNA sequence shows *Pneumocystis carinii* to be a member of the fungi. *Nature* 334:519–522, 1988.
2. ul Haque A, Plattner SB, Cook RT, Hart MN. *Pneumocystis carinii:* Taxonomy as viewed by electron microscopy. *Am J Clin Pathol* 87:504–510, 1987.
3. Meuwissen JH, Tauber I, Leeuwenberg PJ, et al. Parasitologic and serologic observations of infection with pneumocystis in humans. *J Infect Dis* 136:43–49, 1977.
4. Pifer LL, Hughes WT, Stagno S, Woods D. *Pneumocystis carinii* infection: Evidence for high prevalence in normal and immunosuppressed children. *Pediatrics* 61:35–41, 1978.
5. Esterly JA. *Pneumocystis carinii* in lungs of adults at autopsy. *Am Rev Respir Dis* 97:935–937, 1968.
6. Raviglione MC. Extrapulmonary pneumocystosis: The first fifty cases. *Rev Infect Dis* 12:1127–1138, 1990.
7. Northfelt DW, Clement MJ, Safrin S. Extrapulmonary pneumocystosis: Clinical features in human immunodeficiency virus infection. *Medicine* 69:392–398, 1990.
8. Catterall JR, Potasman I, Remington JS. *Pneumocystis carinii* pneumonia in the patient with AIDS. *Chest* 88:758–762, 1985.
9. Engelberg LA, Lerner CW, Tapper ML. Clinical features of *Pneumocystis* pneumonia in the acquired immune deficiency syndrome. *Am Rev Respir Dis* 130:689–694, 1984.
10. Mills J. *Pneumocystis carinii* and *Toxoplasma gondii* infections in patients with AIDS. *Rev Infect Dis* 8:1001–1010, 1986.
11. Murray JF, Felton CP, Garay SM, et al. Pulmonary complications of the acquired immunodeficiency syndrome: report of National Heart, Lung, and Blood Institute Workshop. *N Engl J Med* 310:1682–1688, 1984.
12. Stover DE, White DA, Romano PA, et al. Spectrum of pulmonary diseases associated with the acquired immune deficiency syndrome. *Am J Med* 78:429–437, 1985.
13. Kovacs JA, Hiemenz JW, Macher AM, et al. *Pneumocystis carinii* pneumonia: A comparison between patients with the acquired immunodeficiency syndrome and patients with other immunodeficiencies. *Ann Intern Med* 100:663–671, 1984.
14. Cohen OJ, Stoeckle MY. Extrapulmonary *Pneumocystis carinii* infections in the acquired immunodeficiency syndrome. *Arch Intern Med* 151:1205–1214, 1991.
15. DeLorenzo LJ, Huang CT, Maguire GP, Stone DJ. Roentgenographic patterns of *Pneumocystis carinii* pneumonia in 104 patients with AIDS. *Chest* 91:323–327, 1987.
16. Naidich DP, Garay SM, Leitman BS, McCauley DI. Radiographic manifestations of pulmonary disease in the acquired immunodeficiency syndrome (AIDS). *Semin Roentgenol* 22:14–30, 1987.

17. Suster B, Akerman M, Orenstein M, Wax M. Pulmonary manifestations of AIDS: Review of 106 episodes. *Radiology* 161:87–93, 1986.
18. Jules-Elysee KM, Stover DE, Zaman MB, et al. Aerosolized pentamidine: Effect on diagnosis and presentation of *Pneumocystis carinii* pneumonia. *Ann Intern Med* 112:750–757, 1990.
19. Tietjen PA, Jules-Elysee KM, Stover DE. Increased incidence of pneumothoraces with aerosolized pentamidine. *Chest* 96:187S, 1989.
20. Golden JA, Chernoff D, Hollander H, et al. Prevention of *Pneumocystis carinii* pneumonia by inhaled pentamidine. *Lancet* 1:654–757, 1989.
21. Lowery S, Fallat R, Feigal DW, et al. Changing patterns of *Pneumocystis carinii* pneumonia (PCP) on pentamidine aerosol prophylaxis. Fourth International Conference on AIDS, Stockholm, June 1988.
22. Levine SJ, Masur H, Gill VJ, et al. Effect of aerosolized pentamidine prophylaxis on the diagnosis of *Pneumocystis carinii* pneumonia by induced sputum examination in patients infected with the human immunodeficiency virus. *Am Rev Respir Dis* 144:760–764, 1991.
23. Chaffey MH, Klein JS, Gamsu G, et al. Radiographic distribution of *Pneumocystis carinii* pneumonia in patients with AIDS treated with prophylactic inhaled pentamidine. *Radiology* 175:715–719, 1990.
24. Murphy RL, Lavelle JP, Allan JD, et al. Aerosol pentamidine prophylaxis following *Pneumocystis carinii* pneumonia in AIDS patients: Results of a blinded dose-comparison study using an ultrasonic nebulizer. *Am J Med* 90:418–426, 1991.
25. Curtis J, Goodman P, Hopewell P. Noninvasive tests in the diagnostic evaluation for *P. carinii* pneumonia in patients with or suspected of having AIDS. *Am Rev Respir Dis* 133:A182, 1986.
26. Smith DE, McLuckie A, Wyatt J, et al. Severe exercise hypoxemia with normal or near normal x-rays: A feature of *Pneumocystis carinii* infection. *Lancet* 2:1049–1051, 1988.
27. Stover DE, Greeno RA, Gagliardi AJ. The use of a simple exercise test for the diagnosis of *Pneumocystis carinii* pneumonia in patients with AIDS. *Am Rev Respir Dis* 139:1343–1346, 1989.
28. Barron TF, Birnbaum NS, Shane LB, et al. *Pneumocystis carinii* pneumonia studied by gallium-67 scanning. *Radiology* 154:791–793, 1985.
29. Coleman DL, Hattner RS, Luce JM, et al. Correlation between gallium lung scans and fiberoptic bronchoscopy in patients with suspected *Pneumocystis carinii* pneumonia and the acquired immune deficiency syndrome. *Am Rev Respir Dis* 130:1166–1169, 1984.
30. Kramer EL, Sanger JJ, Garay SM, et al. Gallium-67 scans of the chest in patients with acquired immunodeficiency syndrome. *J Nucl Med* 28:1107–1114, 1987.
31. Woolfenden JM, Carrasquillo JA, Larson SM, et al. Acquired immunodeficiency syndrome: Ga-67 citrate imaging. *Radiology* 162:383–387, 1987.
32. Kim HK, Hughes WT. Comparison of methods for identification of *Pneumocystis carinii* in pulmonary aspirates. *Am J Clin Pathol* 60:464–466, 1973.

33. Broaddus C, Dake MD, Stulbarg MS, et al. Bronchoalveolar lavage and transbronchial biopsy for the diagnosis of pulmonary infections in the acquired immunodeficiency syndrome. *Ann Intern Med* 102:747–752, 1985.
34. Milligan SA, Luce JM, Golden J, et al. Transbronchial biopsy without fluoroscopy in patients with diffuse roentgenographic infiltrates and the acquired immunodeficiency syndrome. *Am Rev Respir Dis* 137:486–488, 1988.
35. Stover DE, White DA, Romano PA, Gellene RA. Diagnosis of pulmonary disease in acquired immune deficiency syndrome (AIDS). *Am Rev Respir Dis* 130:659–662, 1984.
36. Miller RF, Millar AB, Semple SJG. Complications of fiberoptic bronchoscopy in HIV-1 antibody positive patients undergoing investigations for pulmonary disease. *Thorax* 43:847A, 1988.
37. Golden JA, Hollander H, Stulbarg MS, et al. Bronchoalveolar lavage as the exclusive diagnostic modality for *Pneumocystis carinii* pneumonia: A prospective study among patients with acquired immunodeficiency syndrome. *Chest* 90:18–22, 1986.
38. Barrio JL, Harcup C, Baier HJ, et al. Value of repeat fiberoptic bronchoscopies and significance of nondiagnostic bronchoscopic results in patients with the acquired immunodeficiency syndrome. *Am Rev Respir Dis* 135:422–425, 1987.
39. Bigby TD, Margolskee D, Curtis JL, et al. The usefulness of induced sputum in the diagnosis of *Pneumocystis carinii* pneumonia in patients with the acquired immunodeficiency syndrome. *Am Rev Respir Dis* 133:515–518, 1986.
40. Kovacs JA, Ng VL, Masur H, et al. Diagnosis of *Pneumocystis carinii* pneumonia: Improved detection in sputum with use of monoclonal antibodies. *N Engl J Med* 318:589–593, 1988.
41. Ng VL, Gartner I, Weymouth LA, et al. The use of mucolysed induced sputum for the identification of pulmonary pathogens associated with human immunodeficiency virus infection. *Arch Pathol Lab Med* 113:488–493, 1989.
42. Pitchenik AE, Ganjei P, Torres A, et al. Sputum examination for the diagnosis of *Pneumocystis carinii* pneumonia in the acquired immunodeficiency syndrome. *Am Rev Respir Dis* 133:226–229, 1986.
43. Zaman MK, Wooten OJ, Suprahmanya B, et al. Rapid noninvasive diagnosis of *Pneumocystis carinii* from induced liquified sputum. *Ann Intern Med* 109:7–10, 1988.
44. Ng VL, Yajko DM, McPhaul LW, et al. Evaluation of an indirect fluorescent-antibody stain for detection of *Pneumocystis carinii* in respiratory specimens. *J Clin Microbiol* 28:975–979, 1990.
45. Virani N, Ng VL, Chaisson RE, et al. Rapid diagnosis of *Pneumocystis carinii* pneumonia (PCP) in patients with AIDS using a direct fluorescent monoclonal antibody (DFA) assay. Fifth International Conference on AIDS, Montreal, June 1989.
46. Winston DJ, Lau WK, Gale RP, Young LS. Trimethoprim-sulfamethoxa-

zole for the treatment of *Pneumocystis carinii* pneumonia. *Ann Intern Med* 92:762–769, 1980.

47. Small CB, Harris CA, Friedland GH, Klein RS. The treatment of *Pneumocystis carinii* pneumonia in the acquired immunodeficiency syndrome. *Arch Intern Med* 145:837–840, 1985.

48. Efferen LS, Nadarajah D, Palat DS. Survival following mechanical ventilation for *Pneumocystis carinii* pneumonia in patients with the acquired immunodeficiency syndrome: a different perspective. *Am J Med* 87:401–404, 1989.

49. Silverman BA, Rubinstein A. Serum lactate dehydrogenase levels in adults and children with acquired immune deficiency syndrome (AIDS) and AIDS-related complex: Possible indicator of B cell lymphoproliferation and disease activity. *Am J Med* 78:728–736, 1985.

50. Zaman MK, White DA. Serum lactate dehydrogenase levels and *Pneumocystis carinii* pneumonia. *Am Rev Respir Dis* 137:796–800, 1988.

51. Coleman DL, Dodek PM, Golden JA, et al. Correlation between serial pulmonary function tests and fiberoptic bronchoscopy in patients with *Pneumocystis carinii* pneumonia and the acquired immune deficiency syndrome. *Am Rev Respir Dis* 129:491–493, 1984.

52. DeLorenzo LJ, Maguire GP, Wormser GP, et al. Persistence of *Pneumocystis carinii* pneumonia in the acquired immunodeficiency syndrome: Evaluation of therapy by follow-up transbronchial lung biopsy. *Chest* 88:79–83, 1985.

53. Hartmann B, Koss M, Hui A, et al. *Pneumocystis carinii* pneumonia in the acquired immunodeficiency syndrome (AIDS): Diagnosis with bronchial brushings, biopsy, and bronchoalveolar lavage. *Chest* 87:603–607, 1985.

54. Shelhamer JH, Ognibene FP, Macher AM, et al. Persistence of *Pneumocystis carinii* in lung tissue of acquired immunodeficiency syndrome patients treated for pneumocystis pneumonia. *Am Rev Respir Dis* 130:1161–1165, 1984.

55. Colangelo G, Baughman RP, Dohn MN, Frame PT. Follow-up bronchoalveolar lavage in AIDS patients with *Pneumocystis carinii* pneumonia: *Pneumocystis carinii* burden predicts early relapse. *Am Rev Respir Dis* 143:1067–1071, 1991.

56. Brenner M, Ognibene FP, Lack EE, et al. Prognostic factors and life expectancy of patients with acquired immunodeficiency syndrome and *Pneumocystis carinii* pneumonia. *Am Rev Respir Dis* 136:1199–1206, 1987.

57. Haverkos HW. Assessment of therapy for *Pneumocystis carinii* pneumonia: PCP therapy project group. *Am J Med* 76:501–508, 1984.

58. Hughes WT, Feldman S, Chaudhary SC, et al. Comparison of pentamidine isethionate and trimethoprim-sulfamethoxazole in the treatment of *Pneumocystis carinii* pneumonia. *J Pediatr* 92:285–291, 1978.

59. Kales CP, Murren JR, Torres RA, et al. Early predictors of in-hospital mortality for *Pneumocystis carinii* pneumonia in the acquired immunodeficiency syndrome. *Arch Intern Med* 147:1413–1417, 1987.

60. Conte JE, Hollander H, Golden JA. Inhaled or reduced-dose pentamidine for *Pneumocystis carinii* pneumonia: A pilot study. *Ann Intern Med* 107:495–498, 1987.

61. Feigal DW, Edison R, Leoung GS, et al. Recurrent *Pneumocystis carinii* pneumonia (PCP) in 201 patients before AZT or prophylaxis: Implications for clinical trials. Fourth International Conference on AIDS, Stockholm, June 1988.

62. Wachter RM, Luce JM, Turner J, et al. Intensive care of patients with the acquired immunodeficiency syndrome: outcome and changing patterns of utilization. *Am Rev Respir Dis* 134:891–896, 1986.

63. Wachter RM, Russi MB, Bloch DA, et al. *Pneumocystis carinii* pneumonia and respiratory failure in AIDS: Improved outcomes and increased use of intensive care units. *Am Rev Respir Dis* 143:251–256, 1991.

64. Drake S, Lampasona V, Nicks HL, Schwarzmann SW. Pentamidine isethionate in the treatment of *Pneumocystis carinii* pneumonia. *Clin Pharmacol* 4:507–516, 1985.

65. Hughes WT. *Pneumocystis carinii* pneumonitis. *Antibiot Chemother* 30:257–271, 1981.

66. Navin TR, Fontaine RE. Intravenous versus intramuscular administration of pentamidine. *N Engl J Med* 311:1701–1702, 1984.

67. Bennett WM, Muther RS, Parker RA, et al. Drug therapy in renal failure: Dosing guidelines for adults. *Ann Intern Med* 93:62–83, 1980.

68. Conte JE, Chernoff D, Feigal DW, et al. Intravenous or inhaled pentamidine for treating *Pneumocystis carinii* pneumonia in AIDS. *Ann Intern Med* 113:203–209, 1990.

69. Pearson RD, Hewlett EL. Pentamidine for the treatment of *Pneumocystis carinii* pneumonia and other protozoal diseases. *Ann Intern Med* 103:782–786, 1985.

70. Soo Hoo GW, Mohsenifar Z, Meyer RD. Inhaled or intravenous pentamidine therapy for *Pneumocystis carinii* pneumonia in AIDS. *Ann Intern Med* 113:195–202, 1990.

71. Wharton JM, Coleman D, Wofsy C, et al. Trimethoprim-sulfamethoxazole or pentamidine for *Pneumocystis carinii* pneumonia in the acquired immunodeficiency syndrome: a prospective randomized trial. *Ann Intern Med* 105:37–44, 1986.

72. Lachaal M, Venuto RC. Nephrotoxicity and hyperkalemia in patients with acquired immunodeficiency syndrome treated with pentamidine. *Am J Med* 87:260–263, 1989.

73. Polsky B, Dryjanski J, Whimbey E, et al. Severe neutropenia during pentamidine treatment of *Pneumocystis carinii* pneumonia in patients with acquired immunodeficiency syndrome—New York City. *MMWR* 33:65–67, 1984.

74. Bouchard Ph, Sai P, Reach G, et al. Diabetes mellitus following pentamidine-induced hypoglycemia in humans. *Diabetes* 31:40–45, 1982.

75. Gordin FM, Simon GL, Wofsy CB, Mills J. Adverse reactions to trimethoprim-sulfamethoxazole in patients with the acquired immunodeficiency syndrome. *Ann Intern Med* 100:495–499, 1984.

76. Gibbons RB, Lindauer JA. Successful treatment of *Pneumocystis carinii*

pneumonia with trimethoprim-sulfamethoxazole in hypersensitive AIDS patients. *JAMA* 253: 1259–1260, 1985.

77. Finegold I. Oral desensitization to trimethoprim-sulfamethoxazole in a patient with acquired immunodeficiency syndrome. *Allergy Clin Immunol* 78:905–908, 1986.

78. Lau WK, Young LS. Trimethoprim-sulfamethoxazole treatment of *Pneumocystis carinii* pneumonia in adults. *N Engl J Med* 295:716–718, 1976.

79. Sattler FR, Cowan R, Nielsen D, et al. Trimethoprim-sulfamethoxazole compared with pentamidine for the treatment of *Pneumocystis carinii* pneumonia in the acquired immunodeficiency syndrome: A prospective, noncrossover study. *Ann Intern Med* 109:280–287, 1988.

80. Kluge RM, Spaulding DM, Spain AJ. Combination of pentamidine and trimethoprim-sulfamethoxazole in the therapy of *Pneumocystis carinii* pneumonia in rats. *Antimicrob Agents Chemother* 13:975–978, 1978.

81. Mills J, Leoung G, Medina I, et al. Dapsone treatment of *Pneumocystis carinii* pneumonia in the acquired immunodeficiency syndrome. *Antimicrob Agents Chemother* 32: 1057–1060, 1988.

82. Leoung GS, Mills J, Hopewell PC, et al. Dapsone-trimethoprim for *Pneumocystis carinii* pneumonia in the acquired immunodeficiency syndrome. *Ann Intern Med* 105:45–48, 1986.

83. Medina I, Mills J, Leoung G, et al. Oral therapy for *Pneumocystis carinii* pneumonia in the acquired immunodeficiency syndrome: A controlled trial of trimethoprim-sulfamethoxazole versus trimethoprim-dapsone. *N Engl J Med* 323:776–782, 1990.

84. Toma E. Clindamycin/primaquine for treatment of *Pneumocystis carinii* pneumonia in AIDS. *Eur J Clin Microbiol Infect Dis* 10:210–213, 1991.

85. Black JR, Feinberg J, Murphy RL, et al. Clindamycin and primaquine as primary treatment for mild and moderately severe *Pneumocystis carinii* pneumonia in patients with AIDS. *Eur J Clin Microbiol Infect Dis* ;10:204–207, 1991.

86. Ruf B, Rohde I, Pohle HD. Efficacy of clindamycin/primaquine versus trimethoprim/sulfamethoxazole in primary treatment of *Pneumocystis carinii* pneumonia. *Eur J Clin Microbiol Infect Dis* 10:207–210, 1991.

87. Corkery KJ, Luce JM, Montgomery AB. Aerosolized pentamidine for treatment and prophylaxis of *Pneumocystis carinii* pneumonia: An update. *Respir Care* 33:676–685, 1988.

88. Hughes WT, Kennedy W, Shenep JL, et al. Safety and pharmacokinetics of 566C80, a hydroxynaphthoquinone with anti–*Pneumocystis carinii* activity: A phase I study in human immunodeficiency virus (HIV)-infected men. *J Infect Dis* 163:843–848, 1991.

89. Falloon J, Kovacs J, Hughes W, et al. A preliminary evaluation of 566C80 for the treatment of pneumocystis pneumonia in patients with the acquired immunodeficiency syndrome. *N Engl J Med* 325:1534–1538, 1991.

90. Allegra CJ, Chabner BA, Tuazon CU, et al. Trimetrexate for the treatment of *Pneumocystis carinii* pneumonia in patients with acquired immunodeficiency syndrome. *N Engl J Med* 317:978–985, 1987.

91. Sattler FR, Allegra CJ, Verdegem, TD, et al. Trimetrexate-leucovorin dos-

age evaluation study for treatment of *Pneumocystis carinii* pneumonia. *J Infect Dis* 161:91–96, 1990.

92. Clement M, Edison R, Turner J, et al. Corticosteroids as adjunctive therapy in severe *Pneumocystis carinii* pneumonia: A prospective placebo-controlled trial. *Am Rev Respir Dis* 139:A250, 1989.

93. Montaner JSG, Lawson LM, Levitt N, et al. Corticosteroids prevent early deterioration in patients with moderately severe *Pneumocystis carinii* pneumonia and the acquired immunodeficiency syndrome (AIDS). *Ann Intern Med* 113:14–20, 1990.

94. Gagnon S, Boota AM, Fischl MA, et al. Corticosteroids as adjunctive therapy for severe *Pneumocystis carinii* pneumonia in the acquired immunodeficiency syndrome. *N Engl J Med* 323:1444–1450, 1990.

95. Bozzette SA, Sattler FR, Chiu J, et al. A controlled trial of early adjunctive treatment with corticosteroids for *Pneumocystis carinii* pneumonia in the acquired immunodeficiency syndrome. *N Engl J Med* 323:1451–1457, 1990.

96. Gill PS, Loureiro C, Bernstein-Singer M, et al. Clinical effect of glucocorticoids on Kaposi sarcoma related to the acquired immunodeficiency syndrome (AIDS). *Ann Intern Med* 110:937–940, 1989.

97. Real FX, Krown SE, Koziner B. Steroid-related development of Kaposi's sarcoma in a homosexual man with Burkitt's lymphoma. *Am J Med* 80:119–122, 1986.

98. Lambertus MW, Goetz MB, Murthy AR, Mathisen GE. Complications of corticosteroid therapy in patients with the acquired immunodeficiency syndrome and *Pneumocystis carinii* pneumonia. *Chest* 98:38–43, 1990.

99. National Institutes of Health—University of California expert panel for corticosteroids as adjunctive therapy for pneumocystis pneumonia. Special report: Consensus statement on the use of corticosteroids as adjunctive therapy for pneumocystis pneumonia in the acquired immunodeficiency syndrome. *N Engl J Med* 323:1500–1504, 1990.

100. Hughes WT, Kuhn S, Chaudhary S, et al. Successful chemoprophylaxis for *Pneumocystis carinii* pneumonitis. *N Engl J Med* 297:1419–1426, 1977.

101. Hughes WT, Rivera GK, Schell MJ, et al. Successful intermittent chemoprophylaxis for *Pneumocystis carinii* pneumonitis. *N Engl J Med* 316:1627–1632, 1987.

102. Masur H, Ognibene FP, Yarchoan R, et al. CD4 counts as predictors of opportunistic pneumonias in human immunodeficiency virus (HIV) infection. *Ann Intern Med* 111:223–231, 1989.

103. Phair J, Munoz A, Detels R, et al. The risk of *Pneumocystis carinii* pneumonia among men infected with human immunodeficiency virus type I. *N Engl J Med* 322:161–165, 1990.

104. Fischl MA, Dickinson GM, La Voie L. Safety and efficacy of sulfamethoxazole and trimethoprim chemoprophylaxis for *Pneumocystis carinii* pneumonia in AIDS. *JAMA* 259:1185–1189, 1988.

105. Wormser GP, Horowitz HW, Duncanson FP, et al. Low-dose intermittent trimethoprim-sulfamethoxazole for prevention of *Pneumocystis*

carinii pneumonia in patients with human immunodeficiency virus infection. *Arch Intern Med* 151:688–692, 1991.

106. Ruskin J, LaRiviere M. Low-dose co-trimoxazole for prevention of *Pneumocystis carinii* pneumonia in human immunodeficiency virus disease. *Lancet* 337:468–471, 1991.
107. Hirschel B, Lazzarin A, Chopard P, et al. A controlled study of inhaled pentamidine for primary prevention of *Pneumocystis carinii* pneumonia. *N Engl J Med* 324:1079–1083, 1991.
108. Montaner JSG, Lawson LM, Geravais A, et al. Aerosol pentamidine for secondary prophylaxis of AIDS-related *Pneumocystis carinii* pneumonia: A randomized, placebo-controlled study. *Ann Intern Med* 114:948–953, 1991.
109. Leoung GS, Feigal DW, Montgomery AB, et al. Aerosolized pentamidine for prophylaxis against *Pneumocystis carinii* pneumonia: The San Francisco Community Prophylaxis Trial. *N Engl J Med* 323:769–775, 1990.
110. Metroka CE, Braun N, Josefberg H, et al. Successful chemoprophylaxis for *Pneumocystis carinii* pneumonia with dapsone in patients with AIDS and ARC. Fourth International Conference on AIDS, Stockholm, June 1988.
111. Metroka CE, Jacobus D, Lewis N. Successful chemoprophylaxis for pneumocystis with dapsone or Bactrim. Fifth International Conference on AIDS, Montreal, June 1989.
112. Hughes WT, Kennedy W, Dugdale M, et al. Prevention of *Pneumocystis carinii* pneumonitis in AIDS patients with weekly dapsone. *Lancet* 336:1066, 1990.
113. Lavelle J, Falloon J, Morgan A, et al. Weekly dapsone and dapsone/pyrimethamine for PCP prophylaxis. Seventh International Conference on AIDS, Florence, June 1991.
114. Edelson PJ, Metroka CE, Friedman-Kien AF. Dapsone, trimethoprim-sulfamethoxazole, and the acquired immunodeficiency syndrome. *Ann Intern Med* 103:963, 1985.
115. Gottlieb MS, Knight S, Mitsuyasu R, et al. Prophylaxis of *Pneumocystis carinii* infection in AIDS with pyrimethamine-sulfadoxine. *Lancet* 2:398–399, 1984.
116. Madoff LC, Scavuzzo D, Roberts RB. Fansidar secondary prophylaxis of *Pneumocystis carinii* pneumonia in AIDS patients. *Clin Research* 34:524A, 1986.
117. Fischl MA, Dickinson GM. Fansidar prophylaxis of *Pneumocystis* pneumonia in the acquired immunodeficiency syndrome. *Ann Intern Med* 105:629, 1986.
118. Centers for Disease Control. Fansidar-associated fatal reaction in an HIV-infected man. *MMWR* 37:571–577, 1988.
119. Heald A, Flepp M, Chave JP, et al. Treatment for cerebral toxoplasmosis protects against *Pneumocystis carinii* pneumonia in patients with AIDS. *Ann Intern Med* 115:760–763, 1991.
120. Fischl MA, Richman DD, Grieco MH, et al. The efficacy of azidothymidine (AZT) in the treatment of patients with AIDS and AIDS-related com-

plex: A double-blind, placebo-controlled trial. *N Engl J Med* 317:185–191, 1987.

121. Montgomery AB, Leoung GS, Wardlaw LA, et al. Effect of zidovudine on mortality rates and *Pneumocystis carinii* (PCP) incidence in AIDS and ARC patients on aerosol pentamidine. *Am Rev Respir Dis* 139: A250, 1989.

122. Campbell SSW, Carrow MJ, Gold JWM, et al. Comparison of second episodes of *Pneumocystis carinii* pneumonia between AIDS patients treated and not treated with AZT. Fourth International Conference on AIDS, Stockholm, June 1988.

123. Causey DM, Leedom JM, Melancon H. Major opportunistic infections in AIDS patients after eight to one hundred weeks of zidovudine (ZDV) therapy. Fourth International Conference on AIDS, Stockholm, June 1988.

124. Girard PM, Landman R, Gaudebout C, et al. Prevention of *Pneumocystis carinii* pneumonia relapse by pentamidine aerosol in zidovudine-treated AIDS patients. *Lancet* I:1348–1353, 1989.

125. Andrews JC, McManus M, Rogers G, et al. Clinical benefits of concurrent administration of zidovudine and therapy for the suppression of *Pneumocystis carinii*. Fourth International Conference on AIDS, Stockholm, June 1988.

126. Hardy WD. A controlled trial of trimethoprim-sulfamethoxazole or aerolized pentamidine for secondary prophylaxis of *Pneumocystis carinii* pneumonia in patients with the acquired immunodeficiency syndrome. *N Engl J Med* 327:1842–1848, 1992.

127. Schneider MME, et al. A controlled trial of aerolized pentamidine or trimethoprim-sulfamethoxazole as primary prophylaxis against *Pneumocystis carinii* pneumonia in patients with human immunodeficiency virus infection. *N Engl J Med* 327:1836–1841, 1992.

128. Chaisson RE, et al. Pneumocystis prophylaxis and survival in patients with advanced human immunodeficiency virus infection treated with zidovudine. *Arch Intern Med* 152:2009–2013, 1992.

129. Carr A, et al. Low-dose trimethoprim-sulfamethoxazole prophylaxis for toxoplasmic encephalitis in patients with AIDS. *Ann Intern Med* 117:106–111, 1992.

130. Centers for Disease Control. Recommendations for prophylaxis against *Pneumocystis carinii* pneumonia for adults and adolescents infected with human immunodeficiency virus. *MMWR* 41(RR-4):1–11, 1992.

18/Mycobacterial Infections

Harrison W. Farber, Thomas W. Barber

Mycobacteria are responsible for an increasing proportion of the opportunistic infections associated with HIV disease. *Mycobacterium tuberculosis* and *M. avium-intracellulare* (also known as *M. avium* complex [MAC]) are the most common pathogens. *Mycobacterium kansasii* and, perhaps, *M. gordonae* may also infect patients with advanced HIV disease [1–3].

Mycobacterium tuberculosis

Epidemiology

Tuberculosis (TB) is unevenly distributed in the United States. Population groups that are known to have a high incidence of TB include blacks, Latinos, Alaskan natives, prisoners, alcoholics, injection drug users (IDUs), the homeless, the elderly, and foreign-born persons from areas with a high prevalence of TB, including the Caribbean basin, Africa, and Asia [4]. The long-standing downward trend in morbidity from TB in the US reversed and began to rise in the mid-1980s [5]. Current epidemiologic evidence suggests that this resurgence is largely related to the HIV epidemic [6–8].

The greatest increase in reported TB cases has occurred in cities with large numbers of AIDS patients and in groups with the highest rates of TB and AIDS [7, 9–14]. For example, in New York City, the incidence of TB has increased by 68 percent over the past decade. A prospective study of 520 IDUs on methadone maintenance (one third of whom were HIV infected) found that, while 20 percent of both the HIV-positive and HIV-negative groups had a positive TB skin test (purified protein derivative, or PPD), all 8 subsequent cases of active TB were in HIV-infected individuals [15]. Seven of the eight patients with active TB had a positive PPD, and none had received isoniazid (INH) prophylaxis. In a San Francisco study, a greater percentage of HIV-positive heterosexual IDUs were noted to have TB compared to HIV-positive, homosexual, non-IDU control subjects [16]. The increased risk of active TB in Haitians with AIDS appears related to the high prevalence of latent tuberculous infection in this population [7, 17]. In Massachusetts, 33 percent of

263

patients with AIDS and TB are foreign born compared to 3.5 percent of those with AIDS alone [18].

The prevalence of TB in HIV-infected patients ranges from 5 to 35 percent, with affected individuals more likely to be male, African-American, Haitian, or Latino. Extrapulmonary TB has increased sixfold compared to pulmonary TB, reflecting its common association with HIV infection [7, 10, 11, 16]. HIV-infected patients with a positive PPD have an extremely high risk of developing active TB (8% annually vs. 10% lifetime in immunocompetent persons), and clinical disease may develop within months of exposure [15, 19].

Clinical Manifestations

In 70 to 80 percent of cases, the diagnosis of TB coincides with or precedes that of AIDS, suggesting the existence of early defects in cell-mediated immunity [7, 12, 14]. Clinical features may include fever, night sweats, weight loss, and cough, and there is often evidence of dissemination to extrapulmonary sites, including the lymph nodes, liver, bone marrow, and central nervous system [16, 20–22]. Studies demonstrate that 35 to 65 percent of patients with TB and AIDS have extrapulmonary involvement, and 16 to 23 percent have isolated extrapulmonary disease [7, 16, 17, 20, 21]. The chest x-ray (CXR) most often reveals diffuse or miliary infiltrates, focal infiltrates in upper or lower lung fields, and/or mediastinal or hilar adenopathy, but may be unremarkable in up to 10 percent of patients [20, 21, 23, 24]. Compared to HIV-seronegative patients with TB, the CXR in HIV-infected patients is much less likely to show typical cavitary lesions, apical scarring, or pleural effusions [20, 21, 23, 24]. Rapidly evolving radiographic abnormalities generally indicate infection other than TB.

Diagnosis

Tuberculosis is more difficult to diagnose in HIV-infected patients than in the general population. As HIV infection progresses and cellular immunity declines, the PPD often becomes nonreactive, and CXR findings are more nonspecific. Positive sputum smears for acid-fast bacilli (AFB) occur in 31 to 82 percent of TB cases associated with HIV infection, with sensitivity decreasing in more severely immunocompromised individuals, and tissue biopsy specimens less frequently demonstrate granulomas [25, 26]. However, in the appropriate clinical setting, lymph node, bone marrow, or brain biopsy may be diagnostic [12, 26, 27]. Blood cultures using a lysis-centrifugation system are positive in 26 to 42 percent of HIV-infected patients with TB and should be performed whenever disseminated disease is suspected [26, 28, 29]. Because of the difficulty in establishing an early definitive diagnosis of TB, patients in whom there is a high index of suspicion should be treated with anti-mycobacterial therapy pending culture results.

Prognosis

Tuberculosis, both pulmonary and extrapulmonary, is one of the more treatable infectious complications in HIV-infected patients, even in those with severe immunosuppression [16, 17, 21, 30, 31]. Poor outcome is usually associated with medication noncompliance or the presence of disseminated disease [32]. The median survival of HIV-infected patients with TB is significantly reduced compared to individuals with TB who are not HIV-infected [33].

Of great concern are the recent outbreaks of multidrug-resistant TB in HIV-infected patients from hospitals and prisons in Miami and New York City [34–37]. Most patients had advanced immunosuppression (90% had AIDS), and the majority died within 4 months of diagnosis. Several cases were apparently transmitted to health care workers. In many patients, diagnosis was delayed because of unusual clinical presentations, and, in all of the hospitals, AFB isolation precautions were inadequate.

Management

Treatment should be instituted whenever there is a high index of suspicion of TB or whenever AFB are found in a specimen from an HIV-infected patient (Table 18-1). Given that untreated TB is potentially fatal and transmissible to others, all patients with HIV infection and suspected mycobacterial disease of any type should receive empiric treatment that is effective against *M. tuberculosis* [6]. The recent development of DNA probes has expedited the task of distinguishing *M. tuberculosis* from atypical mycobacteria, permitting earlier definitive diagnosis [38]. Pending culture results, initial therapy should consist of INH (300 mg/day), rifampin (600 mg/day), and pyrazinamide (25 mg/kg/day); ethambutol (15 mg/kg/day) is added for the first 2 months if INH resistance is suspected or if there is evidence of central nervous system or disseminated disease [6, 39–41]. Drug susceptibility testing should be performed on all isolates, and therapy adjusted once culture results are available [42]. If multidrug-resistant TB is suspected, patients should be treated with a regimen containing INH, rifampin, pyrazinamide, and at least two other drugs to which the mycobacterial strain is likely susceptible based on local drug sensitivity patterns [34].

The optimal duration of TB therapy in HIV-infected patients is unknown. Current recommendations are for 9 to 12 months (at least 6

Table 18-1 Tuberculosis treatment regimens for the HIV-infected patient

Clinical situation*	Treatment
Initial Therapy	
INH resistance unlikely	INH, RIF, PZA
INH resistance likely	INH, RIF, PZA, EMB
MDR-TB likely	INH, RIF, PZA, 2 others
Therapy after culture results	
Sensitive organism	INH, RIF, PZA (2 mo), then INH, RIF (7 mo) or 6 mo post negative culture (whichever longer)
INH resistance or INH intolerance	RIF, EMB + PZA (18 mo) or 12 mo post negative culture (whichever longer)
RIF intolerance	INH, PZA, EMB (18–24 mo) or 12 mo post negative culture (whichever longer)
MDR-TB	Based on sensitivity (duration unknown)

INH = isoniazid; RIF = rifampin; PZA = pyrazinamide; EMB = ethambutol; MDR-TB = multidrug-resistant TB.
*See text for specific recommendations and dosages for each category.

months after sputum sterilization) in patients with INH-sensitive strains and 18 months (at least 12 months after sputum sterilization) in patients with INH-resistant strains. Following completion of therapy, some authors recommend continuing INH monotherapy indefinitely [41]. In some studies of HIV-infected patients, a higher rate of adverse reactions to antimycobacterial agents, especially rifampin, has been reported [16, 31]. Liver function tests should be closely monitored during therapy, and dosage adjustment of coadministered drugs metabolized in the liver may be necessary.

Prevention

Preliminary evidence suggests that chemoprophylaxis is effective in preventing clinical TB in HIV-infected patients [43]. The high rate of active disease in these patients and public health concerns make this aspect of TB management a priority. All HIV-infected patients should have an intermediate strength (5TU) PPD placed with appropriate controls [44]. Induration of 5 mm or more is considered positive. Recently, the suggestion has been made that lowering the threshold for a positive PPD to 2 mm induration in HIV-infected IDUs may help identify additional patients who have been exposed to TB [45].

Assuming no contraindications, HIV-infected individuals with a positive PPD should receive INH prophylaxis for one year regardless of age once active TB has been excluded [6, 44]. HIV-infected patients who are anergic on skin testing and at high risk for TB, including IDUs, the homeless, past or current prison inmates, or patients from an endemic area, should also receive chemoprophylaxis [6, 44]. Finally, HIV-infected patients with a history of positive PPD who have never been treated with INH or with CXR abnormalities suggestive of prior TB, and close contacts of active cases, should receive prophylaxis as well [6, 40, 44]. When INH resistance is suspected, rifampin should be administered. All patients with HIV infection who have a negative PPD should be regularly screened with repeat skin tests for new exposure to TB.

Mycobacterium avium-intracellulare

Epidemiology

Mycobacterium avium and M. intracellulare are closely related species of nontuberculous or "atypical" mycobacteria, often classified together as M. avium-intracellulare or M. avium complex. HIV seropositivity with disseminated nontuberculous mycobacterial infection constitutes an AIDS-defining diagnosis. MAC accounted for 96.1 percent of such infections in patients with AIDS reported to the Centers for Disease Control between 1981 and 1987 [46].

Before the emergence of HIV, disseminated MAC infection occurred rarely and almost exclusively in individuals with defective cell-mediated immunity. MAC has also been reported to cause lymphadenitis in children and chronic lung infection in adults with underlying obstructive pulmonary disease [47, 48]. Disseminated MAC infection occurs in HIV-infected patients belonging to all risk groups, ages, and races who are at an advanced stage of immunodeficiency (CD4 lymphocyte count $< 100/mm^3$) [49, 50, 51]. The disease has been diagnosed antemortem in approximately 25 percent of AIDS patients and identified at autopsy in up to 50 percent [52, 53].

Patients with AIDS are more likely to develop infection with M. avium than M. intracellulare, while non-AIDS patients are just as likely to become infected with either species [54–56]. MAC is distributed widely in the environment and has been isolated from a number of wild and domestic animals [57]. Suspected modes of acquisition of the organism include inhalation or ingestion of contaminated water, soil, dust, and animal products. It is not known whether person-to-person transmission occurs.

Clinical Manifestations

Disseminated MAC infection produces a nonspecific constellation of symptoms, including fever, night sweats, fatigue, malaise, anorexia, weight loss, abdominal pain, and diarrhea. A malabsorption syndrome has been correlated pathologically with MAC infiltration of the small bowel. Pulmonary symptoms are uncommon. Physical examination reveals cachexia, often with palpable adenopathy and hepatospleno-megaly. Most patients have anemia, thrombocytopenia, leukopenia, and increased liver function tests, especially serum alkaline phosphatase [58]. It is estimated that patients with advanced HIV infection and this clinical profile in whom *Pneumocystis carinii* pneumonia, cytomegalovirus infection, and infectious diarrhea have been excluded are more than 70 percent likely to have disseminated MAC infection [59].

Diagnosis

Diagnosis of disseminated MAC infection is established by a positive culture of blood or other normally sterile body fluid or tissue, such as bone marrow, liver, or lymph node [60]. Blood should be cultured in lysis-centrifugation tubes or using an in vitro radiometric technique. These blood culture systems are highly sensitive, and two blood cultures are almost always sufficient to detect MAC bacteremia [61, 62].

Sputum and stool cultures may reveal MAC but do not dependably indicate or predict disseminated disease. Histopathologic examination of biopsy specimens often shows macrophages, many AFB, and a minimal inflammatory response, with poorly formed epithelioid granulomas and little tissue necrosis or fibrosis [60]. Definitive diagnosis of MAC infection cannot be made based solely on histology. Tuberculosis should always be considered in the differential diagnosis of a positive AFB stain pending culture results.

Prognosis

Disseminated MAC infection is associated with profound immunodeficiency and usually preceded by one or more AIDS-defining illnesses [63]. Recent data suggest that untreated disseminated MAC infection shortens survival by approximately 6 months [46, 64]. The median survival from time of diagnosis of disseminated MAC infection is currently less than 6 months, but it is anticipated that early diagnosis and more effective chemotherapy will improve prognosis [65].

Management

Early reports of treatment for disseminated MAC infection in patients with AIDS were disappointing, but a number of more recent studies evaluating various multidrug regimens with newer agents demonstrate that prolonged therapy may result in reduction or elimination of bacteremia and improvement in constitutional symptoms [49, 50, 66, 67]. A

Table 18-2 Currently available drugs used in the treatment of MAC infection

Drug	Dosage	Major toxicities
Rifampin[a]	600 mg/day	Hepatotoxicity Hematologic toxicity Rash Renal toxicity Orange discoloration of secretions
Clofazimine	50–100 mg/day	Gastrointestinal intolerance Abdominal pain Hepatotoxicity Skin discoloration
Ethambutol	15–25 mg/kg/day	Optic neuritis Rash Gastrointestinal intolerance Hepatotoxicity
Ciprofloxacin	1000–1500 mg/day	Gastrointestinal intolerance Neurotoxicity Rash
Amikacin	7.5 mg/kg q12–24h IM or IV	Nephrotoxicity Ototoxicity
Cycloserine	750–1,000 mg/day	Neurotoxicity Rash
Pyrazinamide	15–30 mg/kg/day	Hepatotoxicity Gastrointestinal intolerance Hyperuricemia Rash
Ethionamide	10–20 mg/kg/day	Gastrointestinal intolerance Neurotoxicity
Rifabutin[a,b]	300–600 mg/day	Gastrointestinal intolerance Leukopenia Rash Hepatotoxicity

[a]This agent may affect the serum levels of coadministered drugs that are hepatically metabolized.
[b]This agent in the dose of 300 mg/day has been shown to be effective in the prophylaxis of MAC infection. See text for details.

retrospective study has suggested that survival of patients treated for MAC may also be improved [68]. However, treatment-limiting drug toxicity is common. Isolates of MAC are often resistant in vitro to first-line antituberculous agents, but antimycobacterial drug susceptibility testing results do not consistently correlate with clinical outcome.

Most conventional regimens now include two to five agents selected from the drugs known to have activity against some isolates of MAC. These include rifampin, rifabutin, ethambutol, clofazimine, ciprofloxacin, and amikacin (Table 18-2). Two new macrolide antibiotics, clarithromycin and azithromycin, also appear to be effective against MAC [69, 70]. Improvement in constitutional symptoms, abdominal pain, and diarrhea usually requires at least several weeks of therapy. If tolerated, treatment is generally continued for the remainder of the patient's life.

Prevention

Knowledge of the ecology and risk factors for acquisition of MAC are inadequate to support specific recommendations for avoidance of infection. As was described previously, disseminated MAC appears to be associated with decreased survival, and current treatment regimens are complex and potentially toxic, and have unpredictable efficacy. Development of useful strategies for prevention of MAC infection is therefore a high priority. Recently, rifabutin has been demonstrated to be an effective prophylactic agent in HIV-infected patients with CD4 cell counts of $200/mm^3$ or less, and has been approved by the Food and Drug Administration for this indication [71, 72]. In these placebo-controlled trials, rifabutin reduced the rate of MAC bacteremia by 50 percent without significant drug toxicity. Although reduced mortality was not demonstrated, there was a trend toward prolonged survival in patients receiving prophylaxis. Surprisingly, MAC isolates from patients on rifabutin therapy were not resistant to the drug in vitro.

References

1. Scherer R, Sable R, Sonnenberg M, et al. Disseminated infection with *Mycobacterium kansasii* in the acquired immunodeficiency syndrome. *Ann Intern Med* 105:710–712, 1986.
2. Levine B, Chaisson RE. *Mycobacterium kansasii*: A cause of treatable pulmonary disease associated with advanced human immunodeficiency virus infection. *Ann Intern Med* 114:861–868, 1991.
3. Barber TW, Craven DE, Farber HW. *Mycobacterium gordonae*: A possible opportunistic respiratory tract pathogen in patients with advanced human immunodeficiency virus, type 1 infection. *Chest* 100:716–720, 1991.
4. Centers for Disease Control. Guidelines for preventing the transmission of tuberculosis in health-care settings, with special focus on HIV-related issues. *MMWR* 39:1–29, 1990.
5. Centers for Disease Control. Update: Tuberculosis elimination—United States. *MMWR* 39:153–156, 1990.
6. Centers for Disease Control. Tuberculosis and human immunodeficiency virus infection: Recommendations of the advisory committee for the elimination of tuberculosis (ACET). *MMWR* 38:236–250, 1989.
7. Rieder HL, Cauthen GM, Bloch AB, et al. Tuberculosis and acquired immunodeficiency syndrome—Florida. *Arch Intern Med* 149:1268–1273, 1989.

8. Chaisson RE, Slutkin G. Tuberculosis and human immunodeficiency virus infection. *J Infect Dis* 159:96–99, 1989.
9. Centers for Disease Control. Tuberculosis—United States, 1985—and the possible impact of the human lymphotropic virus type III/lymphadenopathy-associated virus infection. *MMWR* 35:74–76, 1986.
10. Centers for Disease Control. Tuberculosis and acquired immunodeficiency syndrome—New York City. *MMWR* 36:785–790, 1987.
11. Bloch AB, Reider HL, Kelly GD, et al. The epidemiology of tuberculosis in the United States. *Semin Respir Infect* 4:157–170, 1989.
12. Barnes PF, Bloch AB, Davidson PT, Snider DE, Jr. Tuberculosis in patients with human immunodeficiency virus infection. *N Engl J Med* 324:1644–1650, 1991.
13. Pitchenik AE, Fertel D, Bloch AB. Mycobacterial disease; epidemiology, diagnosis, treatment, and prevention. *Clin Chest Med* 9:425–441, 1988.
14. FitzGerald JM, Grzybowski S, Allen EA. The impact of human immunodeficiency virus infection on tuberculosis and its control. *Chest* 100:191–200, 1991.
15. Selwyn PA, Hartel D, Lewis VA, et al. A prospective study of the risk of tuberculosis among intravenous drug users with human immunodeficiency virus infection. *N Engl J Med* 320:545–550, 1989.
16. Chaisson RE, Schecter GF, Theuer CP, et al. Tuberculosis in patients with the acquired immunodeficiency syndrome: Clinical features, response to therapy, and survival. *Am Rev Respir Dis* 136:570–574, 1987.
17. Pitchenik AE, Burr J, Suarez M, et al. Human T-cell lymphotrophic (virus-III) seropositivity and related disease among 71 nonconsecutive patients in whom tuberculosis was diagnosed. *Am Rev Respir Dis* 135:875–879, 1987.
18. Bernardo J, Murray C, Taylor J, et al. Epidemiology of tuberculosis (TB) and HIV infection in the homeless—Boston, 1989 (abstract). *Am Rev Respir Dis* 141:A260, 1990.
19. Daley CL, et al. An outbreak of tuberculosis with accelerated progression among persons infected with the human immunodeficiency virus. *N Engl J Med* 326:231–235, 1992.
20. Theuer CP, Hopewell PC, Elias D, et al. Human immunodeficiency virus infection in tuberculosis patients. *J Infect Dis* 162:8–12, 1990.
21. Pitchenik AE, Cole C, Russell BW, et al. Tuberculosis, atypical mycobacteriosis, and the acquired immunodeficiency syndrome among Haitian and non-Haitian patients in south Florida. *Ann Intern Med* 101:610–615, 1984.
22. Berenguer J, et al. Tuberculous meningitis in patients infected with the human immunodeficiency virus. *N Engl J Med* 326:668–672, 1992.
23. Pitchenik AE, Rubinson HA. The radiographic appearance of tuberculosis in patients with the acquired immune deficiency syndrome (AIDS) and pre-AIDS. *Am Rev Respir Dis* 131:393–396, 1985.
24. Colebunders RE, Ryder RW, Nzilambi N, et al. HIV infection in patients with tuberculosis in Kinshasa, Zaire. *Am Rev Respir Dis* 139:1082–1085, 1989.
25. Klein NC, Duncanson FP, Lenox TH, III, et al. Use of mycobacterial

smears in the diagnosis of pulmonary tuberculosis in AIDS/ARC patients. *Chest* 95:1190–1192, 1989.

26. Kramer F, Modilevsky T, Waliany AR, et al. Delayed diagnosis of tuberculosis in patients with human immunodeficiency virus infection. *Am J Med* 89:451–456, 1990.

27. Bouchama A, Zuheir Al-Kawi M, Kanaan I, et al. Brain biopsy in tuberculoma: The risks and benefits. *Neurosurgery* 28:405–409, 1991.

28. Shafer RW, Goldberg R, Sierra M, Glatt AE. Frequency of *Mycobacterium tuberculosis* bacteremia in patients with tuberculosis in an area endemic for AIDS. *Am Rev Respir Dis* 140:1611–1613, 1989.

29. Barber TW, Craven DE, McCabe WR. Bacteremia due to *Mycobacterium tuberculosis* in patients with human immunodeficiency virus infection. *Medicine* 69:375–383, 1990.

30. Louie E, Rice L, Holzmann RS. Tuberculosis in non-Haitian patients with the acquired immuno-deficiency syndrome. *Chest* 90:542–545, 1986.

31. Small PM, Schecter GF, Goodman PC, et al. Treatment of tuberculosis in patients with advanced human immunodeficiency virus infection. *N Engl J Med* 324:289–294, 1991.

32. Chaisson RE, Hopewell PC. Survival after active tuberculosis in patients with HIV infection (abstract). *Am Rev Respir Dis* 142:259A, 1990.

33. Stoneburner R. Survival in a cohort of human immunodeficiency virus-infected tuberculosis patients in New York City. *Ann Intern Med* 152:2033–2037, 1992.

34. Centers for Disease Control. Nosocomial transmission of multidrug- resistant tuberculosis among HIV-infected persons—Florida and New York, 1988–1991. *MMWR* 40:586–591, 1991.

35. Edlin BR, et al. An outbreak of multidrug-resistant tuberculosis among hospitalized patients with the acquired immunodeficiency syndrome. *N Engl J Med* 326:1514–1521, 1992.

36. Fischl MA, et al. An outbreak of tuberculosis caused by multiple-drug-resistant tubercle bacilli among patients with HIV infection. *Ann Intern Med* 117:177–183, 1992.

37. Fischl MA, et al. Clinical presentation and outcome of patients with HIV infection and tuberculosis caused by multiple-drug-resistant bacilli. *Ann Intern Med* 117:184–190, 1992.

38. Good RC, Mastro TD. The modern mycobacteriology laboratory: How it can help the clinician. *Clin Chest Med* 10:315–322, 1989.

39. Davidson PT. Treating tuberculosis; what drugs, for how long? *Ann Intern Med* 112:393–395, 1990.

40. American Thoracic Society. Treatment of tuberculosis and tuberculosis infection in adults and children. *Am Rev Respir Dis* 134:355–363, 1986.

41. American Thoracic Society. Mycobacterioses and the acquired immunodeficiency syndrome. *Am Rev Respir Dis* 136:492–496, 1987.

42. American Thoracic Society. Diagnostic standards and classification of tuberculosis. *Am Rev Respir Dis* 142:725–735, 1990.

43. Selwyn PA, et al. High risk of active tuberculosis in HIV-infected drug users with cutaneous anergy. *JAMA* 268:504–509, 1992.

44. Centers for Disease Control. Screening for tuberculosis and tuberculosis

infection in high-risk populations and the use of preventive therapy for tuberculosis infection in the United States: Recommendations of the Advisory Committee for Elimination of Tuberculosis. *MMWR* 39:RR-8:1– 12, 1990.

45. Graham NMH, et al. Prevalence of tuberculin positivity and skin test anergy in HIV-1–seropositive and –seronegative intravenous drug users. *JAMA* 267:369–373, 1992.
46. Horsburgh CR, Selik RM. The epidemiology of disseminated nontuberculous mycobacterial infection in the acquired immunodeficiency syndrome (AIDS). *Am Rev Respir Dis* 139:4–7, 1989.
47. Kinsella JP, Culver K, Jeffrey RB, et al. Extensive cervical lymphadenitis due to *Mycobacterium avium-intracellulare*. *Pediatr Infect Dis* 6:289–291, 1987.
48. Rosenzweig DY, Schlueter DP. Spectrum of clinical disease in pulmonary infection with *Mycobacterium avium-intracellulare*. *Rev Infect Dis* 3:1046– 1051, 1981.
49. Hoy J, Mitch A, Sandland M, et al. Quadruple-drug therapy for *Mycobacterium avium-intracellulare* bacteremia in AIDS patients. *J Infect Dis* 161:801–805, 1990.
50. Chiu J, Nussbaum J, Bozzette S, et al. Treatment of disseminated *Mycobacterium avium* complex infection in AIDS with amikacin, ethambutol, rifampin, and ciprofloxacin. *Ann Intern Med* 113:358–361, 1990.
51. Nightingale SD, et al. Incidence of *Mycobacterium avium-intracellulare* complex bacteremia in human immunodeficiency virus-positive patients. *J Infect Dis* 165:1082–1085, 1992.
52. Wallace JM, Hannah JB. *Mycobacterium avium* complex infection in patients with the acquired immunodeficiency syndrome: A clinicopathologic study. *Chest* 93:926–931, 1988.
53. Hawkins CC, Gold JUM, Whimby E, et al. *Mycobacterium avium* complex infections in patients with the acquired immunodeficiency syndrome. *Ann Intern Med* 105:184–188, 1986.
54. Guthertz LS, Damsker B, Bottone EJ, et al. *Mycobacterium avium* and *Mycobacterium intracellulare* infections in patients with and without AIDS. *J Infect Dis* 160:1037–1041, 1989.
55. Horsburgh CR, Chon DL, Roberts RB, et al. *Mycobacterium avium–Mycobacterium intracellulare* isolates from patients with or without acquired immunodeficiency syndrome. *Antimicrob Agents Chemother* 30:955– 957, 1986.
56. Yakrus MA, Good RC. Geographic distribution, frequency, and specimen source of *Mycobacterium avium* complex serotypes isolated from patients with acquired immunodeficiency syndrome. *J Clin Microbiol* 28:926– 929, 1990.
57. Iseman MC, Corpe RF, O'Brien RJ, et al. Disease due to *Mycobacterium avium-intracellulare*. *Chest* 87:139S-149S, 1985.
58. Horsburgh CR. *Mycobacterium avium* complex infection in the acquired immunodeficiency syndrome. *N Engl J Med* 324:1332–1338, 1991.
59. Young LS. *Mycobacterium avium* complex infection. *J Infect Dis* 157:863– 867, 1988.

60. Klatt EC, Jensen DF, Meyer PR. Pathology of *Mycobacterium avium-intracellulare* infection in acquired immunodeficiency syndrome. *Hum Pathol* 18:709–714, 1987.
61. Yagupsky P, Menegus MA. Cumulative positivity rates of multiple blood cultures for *Mycobacterium avium-intracellulare* and *Cryptococcus neoformans* in patients with the acquired immunodeficiency syndrome. *Arch Pathol Lab Med* 114:923–925, 1990.
62. Wong B, Edwards FF, Kiehn TE, et al. Continuous high-grade *Mycobacterium avium-intracellulare* bacteremia in patients with the acquired immune deficiency syndrome. *Am J Med* 78:35–40, 1985.
63. Modilevsky T, Sattler FR, Barnes PF. Mycobacterial disease in patients with human immunodeficiency virus infection. *Arch Intern Med* 149:2201–2205, 1989.
64. Jacobson MA, Hopewell PC, Yajko DM, et al. Natural history of disseminated *Mycobacterium avium* complex infection in AIDS. *J Infect Dis* 164:994–998, 1991.
65. Horsburgh CR, Havlik JA, Thompson SE. Survival of AIDS patients with disseminated *Mycobacterium avium* complex infection (DMAC): A case-control study. Sixth International Conference on AIDS, San Francisco, June 1990.
66. Agins BC, Berman DS, Spicehandler D, et al. Effect of combined therapy with ansamycin, clofazimine, ethambutol, and isoniazid for *Mycobacterium avium* infection in patients with AIDS. *J Infect Dis* 159:784–787, 1989.
67. Kemper CA, et al. Treatment of *Mycobacterium avium* complex bacteremia in AIDS with a four-drug oral regimen. *Ann Intern Med* 116:466–472, 1992.
68. Kerlinkowske KM, et al. Antimycobacterial therapy for disseminated *Mycobacterium avium* complex infection in patients with acquired immunodeficiency syndrome. *Arch Intern Med* 152:813–817, 1992.
69. Chaisson RE, Benson CA, Dube M, et al. Clarithromycin for disseminated *Mycobacterium avium* complex in AIDS patients. Eighth International Conference on AIDS, Amsterdam, July 1992.
70. Young LS, et al. Azithromycin for treatment of *Mycobacterium avium-intracellulare* complex infection in patients with AIDS. *Lancet* 338:1107–1109, 1991.
71. Cameron W, Sparti P, Pietroski N, et al. Rifabutin therapy for the prevention of MAC bacteremia in patients with AIDS and CD4 ≤ 200. Eighth International Conference on AIDS, Amsterdam, July 1992.
72. Wynne B, et al. The development of *Mycobacterium avium* complex bacteremia in AIDS patients in the placebo-controlled MAC prophylaxis studies. Interscience Conference on Antimicrobial Agents and Chemotherapy (abstract), Anaheim, CA, September 1992.

19/Cryptococcosis

Alan M. Sugar, Carol A. Saunders

Meningitis is the most serious manifestation of infection with the yeast-like organism *Cryptococcus neoformans*. This ubiquitous fungus can cause disease in normal hosts, as well as in those with immunodeficiency [1]. Several reviews of cryptococcosis in AIDS have been published, and there is continuing controversy over the optimal management of patients with acute cryptococcal meningitis [2–7]. This chapter reviews clinical issues related to cryptococcosis and presents an approach to diagnosis and treatment of the disease in patients with AIDS.

Epidemiology

Cryptococcus neoformans is found in all areas of the world; cryptococcosis is not a geographically restricted disease, such as histoplasmosis and coccidioidomycosis. The fungus grows well in soil, especially when enriched with bird droppings. However, it is uncertain if there is a relationship between exposure to birds and clinical disease in patients with AIDS. In Africa, Swinne and associates [8] reported that cultures of dust obtained from 50 percent of the houses of HIV-infected patients with cryptococcosis grew *C. neoformans,* compared to only 20 percent of dust cultures from randomly selected houses in the same area. Moreover, 40 percent of their patients with cryptococcosis claimed contact with pigeons, and pigeon coops frequently harbored the fungus. They suggested that contaminated house dust or exposure to pigeons was a risk factor for cryptococcosis, but similar associations have not been identified in North America.

Cryptococcus neoformans, with a 5 to 10 percent disease rate, is the second most commonly isolated fungal pathogen in AIDS patients. Cryptococcosis was a well-recognized, albeit much less frequent, disease before the advent of AIDS. Patients with impaired cell-mediated immunity resulting from lymphoma or corticosteroid use are at risk for development of the disease, but patients with no known immunologic abnormalities may also develop cryptococcal infection. Under usual circumstances, *C. neoformans* is introduced into the body through the lungs; person-to-person transmission does not occur.

Clinical Manifestations

Pneumonia sometimes occurs as an early manifestation of cryptococcosis, and our local experience includes a number of patients who were hospitalized for treatment of *Pneumocystis carinii* pneumonia and returned approximately 6 weeks later with cryptococcal meningitis. The presumption, still unproven, is that *C. neoformans* was responsible for the pulmonary process. Most patients with cryptococcal meningitis do not have a history of clinically recognized pneumonia. In immunologically intact persons, cryptococcal pneumonia usually resolves spontaneously, and antifungal therapy is not indicated [9]. However, in immunosuppressed patients, dissemination to extrapulmonary sites is frequent, and specific antifungal treatment is necessary. *Cryptococcus neoformans* has a propensity to spread to the central nervous system, but infection of skin, bone, lymph nodes, heart, and other sites has been described as well (see Fig. 9-3).

The clinical presentation of cryptococcal meningitis is variable, ranging from fever and mild constitutional symptoms to seizures and coma. It most often presents insidiously, with symptoms developing over several weeks. The disease has a tendency to wax and wane; symptoms may be dismissed as trivial or indicative of another process. Patients with cryptococcal meningitis often complain of headache, nausea, and vomiting, reflecting increased intracranial pressure [10]. Photophobia may occur, and signs suggestive of meningeal irritation are sometimes found. Changes in personality and alterations in level of consciousness have also been described.

Diagnosis

The diagnosis of cryptococcal meningitis can be made using three complementary methods: microscopy, antigen detection, and culture. Before a lumbar puncture is performed, a complete history and physical examination should be done, with particular attention to the patient's neurologic status and to other possible sites of dissemination (Table 19-1). Since cryptococcal infection of the central nervous system involves the brain parenchyma as well as meninges, computed tomography (CT) scan or magnetic resonance imaging of the brain may show mass lesions, even in patients without focal neurologic findings.

The patient with suspected cryptococcal meningitis should undergo lumbar puncture; if papilledema or focal neurologic deficits are present, a CT scan of the brain should be performed first. Cerebrospinal fluid (CSF) should be sent for India ink examination, fungal culture, and cryptococcal antigen assay, in addition to the usual studies. Cryptococcal meningitis in AIDS is characterized by a large number of organisms in

Table 19-1 *Evaluation of patients with cryptococcosis*

History
    Antecedent respiratory symptoms
    Fever, malaise, anorexia
    Headache
    Visual disturbances
    Change in personality or behavior

Physical examination
    Pneumonia
    Focal neurologic abnormalities
    Altered mental status
    Papilledema
    Skin lesions

Laboratory tests
    Cerebrospinal fluid analysis
        Opening pressure
        Cell count, glucose, protein
        India ink preparation
        Culture
        Cryptococcal antigen
    CT scan of brain
    Serum cryptococcal antigen
    Blood and urine cultures

the CSF and a minimal host inflammatory response. Organisms are readily observed under the microscope, even in uncentrifuged specimens.

The most immediate method for diagnosing cryptococcal meningitis is by mixing CSF or its sediment with India ink. A drop of CSF is placed on the microscope slide adjacent to a drop of India ink, and a cover slip is then positioned over them. A positive test shows clearly demarcated circular organisms with a smooth perimeter, a surrounding clear zone (capsule), and a visible internal anatomy (organelles) (Fig. 19-1). False–positive India ink preparations occur when host white blood cells are confused with the fungus. White blood cells typically have a hazy and poorly demarcated periphery, and no internal structures are seen. Occasionally, adjacent cells touch, giving the appearance of budding yeast.

Capsule-deficient *C. neoformans* has been described in patients with AIDS. The meaning of this observation is not entirely clear, but may merely reflect rapid growth of the organism with less time for each yeast to produce capsular material. An alternative hypothesis is that relatively avirulent environmental isolates, not normally encapsulated, may cause disease in sufficiently immunosuppressed hosts.

The cryptococcal antigen latex agglutination test remains an important tool for diagnosis of cryptococcosis. This assay detects the presence

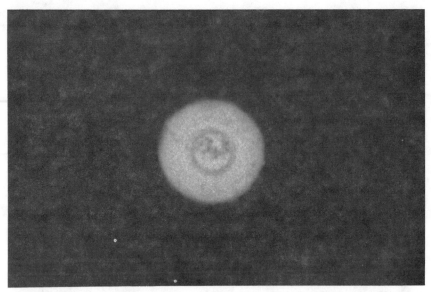

Figure 19-1. Cryptococcus neoformans *demonstrated on India ink preparation.*

of cryptococcal polysaccharide in serum or CSF using antibody-coated particles to trap the antigen. In studies of patients without HIV infection, cryptococcal antigen titers have been useful prognostically, as well as diagnostically [11, 12]. However, in AIDS patients, extraordinarily high titers have been noted, and unpredictable fluctuations in serum titer may occur during the course of treatment, as may false-positive tests. Thus, cryptococcal antigen titers are not recommended for determining prognosis or duration of therapy in AIDS patients.

The mainstay for diagnosis remains the CSF culture. Since the organism enters the body through the lungs and disseminates hematogenously, sputum and blood cultures should also be performed. *Cryptococcus neoformans* readily grows in standard blood culture media, provided that the bottles have been vented to room air, as well as on blood agar. Within 2 to 5 days, yeast-like colonies are generally visible. Definitive microbiologic identification relies on the organism producing a brownish color when cultured on birdseed agar, a result of its intrinsic phenol oxidase activity and the production of melanin.

Management

In the AIDS patient, treatment of cryptococcal meningitis can be divided into two phases: (1) primary or acute therapy and (2) maintenance or suppressive therapy.

Primary Therapy

In the largest study to date, a collaborative effort of the Mycoses Study Group (MSG), AIDS Clinical Trials Group (ACTG), and independent physicians, amphotericin B, in a dose of at least 0.3 mg/kg/day, was compared to fluconazole, initial dose of 200 mg per day, with escalation to 400 mg per day if the patient did not respond [13]. After 10 weeks of therapy, only 40 percent of amphotericin-B–treated patients and 34 percent of fluconazole-treated patients were successfully treated. Approximately 25 percent of patients in both treatment groups were classified as clinical responders, but their CSF could not be sterilized.

Evidence derived from this study suggests that it is critical to stratify patients into risk groups before embarking on any treatment course. Altered mental status was predictive of poor outcome. A CSF cryptococcal antigen titer greater than 1:1,024 and CSF white blood cell count less than $20/mm^3$, reflecting high fungal burden and little host inflammatory response, were also important negative prognostic indicators. Over 90 percent of patients without these findings responded to therapy with either amphotericin B or fluconazole. In contrast, in patients with these findings, mortality was high for treatment both with amphotericin B (33%) and fluconazole (44%).

Thus, in patients with predictors of poor outcome, either amphotericin B or fluconazole therapy is reasonable. Based on information from several studies in AIDS patients, CSF cultures become negative after approximately 1 month in patients treated with amphotericin B and in approximately 2 months with fluconazole. In patients with negative prognostic indicators, response to therapy is poor and mortality is high. For this group, consideration should be given to using high doses of amphotericin B with or without flucytosine. Many investigators recommend reduced doses of flucytosine (75–100 mg/kg/day in four divided doses vs. the usual dose of 150 mg/kg/day) in patients with AIDS. However, even at reduced doses, the hematologic toxicity of flucytosine may still be significant in this patient population.

The optimal duration of primary therapy has not been well defined. Ideally, there should be resolution of symptoms and signs of disease and no evidence of growth of the fungus from infected sites. Six to 10 weeks of therapy, and sometimes more, is usually administered before maintenance therapy is begun [12]. Persistence of C. neoformans in the prostate has been described and hypothesized as a potential source of reinfection following successful treatment of meningitis [14]. It may be prudent to culture urine and prostatic secretions before and after primary therapy for cryptococcosis.

Maintenance Therapy

HIV-infected patients with cryptococcal meningitis require lifelong suppressive antifungal therapy. Two open-label studies have been performed to evaluate the role of fluconazole as suppressive therapy for cryptococcal meningitis in AIDS patients [15, 16]. Both have shown that the relapse rate in patients treated with this drug can be decreased to about 10 percent, compared to 50 to 90 percent in those not receiving suppressive therapy. Subsequently, a placebo-controlled study and a large multicenter study have confirmed fluconazole as the drug of choice for maintenance therapy of cryptococcal meningitis [17, 18]. A dose of 200 mg per day is adequate in most instances.

Monitoring Patients

Once patients have clinically improved on primary therapy, they should be evaluated every 4 to 6 weeks for symptoms and signs of relapse and toxicity related to treatment. Because the first evidence for relapse is often a positive culture, lumbar puncture with CSF culture is recommended on a periodic basis. Routine lumbar puncture is not indicated during primary therapy, since negative CSF culture is unusual regardless of the drug used. Fluctuations in CSF cryptococcal antigen titers usually have no correlation with the disease course, and clinicians should not rely on titer results to determine patient management. Rather, such decisions should be based on clinical parameters and CSF culture results.

Specific Treatment Recommendations

Amphotericin B, at a dose of 0.6 to 1.0 mg/kg/day, is the preferred drug in severely ill patients. The addition of flucytosine, 75 to 150 mg/kg/day in four divided doses, can also be considered in this group if the capacity for monitoring flucytosine serum concentrations is available. The role of high-dose fluconazole (800–1,000 mg/day) in primary therapy is uncertain.

In patients without mental status changes or focal neurologic deficits, the choice of appropriate primary therapy is less clear. Fluconazole may be preferable to amphotericin B because of its ease of administration. It can be given as a single oral dose of 400 mg/day. On the basis of anecdotal reports, this dose should probably be continued for at least 10 weeks following the first negative CSF culture. In most cases, there is no need for determination of fluconazole serum concentrations.

Fluconazole in a dose of 200 mg per day is the drug of choice for maintenance therapy. Most patients do well on this regimen, although a small number will relapse. Patients with relapsing infection can be managed by switching from fluconazole to amphotericin B or by increasing the dose of fluconazole to 600 to 800 mg per day in those who cannot tolerate amphotericin B.

Prognosis

Most AIDS patients respond to therapy for an initial episode of cryptococcal meningitis, but relapse following apparently successful primary therapy is frequent. From studies in the pre-AIDS era, we know that patients with positive India ink smears after completion of therapy, those with high CSF cryptococcal antigen titers, and those with cultures positive for C. neoformans at extraneural sites are all at high risk of relapse. Since these characteristics are found in the majority of AIDS patients with cryptococcal infection, all such individuals should be placed on chronic maintenance therapy.

The overall prognosis for AIDS patients with cryptococcosis is guarded. In a retrospective series, Chuck and Sande [6] found mean survival to be approximately 8 months in those receiving long-term antifungal treatment and 5 months in those not receiving maintenance therapy. Similarly, in another retrospective review, mean survival time for the 47 of 68 who died was 5 months [5]. Bozzette and associates [17] found that about two thirds of their patients died after a mean of approximately 9 months. This was true whether placebo or fluconazole was used during the maintenance phase of treatment.

Prevention

There are no currently recognized means for preventing acquisition of cryptococcal infection. As the organism is ubiquitous, it is not feasible to limit exposure. Moreover, some of the cryptococcal disease occurring in patients with AIDS may represent reactivation of previously acquired infection. The role of antifungal prophylaxis for cryptococcosis remains undefined, but, with the introduction of newer agents such as fluconazole and itraconazole, successful preventive therapy may be possible. Clinical studies are under way to address this issue.

References

1. Diamond RD. Cryptococcus neoformans. In: GL Mandell, RG Douglas, Jr, JE Bennett (eds), Principles and Practice of Infectious Diseases, (3rd ed). New York: Churchill Livingstone, 1990.

2. Kovacs JA, Kovacs AA, Polis M, et al. Cryptococcosis in the acquired immunodeficiency syndrome. *Ann Intern Med* 103:533–538, 1985.
3. Zuger A, Louie E, Holzman RS, et al. Cryptococcal disease in patients with the acquired immunodeficiency syndrome. *Ann Intern Med* 104:234–240, 1986.
4. Dismukes WE. Cryptococcal meningitis in patients with AIDS. *J Infect Dis* 157:624–628, 1988.
5. Clark RA, Greer D, Atkinson W, et al. Spectrum of *Cryptococcus neoformans* infection in 68 patients infected with human immunodeficiency virus. *Rev Infect Dis* 12:768–778, 1990.
6. Chuck SL, Sande MA. Infections with *Cryptococcus neoformans* in the acquired immunodeficiency syndrome. *N Engl J Med* 321:794–799, 1989.
7. Sugar AM, Stern JJ, Dupont B. Overview: Treatment of cryptococcal meningitis. *Rev Infect Dis* 12:S338–S348, 1990.
8. Swinne D, Deppner M, Maniratunga S, et al. AIDS-associated cryptococcosis in Bujumbura, Burundi: An epidemiological study. *J Med Vet Mycol* 29:25–30, 1991.
9. Kerkering TM, Duma RJ, Shadomy S. The evolution of pulmonary cryptococcosis: Clinical implications from a study of 41 patients with and without compromising host factors. *Ann Intern Med* 94:611–616, 1981.
10. Denning DW, Armstrong RW, Lewis BH, Stevens DA. Elevated cerebrospinal fluid pressures in patients with cryptococcal meningitis and acquired immunodeficiency syndrome. *Am J Med* 91:267–272, 1991.
11. Diamond RD, Bennett JE. Prognostic factors in cryptococcal meningitis: A study of 111 cases. *Ann Intern Med* 80:176–181, 1974.
12. Dismukes WE, Cloud G, Gallis HA, et al. Treatment of cryptococcal meningitis with combination amphotericin B and flucytosine for four as compared with six weeks. *N Engl J Med* 317:334–341, 1987.
13. Saag MS, Powderly WG, Cloud GA, et al. Treatment of acute AIDS-associated cryptococcal meningitis with amphotericin B or fluconazole: Results of a randomized clinical trial. *N Engl J Med* 326:83–89, 1992.
14. Larsen RA, Bozzette S, McCutchan JA, et al. Persistent *Cryptococcus neoformans* infection of the prostate after successful treatment of meningitis. *Ann Intern Med* 111:125–128, 1989.
15. Stern JJ, Hartman BJ, Sharkey P, et al. Oral fluconazole therapy for patients with acquired immunodeficiency syndrome and cryptococcosis: Experience with 22 patients. *Am J Med* 85:477–480, 1988.
16. Sugar AM, Saunders C. Oral fluconazole as suppressive therapy of disseminated cryptococcosis in patients with acquired immunodeficiency syndrome. *Am J Med* 85:481–489, 1988.
17. Bozzette SA, Larsen RA, Chiu J, et al. A placebo-controlled trial of maintenance therapy with fluconazole after treatment of cryptococcal meningitis in the acquired immunodeficiency syndrome. *N Engl J Med* 324:580–584, 1991.
18. Powderly WG, et al. A controlled trial of fluconazole or amphotericin B to prevent relapse of cryptococcal meningitis in patients with the acquired immunodeficiency syndrome. *N Engl J Med* 326:793–798, 1992.

20/Toxoplasmosis

Carol A. Sulis

Toxoplasmosis is a common central nervous system (CNS) infection in patients with advanced HIV disease, and presumptive toxoplasmic encephalitis is an AIDS-defining diagnosis [1]. Toxoplasmic encephalitis accounts for approximately 15 percent of CNS infection in patients with AIDS [2–10].

Epidemiology

Toxoplasma gondii is an obligate intracellular parasite with worldwide distribution. Developmental forms include the oocyst, trophozoite, and tissue cyst. Organisms reproduce sexually in the intestinal mucosa of cats, the only definitive host, to form oocysts, which are excreted in the stool. Oocysts become infectious once they undergo sporogony outside the body. Humans are infected following ingestion of oocysts from dried cat feces or tissue cysts from contaminated food, especially undercooked meat. Serologic evidence of toxoplasmosis is found in 15 to 70 percent of the United States population and increases with age. High rates are associated with tropical climate, poor sanitary conditions, and prevalence of cats.

Pathogenesis

Following the ingestion of *T. gondii*, trophozoites disseminate throughout the body via the lymphatics and bloodstream. Organisms invade nucleated cells and multiply, resulting in cell death and progressive tissue necrosis [11]. In the immunocompetent patient, host defenses, including T lymphocytes, activated macrophages, gamma-interferon, and type-specific antibody, generally control the primary infection. Most organisms are killed, and the remainder encyst and become latent. Cysts, containing several thousand slowly growing organisms, may develop in any tissue, but are especially common in the CNS, myocardium, and skeletal muscle. Through an unknown mechanism, HIV-induced immunosuppression permits reactivation and dissemination of latent infection, producing symptomatic disease [5, 12, 13]. Animal studies suggest that the development of encephalitis during chronic infection may be related to strain-specific virulence factors [14].

Congenital toxoplasmosis occurs following transplacental passage of parasites during acute infection in the pregnant woman. A recent case report describes four children congenitally infected with both toxoplasmosis and HIV [15]. One of the HIV-infected mothers had symptomatic reactivation of toxoplasmic encephalitis at the time of delivery; the others had a positive *Toxoplasma* serology but no clinical history of active toxoplasmosis. The authors speculated that the mothers had either chronic or intermittent parasitemia during gestation.

Clinical Manifestations

In the normal host, most primary *T. gondii* infection is either subclinical or produces a mild, self-limited illness characterized by fever, malaise, and regional adenopathy. The majority of cases of toxoplasmic chorioretinitis are late sequelae of congenital infection. CNS toxoplasmosis is usually the result of reactivated latent infection.

Toxoplasmic encephalitis often presents with focal or generalized neurologic abnormalities. A prodrome of frontal headache, low-grade fever, lethargy, and confusion or disorientation is common. Focal findings, including seizures or a stroke syndrome, occur as lesions become necrotic and the surrounding brain becomes edematous. Meningismus is infrequent. Other neuropsychological symptoms reported include diplopia, homonymous hemianopsia, blindness, unsteady gait, conus medullaris syndrome, myoclonus, tremor, personality change, hallucinosis, and syncope. Without treatment, rapid neurologic deterioration ensues, followed by coma and death. Even with effective therapy, mean survival following diagnosis is less than one year [2, 4–10, 16–20].

Although encephalitis is the most common presentation of toxoplasmosis in the AIDS patient, reports of severe or disseminated extraneural disease have become more frequent. Clinical manifestations reflect the organ system involved and may be associated with fever, maculopapular rash, generalized adenopathy, and hepatosplenomegaly. Fulminant infections of the eye, heart, lung, gut, and testes have been described [15, 21–24].

Diagnosis

Definitive diagnosis of toxoplasmosis requires demonstration of free or intracellular trophozoites in tissue, nucleated cells, or body fluids. Even

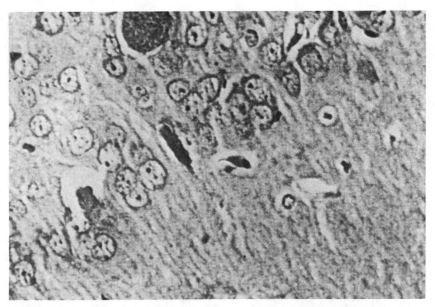

Figure 20-1. *Brain biopsy showing* Toxoplasma gondii *encephalitis. (Reprinted with permission of* Fam Pract Recert 9:84–118, 1987.)

with the use of special stains, trophozoites are difficult to identify on histologic evaluation because of their small size, their location at the periphery of necrotic lesions, and the presence of inflammatory debris and mononuclear cells (Fig. 20-1). Pathologic findings in the brain range from focal necrotic abscesses to diffuse meningoencephalitis. Identification of cyst forms or culture of organisms from tissue is consistent with prior infection, but does not necessarily indicate the presence of active disease.

Cerebrospinal fluid analysis may be abnormal but nonspecific, with mild pleocytosis, normal glucose, and mild protein elevation [4–6]. Microscopic detection of *Toxoplasma* trophozoites in body fluids has proven a reliable means of diagnosis [5, 15, 21, 23, 25]. Other diagnostic modalities, including DNA probes, *Toxoplasma* tissue culture methods, and a *Toxoplasma*-specific antigen test, are currently being evaluated [12, 21, 26].

When brain biopsy is not feasible, patients with clinically suspected toxoplasmic encephalitis can be treated empirically [27, 28]. Presumptive diagnosis is based on the combination of clinical manifestations, neuroradiologic findings, and response to empiric therapy [1]. Cranial computed tomography (CT) scans are usually abnormal, revealing one or more hypodense lesions that enhance in a ring or nodular pattern following the administration of contrast [2, 3] (see Fig. 15-3). Lesions are often located in the basal ganglia but may be scattered throughout the brain parenchyma [2, 3, 6, 29, 30]. Magnetic resonance imaging (MRI) may be more sensitive and depict lesions before the CT is abnormal [4, 29, 31]. Serial neuroradiologic examinations demonstrating improvement of lesions within 10 to 14 days following the initiation of specific therapy support the diagnosis of toxoplasmic encephalitis [1, 3, 5]. Absence of improvement suggests an alternative diagnosis and is an indication for brain biopsy [27, 28, 32].

Primary infection with *T. gondii* in the normal host generally results in seroconversion. Antibody is measured by the Sabin-Feldman dye exclusion test or with an indirect fluorescent antibody (IFA) test. The peak level of immunoglobulin G (IgG) is usually 1:1,000 or greater. Immunoglobulin G levels gradually fall, but a low level of antibody (1:16–1:64) persists for years. Although helpful in screening large numbers of patients, the use and interpretation of serologic tests to diagnose active toxoplasmosis in HIV-infected patients are controversial [33–35]. Because toxoplasmosis in this population usually results from reactivation of latent infection, serum immunoglobulin M (IgM) *Toxoplasma* antibodies are not present. Serum IgG antibodies are often detectable, but fewer than one third of patients achieve the high titers (IFA ≥ 1:1,000) indicative of active infection. Some clinicians obtain a serum IgG *Toxoplasma* antibody assay as part of the initial laboratory evaluation of the HIV-infected patient; others reserve the test for use in patients with a neurologic syndrome consistent with toxoplasmosis [36]. A negative test, while suggesting an alternative diagnosis, does not exclude the possibility of toxoplasmosis [37]. The clinical significance of *Toxoplasma* antibody in cerebrospinal fluid has not been established [6].

Other neurologic conditions in the HIV-infected patient may present in a manner similar to that of CNS toxoplasmosis. Differential diagnosis of toxoplasmic encephalitis includes cryptococcal meningitis, mycobacterial infection, syphilis, pyogenic brain abscess, progressive multifocal leukoencephalopathy, viral encephalitis, Kaposi's sarcoma, primary CNS lymphoma, and HIV encephalopathy.

Treatment

A combination of pyrimethamine and sulfadiazine is the treatment of choice for toxoplasmosis [18, 38, 39] (Table 20-1). This regimen inhibits replication of the trophozoite by blocking folate metabolism, but the drugs do not kill the trophozoite and have no effect on encysted organisms. Toxicity of pyrimethamine includes neutropenia and thrombocytopenia; the oral administration of folinic acid minimizes its myelosup-

Table 20-1 Treatment of toxoplasmic encephalitis

Drug	Primary therapy	Maintenance therapy
First choice		
Pyrimethamine[a] and	100–200 mg loading dose, then 50–100 mg/day po	25–50 mg/day po or 0.25 mg/kg po twice a week
Sulfadiazine[b] plus	1–2 gm q6h po (100 mg/kg/day)	0.5–1.0 gm q6h po or 75 mg/kg po twice a week
Folinic acid[c]	5–10 mg/day	5–10 mg/day po
Alternative		
Pyrimethamine and	100–200 mg loading dose, then 50–100 mg/day po	25–50 mg/day po or 0.25 mg/kg po twice a week
Clindamycin[d] plus	600–1,200 mg q6–8h IV/po	300–450 mg q6–8h po
Folinic acid	5–10 mg/day	5–10 mg/day po

[a]Side effects—occasional: blood dyscrasias, folic acid deficiency; rare: rash, vomiting, convulsions, shock.
[b]Side effects—frequent: rash, photosensitivity, drug fever; occasional: renal toxicity, hepatotoxicity, Stevens-Johnson syndrome, blood dyscrasias, hemolytic anemia, vasculitis; rare: myopia, pseudomembranous colitis, crystalluria with stone formation.
[c]The dose should be titrated as necessary to minimize bone marrow toxicity. Higher doses (up to 50 mg) are sometimes needed.
[d]Side effects—frequent: diarrhea, allergic reactions; occasional: pseudomembranous colitis; rare: blood dyscrasias, hepatotoxicity.

pressive effect. Pyrimethamine is teratogenic and should not be used in pregnant women. Side effects of sulfadiazine include fever, rash, and nephrolithiasis. Clindamycin with pyrimethamine is an effective alternative regimen for patients who are intolerant to sulfadiazine [40–42].

High-dose combination primary therapy is continued for 4 to 6 weeks, with drug dosage titrated to minimize toxicity. Corticosteroid therapy can be used adjunctively if there is evidence of cerebral edema [5, 18]. Maintenance therapy using reduced doses of the same agents is continued indefinitely [27, 33, 38, 39, 43]. Symptoms that recur during maintenance therapy may reflect reactivation of toxoplasmosis or signify a new neurologic process. In this setting, primary therapy should be reinstituted until a diagnostic evaluation has been completed.

A toxoplasmosis drug therapy that eradicates tissue cysts and causes fewer side effects is needed [44–46]. Clinical trials of treatment regimens currently in progress include: (1) a study comparing the efficacy of various doses of pyrimethamine with or without folinic acid; (2) an evaluation of oral azithromycin plus pyrimethamine; and (3) an assessment of atovaquone, an oral hydroxynaphthoquinone, for treatment of toxoplasmosis and *Pneumocystis carinii* pneumonia (PCP) in patients who have failed or cannot tolerate standard therapy [45, 47, 48].

Prevention

Individuals who are seronegative for toxoplasmosis should avoid exposure to infective forms of *T. gondii*. Meat should be frozen to $-20°C$ or cooked to $60°C$ to kill tissue cysts [9]. Pet cats should remain indoors to avoid exposure to potentially infected wild animals and should not be fed raw meat products. Litter boxes should be cleaned regularly using gloved hands; oocysts require 1 to 21 days to undergo sporogony and become infectious. Other areas where cats defecate (e.g., sandboxes, moist soil) should be avoided. Recently, low-dose trimethoprim-sulfamethoxazole used for the prevention of PCP in patients with AIDS has also been shown to afford protection against toxoplasmosis [49]. A placebo-controlled trial evaluating pyrimethamine for primary prophylaxis of toxoplasmic encephalitis has been discontinued because of increased mortality in the pyrimethamine-treated group [50].

References

1. Centers for Disease Control. Revision of surveillance case definition for acquired immunodeficiency syndrome. *MMWR* 36 (suppl):1–15, 1987.
2. Levy RM, Bredesen DE, Rosenblum ML. Neurological manifestations of the acquired immunodeficiency syndrome (AIDS): Experience at UCSF and review of the literature. *J Neurosurg* 62:475–495, 1985.
3. Post MJD, Kursunoglu SJ, Hensley GT, et al. Cranial CT in acquired immunodeficiency syndrome: Spectrum of diseases and optimal contrast enhancement technique. *Am J Radiol* 145:929–940, 1985.
4. Levy RM, Bredesen DE. Central nervous system dysfunction in acquired immunodeficiency syndrome. *J AIDS* 1:41–64, 1988.
5. Israelski DM, Remington JS. Toxoplasmic encephalitis in patients with AIDS. *Infect Dis Clin North Am* 2:429–445, 1988.
6. Luft BJ, Remington JS. Toxoplasmic encephalitis. *J Infect Dis* 157:1–6, 1988.
7. Elder GA, Sever JL. Neurologic disorders associated with AIDS retroviral infection. *Rev Infect Dis* 10:286–302, 1988.
8. Esiri MM, Scaravilli F, Millard PR, Harcourt-Webster JN. Neuropathology of HIV infection in haemophiliacs: Comparative necropsy study. *Br Med J* 299:1312–1315, 1989.
9. Reinis-Lucey C, Sande MA, Gerberding JL. Toxoplasmosis. In: PT Cohen, MA Sande, PA Volberding (eds), *The AIDS Knowledge Base*. Waltham, MA: The Medical Publishing Group, Pp 6.5.6.1–6.5.6.15, 1990.
10. Laughon BE, Allaudeen HS, Becker JM, et al. Summary of the workshop

on future directions in discovery and development of therapeutic agents for opportunistic infections associated with AIDS. *J Infect Dis* 164:244–251, 1991.

11. Werk R. How does *Toxoplasma gondii* enter host cells? *Rev Infect Dis* 7:449–457, 1985.

12. Tirard V, Niel G, Rosenheim M, et al. Diagnosis of toxoplasmosis in patients with AIDS by isolation of the parasite from the blood (letter). *N Engl J Med* 324:634, 1991.

13. Crowe SM, Carlin JB, Stewart KI, et al. Predictive value of CD4 lymphocyte numbers for the development of opportunistic infections and malignancies in HIV-infected persons. *J AIDS* 4:770–776, 1991.

14. Suzuki Y, Conley FK, Remington JS. Differences in virulence and development of encephalitis during chronic infection vary with the strain of *Toxoplasma gondii*. *J Infect Dis* 159:790–794, 1989.

15. Mitchell CD, et al. Congenital toxoplasmosis occurring in infants perinatally infected with human immunodeficiency virus 1. *Pediatr Infect Dis J* 9:512–518, 1990.

16. Engstrom JW, Lowenstein DH, Bredesen DE. Cerebral Infarctions and transient neurologic deficits associated with acquired immunodeficiency syndrome. *Am J Med* 86:528–532, 1989.

17. Overhage JM, Greist A, Brown DR. Conus medullaris syndrome resulting from *Toxoplasma gondii* infection in a patient with the acquired immunodeficiency syndrome. *Am J Med* 89:814–815, 1990.

18. Haverkos HW. Assessment of therapy for toxoplasma encephalitis. *Am J Med* 82:907–914, 1987.

19. Turner BJ, Markson LE, McKee L, et al. The AIDS-defining diagnosis and subsequent complications: A survival based severity index. *J AIDS* 4:1059–1071, 1991.

20. Friedland GH, Saltzman B, Vileno J, et al. Survival differences in patients with AIDS. *J AIDS* 4:144–153, 1991.

21. Israelski DM, et al. Toxoplasma peritonitis in a patient with acquired immunodeficiency syndrome. *Arch Intern Med* 148:1655–1657, 1988.

22. Schnapp LM, et al. *Toxoplasma gondii* pneumonitis in patients infected with the human immunodeficiency virus. *Arch Intern Med* 152:1073–1077, 1992.

23. Oksenhendler E, Cadranel J, Sarfati C, et al. *Toxoplasma gondii* pneumonia in patients with the acquired immunodeficiency syndrome. *Am J Med* 88 (suppl 5):18–21, 1990.

24. Tschirart D, Klatt EC. Disseminated toxoplasmosis in the acquired immunodeficiency syndrome. *Arch Pathol Lab Med* 112:1237–1241, 1988.

25. Threlkeld MG, Graves AH, Cobbs CG. Cerebrospinal fluid staining for the diagnosis of toxoplasmosis in patients with the acquired immunodeficiency syndrome. *Am J Med* 83:599–600, 1987.

26. Weiss LM, Udem SA, Salgo M, et al. Sensitive and specific detection of toxoplasma DNA in an experimental murine model: Use of *Toxoplasma gondii*-specific cDNA and the polymerase chain reaction. *J Infect Dis* 163:180–186, 1991.

27. Cohn JA, McMeeking A, Cohen W, et al. Evaluation of the policy of

empiric treatment of suspected toxoplasma encephalitis in patients with the acquired immunodeficiency syndrome. *Am J Med* 86:521–527, 1989.

28. Cimino C, Lipton RB, Williams A, et al. The evaluation of patients with human immunodeficiency virus–related disorders and brain mass lesions. *Arch Intern Med* 151:1381–1384, 1991.

29. Levy RM, Rosenbloom S, Perrett LV. Neuroradiological findings in the acquired immunodeficiency syndrome (AIDS): A review of 200 cases. *Am J Radiol* 147:977–983, 1986.

30. Carrazana EJ, Rossitch E, Schachter S. Cerebral toxoplasmosis masquerading as herpes encephalitis in a patient with the acquired immunodeficiency syndrome. *Am J Med* 86:730–732, 1989.

31. Levy RM, Mills CM, Posin JP, et al. The efficacy and clinical impact of brain imaging in neurologically symptomatic AIDS patients: A prospective CT/MRI study. *J AIDS* 3:461–471, 1990.

32. Bishburg E, Eng RHK, Slim J, et al. Brain lesions in patients with acquired immunodeficiency syndrome. *Arch Intern Med* 149:941–943, 1989.

33. Potasman I, Resnick L, Luft BJ, Remington JA. Intrathecal production of antibodies against *Toxoplasma gondii* in patients with toxoplasmic encephalitis and the acquired immunodeficiency syndrome (AIDS). *Ann Intern Med* 108:49–51, 1988.

34. Stepick-Biek P, Thulliez P, Araujo FG, Remington JS. IgA antibodies for diagnosis of acute congenital and acquired toxoplasmosis. *J Infect Dis* 162:270–273, 1990.

35. Hedman K, Lappalainen M, Seppaia I, Makela O. Recent primary toxoplasma infection indicated by a low avidity of specific IgG. *J Infect Dis* 159:736–740, 1989.

36. Grant IH, Gold JWM, Rosenblum M, et al. *Toxoplasma gondii* serology in HIV-infected patients: the development of central nervous system toxoplasmosis in AIDS. *AIDS* 4:519–521, 1990.

37. Porter SB, Sande MA. Toxoplasmosis of the central nervous system in the acquired immunodeficiency syndrome. *N Engl J Med* 327:1643–1648, 1992.

38. Leport C, Raffi F, Matheron S, et al. Treatment of central nervous system toxoplasmosis with pyrimethamine/sulfadiazine combination in 35 patients with the acquired immunodeficiency syndrome: Efficacy of long-term continuous therapy. *Am J Med* 84:94–100, 1988.

39. Sanford JP. *Guide to Antimicrobial Therapy.* West Bethesda, MD: Antimicrobial Therapy, Inc, 1991. P 78.

40. Dannemann BR, Israelski DM, Remington JS. Treatment of toxoplasmic encephalitis with intravenous clindamycin. *Arch Intern Med* 148:2477–2482, 1988.

41. Dannemann B, et al. Treatment of toxoplasmic encephalitis in patients with AIDS; a randomized trial comparing pyrimethamine plus clindamycin to pyrimethamine plus sulfadiazine. *Ann Intern Med* 116:33–43, 1992.

42. Remington JS, Vilde JL. Clindamycin for toxoplasma encephalitis in AIDS (letter). *Lancet* 338:1142–1143, 1991.

43. Weiss LM, Harris C, Berger M, et al. Pyrimethamine concentrations in

serum and cerebrospinal fluid during treatment of acute toxoplasma encephalitis in patients with AIDS. *J Infect Dis* 157:580–583, 1988.

44. Leport C, Bastuji-Garin S, Perronne C, et al. An open study of the pyrimethamine-clindamycin combination in AIDS patients with brain toxoplasmosis. *J Infect Dis* 160:557–558, 1989.

45. Chang HR, Pechere JCF. In vitro effects of four macrolides (roxithromycin, spiramycin, azithromycin [CP-62,993], and A-56268) on *Toxoplasma gondii*. *Antimicrob Agents Chemother* 32:524–529, 1988.

46. Huskinson-Mark J, Araujo FG, Remington JS. Evaluation of the effect of drugs on the cyst form of *Toxoplasma gondii*. *J Infect Dis* 164:170–177, 1991.

47. Hughes WT, Kennedy W, Shenep JL, et al. Safety and pharmacokinetics of 566C80, a hydroxynaphthoquinone with anti-*Pneumocystis carinii* activity: A phase I study in human immunodeficiency virus (HIV)-infected men. *J Infect Dis* 163:843–848, 1991.

48. Kovacs JA, et al. Efficacy of atovaquone in treatment of toxoplasmosis in patients with AIDS. *Lancet* 340:637–638, 1992.

49. Carr A, Tindall B, Brew BJ, et al. Low-dose trimethoprim-sulfamethoxazole prophylaxis for toxoplasmic encephalitis in patients with AIDS. *Ann Intern Med* 117:106–111, 1992.

50. Burroughs Wellcome Company. Letter to physicians. August 10, 1992.

21/Syphilis

Judith L. Steinberg

Epidemiology

In 1990, the incidence of primary and secondary syphilis in the United States was 20 cases per 100,000 persons, which represented a 75 percent increase over 5 years and the highest rate since 1949 [1]. Rising rates of syphilis over the past decade have been associated with a change in its epidemiology. Whereas in the 1970s the disease occurred most commonly in homosexual or bisexual men, the current epidemic involves primarily heterosexual men and women, with the highest rate in the black population.

From 1985 through 1990, rates of primary and secondary syphilis for black men increased from 69 to 156 per 100,000 (126%) and for black women from 35 to 116 per 100,000 (231%) [1]. Concurrently, the incidence of syphilis has decreased among white men, probably because of recent sexual behavioral changes among homosexual and bisexual men. The changing epidemiology of syphilis has paralleled that of the AIDS epidemic, with increasing involvement of drug users, heterosexuals, and minorities [2–4].

Many retrospective studies have linked HIV seropositivity with historical or serologic evidence of syphilis and other genital ulcer diseases [5–13]. For example, among patients in Baltimore sexually transmitted disease clinics, the HIV seroprevalence rate was 24.3 percent in those with reactive syphilis serologies, compared to 3.5 percent in those with nonreactive tests [14]. Several prospective studies have linked the presence of genital ulcer disease with HIV seroconversion [15–17]. One study showed a significant association between genital ulcer disease in HIV-infected men and the transmission of HIV to their female partners [18].

Syphilis and HIV infection are related in several ways: (1) They are both acquired through high-risk sexual behaviors; (2) genital ulceration may be an important factor in the transmission and acquisition of HIV; (3) HIV infection may increase susceptibility to other sexually transmitted diseases (STDs), including genital ulcer diseases; and (4) concurrent HIV infection may alter the clinical presentation, disease severity, and treatment response of STDs [7, 19, 20].

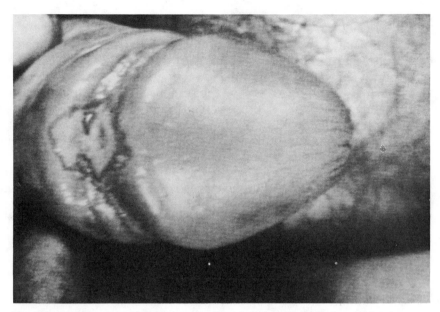

Figure 21-1. *Primary syphilitic chancre. (Reprinted with permission of Upjohn Company.)*

Clinical Manifestations

Our current knowledge of syphilis in the context of HIV infection is based on numerous case reports and series but few prospective data. These cases have suggested that HIV-infected patients with syphilis may have atypical clinical presentations, altered serologic response to infection, an increased frequency of neurosyphilis, and an inadequate clinical response to standard therapy. Given that cell-mediated immunity is important in the host response to syphilis, it is understandable that concurrent HIV infection might alter its course [21–23]. However, it is important to emphasize that most HIV-infected patients with syphilis probably have typical disease manifestations [24–26] (Fig. 21-1; see Plate 13).

Reported atypical presentations of syphilis in HIV-infected patients include fever of unknown origin, lues maligna (a rare form of secondary syphilis manifested by skin ulcerations and severe constitutional symptoms), uveitis, atypical oral ulcerations with gummatous perforation, oral hairy leukoplakia, Kaposi's sarcoma–like skin lesions, giant nodular skin lesions, and Reiter's syndrome (Centers for Disease Control [CDC], personal communication; [27–33]).

Serologic Response

There have been case reports of delayed serologic response and unusually high nontreponemal serologic titers in patients with HIV infection and syphilis [25, 26, 34–36]. However, recently a case series and comparative study suggested that the serologic response to syphilis in HIV-infected individuals is preserved and comparable to that of HIV-seronegative patients [35, 37]. Increased nontreponemal titers may be a manifestation of the polyclonal B-cell activation that occurs in HIV infection. Some studies have documented the loss of treponemal test reactivity in HIV-infected patients, which may be related to immune compromise [38, 39]. There may also be an increased frequency of biologically false-positive serologic tests for syphilis in HIV-infected patients and falsely rising titers in individuals with previously treated syphilis, especially among those with *Pneumocystis carinii* pneumonia (CDC, personal communication); [40]).

Neurosyphilis

Central nervous system (CNS) involvement is common in the early stages of syphilis and is usually asymptomatic. Early investigators documented CNS involvement in up to 13 percent of patients with primary syphilis and 40 percent of those with secondary syphilis [41]. Recently, Lukehart and associates [42] isolated *Treponema pallidum* from the cerebrospinal fluid (CSF) in 30 percent of patients with primary and secondary syphilis. The rate of CNS involvement was similar in HIV-infected and uninfected patients.

The clinical significance of early asymptomatic CNS syphilis is unclear; only 5 to 10 percent of untreated patients develop clinically recognizable neurosyphilis [35]. The currently recommended therapy for early and latent syphilis, benzathine penicillin G, does not achieve treponemicidal levels in the CSF [43, 44]. Although case reports of neurologic relapse following benzathine penicillin G therapy appeared in the pre-AIDS era, several studies have shown that progression to neurosyphilis rarely occurs following standard treatment [35, 45, 46].

There have been numerous case reports of neurosyphilis or neurologic relapse following standard therapy for syphilis in HIV-infected patients. Most commonly described is early symptomatic neurosyphilis, including aseptic meningitis, cranial nerve abnormalities, or meningovascular disease. Other reported manifestations of neurosyphilis in this population have included necrotizing encephalitis, tabes dorsalis, meningomyelitis, lumbosacral polyradiculopathy, otosyphilis, and ocular disease (chorioretinitis, optic neuritis) [32, 47–56].

In a retrospective study, Katz and Berger [57] found that 44 percent of all cases of neurosyphilis occurred in the context of HIV infection, representing 1.5 percent of all patients hospitalized with AIDS. Musher [58] reviewed 42 cases of neurosyphilis in HIV-infected patients and found optic neuritis or neuroretinitis to be the most frequent manifestation. This retrospective study also demonstrated the common occurrence of neurosyphilis in early HIV infection, neurosyphilis as a sentinel disease of HIV infection, and the frequency with which neurosyphilis occurs following standard treatment of syphilis. A recent prospective study documented neurosyphilis in 13 percent of HIV-infected patients with latent syphilis; 42 percent of patients had abnormal CSF findings [59]. A positive CSF Venereal Disease Research Laboratory test (VDRL) was associated with an increased titer of the serum nontreponemal test and advancing age.

Based on these data, some authorities have concluded that the incidence of neurosyphilis is increased in HIV-infected patients [35]. Others have argued that the observations are consistent with the natural variability of syphilis and may represent an ascertainment bias [60]. Prospective studies are necessary to resolve this issue.

Diagnosis

The current CDC recommendations for the diagnosis of syphilis in HIV-infected patients are as follows: (1) HIV counseling and testing should be encouraged for all sexually active patients with syphilis; (2) when clinical findings suggest a diagnosis of syphilis, but serologic tests are negative or confusing, alternative tests, such as biopsy, dark-field examination, or direct fluorescent antibody staining of lesions, should be used; and (3) CSF examination is indicated for HIV-infected patients with syphilis of more than one year's duration. CSF examination is recommended in HIV-infected patients with early syphilis only if clinical evidence of neurologic involvement is found [61].

The diagnosis of neurosyphilis is often difficult in HIV-infected patients. Traditional diagnostic criteria include a positive CSF VDRL in combination with an elevated CSF white blood cell count or protein level, or both [62]. Tramont [63] requires only one of these CSF abnormalities. Jordan [64] also includes a reactive serum treponemal test to confirm that the CSF VDRL does not represent a biologic false positive. Spirochetes have been isolated from the CSF of patients who have no abnormalities on CSF analysis, and there is evidence suggesting that the CSF may be entirely normal in up to 25 percent of patients with neurosyphilis [42, 65]. Moreover, in symptomatic neurosyphilis, the sensitivity of the CSF VDRL is only 22 to 69 percent [66]. Therefore, a diagnosis of presumptive neurosyphilis should be made in the absence of a reactive CSF VDRL if symptoms and signs consistent with neurosyphilis are present and no alternative diagnosis is evident [64].

Retrospective reviews of neurosyphilis in HIV-infected patients have shown that the serum treponemal and nontreponemal tests are commonly reactive, the latter often in high titer [57, 67]. In his review, Musher [58] found that CSF parameters were frequently abnormal, including a positive CSF VDRL in 79 percent of cases. Feraru and associates [68] reported delayed reactivity of the CSF VDRL in patients with neurosyphilis and AIDS. Computed tomographic scans were abnormal in 5 of 10 patients with neurosyphilis and AIDS in another series [57]. Findings included cerebral atrophy, multiple infarctions, nodular enhancing lesions, meningeal enhancement, and lobar hemorrhage. Angiography may demonstrate multiple areas of narrowing of the cerebral arteries [58].

Some authorities have argued that lumbar puncture is indicated in all HIV-infected patients with syphilis regardless of the stage of disease [35]. However, interpretation of CSF results in neurologically asymptomatic HIV-infected patients with syphilis is difficult because 40 to 60 percent of HIV-infected patients without syphilis have an elevated CSF white blood cell count or protein level [69]. Thus, while the finding of a positive CSF VDRL in an HIV-infected patient establishes the diagnosis of neurosyphilis, the presence of nonspecific CSF abnormalities is uninterpretable. Because of case reports suggesting more frequent and fulminant neurologic involvement in HIV-infected patients with syphilis, some clinicians treat for neurosyphilis even if only nonspecific CSF abnormalities are present.

Prognosis

Several reports have documented a poor clinical response to standard therapy in HIV-infected patients with syphilis. Thirty-three and 38 percent of patients with neurosyphilis and HIV infection reviewed by Katz and Berger [57] and Musher [58], respectively, had been previously treated for syphilis; other authors have reported similar results [70, 71]. Lukehart and associates [42] found that three HIV-infected patients treated for secondary syphilis with 2.4 mIU benzathine penicillin G did not clear the CSF of spirochetes or improve other CSF parameters. These reports have fostered the view that a therapeutic response to the currently recommended benzathine penicillin G regimen may require normal host immunity.

Frederick and associates [72] documented delayed lesion healing and serologic response in 7 of 16 HIV-infected patients treated for secondary syphilis. In a case-control study, Telzak and colleagues [73]

Table 21-1 *CDC guidelines for the treatment of syphilis*

Primary, secondary, and early latent (< 1 yr duration) syphilis
Recommended regimen: 2.4 mIU benzathine penicillin G IM once
Doxycycline, 100 mg po bid × 2 wk, if penicillin allergic

Late latent (> 1 yr duration) and cardiovascular syphilis
Recommended regimen: 2.4 mIU benzathine penicillin G IM weekly × 3 wk
(total 7.2 mIU)
Doxycycline, 100 mg po bid × 4 wk, if penicillin allergic

Neurosyphilis*
Recommended regimen: 12–24 mIU aqueous penicillin G IV daily × 10–14
days
Alternative: 2.4 mIU procaine penicillin IM daily plus 500 mg probenecid po
qid × 10–14 days
If patient is penicillin allergic, skin test and desensitize if necessary

*Note: Following completion of a neurosyphilis regimen, many authorities
recommend the administration of 2.4 mIU benzathine penicillin G weekly
× 3 wk.

Source: Adapted from Centers for Disease Control, Sexually transmitted diseases treatment guidelines, 1989. *MMWR* 38 (suppl 8):1–43, 1989.

found that HIV-infected patients with primary syphilis were significantly less likely than seronegative control subjects to have a fourfold or greater rapid plasma reagin (RPR) test decrease or seroreversion within 6 months of treatment. However, other studies have shown no major differences in the response to treatment between HIV-infected patients with syphilis and control subjects [26, 74].

Management

The most recent CDC guidelines for the treatment of syphilis are presented in Table 21-1 [61]. As part of its recommendations, the CDC adds the following two caveats regarding HIV-infected patients: (1) Penicillin regimens should be used whenever possible for all stages of syphilis in HIV-infected patients. Skin testing to confirm penicillin allergy can be used if minor and major determinants are available. However, data on its use in HIV-infected individuals are inadequate. Patients can be desensitized and treated with penicillin. (2) No change in therapy for syphilis in HIV-infected patients is recommended. In all cases, careful follow-up study is necessary to ensure adequacy of treatment.

Some authorities disagree with these recommendations and have advocated the use of higher doses of benzathine penicillin G. Fiumara [75] has recommended a regimen of 2.4 mIU benzathine penicillin G administered weekly for 2 weeks (total dose 4.8 mIU) for all patients with early syphilis, including HIV-infected patients. Others have advocated treating HIV-infected patients with early syphilis with a total dose of 7.2 mIU benzathine penicillin G: 2.4 mIU administered weekly for 3 weeks or 1.2 mIU twice a week for 3 consecutive weeks [35, 76, 77]. Tramont [78] has suggested that neurosyphilis regimens should be used for all HIV-infected individuals with syphilis, regardless of the stage of disease.

Several alternative antibiotic regimens aimed at increasing CSF drug levels have been proposed. These include: (1) 1.2 mIU procaine penicillin intramuscularly daily for 10 to 14 days, (2) the use of high-dose oral amoxicillin (up to 6 gm/day), (3) the addition of probenecid to penicillin regimens, (4) the addition of oral penicillin or amoxicillin to benzathine penicillin G regimens, and (5) the use of ceftriaxone [79]. A multicenter trial is in progress comparing the efficacy of standard therapy with 2.4 mIU benzathine penicillin G to a regimen supplemented with high-dose amoxicillin and probenecid. Clinical studies have documented the efficacy of ceftriaxone in the treatment of incubating and early syphilis, and the drug has also been used successfully to treat asymptomatic neurosyphilis [80–82]. However, its optimal dose and duration are unknown.

Close clinical and serologic observation is necessary following treatment of HIV-infected patients with syphilis. The CDC recommends follow-up evaluation at 1, 2, 3, 6, 9, and 12 months after treatment [61]. Others have recommended obtaining nontreponemal tests on a monthly basis for at least the first 6 months [24]. An adequate response to therapy is defined as a fourfold decline in nontreponemal antibody titer by 3 months for primary and secondary syphilis and by 6 months for early latent syphilis [61, 83]. If this does not occur or if there is a sustained rise in nontreponemal antibody titer, then reevaluation with lumbar puncture is indicated, followed by retreatment [61]. The same is true if, after treatment of late latent syphilis, there is a sustained fourfold rise in nontreponemal antibody titer or if an initially high titer ($\geq$1:32) fails to decline over a period of 6 to 12 months.

Of note, a recent study showed that the usual serologic response to treatment of syphilis may be slower than that described above [84]. Romanowski and associates [84] found that successful treatment of primary and secondary syphilis results in a four- and eightfold decline in RPR titer by 6 and 12 months, respectively. A fourfold decline in titer was seen by 12 to 24 months in patients treated for early latent syphilis. Thus, the standard criteria to assess response of early syphilis to therapy may be too stringent.

Recommendations for the follow-up and expected CSF response of patients treated for neurosyphilis vary [61, 64, 85, 86]. According to Simon [85] and Swartz [86], repeat CSF examinations should be performed at 3 to 6 months after treatment and at 6-month intervals thereafter for 2 years or until the CSF cell count and protein level return to normal. An adequate therapeutic response is defined as a normal CSF cell count and a falling protein level (if it was initially elevated) at 6 months after treatment. The CSF VDRL titer generally declines but may not become nonreactive. If the CSF cell count is not normal by 3 to 6 months or, if having normalized, the cell count rises, retreatment is necessary. Swartz [86] recommends annual lumbar puncture for several years after the normalization of CSF values. The CDC recommends consideration of retreatment if the CSF cell count does not decline by 6 months or if the count has not normalized by 2 years [61]. However, given the frequency of CSF abnormalities in HIV-infected patients without syphilis and of neurologic disease in AIDS, changes in these nonspecific parameters may not be indicative of therapeutic response or lack thereof [69].

Prevention

The prevention and control of syphilis and other STDs require primary, secondary, and tertiary strategies [87]. Disease avoidance (primary prevention) includes health education and interventions to promote safer sexual behaviors. Because the acquisition of syphilis and HIV infection are behaviorally related, such primary prevention strategies may affect the occurrence of both diseases.

The prevention of disease sequelae and transmission of infection (secondary prevention) requires early diagnosis and treatment, including screening of high-risk individuals and partner notification. Targeted syphilis screening and treatment in locations such as crack houses or jails may be required to improve the efficacy of these efforts [88–90].

Tertiary prevention (efforts to minimize the effects of disease sequelae) may be especially important in HIV-infected patients with syphilis. This includes intensive antibiotic therapy as described previously, with repeated follow-up evaluations. Some clinicians have suggested that suppressive therapy may be indicated to prevent relapse of syphilis in HIV-infected patients. Musher [58] argues against this, citing that neurologic relapse is rare when three doses of benzathine penicillin are used and chronic oral therapy is unlikely to achieve significant levels in the CSF.

References

1. Centers for Disease Control. Primary and secondary syphilis—United States, 1981–1990. *MMWR* 40:314–315, 321–323, 1991.

2. Rolfs RT, Goldberg M, Sharrar RG. Risk factors for syphilis: cocaine use and prostitution. *Am J Public Health* 80:853–857, 1990.
3. Minkoff HL, McCalla S, Delke I, et al. The relationship of cocaine use to syphilis and human immunodeficiency virus infections among inner city parturient women. *Am J Obstet Gynecol* 163:521–526, 1990.
4. Centers for Disease Control. The HIV/AIDS epidemic: The first 10 years. *MMWR* 40:357–363, 369, 1991.
5. Kreiss JK, Koech D, Plummer FA, et al. AIDS virus infection in Nairobi prostitutes: spread of the epidemic to east Africa. *N Engl J Med* 314:414–418, 1986.
6. Quinn TC, Glasser D, Cannon RO, et al. Human immunodeficiency virus infection among patients attending clinics for sexually transmitted diseases. *N Engl J Med* 318:197–203, 1988.
7. Stamm WE, Handsfield HH, Rompalo AM, et al. The association between genital ulcer disease and acquisition of HIV infection in homosexual men. *JAMA* 260:1429–1433, 1988.
8. Greenblatt RM, Lukehart SL, Plummer FA, et al. Genital ulceration as a risk factor for human immunodeficiency virus infection in Kenya. Third International Conference on AIDS, Washington, DC, June 1987.
9. Levine WC, McKinley TW, Smith JD, et al. HIV seroprevalence and drug use among patients with syphilis attending sexually transmitted disease clinics in Georgia. Seventh International Conference on AIDS, Florence, June 1991.
10. Valdespino JL, Loo E, Cruz C, et al. Risk factors interrelated between AIDS and STD among female prostitutes in Mexico. Seventh International Conference on AIDS, Florence, June 1991.
11. Larco P, Metelus-Chalumeau E, Poumerol G. Evaluation of HIV infection, hepatitis B and syphilis among blood donors in Haiti (1986–1990). Seventh International Conference on AIDS, Florence, June 1991.
12. Evans BA, McLean KA, Dawson SG, et al. Trends in sexual behaviour and risk factors for HIV infection among homosexual men, 1984–7. *Br Med J* 298:215–218, 1989.
13. Harkess JR, Kudlac J, Istre GR. Syphilis, human immunodeficiency virus infection, and targeting prevention. *South Med J* 83:1253–1255, 1990.
14. Quinn TC, Cannon RO, Glasser D, et al. The association of syphilis with risk of human immunodeficiency virus infection in patients attending sexually transmitted disease clinics. *Arch Intern Med* 150:1297–1302, 1990.
15. Plummer F, Cameron W, Simonsen N, et al. Co-factors in male-female transmission of HIV. Fourth International Conference on AIDS, Stockholm, June 1988.
16. Cameron DW, D'Costa LJ, Ndinya-Achola JO, et al. Incidence and risk factors for female to male transmission of HIV. Fourth International Conference on AIDS, Stockholm, June 1988.
17. Cameron DW, Simonsen JN, D'Costa LJ, et al. Genital ulcer disease and lack of circumcision are cofactors in female to male sexual transmission of human immunodeficiency virus. *Lancet* 2:403–408, 1989.
18. Katzenstein DA, Latif A, Bassett MT, Emmanuel JC. Risks for heterosexual

transmission of HIV in Zimbabwe. Third International Conference on AIDS, Washington, DC, June 1987.

19. Malele B, Manoka T, Kivuvu M, et al. The impact of HIV infection on the incidence of STD in high risk women. Seventh International Conference on AIDS, Florence, June 1991.
20. Plummer FA. The role of sexually transmitted disease in human immunodeficiency virus type 1 transmission. 31st Interscience Conference on Antimicrobial Agents and Chemotherapy, Chicago, 1991.
21. Lukehart SA, Baker-Zander SA, Sell S. Characterization of lymphocyte responsiveness in early experimental syphilis. I. *In vitro* response to mitogens and *Treponema pallidum* antigens. *J Immunol* 124:454–460,1980.
22. Lukehart SA, Baker-Zander SA, Lloyd RM, Sell S. Characterization of lymphocyte responsiveness in early experimental syphilis: Nature of cellular infiltration and *Treponema pallidum* distribution in testicular infection. *J Immunol* 124:461–467, 1980.
23. Pavia CS, Folds JD, Baseman JB. Cell-mediated immunity during syphilis: A review. *Br J Vener Dis* 54:144–150, 1978.
24. Hook EW, III. Syphilis and HIV infection. *J Infect Dis* 160:530–534, 1989.
25. Hutchinson CM, Rompalo AM, Reichart CA, Hook EW, III. Characteristics of patients with syphilis attending Baltimore STD clinics. *Arch Intern Med* 151:511–516, 1991.
26. Gourevitch MN, Selwyn PA, Davenny K, et al. Syphilis among intravenous drug users (IVDU's) in a prospective cohort study in a New York City methadone treatment program. Seventh International Conference on AIDS, Florence, June 1991.
27. Shulkin D, Tripoli L, Abell E. Lues maligna in a patient with human immunodeficiency virus infection. *Am J Med* 85:425–427, 1988.
28. Chung WM, Pien FD, Grekin JL. Syphilis: A cause of fever of unknown origin. *Cutis* 31:537–540, 1983.
29. Gregory N, Sanchez M, Buchness MR. The spectrum of syphilis in patients with human immunodeficiency virus infection. *J Am Acad Dermatol* 22:1061–1067, 1990.
30. Radolf JD, Kaplan RP. Unusual manifestations of secondary syphilis and abnormal humoral immune response to *Treponema pallidum* antigens in a homosexual man with asymptomatic human immunodeficiency virus infection. *J Am Acad Dermatol* 18:423–428, 1988.
31. Cusini M, Zerboni R, Muratori S, et al. Atypical early syphilis in an HIV-infected homosexual male. *Dermatologica* 177:300–304, 1988.
32. Becerra LI, Ksiazek SM, Savino PJ, et al. Syphilitic uveitis in human immunodeficiency virus–infected and noninfected patients. *Ophthalmology* 96:1727–1730, 1989.
33. Richards BW, Hessburg TJ, Nussbaum JN. Recurrent syphilitic uveitis. *N Engl J Med* 320:62, 1989.
34. Hicks CB, Benson PM, Lupton GP, Tramont EC. Seronegative secondary syphilis in a patient infected with the human immunodeficiency virus (HIV) with Kaposi's sarcoma. *Ann Intern Med* 107:492–495, 1988.
35. Musher DM, Hamill RJ, Baughn RE. Effect of human immunodeficiency

virus (HIV) infection on the course of syphilis and on the response to treatment. *Ann Intern Med* 113:872–881, 1990.

36. Centers for Disease Control. Recommendations for diagnosing and treating syphilis in HIV-infected patients. *MMWR* 37:600–608, 1988.

37. Terry PM, Page ML, Goldmeier LD. Are serological tests of value in diagnosing and monitoring response to treatment of syphilis in patients infected with human immunodeficiency virus? *Genitourin Med* 64:219–222, 1988.

38. Haas JS, Bolan G, Larsen SA, et al. Sensitivity of treponemal tests for detecting prior treated syphilis during human immunodeficiency virus infection. *J Infect Dis* 162:862–866, 1990.

39. Johnson PDR, Graves SR, Stewart L, et al. Specific syphilis serological tests may become negative in HIV infection. *AIDS* 5:419–423, 1991.

40. Rompalo AM, et al. Association of biologic false-positive reactions for syphilis with human immunodeficiency virus infection. *J Infect Dis* 165:1124–1126, 1992.

41. Mills CH. Routine examination of the cerebro-spinal fluid in syphilis: Its value in regard to more accurate knowledge, prognosis, and treatment. *Br Med J* 2:527–532, 1927.

42. Lukehart SA, Hook EW, Baker-Zander SA, et al. Invasion of the central nervous system by *Treponema pallidum*: Implications for diagnosis and treatment. *Ann Intern Med* 109:855–862, 1988.

43. Mohr JA, Griffiths W, Jackson R, et al. Neurosyphilis and penicillin levels in cerebrospinal fluid. *JAMA* 236:2208–2209, 1976.

44. Dunlop EMC, Al-Egaily SS, Houang ET. Penicillin levels in blood and CSF achieved by treatment of syphilis. *JAMA* 241:2538–2540, 1979.

45. Moskovitz BL, Klimek JJ, Goldman RL, et al. Meningovascular syphilis after "appropriate" treatment of primary syphilis. *Arch Intern Med* 142:139–140, 1982.

46. Tramont EC. Persistence of *Treponema pallidum* following penicillin G therapy: Report of two cases. *JAMA* 236:2206–2207, 1976.

47. Morgella S, Laufer H. Quaternary neurosyphilis in a Haitian man with human immunodeficiency virus infection. *Hum Pathol* 20:808–811, 1989.

48. Calderon W, Douville H, Nigro M, et al. Concomitant syphilitic and HIV infection: A case report. *Acta Neurologica* 12:132–137, 1990.

49. Strom, T, Schneck SA. Syphilitic meningomyelitis. *Neurology* 41:325–326, 1991.

50. Lanska MJ, Lanska DJ, Schmidley JW. Syphilitic polyradiculopathy in an HIV-positive man. *Neurology* 38:1297–1301, 1988.

51. Smith ME, Canalis RF. Otologic manifestations of AIDS: The otosyphilis connection. *Laryngoscope* 99:365–372, 1989.

52. Passo MS, Rosenbaum JT. Ocular syphilis in patients with human immunodeficiency virus infection. *Am J Ophthalmol* 106:1–6, 1988.

53. Zambrano W, Perez GM, Smith JL. Acute syphilitic blindness in AIDS. *J Clin Neuro Ophthalmol* 7:1–5, 1987.

54. McLeish WM, Pulido JS, Holland S, et al. The ocular manifestations of syphilis in the human immunodeficiency virus type 1–infected host. *Ophthalmology* 97:196–203, 1990.

55. Levy JH, Liss RA, Maguire AM. Neurosyphilis and ocular syphilis in patients with concurrent human immunodeficiency virus infection. *Retina* 9:175–180, 1989.
56. Tamesis RR, Foster CS. Ocular syphilis. *Ophthalmology* 97:1281–1287, 1990.
57. Katz DA, Berger JR. Neurosyphilis in acquired immunodeficiency syndrome. *Arch Neurol* 46:895–898, 1989.
58. Musher DM. Syphilis, neurosyphilis, penicillin, and AIDS. *J Infect Dis* 163:1201–1206, 1991.
59. Kemper C, Holtom P, Feigal D, et al. RPR, CD4 and CSF findings in HIV infection and syphilis. 31st Interscience Conference on Antimicrobial Agents and Chemotherapy, Washington, DC, 1991.
60. Zenker PN, Rolfs RT. Treatment of syphilis, 1989. *Rev Infect Dis* 12 (suppl 6):S590–S609, 1990.
61. Centers for Disease Control. Sexually transmitted diseases treatment guidelines, 1989. *MMWR* 38 (suppl 8):1–43, 1989.
62. Wolters EC, Hische EAH, Tutuarima JA, et al. Central nervous system involvement in early and late syphilis: The problem of asymptomatic neurosyphilis. *J Neurol Sci* 88:29–39, 1988.
63. Tramont EC. *Treponema pallidum* (syphilis). In Mandell, Douglas, Bennett (eds), *Principles and Practice of Infectious Diseases*. New York: Churchill Livingstone, 1990. Pp. 1794–1808.
64. Jordan KG. Modern neurosyphilis: A critical analysis. *West J Med* 149:47–57, 1988.
65. Musher DM. How much penicillin cures early syphilis? *Ann Intern Med* 109:849–851, 1988.
66. Hart G. Syphilis tests in diagnostic and therapeutic decision making. *Ann Intern Med* 104:368–376, 1986.
67. Matlow AG, Rachlis AR. Syphilis serology in human immunodeficiency virus–infected patients with symptomatic neurosyphilis: Case report and review. *Rev Infect Dis* 12:703–707, 1990.
68. Feraru ER, Aronow HA, Lipton RB. Neurosyphilis in AIDS patients: Initial CSF VDRL may be negative. *Neurology* 40:541–543, 1990.
69. Hollander H. Cerebrospinal fluid normalities and abnormalities in individuals infected with human immunodeficiency virus. *J Infect Dis* 158:855–858, 1988.
70. Johns DR, Tierney M, Felsenstein D. Alteration in the natural history of neurosyphilis by concurrent infection with the human immunodeficiency virus. *N Engl J Med* 316:1569–1572, 1987.
71. Berry CD, Hooton TM, Collier AC, Lukehart SA. Neurologic relapse after benzathine penicillin therapy for secondary syphilis in a patient with HIV infection. *N Engl J Med* 316:1587–1589, 1987.
72. Frederick WR, Delapenha R, Barnes S, et al. Secondary syphilis and HIV infection. 28th Interscience Conference on Antimicrobial Agents and Chemotherapy, Washington, DC, 1988.
73. Telzak EE, Zweig Greenberg MS, Harrison J, et al. Syphilis treatment response in HIV-infected individuals. *AIDS* 5:591–595, 1991.
74. Manoka AT, Laga M, Kivuvu M, et al. Syphilis among HIV positive and HIV

negative prostitutes in Kinshasa: prevalence and serologic response to treatment. Sixth International Conference on AIDS, San Francisco, June 1990.

75. Fiumara N. Human immunodeficiency virus infection and syphilis. *J Am Acad Dermatol* 21:141–142, 1989.

76. Felman YM. Recent developments in the diagnosis and treatment of sexually transmitted diseases: Infectious syphilis and acquired immunodeficiency syndrome. *Cutis* 44:288–290, 1989.

77. Manganoni AM, Graifemberghi S, Facchetti F, et al. Effectiveness of penicillin G benzathine therapy for primary and secondary syphilis in HIV infection. *J Am Acad Dermatol* 23:1185–1186, 1990.

78. Tramont EC. Syphilis in the AIDS era. *N Engl J Med* 316:1600–1601, 1987.

79. Dowell ME, et al. Response of latent syphilis or neurosyphilis to ceftriaxone therapy in persons infected with human immunodeficiency virus. *Am J Med* 93:481–488, 1992.

80. Hook EW, III, Roddy RE, Handsfield HH. Ceftriaxone therapy for incubating and early syphilis. *J Infect Dis* 158:881–884, 1988.

81. Schofer H, Vogt HJ, Milbrodt R. Ceftriaxone for the treatment of primary and secondary syphilis. *Chemotherapy* 35:140–145, 1989.

82. Hook EW, III, Baker-Zander SA, Moskovitz BL, et al. Ceftriaxone therapy for asymptomatic neurosyphilis: Case report and Western blot analysis of serum and cerebrospinal fluid IgG response to therapy. *Sex Transm Dis* 13:185–188, 1986.

83. Brown ST, Zaidi A, Larsen SA, Reynolds GH. Serological response to syphilis treatment: A new analysis of old data. *JAMA* 253:1296–1299, 1985.

84. Romanowski B, Sutherland R, Fick GH, et al. Serologic response to treatment of infectious syphilis. *Ann Intern Med* 114:1005–1009, 1991.

85. Simon RP. Neurosyphilis. *Arch Neurol* 42:606–613, 1985.

86. Swartz MN. Neurosyphilis. In Holmes, Mardh, Sparling, Wiesner (eds), *Sexually Transmitted Diseases*. New York: McGraw-Hill, 1984. Pp 318–334.

87. Report of the NIAID Study Group on integrated behavioral research for prevention and control of sexually transmitted diseases. *Sex Transm Disease* 17:200–210, 1990.

88. Andrus JK, Fleming DW, Harger DR, et al. Partner notification: Can it control epidemic syphilis? *Ann Intern Med* 112:539–543, 1990.

89. Centers for Disease Control. Epidemic early syphilis—Escambia County, Florida, 1987 and July 1989–June 1990. *MMWR* 40:323–325, 1991.

90. Centers for Disease Control. Alternative case-finding methods in a crack-related syphilis epidemic—Philadelphia. *MMWR* 40:77–80, 1991.

22 / Cytomegalovirus Infection

Lawrence M. Barat, Donald E. Craven

Cytomegalovirus (CMV) is a ubiquitous DNA virus belonging to the family of human herpesviruses that includes herpes simplex virus, Epstein-Barr virus, and varicella-zoster virus. The virion ranges in size from 180 to 250 nm in diameter and has a genome in the range of 150 million daltons.

Epidemiology

Most people are infected with CMV sometime during their life. Seroprevalence studies indicate that 40 to 60 percent of healthy blood donors in industrialized nations have evidence of CMV infection, and rates in developing countries are even higher [1–4]. Antibody to CMV has been detected in over 90 percent of homosexual men and 60 percent of women attending sexually transmitted disease clinics in the United States [2–4]. The high prevalence of CMV infection is attributable in part to its ease of transmission. Cytomegalovirus can be cultured from saliva, semen, vaginal secretions, blood, or infected tissues [5]. Common modes of transmission include sexual intercourse, sharing contaminated drug injection paraphernalia, blood transfusion, and perinatal (vertical) transmission [4, 6–8]. Vertical transmission may occur at delivery through contact with infected secretions or postpartum via contaminated breast milk [5]. Infected organs used for transplantation are also a potential source of CMV infection [9–11].

Remarkable variability is found among CMV strains examined by restriction endonuclease analysis (REA). Epidemiologic tracking by REA has demonstrated that individuals can be reinfected with new, antigenically distinct strains of the virus [12–14]. Strains of CMV appear to vary in their cytopathic effect in tissue culture.

The rate of symptomatic CMV infection in the HIV-infected population based on clinical case reporting may be grossly underestimated. According to the Centers for Disease Control, CMV accounts for fewer than 10 percent of opportunistic infections in patients with AIDS. In contrast, autopsy series report evidence of CMV infection in more than 50 percent of cases, making it one of the most common opportunistic

305

diseases [15–17]. Between 1981 and 1989, there was a sixfold increase in the rate of CMV retinitis reported as an AIDS-defining diagnosis, and it is likely that this trend will continue as HIV-infected patients live longer with profound immunodeficiency [18].

CMV and Immune Function

Humoral immunity to CMV does not prevent infection, but the presence of specific antibody does appear to improve prognosis [19]. Cytotoxic T lymphocytes and natural killer cells play an integral role in the immune response to CMV, and severe disease occurs almost exclusively in individuals with profound impairment of cell-mediated immunity [19, 20].

Cytomegalovirus may serve as a cofactor in HIV disease progression. Mononuclear leukocytes in primary CMV infection have a diminished proliferative response to mitogens and herpesvirus antigens, and the CD4 lymphocyte count may also decline in primary CMV infection [21, 22]. A clinical study of HIV-infected hemophiliacs showed that CMV-infected patients were more likely to develop AIDS than their CMV-negative counterparts [23]. Some investigators theorize that CMV may augment HIV replication by cytokine-mediated activation of HIV regulatory genes and enhancement of cellular tropism [24].

Clinical Manifestations

Cytomegalovirus disease in HIV-infected patients usually results from reactivation of latent infection, but both primary infection and reinfection have also been documented. The CMV mononucleosis syndrome, consisting of fever, malaise, fatigue, lymphadenopathy, hepatosplenomegaly, and atypical lymphocytosis, has been described in patients with early HIV disease [25]. In patients with advanced immunodeficiency (CD4 cell count $\leq 100/mm^3$), disseminated infection occurs, and the clinical presentation varies with the specific organ system(s) involved [26, 27] (Table 22-1).

Retinitis

Cytomegalovirus retinitis occurs in 20 to 30 percent of AIDS patients and is the leading cause of visual loss in this population [28–30]. Early retinitis is often asymptomatic, but patients may complain of "floaters" or photopsia. Visual disturbances occur only if the fovea is involved. On funduscopic examination, early lesions appear as small, multifocal, yellow-white patches with a granular appearance [28–32] (see Plate 8).

Table 22-1 *Sites of cytomegalovirus infection in the HIV-infected patient*

Organ system	Reference(s)
Ophthalmologic	
Retinitis	28–33
Uveitis	35
Conjunctivitis	34
Neurologic	
Encephalitis	36
Myelitis	37
Radiculitis	37–39
Neuropathy	40, 41
Gastrointestinal	
Oropharyngeal ulcers	42
Esophagitis	44
Gastritis/duodenitis	44
Colitis/ileitis	45–48
Anal ulcers	43
Hepatobiliary	
Cholecystitis	50–52
Cholangitis	53–56
Hepatitis	49, 50
Pancreatitis	57
Pulmonary	
Pneumonitis	58–61
Bronchiolitis	62
Tracheitis	63
Other	
Adrenalitis	64
Cystitis	67
Dermatitis	65
Pericarditis	66
Thrombophlebitis	68

Lesions are usually located contiguous to blood vessels but can be found anywhere in the retina. Associated hemorrhage is a distinctive feature of CMV retinitis and helps differentiate it from cotton-wool spots [30, 33] (see Plate 7). Cytomegalovirus disease usually presents unilaterally but may later spread to the other eye. Untreated CMV disease progresses to hemorrhagic necrosis of the entire retina over a 2- to 6-month period, resulting in blindness. In addition to retinitis, CMV conjunctivitis and uveitis have also been reported [34, 35].

Neurologic Disease

Autopsy studies demonstrate CMV infection of the central nervous system (CNS) in up to 33 percent of patients with AIDS [36]. Clinically,

CMV encephalitis may be indistinguishable from other types but tends to be rapidly progressive. Cytomegalovirus can infect neurons, glial cells, and endothelial cells. Two distinctive histologic patterns have been observed: (1) microglial nodules with cytomegalic cells scattered throughout the brain, predominantly in the gray matter, and (2) microscopic infarctions, presumably due to vessel occlusion by CMV-infected endothelial cells [36]. In severe cases, extensive necrosis of brain tissue and focal areas of demyelination may develop.

Acute polyradiculomyelitis is a well-described neurologic manifestation of CMV infection, presenting with paresis, which may progress rapidly to flaccid paralysis [37, 38]. Bowel and bladder incontinence may also occur. Cerebrospinal fluid pleocytosis is common [39]. Characteristic pathologic changes associated with a mononuclear cell infiltrate are seen in the ventral horn of the spinal cord.

Cytomegalovirus may also cause a rapidly progressive mixed motor and sensory neuropathy [40]. An association between CMV infection and chronic painful peripheral neuropathy in AIDS patients has also been described [41]. In general, CMV-related neurologic disease carries a poor prognosis and is not responsive to antiviral therapy.

Gastrointestinal Disease

Cytomegalovirus infection may involve any part of the gastrointestinal tract. Oral, labial, or perirectal ulcers due to CMV are clinically indistinguishable from those of herpes simplex infection; the diagnosis of CMV mucositis should be considered when such lesions fail to respond to acyclovir therapy [42, 43]. Cytomegalovirus esophagitis presents most often with odynophagia; lesions are generally solitary, large, shallow, and localized to the distal esophagus [44]. The diagnosis of CMV disease should be considered when presumptive candidal esophagitis does not respond to antifungal therapy. Cytomegalovirus involvement of the gastric and duodenal mucosa may mimic the symptoms of peptic ulcer disease, with ulcerations most frequently located in the fundus and antrum.

Cytomegalovirus localizes to the colon and terminal ileum more commonly than any other site in the gastrointestinal tract [45]. In many HIV-infected patients, viral inclusions can be found even in the absence of symptoms or evidence of inflammation on colonoscopy [45, 46]. When symptoms do occur, diarrhea and weight loss predominate. The diarrhea of CMV, which may be intermittent or chronic, is indistinguishable from that caused by mycobacteria and cryptosporidia [45, 47]. Cytomegalovirus colitis should be considered in the differential diagnosis of diarrhea and wasting syndrome in AIDS patients. In more severe cases, extensive ulcerations may develop, with risk of colonic perforation and peritonitis requiring operative intervention [48]. Radiographic studies are often nondiagnostic, and lesions seen on endoscopy may suggest inflammatory bowel disease or pseudomembranous colitis. Endoscopic biopsy and histopathologic examination of suspicious lesions are necessary for definitive diagnosis of CMV colitis.

Hepatobiliary Disease

Although CMV inclusions can often be found on examination of liver tissue from biopsy or necropsy, clinical hepatitis is rare in patients with advanced HIV disease. Pancreatitis and focal fatty infiltrates mimicking hepatic metastases have been reported in association with CMV [49, 50]. Two important syndromes related to CMV, often in association with cryptosporidia, are acalculous cholecystitis and sclerosing cholangitis.

Patients with acalculous cholecystitis usually have fever, right upper quadrant pain and tenderness, and increased serum alkaline phosphatase [51–53]. The gallbladder is not visualized on radionucleotide cholecystogram, and ultrasound and computed tomography of the abdomen demonstrate an enlarged, thickened gallbladder without stones or sludge. Cholecystectomy may be necessary to avert rupture and ensuing peritonitis. The clinical presentation of sclerosing cholangitis includes fever, abdominal pain, increased serum alkaline phosphatase, and sometimes increased serum bilirubin [54–57]. Endoscopic cholangiography demonstrates intra- and extrahepatic biliary strictures and/or papillary stenosis.

Pulmonary Disease

Cytomegalovirus is second only to *Pneumocystis carinii* as a cause of pulmonary infection in AIDS and is found postmortem in 50 to 90 percent of cases, but its clinical significance is uncertain [16]. Cytomegalovirus has been isolated from up to 50 percent of bronchoalveolar lavage specimens from HIV-infected patients, often in association with other pathogens, but its presence does not appear to alter prognosis [58–61]. Cytoplasmic inclusions may be found in endothelial, epithelial, and pulmonary parenchymal cells and macrophages. In addition to pneumonitis, CMV tracheitis and bronchiolitis have also been described [62, 63].

Other Manifestations

Cytomegalovirus adrenalitis has been reported at autopsy in 40 to 90 percent of AIDS patients. Involvement varies from focal necrosis to hemorrhage and infarction of the entire adrenal gland, but clinical adrenal insufficiency is uncommon [64]. However, when hypoadrenalism is identified in a patient with AIDS, CMV infection should be considered in the differential diagnosis. Cytomegalovirus has been reported to be the cause of skin lesions in AIDS patients [65]. Single or multiple verrucous or ulcerative lesions with a translucent base have been described. Other unusual manifestations of CMV infection include pericarditis, cystitis, and septic thrombophlebitis [66–68].

Diagnosis

The diagnosis of active CMV infection is often difficult and usually requires documentation by histology, tissue culture, or both. One important exception is CMV retinitis, which is diagnosed presumptively by funduscopic examination alone.

Histology

Histologic examination of biopsy specimens may demonstrate typical CMV inclusions, tissue necrosis, or both. Definitive histologic diagnosis of CMV infection requires the presence of characteristic "owl's eye" cells, with cytomegaly and large intranuclear or intracytoplasmic inclusions surrounded by a halo. Touch preparations and immunofluorescent staining of frozen sections using an anti-CMV monoclonal antibody may facilitate diagnosis and increase the sensitivity of cytologic examination [69, 70].

Culture

Culture for CMV is expensive, and the virus may require up to three weeks to grow. Identification of CMV in blood or urine does not establish the presence of symptomatic CMV disease. However, a positive blood or urine culture can be used to confirm the presence of symptomatic infection in the patient with a characteristic clinical syndrome. Culture of biopsy tissue for CMV is preferable to blood or urine culture but must be correlated with histologic findings.

Serology

A variety of serologic tests for CMV antibody are available, including specific anti-CMV immunoglobulin M (IgM) and immunoglobulin G (IgG) assays. Antibodies may be absent in AIDS patients with severe CMV infection, and a negative titer does not exclude the possibility of active disease [71]. Therefore, serologic testing for CMV is of little diagnostic utility in HIV-infected patients.

Management

Treatment of CMV infection has been less satisfactory than that for other herpesviruses. Presently, two compounds have been proven effective for the management of clinically significant CMV infection: ganciclovir and foscarnet. Agents under investigation for the primary prevention of CMV disease include an acyclovir prodrug and oral ganciclovir.

Ganciclovir

Dihydroxypropoxymethylguanine (DHPG), or ganciclovir, is closely related to acyclovir, differing structurally in a 3′ carbon and hydroxyl group substitution on the acyclic side chain. This minor change confers markedly increased activity against CMV, with CMV-infected cells able to produce high concentrations of the active triphosphate form. Like acyclovir, ganciclovir acts as an inhibitor of viral DNA polymerase, as well as a false substrate, causing chain termination. In vitro studies show ganciclovir to have 25- to 100-fold increased activity against CMV compared to acyclovir [72, 73].

Data from clinical trials strongly support the use of ganciclovir therapy for CMV infection in HIV-infected patients (Table 22-2). The recommended ganciclovir dosage for primary therapy is 10 mg/kg/day intravenously in two divided doses for 14 to 21 days; patients with renal dysfunction require dosage adjustment (Table 22-3). The most promising results have been in the treatment of retinitis; clinical improvement, documented by resolution of lesions on funduscopy, has been reported in 54 to 100 percent of patients [74–78]. Response rates in ganciclovir treatment of CMV gastrointestinal disease range from 60 to 100 percent, depending on the specific site of infection [74–76, 78–80]. Treatment of CMV pneumonitis has been less encouraging, with clinical improvement in 40 to 80 percent of patients [75, 76, 78]. Cytomegalovirus encephalitis appears to respond poorly to ganciclovir [75–78].

Unfortunately, clinical responses to primary ganciclovir therapy are often short lived [75, 78]. However, maintenance therapy with 5 mg/kg/day intravenously five to seven times a week appears to delay or prevent recurrence of CMV retinitis [78, 81, 82]. Lower doses and less frequent dosing schedules have high breakthrough rates. The development of ganciclovir-resistant isolates has been reported in patients receiving long-term maintenance therapy [83].

Table 22-2 Response of cytomegalovirus infection to treatment

Reference	Site	No. of patients treated	% improved or stabilized
Ganciclovir			
Masur et al. [74]	Retina	7	85
	Colon	1	100
DHPG Treatment Group [75]	Retina	13	84
	Colon	8	62
	Lung	7	42
Laskin et al. [76][a]	Retina	5	60
	GI	5	80
	Lung	2	50
	CNS	2	0
Laskin et al. [76][b]	Retina	12	100
	GI	13	100
	Lung	4	100
Holland et al. [77]	Retina	24	54
Buhles et al. [78]	Retina	105	84
	Lower GI	31	87
	Upper GI	8	75
	Lung	23	78
Chachoua et al. [79]	Colon	31	74
	Esophagus	4	100
	Rectum	4	75
	Ileum	1	0
Dieterich et al. [80]	Colon	46	91
	Esophagus	15	86
	Rectum	5	80
	Liver	2	100
	Ileum	1	0
Foscarnet			
Pelletier et al. [92]	Retina	12	100
Jacobson et al. [94]	Retina	10	90
Fanning et al. [90]	Retina	17	94
Lehoang et al. [93]	Retina	31	93

[a]Drug dose: 3 mg/kg/day.
[b]Drug dose: 7.5 mg/kg/day.

Toxicity to ganciclovir is relatively common. Neutropenia develops in 15 to 70 percent of patients, often requiring dose adjustment or cessation of therapy [75, 78, 80, 81]. Anemia and thrombocytopenia may occur as well. Less frequent side effects include gastrointestinal intolerance, azoospermia, hepatocellular dysfunction, thrombophlebitis at the infusion site, and CNS disturbances. Concomitant use of granulocyte/macrophage colony stimulating factor (GM-CSF) or granulocyte colony stimulating factor (G-CSF) may alleviate the myelosuppressive

Table 22-3 Dosing and toxicity of therapies for cytomegalovirus infection

Drug	Dose*	Toxicity
Ganciclovir		
Induction	5.0 mg/kg q12h	Leukopenia
		Anemia
Maintenance	5.0 mg/kg q day,	Thrombocytopenia
	5–7 days/wk	GI disturbances
		Azoospermia
		Hepatitis
		CNS disturbances
		Thrombophlebitis
Foscarnet		
Induction	60 mg/kg q8h	Azotemia
		Hypocalcemia
Maintenance	90 mg/kg q day	Hyperphosphatemia
		Hypomagnesemia
		Myalgias
		Anemia
		Thrombophlebitis
		GI disturbances

*Doses require adjustment for renal failure.

effects of ganciclovir [84, 85]. Ganciclovir is not recommended for use with zidovudine (ZDV), as marrow suppression is a frequent side effect of both drugs [86, 87]. Didanosine (ddI) should be considered as an alternative antiretroviral agent in patients receiving ganciclovir.

Intravitreal injection of ganciclovir for primary and maintenance therapy of CMV retinitis has been performed with good clinical response and no systemic toxicity, although it may not be available at all institutions [88, 89]. Bacterial endophthalmitis is a reported complication.

Foscarnet

Phosphonoformate, or foscarnet, is presently the most active agent against CMV in vitro. Its mechanism of action is reversible, noncompetitive inhibition of CMV-specific DNA polymerase [90]. It also inhibits the reverse transcriptase of many retroviruses including HIV [91]. Open-label, noncomparative studies of foscarnet in the treatment of CMV retinitis in AIDS patients have shown clinical response rates of over 90 percent [90, 92–94] (see Table 22-2). One randomized study comparing foscarnet to no treatment in patients with non–sight-threatening CMV retinitis demonstrated a significant delay in progression of disease in the treated group [95].

Primary foscarnet therapy is given at a dose of 60 mg/kg intravenously every 8 hours for 14 to 21 days (see Table 22-3). Dose adjustment is necessary in patients with compromised renal function [95]. Maintenance therapy using one third to one half of the total daily dose, given over 2 or 3 hours five times a week, has had limited success, with approximately 50 percent of patients relapsing within 2 months [90, 92–94].

The toxicity profile of foscarnet differs from that of ganciclovir. Serious side effects may occur in up to 50 percent of patients. Nephrotoxicity, including acute renal failure, is common and often dose limiting. Electrolyte abnormalities, including hypocalcemia, hyperphosphatemia, and hypomagnesemia, are frequent, can be life-threatening, and are often refractory to replacement therapy. Seizures have been reported in over 10 percent of patients, and gastrointestinal disturbances and anemia are common. Phlebitis at the infusion site and low back pain have also been reported.

Data from a recent comparative study conducted by the National Eye Institute indicate that patients treated with foscarnet for CMV retinitis survive an average of 4 months longer than those treated with ganciclovir [96]. No difference was seen in the median time (2 months) to progression of retinitis. The survival advantage of foscarnet could not be explained by the concurrent use of antiretroviral therapy and may be the result of its anti-HIV activity. While foscarnet treatment for CMV retinitis may confer a survival advantage over ganciclovir, drug intolerance remains a problem.

References

1. Drew WL. Cytomegalovirus infection in patients with AIDS. *J Infect Dis* 158:449–455, 1988.
2. Drew WL, Mills J, Hauer LB, et al. Declining prevalence of Kaposi's sarcoma in homosexual AIDS patients paralleled by fall in cytomegalovirus transmission. *Lancet* 1:66, 1988.
3. Mintz L, Drew WL, Miner RC, Braff EH. Cytomegalovirus infections in homosexual men: An epidemiological study. *Ann Intern Med* 99:326–329, 1983.
4. Handsfield HH, Chandler SH, Caine VA, et al. Cytomegalovirus infection in sex partners: Evidence for sexual transmission. *J Infect Dis* 151:344–348, 1985.
5. Cohen JI, Corey GR. Cytomegalovirus infection in the normal host. *Medicine* 64:100–114, 1985.
6. Chretien JH, McGinniss CG, Muller A. Venereal causes of cytomegalovirus mononucleosis. *JAMA* 238:1644–1645, 1977.
7. Jordan MC, Rousseau WE, Noble GR, et al. Association of cervical cytomegalovirus with venereal disease. *N Engl J Med* 288:932–934, 1973.

8. Lang DJ, Kummer JF. Demonstration of cytomegalovirus in semen. *N Engl J Med* 287:756–758, 1972.
9. Peterson PK, Balfour HH, Jr, Marker SC, et al. Cytomegalovirus disease in renal allograft recipients: A prospective study of the clinical features, risk factors and impact of renal transplantation. *Medicine* 59:283–299, 1980.
10. Pass RF, Long WK, Whitley RJ, et al. Productive infection with cytomegalovirus and herpes simplex virus in renal transplant recipients: Role of source of kidney. *J Infect Dis* 137:556–562, 1978.
11. Marker SC, Howard RJ, Simmons RL, et al. Cytomegalovirus infection: A quantitative prospective study of three hundred twenty consecutive renal transplants. *Surgery* 89:660–671, 1981.
12. Drew WL, Sweet ES, Miner RC, Mocarski ES. Multiple infections by cytomegalovirus in patients with acquired immunodeficiency syndrome: Documentation by Southern blot hybridization. *J Infect Dis* 150:952–953, 1984.
13. Spector SA, Hirata KK, Neuman TR. Identification of multiple cytomegalovirus strains in homosexual men with acquired immunodeficiency syndrome. *J Infect Dis* 150:953–956, 1984.
14. Grundy JE, Super M, Griffiths PD. Reinfection of a seropositive allograft recipient by cytomegalovirus from donor kidney. *Lancet* 1:159–160, 1986.
15. Niedt GW, Schinella RA. Acquired immunodeficiency syndrome: Clinicopathologic study of 56 autopsies. *Arch Pathol Lab Med* 109:727–734, 1985.
16. Macher AM, Reichert CM, Straus SE, et al. Death in the AIDS patient: Role of cytomegalovirus. *N Engl J Med* 309:1454, 1983.
17. Klatt EC, Shibata D. Cytomegalovirus infection in the acquired immunodeficiency syndrome. *Arch Pathol Lab Med* 112:540–544, 1988.
18. Crumpacker CS, Heath-Chiozzi M. Overview of cytomegalovirus infections in HIV-infected patients: Current therapies and future strategies. *J AIDS* 4 (suppl 1):S1–S5, 1991.
19. Rook AH, Quinnan GV, Jr, Frederick WJR, et al. Importance of cytotoxic lymphocytes during cytomegalovirus infection in renal transplant recipients. *Am J Med* 76:385–392, 1984.
20. Quinnan GV, Jr, Kirmani N, Rook AH, et al. Cytotoxic T cells in cytomegalovirus infection: HLA-restricted T-lymphocyte and non–T-lymphocyte cytotoxic responses correlate with recovery from cytomegalovirus infection in bone-marrow–transplant recipients. *N Engl J Med* 307:7–13, 1982.
21. Rinaldo CR, Jr, Carney WP, Richter BS, et al. Mechanisms of immunosuppression in cytomegaloviral mononucleosis. *J Infect Dis* 141:488–495, 1980.
22. Carney WP, Rubin RH, Hoffman RA, et al. Analysis of T lymphocyte subsets in cytomegalovirus mononucleosis. *J Immunol* 126:2114–2116, 1981.
23. Webster A, Lee CA, Cook DG, et al. Cytomegalovirus infections and progression towards AIDS in haemophiliacs with human immunodeficiency virus. *Lancet* 2:63–66, 1989.
24. Webster A. Cytomegalovirus as a possible cofactor in HIV disease progression. *J AIDS* 4 (suppl 1):S47–S52, 1991.

25. Leport C, Harzic M, Pignon JM, et al. Benign cytomegalovirus mononucleosis in non-AIDS, HIV-infected patients. *Lancet* 2:214, 1987.
26. Gallant JE, et al. Incidence and natural history of cytomegalovirus disease in patients with advanced human immunodeficiency virus disease treated with zidovudine. *J Infect Dis* 166:1223–1227, 1992.
27. Peter P, et al. Risk of developing cytomegalovirus retinitis in persons infected with human immunodeficiency virus. *J AIDS* 5:1069–1074, 1992.
28. Culbertson WW. Infections of the retina in AIDS. *Int Ophthalmol Clin* 29:108–118, 1989.
29. Jabs DA, Enger C, Bartlett JG. Cytomegalovirus retinitis and acquired immunodeficiency syndrome. *Arch Ophthalmol* 107:75–80, 1989.
30. Jabs DA, Green WR, Fox R, et al. Ocular manifestations of acquired immune deficiency syndrome. *Ophthalmology* 96:1092–1099, 1989.
31. Henderley DE, Freeman WR, Smith RE, et al. Cytomegalovirus retinitis as the initial manifestation of the acquired immune deficiency syndrome. *Am J Ophthalmol* 103:316–320, 1987.
32. Henderley DE, Jampol LM. Diagnosis and treatment of cytomegalovirus retinitis. *J AIDS* 4 (suppl 1):S6–S10, 1991.
33. O'Donnell JJ, Jacobson MA. Cotton-wool spots and cytomegalovirus retinitis in AIDS. *Int Ophthalmol Clin* 29:105–107, 1989.
34. Brown HH, Glasgow BJ, Holland GN, Foos RY. Cytomegalovirus infection of the conjunctiva in AIDS. *Am J Ophthalmol* 106:102–104, 1988.
35. Daicker B. Cytomegalovirus panuveitis with infection of corneo-trabecular endothelium in AIDS. *Ophthalmologica* 197:169–175, 1988.
36. Wiley CA, Nelson JA. Role of human immunodeficiency virus and cytomegalovirus in AIDS encephalitis. *Am J Pathol* 133:73–81, 1988.
37. Mahieux F, Gray F, Fenelon G, et al. Acute myeloradiculitis due to cytomegalovirus as the initial manifestation of AIDS. *J Neurol Neurosurg Psychiat* 52:270–274, 1989.
38. Behar R, Wiley C, McCutchan JA. Cytomegalovirus polyradiculoneuropathy in acquired immune deficiency syndrome. *Neurology* 37:557–561, 1987.
39. deGans J, Tiessens G, Portegies P, et al. Predominance of polymorphonuclear leukocytes in cerebrospinal fluid of AIDS patients with cytomegalovirus polyradiculomyelitis. *J AIDS* 3:1155–1158, 1990.
40. Said G, Lacroix C, Chemouilli P, et al. Cytomegalovirus neuropathy in acquired immunodeficiency syndrome: A clinical and pathological study. *Ann Neurol* 29:139–146, 1991.
41. Fuller GN, Jacobs JM, Guiloff RJ. Association of painful peripheral neuropathy in AIDS with cytomegalovirus infection. *Lancet* 2:937–941, 1989.
42. Kanas RJ, Jensen JL, Abrams AM, Wuerker RB. Oral mucosal cytomegalovirus as a manifestation of the acquired immune deficiency syndrome. *Oral Surg* 64:183–189, 1987.
43. Puy-Montbrun T, Ganansia R, Lemarchand N, et al. Anal ulcerations due to cytomegalovirus in patients with AIDS: Report of six cases. *Dis Colon Rectum* 33:1041–1043, 1990.
44. Wilcox CM, Diehl DL, Cello JP, et al. Cytomegalovirus esophagitis in

patients with AIDS: A clinical, endoscopic, and pathologic correlation. *Ann Intern Med* 113:589–593, 1990.

45. Dieterich DT, Rahmin M. Cytomegalovirus colitis in AIDS: Presentation in 44 patients and a review of the literature. *J AIDS* 4 (suppl 1):S29–S35, 1991.

46. Laughon BE, Druckman DA, Vernon A, et al. Prevalence of enteric pathogens in homosexual men with and without acquired immunodeficiency syndrome. *Gastroenterology* 94:984–993, 1988.

47. Kotler DP. Cytomegalovirus colitis and wasting. *J AIDS* 4 (suppl 1):S36–S41, 1991.

48. Kram HB, Shoemaker WC. Intestinal perforation due to cytomegalovirus infection in patients with AIDS. *Dis Colon Rectum* 33:1037–1040, 1990.

49. Vieco PT, Rochon L, Lisbona A. Multifocal cytomegalovirus-associated hepatic lesions simulating metastases in AIDS. *Radiology* 176:123–124, 1990.

50. Wilcox CM, Forsmark CE, Grendell JH, et al. Cytomegalovirus-associated acute pancreatic disease in patients with acquired immunodeficiency syndrome: Report of two patients. *Gastroenterology* 99:263–267, 1990.

51. Kahn DG, Garfinkle JM, Klonoff DC, et al. Cryptosporidial and cytomegaloviral hepatitis and cholecystitis. *Arch Pathol Lab Med* 111:879–881, 1987.

52. Kavin H, Jonas RB, Chowdhury L, Kabins S. Acalculous cholecystitis and cytomegalovirus infection in the acquired immunodeficiency syndrome. *Ann Intern Med* 104:53–54, 1986.

53. Aaron JS, Wynter CD, Kirton OC, Simko V. Cytomegalovirus associated with acalculous cholecystitis in a patient with acquired immune deficiency syndrome. *Am J Gastroenterol* 83:879–881, 1988.

54. Cello JP. Acquired immunodeficiency syndrome cholangiopathy: Spectrum of disease. *Am J Med* 86:539–546, 1989.

55. Schneiderman DJ, Cello JP, Laing FC. Papillary stenosis and sclerosing cholangitis in the acquired immunodeficiency syndrome. *Ann Intern Med* 106:546–549, 1987.

56. Margulis SJ, Honig CL, Soave R, et al. Biliary tract obstruction in the acquired immunodeficiency syndrome. *Ann Intern Med* 105:207–210, 1986.

57. Jacobson MA, Cello JP, Sande MA. Cholestasis and disseminated cytomegalovirus disease in patients with the acquired immunodeficiency syndrome. *Am J Med* 84:218–224, 1988.

58. Millar AB, Patou G, Miller RF, et al. Cytomegalovirus in the lungs of patients with AIDS: Respiratory pathogen or passenger? *Am Rev Respir Dis* 141:1474–1477, 1990.

59. Miles PR, Baughman RP, Linnemann CC, Jr. Cytomegalovirus in the bronchoalveolar lavage fluid of patients with AIDS. *Chest* 97:1072–1076, 1990.

60. Bower M, Barton SE, Nelson MR, et al. The significance of the detection of cytomegalovirus in the bronchoalveolar lavage fluid in AIDS patients with pneumonia. *AIDS* 4:317–320, 1990.

61. Bozzette et al. Impact of *Pneumocystis carinii* and cytomegalovirus on the course and outcome of atypical pneumonia in advanced human immunodeficiency virus disease. *J Infect Dis* 165:93–98, 1992.

62. Vasudevan VP, Mascarenhas DAN, Klapper P, Lomvardias S. Cytomegalovirus necrotizing bronchiolitis with HIV infection. *Chest* 97:483–484, 1990.

63. Imoto EM, Stein RM, Shellito JE, Curtis JL. Central airway obstruction due to cytomegalovirus-induced necrotizing tracheitis in a patient with AIDS. *Am Rev Respir Dis* 142:884–886, 1990.

64. Pulakhandam U, Dincsoy HP. Cytomegaloviral adrenalitis and adrenal insufficiency in AIDS. *Am J Clin Pathol* 93:651–656, 1990.

65. Bournerias I, Boisnic S, Patey O, et al. Unusual cutaneous cytomegalovirus involvement in patients with acquired immunodeficiency syndrome. *Arch Dermatol* 125:1243–1246, 1989.

66. Nathan PE, Arsura EL, Zappi M. Pericarditis with tamponade due to cytomegalovirus in the acquired immunodeficiency syndrome. *Chest* 99:765–766, 1991.

67. Benson MC, Kaplan MS, O'Toole K, Romagnoli M. A report of cytomegalovirus cystitis and a review of other genitourinary manifestations of the acquired immune deficiency syndrome. *J Urol* 140:153–154, 1988.

68. Peterson P, Stahl-Bayliss CM. Cytomegalovirus thrombophlebitis after successful DHPG therapy. *Ann Intern Med* 106:632–633, 1987.

69. Hackman RC, Myerson D, Meyers JD, et al. Rapid immunodiagnosis of cytomegaloviral pneumonia by tissue immunofluorescence with a murine monoclonal antibody. *J Infect Dis* 151:325–329, 1985.

70. Emanuel D, Peppard J, Stover D, et al. Rapid immunodiagnosis of cytomegalovirus pneumonia by bronchoalveolar lavage using human and murine monoclonal antibodies. *Ann Intern Med* 104:476–481, 1986.

71. Dylewski J, Chou S, Merigan TC. Absence of detectable IgM antibody during cytomegalovirus disease in patients with AIDS. *N Engl J Med* 309:493, 1983.

72. Freitas VR, Smee DF, Chernow M, et al. Activity of 9-(1,dihydroxy-2-propoxymethyl)guanine compared with that of acyclovir against human, monkey, and rodent cytomegalovirus. *Antimicrob Agents Chemother* 24:240–245, 1985.

73. Balfour HH, Jr. Management of cytomegalovirus disease with antiviral drugs. *Rev Infect Dis* 12 (suppl 7):S849–S860, 1990.

74. Masur H, Lane HC, Palestine A, et al. Effect of 9-(1,3-dihydroxy-2-propoxymethyl) guanine on serious cytomegalovirus disease in eight immunosuppressed homosexual men. *Ann Intern Med* 104:41–44, 1986.

75. Collaborative DHPG Treatment Study Group. Treatment of serious cytomegalovirus infections with 9-(1,3-dihydroxy-propoxymethyl) guanine in patients with AIDS and other immunodeficiencies. *N Engl J Med* 314:801–805, 1986.

76. Laskin OL, Stahl-Bayliss CL, Kalman CM, Rosecan LR. Use of ganciclovir to treat serious cytomegalovirus infections in patients with AIDS. *J Infect Dis* 155:323–327, 1987.

77. Holland GN, Buhles WC, Jr, Mastre B, Kaplan HJ. The UCLA CMV Retinopathy Study Group: A controlled retrospective study of ganciclovir treatment for cytomegalovirus retinopathy. *Arch Ophthalmol* 107:1759–1766, 1989.
78. Buhles WC, Mastre BJ, Tinker AJ, et al. Ganciclovir treatment of life- or sight-threatening cytomegalovirus infection: Experience in 314 immunocompromised patients. *Rev Infect Dis* 10 (suppl 3):S495–S503, 1988.
79. Chachoua A, Dieterich D, Krasinski K, et al. 9-(1,3-dihydroxy- 2-propoxymethyl)guanine (ganciclovir) in the treatment of cytomegalovirus gastrointestinal disease with the acquired immunodeficiency syndrome. *Ann Intern Med* 107:133–137, 1987.
80. Dieterich DT, Chachoua A, Lafleur F, Worrell C. Ganciclovir treatment of gastrointestinal infections caused by cytomegalovirus in patients with AIDS. *Rev Infect Dis* 10 (suppl 3):S532–S537, 1988.
81. Weisenthal RW, Sinclair SH, Frank I, Rubin DH. Long-term outpatient treatment of CMV retinitis with ganciclovir in AIDS patients. *Br J Ophthalmol* 73:996–1001, 1989.
82. Gross JG, Bozzette SA, Mathews WC, et al. Longitudinal study of cytomegalovirus retinitis in acquired immune deficiency syndrome. *Ophthalmology* 97:681–686, 1990.
83. Drew WL, Miner RC, Busch DF, et al. Prevalence of resistance in patients receiving ganciclovir for serious cytomegalovirus infection. *J Infect Dis* 163:716–719, 1991.
84. Hardy WD. Combined ganciclovir and recombinant human granulocyte-macrophage colony-stimulating factor in the treatment of cytomegalovirus retinitis in AIDS patients. *J AIDS* 4 (suppl 1):S22–S28, 1991.
85. Grossberg HS, Bonnem EM, Buhles WC, Jr. GM-CSF with ganciclovir for the treatment of CMV retinitis in AIDS. *N Engl J Med* 320:1560, 1989.
86. Causey D. Concomitant ganciclovir and zidovudine treatment for cytomegalovirus retinitis in patients with HIV infection: An approach to treatment. *J AIDS* 4 (suppl 1):S16–S21, 1991.
87. Hochster H, Dieterich D, Bozzette S, et al. Toxicity of combined ganciclovir and zidovudine for cytomegalovirus disease associated with AIDS. *Ann Intern Med* 113:111–117, 1990.
88. Cantrill HL, Henry K, Melroe NH, et al. Treatment of cytomegalovirus retinitis with intravitreal ganciclovir: Long term results. *Ophthalmology* 96:367–374, 1989.
89. Heinemann MH. Long-term intravitreal ganciclovir therapy for cytomegalovirus retinopathy. *Arch Ophthalmol* 107:1767–1772, 1989.
90. Fanning MM, Read SE, Benson M, et al. Foscarnet therapy of cytomegalovirus retinitis in AIDS. *J AIDS* 3:472–479, 1990.
91. Sandstrom EG, Byington RE, Kaplan JC, Hirsch MS. Inhibition of human T-cell lymphotropic virus type III in vitro by phosphonoformate. *Lancet* 1:1480–1482, 1985.
92. Pelletier LL, Baker CB, Gam AA, et al. Treatment of cytomegalovirus retinitis with trisodium phosphonoformate hexahydrate (foscarnet). *J Infect Dis* 157:569–576, 1988.

93. Lehoang P, Girard B, Robinet M, et al. Foscarnet in the treatment of cytomegalovirus retinitis in acquired immune deficiency syndrome. *Ophthalmology* 96:865–874, 1989.
94. Jacobson MA, O'Donnell JJ, Mills J. Foscarnet treatment of cytomegalovirus retinitis in patients with the acquired immunodeficiency syndrome. *Antimicrob Agents Chemother* 33:736–741, 1989.
95. Palestine AG, Polis PA, DeSmet MD, et al. A randomized, controlled trial of foscarnet in the treatment of cytomegalovirus retinitis in patients with AIDS. *Ann Intern Med* 115:665–673, 1991.
96. Studies of Ocular Complications of AIDS Research Group and AIDS Clinical Trials Group. Mortality in patients with the acquired immunodeficiency syndrome treated with either foscarnet or ganciclovir for cytomegalovirus retinitis. *N Engl J Med* 326:213–220, 1992.

23/Herpes Simplex and Varicella-Zoster Virus Infections

Carol A. Sulis

Primary or recurrent infection with herpes simplex virus (HSV) and varicella-zoster virus (VZV) is common in the HIV-infected patient. Illness is often more severe, more invasive, and of longer duration than disease in the immunocompetent host. Both viruses cause painful mucocutaneous lesions and may disseminate, with significant visceral involvement [1-3].

Herpes Simplex Virus

Epidemiology

Herpes simplex virus is ubiquitous. Primary infection occurs 2 to 12 days after the introduction of infectious secretions into the oral cavity (HSV-1), genital area (HSV-2), skin, or eye. Thirty to fifty percent of adults have antibody to HSV, with a higher prevalence in certain populations, including male homosexuals, urbanites, and those from developing countries. Anal or perianal HSV-2 infection, with autoinoculation to thigh and hand, is especially common among male homosexuals. Up to 90 percent of women who are seropositive for HSV-2 deny a history of genital herpes. Twenty-five percent of women presenting with what they describe as their first episode of genital HSV infection have serologic evidence of prior exposure [4-6]. Recurrent HSV infection, usually due to reactivation of latent virus, occurs with variable frequency and severity. Rarely, recurrence is the result of exogenous reinfection. Several studies have noted an association between genital HSV infection and acquisition of HIV [6-10]. Others have clarified the mechanisms by which acute and reactivated HSV infection induces HIV expression, modifying and potentially accelerating the course of disease [11, 12].

Pathogenesis

Herpes simplex virus replicates in, then lyses, epithelial cells. The characteristic thin-walled vesicle on an erythematous base is the result of a local inflammatory response. Histologic examination reveals multinucleated giant cells, marked edema, and Cowdry type A intranuclear inclusions. As nerve endings become infected, the virus is transported intraaxonally to ganglia, where it remains latent. In the normal host, infection is contained locally by cell-mediated immunity, with only a minor contribution from neutralizing antibody [13, 14]. With reactivation, the virus moves back along sensory nerves to the skin [15]. In neonates and immunocompromised hosts, viremia and visceral dissemination may ensue.

Clinical Manifestations

Primary Infection

In the normal host, primary HSV-1 infection generally occurs during childhood and is asymptomatic. Some children have gingivostomatitis, characterized by fever, leukocytosis, intensely painful oral lesions, and foul breath. Vesicles begin on the buccal or gingival mucosa or tongue, coalesce, and rupture, leaving ulcers with an erythematous margin and a white-yellow necrotic membrane. The course varies in severity and duration but is generally self-limited, with complete healing without scar formation in 2 weeks. Differential diagnosis includes aphthous stomatitis, Stevens-Johnson syndrome, and herpangina. Adolescents with symptomatic primary HSV-1 infection often have constitutional symptoms, exudative pharyngitis, cervical adenopathy, headache, and leukocytosis. HSV-1 infection of the eye may cause acute, self-limited keratoconjunctivitis or progress to corneal ulceration with scarring. Herpetic "whitlow" is an infection of the skin, usually the finger.

Primary infection with HSV-2 usually occurs during adolescence or adulthood. It is manifested by constitutional symptoms and exquisitely tender vesicular lesions in the genital area. Vesicles ulcerate rapidly and become covered with a grayish-white exudate, requiring several weeks to heal completely. HSV-2 is a common cause of nongonococcal proctitis in sexually active homosexual men. Symptoms of primary perianal/rectal HSV-2 infection include painful ulcers and tenesmus associated with constitutional symptoms. Difficulty in urinating, constipation, sacral paresthesias, radiculopathy, impotence, and neurogenic bladder occur less frequently. In the normal host, disease is usually self-limited [15, 16]. Chronic aggressive perianal HSV infection was among the first opportunistic diseases described with AIDS [17]. Perianal ulcers may occur without true proctitis; lesions coalesce, extend along the gluteal crease resembling a decubitus ulcer or anal fissure, and may become superinfected [18].

Reactivation Infection

Herpes labialis ("cold sore" or "fever blister") is the most common presentation of recurrent HSV-1 infection. Patients describe several hours of burning, tingling, itching, or localized hyperesthesia or pain before eruption of lesions at the mucocutaneous junction of the lip. In the normal host, recurrent HSV-1 rarely involves oral mucosa. Painful vesicles appear, ulcerate, crust within 48 hours, and heal in 8 to 10 days. Recurrent HSV-1 infection in the context of HIV disease manifests more like primary infection [19]. Oral ulcers may progress to frank gingivostomatitis, with extensive tissue destruction and prolonged viral shedding. Orolabial recurrences increase in frequency and severity as immunosuppression worsens. Mucocutaneous HSV infection that persists longer than 4 weeks in an HIV-infected patient fulfills the current Centers for Disease Control (CDC) case definition for AIDS [20]. In the normal host, recurrent HSV-2 genital disease is associated with milder systemic symptoms and less extensive local involvement than first attacks [15, 16, 21]. HIV-infected patients may have prolonged formation of new, exquisitely painful lesions, continued tissue destruction, and persistent viral shedding (see Plate 9).

Encephalitis is a rare complication of primary or recurrent infection with HSV-1 or HSV-2 [22]. Headache, meningismus, and personality changes may develop gradually, or the onset may be abrupt, with fever, headache, nausea, and rapidly progressive neurologic abnormalities, including altered mental status, cranial nerve deficits, aphasia, and seizures. Rarely, aseptic meningitis complicates primary HSV-2 genital infection.

In the HIV-infected patient, diagnosis of herpetic esophagitis, tracheobronchitis, or pneumonia meets the current CDC case definition for AIDS [20]. Herpes simplex virus esophagitis is manifested by retrosternal pain and odynophagia; bacterial or fungal superinfection of ulcers may occur [23]. HIV-infected patients do not have an increased frequency of the more unusual syndromes caused by HSV, such as erythema multiforme, hepatitis, monoarticular arthritis, adrenal necrosis, and glomerulonephritis.

Diagnosis

Although the presence of HSV infection is often determined clinically, isolation of virus is required for definitive diagnosis. Optimally, fluid should be cultured from an intact vesicle or the epithelial cells scraped from the base of a freshly unroofed ulcer. Because as many as 15 percent of normal adults shed HSV in oral or genital secretions, a positive culture from these sites may not reflect active disease. Specimens can be stored for a few hours at 4°C but should be inoculated as soon as possible into tissue culture. HSV-induced cytopathic changes are generally seen within 24 to 48 hours. Tzanck smear of specimens is prepared with Wright's, Gram's, or Papanicolaou's stains. Multinucleated giant cells and intranuclear inclusions, suggestive of HSV infection, can also be seen with VZV. Most commercially available immunoassays are not sufficiently sensitive or specific to be diagnostically useful, and the utility of polymerase chain reaction testing is currently under investigation [24, 25].

Esophagitis occurs commonly in the AIDS patient. Neither symptoms nor the finding of cobblestone mucosa on barium swallow permits differentiation between candidal, viral (HSV, cytomegalovirus), and malignant (Kaposi's sarcoma) esophagitis. Definitive diagnosis requires endoscopic visualization with biopsy and culture [23, 26]. Dendritic corneal ulcers that stain with fluorescein in a patient with keratitis strongly suggest HSV infection, but can also be caused by VZV. Herpes simplex virus infection of the skin can be distinguished from VZV by the absence of dermatomal distribution and by culture. Definitive diagnosis of HSV encephalitis requires brain biopsy, as the virus cannot be cultured from cerebrospinal fluid [22, 27–29]. Histopathologic findings seen in the normal host, such as hemorrhagic cortical necrosis and lymphocytic infiltration, may be sparse or absent in the AIDS patient.

Treatment

The antiviral drug acyclovir, a nucleoside analogue, is currently the treatment of choice for HSV infection [2, 6, 21, 30–37]. Acyclovir penetrates virus-infected cells, undergoes monophosphorylation by virus-specific thymidine kinase, and is phosphorylated to an active triphosphate by cellular enzymes. The activated drug selectively inhibits viral DNA polymerase, causing early termination of DNA chain synthesis. Acyclovir distributes into all tissues including the central nervous system. It is cleared by the kidney and has a half-life of 2 to 3 hours; the dose must be adjusted for patients with renal insufficiency. Acyclovir is available in topical, oral, and intravenous preparations. Route, dosage, and duration of therapy depend on the type and severity of HSV infection (Table 23-1).

Topical acyclovir is not effective for recurrent herpes labialis but is occasionally useful in primary genital HSV infection [33, 38]. Oral acyclovir in a dose of 200 to 400 mg five times a day is indicated for mucocutaneous disease associated with HIV infection. Anecdotal reports that larger doses are more effective in this population are currently under

Table 23-1 Treatment of HSV and VZV infections associated with HIV disease

HSV infection	
Primary or recurrent mucocutaneous disease	Acyclovir, 200–400 mg po q4h while awake × 7 days[a,b]
Extensive mucocutaneous disease or Disseminated infection	Acyclovir, 5 mg/kg IV q8h × 7–14 days
Encephalitis	Acyclovir, 10 mg/kg IV q8h × 14–21 days
Prevention of relapse	Oral acyclovir at reduced dose
Infection with acyclovir-resistant HSV strain	Foscarnet[c], 40 mg/kg IV q8h
VZV infection	
Localized infection (shingles)	Acyclovir, 800 mg po q4h while awake × 7 days[a]
Disseminated infection (cutaneous or visceral)	Acyclovir, 10 mg/kg IV q8h × 7 days
Prevention of relapse	No therapy indicated
Infection with acyclovir-resistant VZV stain	Foscarnet[c], 40 mg/kg IV q8h

[a]Side effects of acyclovir—frequent: phlebitis (IV preparation); occasional: headache, rash, gastrointestinal intolerance, vertigo, renal dysfunction, bone marrow depression, hepatic dysfunction; rare: encephalopathy.
[b]Dose of acyclovir should be decreased in the presence of renal dysfunction.
[c]See Chap. 22 for additional information.

investigation [36, 37]. Therapy is continued until all lesions have crusted, usually 7 to 10 days; there are no data available to support longer regimens. Intravenous acyclovir should be used in patients with severe mucocutaneous HSV disease; involvement of viscera, such as brain, eye, or esophagus; or neurologic complications, such as transverse myelitis or atonic bladder. Patients with suspected HSV encephalitis should be treated empirically with intravenous acyclovir; brain biopsy is generally not necessary [28, 29, 39]. Ocular HSV infection is treated with trifluridine. Acyclovir cannot eliminate latent virus from ganglia, and severe, prolonged, and frequent recurrences may occur after discontinuation of therapy [34, 35].

Acyclovir-resistant strains of HSV with thymidine kinase or DNA polymerase mutations are being reported with increasing frequency; viral culture and sensitivity testing should be performed in patients whose symptoms do not improve on standard therapy [40–48]. In most reports, acyclovir-resistant HSV isolates have been sensitive to either foscarnet or vidarabine.

Foscarnet is a pyrophosphate analogue that directly inhibits DNA polymerase. Side effects are common and include renal insufficiency, alterations in serum calcium and phosphorus, anemia, and leukopenia [37]. Vidarabine, which is activated to a triphosphate by cellular enzymes, also inhibits viral DNA polymerase, but is generally less active than acyclovir against HSV and has numerous side effects. The usual dose is 15 mg/kg/day.

The combined administration of zidovudine and acyclovir for the treatment of HIV infection is currently being evaluated in clinical trials, but there are insufficient data to determine if such therapy is useful for the treatment of HSV [49]. Trials using systemic beta-interferon, topical 15% idoxuridine in 80% dimethyl sulfoxide (DMSO), topical 3% edoxudine cream, topical alpha-interferon (10^6 IU/gm with 1% nonoxynol 9 in 3.5% methylcellulose), and foscarnet cream for the treatment of HSV infection have been promising [50–53]. Recent AIDS Clinical Trials Group protocols include a comparison of acyclovir and 256U87 to treat recurrent anogenital HSV infection [54], the use of trifluridine to treat acyclovir-resistant mucocutaneous HSV infection, and an evaluation of fialuridine, a nucleoside analogue with good bioavailability that is thought to inhibit viral replication.

Prevention

There is no evidence that primary prophylaxis against HSV is effective in HIV-infected patients. The efficacy of secondary prophylaxis is being evaluated, but it appears that AIDS patients who have frequently recurrent or chronic HSV infection benefit from suppressive acyclovir therapy [21, 36, 37, 55–57]. Recurrence during therapy may represent the development of viral resistance. Patients who are receiving long-term suppressive therapy should be warned that discontinuation of the drug may be associated with a severe exacerbation of their condition. Condom use is effective in preventing the spread of HSV infection. Health care workers should avoid contact with potentially infectious lesions by wearing gloves or employing barrier precautions, and patients with extensive herpetic lesions should be isolated. No effective vaccine is available for the prevention of HSV infection [58].

Varicella-Zoster Virus

Herpes zoster (shingles) is a dermatomal cutaneous eruption caused by reactivation of the varicella-zoster virus. This virus remains latent in sensory ganglia after infection with varicella (chickenpox). While chickenpox is generally a mild disease in children, visceral dissemination occurs in one third of normal adults and develops at an even higher frequency in immunocompromised hosts [58]. Since 90 percent of adults have prior infection with VZV, most HIV-infected patients are not at risk for primary VZV infection [60–62].

Epidemiology

The overall annual incidence of zoster is 3.4 in 1,000, with the highest rates in the elderly and immunosuppressed. Zoster occurs with an increased frequency in patients with early HIV infection, and recurrences are common [63–67]. Immunosuppression predisposes to systemic and central nervous system dissemination.

Pathogenesis

Studies have clarified the mechanism of viral dissemination during primary varicella infection in normal children, as well as VZV reactivation in adult cancer patients and HIV-infected children [68–72]. Few data are available regarding primary, recurrent, and disseminated VZV infection in HIV-infected adults.

Clinical Manifestations

Shingles occurs when latent VZV is reactivated, travels along the peripheral sensory nerve, and seeds the skin. Most patients have a prodrome of dermatomal pain (sometimes mistaken as visceral in origin), itching, or paresthesias several days before eruption of the characteristic vesicular rash. The rash begins as erythematous macules, and clustered vesicles appear over the next 24 hours (see Plate 10). Lesions dry during the first week and crust during the second week; residual scarring is variable. While zoster may affect any of the cranial nerves, involvement of the first branch of the trigeminal nerve is most common. Acute retinal necrosis may occur as a complication of ophthalmic zoster [73–76]. Facial palsy, with the loss of taste on the anterior two thirds of the tongue, is seen with both otic zoster (Ramsay Hunt syndrome) and C2–3 (cervical collar) zoster. Segmental weakness, sometimes associated with zoster of the extremities or trunk, corresponds to the involved cutaneous dermatome(s).

Zoster may occur recurrently and with more frequent cutaneous and visceral dissemination in HIV-infected patients [59, 63–65, 77–79]. Acyclovir-resistant virus has been isolated from skin lesions in patients with VZV infection who are maintained on chronic oral acyclovir prophylaxis [80–83]. Mild diffuse meningoencephalitis sometimes accompanies acute zoster. A more severe form with delirium and cerebrospinal fluid pleocytosis has been described 3 to 8 days after the onset of chickenpox and 1 to 2 weeks after the onset of zoster [84–86]. Focal VZV encephalitis is a rare complication seen primarily in the immunosuppressed host. It is characterized by cerebral white matter lesions that resemble progressive multifocal leukoencephalopathy. Onset may be months after the cutaneous rash, and definitive diagnosis requires brain biopsy. Myelitis is a late complication of VZV infection that is sometimes seen in the immunosuppressed patient, usually presenting with bladder dysfunction, transient mild asymmetry of reflexes, and lower-extremity weakness or sensory deficits. Cerebral vasculitis has also been described in association with VZV infection [87].

Diagnosis

Clinical diagnosis of zoster is based on the presence of a dermatomal vesicular rash and a positive Tzanck smear. Definitive diagnosis requires direct culture or immunohistochemical stain of biopsied tissue. Serologic tests are not diagnostically helpful. The use of polymerase chain reaction testing is under investigation [72].

Treatment

The main goals of therapy for VZV infection are to abort cutaneous infection and prevent dissemination. Acyclovir is the treatment of choice [30, 88, 89] (see Table 23-1). Small trials have evaluated the efficacy of acyclovir in the treatment of primary varicella in normal adults and immunocompromised children, varicella pneumonia in normal adults, and acute zoster [90–95]. Although clinical experience suggests that acyclovir is effective for the treatment of shingles in HIV-infected patients, this has not been demonstrated in a controlled clinical trial.

Standard doses of oral acyclovir do not achieve sufficient serum levels to inhibit VZV in tissue culture. A higher dose (800 mg five times a day) may be necessary for satisfactory clinical response, but is expensive and may be associated with gastrointestinal toxicity. Acyclovir resistance remains a concern, especially in patients treated for an extended period of time [96]. In one uncontrolled study, 4 of 5 patients with painful cutaneous acyclovir-resistant zoster had healing in response to foscarnet [83]. Zoster lesions may become secondarily infected and require antibiotic or antifungal therapy; necrotic lesions sometimes require debridement.

Intravenous acyclovir is recommended for VZV infection that is severe, disseminated, or associated with local complications [97, 98]. Patients treated with intravenous acyclovir have reduced new lesion formation, shorter duration of viral shedding, and a lower incidence of dissemination [99]. The optimal duration of therapy is unknown. The question of whether corticosteroids decrease the incidence of postherpetic neuralgia in the normal host is controversial. HIV-infected patients, because of their relatively young age, appear to have a low frequency of postherpetic neuralgia. In this population, empiric steroid use is generally discouraged because of its potential immunosuppressive effect.

Prevention

There have been no studies on the use of antiviral therapy to prevent primary or recurrent varicella-zoster infection. VZV is easily spread, and isolation with the use of barrier precautions is strongly recommended to prevent nosocomial transmission, especially on wards with immunocompromised patients [100]. Vaccination with live attenuated VZV has been shown to be safe and effective in preventing severe or fatal infection in children with leukemia [101, 102]. However, the vaccine is less immunogenic in adults, and its safety and efficacy in HIV-infected patients is unknown. The CDC recommends that varicella-zoster immune globulin (VZIG) be given to susceptible immunocompromised hosts within 96 hours of exposure to VZV, although its benefit in preventing or modifying infection in this population is uncertain.

References

1. Armstrong D, Gold JWM, Dryjanski J, et al. Treatment of infections in patients with the acquired immunodeficiency syndrome. *Ann Intern Med* 103:738–743, 1985.
2. Drew WL, Buhles W, Erlich KS, et al. Herpes virus infections (cytomegalovirus, herpes simplex virus, varicella zoster virus): How to use gancyclovir (DHPG) and acyclovir. *Infect Dis Clin North Am* 2:495–509, 1988.
3. Quinnan GV, Masur H, Rook AH, et al. Herpes virus infections in the acquired immunodeficiency syndrome. *JAMA* 252:72–77, 1984.
4. Breinig MK, Kingsley LA, Armstrong JA, et al. Epidemiology of genital herpes in Pittsburgh: Serologic, sexual, and racial correlates of apparent and inapparent herpes simplex infections. *J Infect Dis* 162:299–305, 1990.
5. Lafferty WE, Coombs RW, Benedetti J, et al. Recurrences after oral and genital herpes simplex virus infection. *N Engl J Med* 316:1444–1449, 1987.
6. Mertz GJ. Genital herpes simplex virus infections. *Med Clin North Am* 74:1433–1454, 1990.
7. Holmberg SD, Stewart JA, Gerber AR, et al. Prior herpes simplex virus type 2 infection as a risk factor for HIV infection. *JAMA* 259:1048–1050, 1988.
8. Stamm WE, Handsfield HH, Rompalo AM, et al. The association between genital ulcer disease and acquisition of HIV infection in homosexual men. *JAMA* 260:1429–1433, 1988.

9. Kuiken CL, van Griensven GJP, de Vroome EMM, Coutinho RA. Risk factors and changes in sexual behavior in male homosexuals who seroconverted for human immunodeficiency virus antibodies. *Am J Epidemiol* 132:523–530, 1990.
10. Keet IPM, Lee FK, van Griensven GJP, et al. Herpes simplex virus type 2 and other genital ulcerative infections as a risk factor for HIV-1 acquisition. *Genitourin Med* 66:330–333, 1990.
11. Stevens JG. Human herpesviruses: A consideration of the latent state. *Micro Rev* 53:318–332, 1989.
12. Laurence J. Molecular interactions among herpesviruses and human immunodeficiency viruses. *J Infect Dis* 162:338–346, 1990.
13. Kohl S. Role of antibody-dependent cellular cytotoxicity in defense against herpes simplex virus infections. *Rev Infect Dis* 13:108–114, 1991.
14. Mester JC, Glorioso JC, Rouse BT. Protection against zosteriform spread of herpes simplex virus by monoclonal antibodies. *J Infect Dis* 163:263–269, 1991.
15. Corey L, Spear PG. Infections with herpes simplex viruses. *N Engl J Med* 314:686–691, 749–757, 1986.
16. Corey L, Adams HG, Brown ZA, et al. Genital herpes simplex virus infections: Clinical manifestations, course, and complications. *Ann Intern Med* 98:958–972, 1983.
17. Siegal FP, Lopez C, Manner GS, et al. Severe acquired immunodeficiency in male homosexuals manifested by chronic perianal ulcerative herpes simplex lesions. *N Engl J Med* 305:1439–1444, 1981.
18. Goodell SE, Quinn TC, Mkrtichian E, et al. Herpes simplex virus proctitis in homosexual men: Clinical, sigmoidoscopic, and histopathological features. *N Engl J Med* 308:868–871, 1983.
19. Safrin S, Ashley R, Houlihan C, et al. Clinical and serologic features of herpes simplex virus infection in patients with AIDS. *AIDS* 5:1107–1110, 1991.
20. Centers for Disease Control. Revision of the CDC surveillance case definition for acquired immunodeficiency syndrome. *MMWR* 36 (suppl):1–15, 1987.
21. Mertz GJ. Diagnosis and treatment of genital herpes infections. *Infect Dis Clin North Am* 1:341–366, 1987.
22. Nahmias AJ, Whitley RJ, Visintine AN, et al. Herpes simplex virus type 2 encephalitis: Laboratory evaluations and their diagnostic significance. *J Infect Dis* 146:829–836, 1982.
23. Gould E, Kory WP, Raskin JB, et al. Esophageal biopsy findings in the acquired immunodeficiency syndrome (AIDS): Clinicopathologic correlation in 20 patients. *South Med J* 81:1392–1395, 1988.
24. Ashley R, Cent A, Maggs V, et al. Inability of enzyme immunoassays to discriminate between infections with herpes simplex virus types 1 and 2. *Ann Intern Med* 115:520–526, 1991.
25. Cone RW, Hobson AC, Palmer J, et al. Extended duration of herpes simplex virus DNA in genital lesions detected by the polymerase chain reaction. *J Infect Dis* 164:757–760, 1991.
26. Bonacini M, Young T, Laine L. The causes of esophageal symptoms in

human immunodeficiency virus infection. *Arch Intern Med* 151:1567–1572, 1991.

27. Kahlon J, Chatterjee S, Lakeman FD, et al. Detection of antibodies to herpes simplex virus in the cerebrospinal fluid of patients with herpes simplex encephalitis. *J Infect Dis* 155:38–44, 1987.
28. Soong S, Watson NE, Caddell GR, et al. Use of brain biopsy for diagnostic evaluation of patients with suspected herpes simplex encephalitis: A statistical model and its clinical implications. *J Infect Dis* 163:17–22, 1991.
29. Quintiliani R, Levitz RE. Herpes simplex encephalitis: The case against brain biopsy (letter). *J Infect Dis* 164:426, 1991.
30. Dorsky DI, Crumpacker CS. Drugs five years later: Acyclovir. *Ann Intern Med* 107:859–874, 1987.
31. Stone KM, Whittington WL. Treatment of genital herpes. *Rev Infect Dis* 12 (suppl 6):S610–S619, 1990.
32. Spruance SL, Stewart JCB, Rowe NH, et al. Treatment of recurrent herpes simplex labialis with oral acyclovir. *J Infect Dis* 161:185–190, 1990.
33. Whitley RJ, Levin M, Barton N, et al. Infections caused by herpes simplex virus in the immunocompromised host: Natural history and topical acyclovir therapy. *J Infect Dis* 150:323–329, 1984.
34. Nusinoff-Lehrman S, Douglas JM, Corey L, et al. Recurrent genital herpes and suppressive oral acyclovir therapy: Relation between clinical outcome and in-vitro sensitivity. *Ann Intern Med* 104:786–790, 1986.
35. Thin RN. Management of genital herpes simplex infections. *Am J Med* 85(2A):3–6, 1988.
36. Shepp DH, Newton BA, Dandliker PS, et al. Oral acyclovir therapy for mucocutaneous herpes simplex virus infections in immunocompromised marrow transplant recipients. *Ann Intern Med* 102:783–785, 1985.
37. Straus SE, Seidlin M, Takiff H, et al. Oral acyclovir to suppress recurring herpes simplex virus infections in immunodeficient patients. *Ann Intern Med* 100:522–524, 1984.
38. Spruance SL, Freeman DJ, Stewart JCB, et al. The natural history of ultraviolet radiation–induced herpes simplex labialis and response to therapy with peroral and topical formulations of acyclovir. *J Infect Dis* 163:728–734, 1991.
39. Whitley RJ, Alford CA, Hirsch MS, et al. Vidarabine versus acyclovir therapy in herpes simplex encephalitis. *N Engl J Med* 314:144–149, 1986.
40. Sacks SL, Wanklin RJ, Reece DE, et al. Progressive esophagitis from acyclovir-resistant herpes simplex: Clinical roles for DNA polymerase mutants and viral heterogeneity? *Ann Intern Med* 111:893–899, 1989.
41. Birch CJ, Tachedjian G, Doherty RR, et al. Altered sensitivity to antiviral drugs of herpes simplex virus isolates from a patient with acquired immunodeficiency syndrome. *J Infect Dis* 162:731–734, 1990.
42. Ljungman P, Ellis MN, Hackman RC, et al. Acyclovir-resistant herpes simplex virus causing pneumonia after marrow transplantation. *J Infect Dis* 162:244–248, 1990.
43. Gateley A, Gander RM, Johnson PC, et al. Herpes simplex virus type 2

meningoencephalitis resistant to acyclovir in a patient with AIDS. *J Infect Dis* 161:711–715, 1990.

44. Englund JA, Zimmerman ME, Swierkosz EM, et al. Herpes simplex virus resistant to acyclovir: A study in a tertiary care center. *Ann Intern Med* 112:416–422, 1990.

45. Chatis PA, Miller CH, Schrager LE, Crumpacker CS. Successful treatment with foscarnet of an acyclovir-resistant mucocutaneous infection with herpes simplex virus in a patient with acquired immunodeficiency syndrome. *N Engl J Med* 320:297–300, 1989.

46. Erlich KS, Mills J, Chatis P, et al. Acyclovir-resistant herpes simplex virus infections in patients with the acquired immunodeficiency syndrome. *N Engl J Med* 320:293–296, 1989.

47. Safrin S, Assaykeen T, Follansbee S, Mills J. Foscarnet therapy for acyclovir-resistant mucocutaneous herpes simplex virus infection in 26 AIDS patients: Preliminary data. *J Infect Dis* 161:1078–1084, 1990.

48. Safrin S, Crumpacker C, Chatis P, et al. A controlled trial comparing foscarnet with vidarabine for acyclovir-resistant mucocutaneous herpes simplex in the acquired immunodeficiency syndrome. *N Engl J Med* 325:551–555, 1991.

49. Cooper DA, Pedersen C, Aiuti F, et al. The efficacy and safety of zidovudine with or without acyclovir in the treatment of patients with AIDS-related complex. *AIDS* 5:933–943, 1991.

50. Spruance SL, Stewart JCB, Freeman DJ, et al. Early application of topical 15% idoxuridine in dimethyl sulfoxide shortens the course of herpes simplex labialis: A multicenter placebo-controlled trial. *J Infect Dis* 161:191–197, 1990.

51. Sacks SL, Tyrrell LD, Lawee D, et al. Randomized, double-blind, placebo-controlled, clinic initiated Canadian multicenter trial of topical edoxudine 3% cream in the treatment of recurrent genital herpes. *J Infect Dis* 164:665–672, 1991.

52. Sacks SL, Varner TL, Davies KS, et al. Randomized, double-blind, placebo-controlled, patient initiated study of topical high- and low-dose interferon-alpha with nonoxynol-9 in the treatment of recurrent genital herpes. *J Infect Dis* 161:692–698, 1990.

53. Sacks SL, Portnoy J, Lawee D, et al. Clinical course of recurrent genital herpes and treatment with foscarnet cream: Results of a Canadian multicenter trial. *J Infect Dis* 155:178–186, 1987.

54. Kessler, IA, et al. Treatment of acyclovir-resistant mucocutaneous herpes simplex virus infection in patients with AIDS: Open label pilot study of topical trifluridine (abstract). Eighth International Conference on AIDS, Amsterdam, July 1992.

55. Kaplowitz LG, Baker D, Gelb L, et al. Prolonged continuous acyclovir treatment of normal adults with frequently recurring genital herpes simplex virus infection. *JAMA* 265:747–751, 1991.

56. Klein RS. Prophylaxis of opportunistic infections in individuals infected with HIV. *AIDS* 3 (suppl 1):S161–S173, 1989.

57. Gold D, Corey L. Acyclovir prophylaxis for herpes simplex virus infection. *Antimicrob Agents Chemother* 31:361–367, 1987.

58. Mertz GJ, Ashley R, Burke RL, et al. Double-blind, placebo controlled trial of a herpes simplex virus type 2 glycoprotein vaccine in persons at high risk for genital herpes infection. *J Infect Dis* 161:653–660, 1990.
59. Cohen PR, Beltrani VP, Grossman ME. Disseminated herpes zoster in patients with human immunodeficiency virus infection. *Am J Med* 84:1076–1080, 1988.
60. Dolin R, Reichman RC, Mazur MH, et al. Herpes zoster and varicella infections in immunosuppressed patients. *Ann Intern Med* 89:375–388, 1978.
61. Straus SE (moderator). Varicella-zoster virus infection: Biology, natural history, treatment, and prevention. *Ann Intern Med* 108:221–237, 1988.
62. Weller TH. Varicella and herpes zoster: Changing concepts of the natural history, control, and importance of a not-so-benign virus. *N Engl J Med* 309:1362–1368, 1434–1440, 1983.
63. Colebunders R, Mann JM, Francis H, et al. Herpes zoster in African patients: A clinical predictor of human immunodeficiency virus infection. *J Infect Dis* 157:314–318, 1988.
64. Cone LA, Schiffman MA. Herpes zoster and the acquired immunodeficiency syndrome (letter). *Ann Intern Med* 100:462, 1984.
65. Van de Perre P, Bakkers E, Batungwanayo J, et al. Herpes zoster in African patients: An early manifestation of HIV infection. *Scand J Infect Dis* 20:277–282, 1988.
66. Friedman-Kien AE, Lafleur FL, Gendler E, et al. Herpes zoster: A possible early clinical sign for the development of acquired immunodeficiency syndrome in high risk individuals. *J Am Acad Dermatol* 14:1023–1028, 1986.
67. Melbye M, Grossman RJ, Goedert JJ, et al. Risk of AIDS after herpes zoster. *Lancet* 1:728–730, 1987.
68. Asano Y, Itakura N, Kajita Y, et al. Severity of viremia and clinical findings in children with varicella. *J Infect Dis* 161:1095–1098, 1990.
69. Rusthoven JJ, Ahlgren P, Elhakim T, et al. Varicella-zoster infection in adult cancer patients. *Arch Intern Med* 148:1561–1566, 1988.
70. Jura E, Chadwick EG, Josephs SH, et al. Varicella-zoster virus infections in children infected with human immunodeficiency virus. *Pediatr Infect Dis J* 8:586–590, 1989.
71. Patterson LE, Butler KM, Edwards MS. Clinical herpes zoster shortly following primary varicella in two HIV-infected children. *Clin Pediatr* 28:354, 1989.
72. Koropchak CM, Graham G, Palmer J, et al. Investigation of varicella-zoster virus infection by polymerase chain reaction in the immunocompetent host with acute varicella. *J Infect Dis* 163:1016–1022, 1991.
73. Chess J, Marcus DM. Zoster-related bilateral acute retinal necrosis syndrome as presenting sign in AIDS. *Ann Ophthalmol* 20:431–435, 438, 1988.
74. Sandor E, Croxson TS, Millman A, et al. Herpes zoster ophthalmicus in patients at risk for AIDS (letter). *N Engl J Med* 310:1118–1119, 1984.
75. Sandor E, Croxson TS, Millman A, et al. Herpes zoster ophthalmicus in

patients at risk for the acquired immunodeficiency syndrome (AIDS). *Am J Ophthalmol* 101:153–155, 1986.

76. Cole EL, Meisler DM, Calabrese LM, et al. Herpes zoster ophthalmicus and acquired immune deficiency syndrome. *Arch Ophthalmol* 102:1027–1029, 1984.

77. Gilson IH, Barnett JH, Conant MA, et al. Disseminated ecthymatous herpes varicella-zoster virus infection in patients with acquired immunodeficiency syndrome. *J Am Acad Dermatol* 20:637–642, 1989.

78. Gilden DH, Murray RS, Wellish M, et al. Chronic progressive varicella-zoster virus encephalitis in an AIDS patient. *Neurology* 38:1150–1153, 1988.

79. Perronne C, Lazanas M, Leport C, et al. Varicella in patients infected with the human immunodeficiency virus. *Arch Dermatol* 126:1033–1036, 1990.

80. Jacobson MA, Berger TG, Fikrig S, et al. Acyclovir-resistant varicella zoster virus infection after chronic oral acyclovir therapy in patients with acquired immunodeficiency syndrome (AIDS). *Ann Intern Med* 112:187–191, 1990.

81. Hoppenjans WB, Bibler MR, Orme RL, Solinger AM. Prolonged cutaneous herpes zoster in acquired immunodeficiency syndrome. *Arch Dermatol* 126:1048–1050, 1990.

82. Disler RS, Dover JS. Chronic localized herpes zoster in the acquired immunodeficiency syndrome. *Arch Dermatol* 126:1105–1106, 1990.

83. Safrin S, Berger TG, Gilson I, et al. Foscarnet therapy in five patients with AIDS and acyclovir-resistant varicella-zoster virus infection. *Ann Intern Med* 115:19–21, 1991.

84. Jemsek J, Greenberg SB, Taber L, et al. Herpes zoster–associated encephalitis: Clinicopathologic report of 12 cases and a review of the literature. *Medicine* 62:81–97, 1983.

85. Rostad SW, Olson K, McDougall J, et al. Transsynaptic spread of varicella zoster virus through the visual system: A mechanism of viral dissemination in the central nervous system. *Hum Pathol* 20:174–179, 1989.

86. Ryder JW, Croen K, Kleinschmidt-De-Masters BK, et al. Progressive encephalitis three months after resolution of cutaneous zoster in a patient with AIDS. *Ann Neurol* 19:182–188, 1986.

87. Verghese A, Sugar AM. Herpes zoster ophthalmicus and granulomatous angiitis: An ill-appreciated cause of stroke. *J Am Geriatr Soc* 34:309–312, 1986.

88. Shepp DH, Dandliker PS, Meyers JD. Treatment of varicella zoster virus infection in severely immunocompromised patients. *N Engl J Med* 314:208–212, 1986.

89. Straus SE. The management of varicella and zoster infections. *Infect Dis Clin North Am* 1:367–383, 1987.

90. Feder HM. Treatment of adult chickenpox with oral acyclovir. *Arch Intern Med* 150:2061–2065, 1990.

91. Nyerges G, Meszner Z, Gyarmati E, Kerpel-Fronius S. Acyclovir prevents dissemination of varicella in immunocompromised children. *J Infect Dis* 157:309–313, 1988.

92. Haake DA, Zakowski PC, Haake DL, Bryson YL. Early treatment with acyclovir for varicella pneumonia in otherwise healthy adults: Retrospective controlled study and review. *Rev Infect Dis* 12:788–798, 1990.
93. Huff JC, Bean B, Balfour HH, et al. Therapy of herpes zoster with oral acyclovir. *Am J Med* 85 (suppl 2A):84–89, 1988.
94. Wood MJ, Ogan PH, McKendrick MW, et al. Efficacy of oral acyclovir treatment of acute herpes zoster. *Am J Med* 85 (suppl 2A):79–84, 1988.
95. McKendrick MW, McGill JI, White JE, et al. Oral acyclovir and herpes zoster. *Br Med J* 293:1529–1532, 1986.
96. Pahwa S, Biron K, Lim W, et al. Continuous varicella-zoster infection associated with acyclovir resistance in a child with AIDS. *JAMA* 260:2879–2882, 1988.
97. Schulman JA, Peyman GA. Management of viral retinitis. *Ophthalmic Surg* 19:876–884, 1988.
98. Seiff SR, Margolis T, Graham SH, O'Donnell JJ. Use of intravenous acyclovir for treatment of herpes zoster ophthalmicus in patients at risk for AIDS. *Ann Ophthalmol* 20:480–482, 1988.
99. Balfour HH, Bean B, Laskin OL, et al. Acyclovir halts progression of herpes zoster in immunocompromised patients. *N Engl J Med* 308:1448–1453, 1983.
100. Josephson A, Gombert ME. Airborne transmission of nosocomial varicella from localized zoster. *J Infect Dis* 158:238–241, 1988.
101. Gershon AA, Steinberg SP, National Institute of Allergy and Infectious Diseases Varicella Vaccine Study Group. Live attenuated varicella vaccine: Protection in healthy adults compared with leukemic children. *J Infect Dis* 161:661–666, 1990.
102. Lawrence R, Gershon AA, Holzman R, Steinberg SP, NIAID Varicella Vaccine Collaborative Study Group. The risk of zoster after varicella vaccination in children with leukemia. *N Engl J Med* 318:543–548, 1988.

24 / Candidiasis

Carol A. Sulis

Candidiasis is a superficial mucocutaneous or invasive visceral infection caused by *Candida albicans* and other species that commonly occurs in HIV-infected patients.

Epidemiology

Candida species are ubiquitous. In the normal host, they colonize the skin, mucosa, and gastrointestinal tract, and they are probably transmitted from person to person without an environmental reservoir. Colonization at all sites is increased by the use of antibiotics and corticosteroids.

Pathogenesis

Candida attach to tissues using fungal synthetic products such as "adhesin." Infection occurs when the skin or mucosa is disrupted; the adherent *Candida* then invade the superficial epithelium and/or disseminate hematogenously. In the normal host, polymorphonuclear leukocytes and cellular immune mechanisms limit the extent and severity of infection. Disseminated infection is associated with neutropenia, and an increased incidence of mucocutaneous disease occurs in the context of defective cell-mediated immunity. While HIV-induced suppression of the immune system facilitates candidal infection, there are also data suggesting that candidiasis itself may induce T- and B-lymphocyte defects that enhance bacterial superinfection [1, 2]. New or unusually virulent candidal strains have not been identified in HIV-infected patients [3].

Clinical Manifestations

Mucocutaneous Infection

Thrush, the most common fungal disease associated with HIV infection, was described early in the HIV epidemic and is independently predictive of progression to AIDS [4-7]. The most common manifestation is white patches or "pseudomembranes" on the tongue or oral mucosa (see Plate 1). Removal of this material leaves an erythematous base that may ooze or bleed. Clinical variants include an atrophic form (smooth red patches anywhere in the mouth), *Candida* leukoplakia (firm, adherent white patches that are difficult to remove), and angular cheilitis (erythema and fissures at the corner of the mouth) [8]. Thrush may be asymptomatic or present with pain or a bad taste in the mouth [9]. Hairy leukoplakia, an oral lesion caused by Epstein-Barr virus, is distinguished from thrush by its papilliform appearance and location on the lateral aspect of the tongue (see Plate 3).

Candidal esophagitis is a frequent AIDS-defining diagnosis, occurring most often when the CD4 lymphocyte count is below 100 cells/mm^3 [10-15]. Patients may complain of dysphagia, retrosternal pain, and odynophagia. However, odynophagia associated with herpes simplex virus or cytomegalovirus esophagitis is generally more severe [16, 17].

Recurrent or chronic vulvovaginal candidiasis is a common early manifestation of HIV infection in women, although it may occur in immunocompetent hosts as well [13, 18, 19]. Occasional cases of cutaneous and gastrointestinal infection with *C. albicans* have also been associated with HIV infection, but dissemination is uncommon in the absence of other predisposing factors [20]. Candidal balanitis, cystitis, intertrigo, and paronychia do not appear to occur with increased frequency in the context of HIV infection [19, 21].

Hematogenously Disseminated Candidiasis

Candidal endophthalmitis, meningitis, brain abscess, endocarditis, pneumonia, and infections of the liver and kidney are unusual in AIDS patients; other risk factors, such as neutropenia, diabetes mellitus, central intravascular lines, and high-dose corticosteroid therapy, are generally present [21-26]. Diagnosis of candidiasis of the trachea, bronchi, or lungs meets the Centers for Disease Control case definition for AIDS, although these conditions are relatively rare [11].

Diagnosis

Mucocutaneous lesions can be scraped or biopsied. The specimen should be suspended in 10% potassium hydroxide (KOH), which dissolves squamous cells and leukocytes, and examined microscopically for the presence of hyphae, pseudohyphae, and budding yeast. Neither symptoms nor radiographic appearance of "cobblestone mucosa" on barium swallow are sufficient to differentiate candidal esophagitis

(>50% of cases) from viral infection or malignancy. Definitive diagnosis of candidal esophagitis requires the demonstration of tissue-invasive mycelia on endoscopic biopsy, although a presumptive diagnosis can be made if odynophagia and thrush are present [11, 16, 27–30]. Disseminated candidal infection may be extremely difficult to document and requires biopsy evidence of tissue invasion or isolation of fungus from a normally sterile body site. Positive blood cultures may reflect a removable intravascular focus of candidal infection, such as a central venous line, or indicate disseminated candidiasis [31, 32]. Skin tests and serologic studies for candidal antibody or antigen show inconsistent results and are not recommended for diagnosis.

Treatment

Superficial mucous membrane infection may respond to topical therapy with nystatin, a polyene antifungal drug that is available in oral suspension, or clotrimazole, an imidazole available in troche form (Table 24-1). Vaginal and cutaneous infections generally respond well to antifungal creams. If mucocutaneous candidal infection fails to respond to topical therapy or if esophagitis is suspected because of the presence of odynophagia, treatment with ketoconazole is indicated.

Ketoconazole is an oral imidazole metabolized by the liver [33]. Absorption requires an acid pH; levels are greatly diminished in patients with achlorhydria or those receiving H_2 blockers or antacids. Ketoconazole has been associated with hepatic necrosis, interference with oral anticoagulants, and inhibition of steroidogenesis [34–37]. Patients receiving ketoconazole should not be treated concurrently with the antihistamine terfenadine because of an increased risk of serious cardiac dysrhythmias [38]. Ketoconazole is embryotoxic in animals and is contraindicated in pregnancy.

Therapy with ketoconazole is usually continued for 1 to 2 weeks, although longer regimens are sometimes required. Experience suggests that maintenance therapy is often necessary to prevent recurrence; antimicrobial resistance and the emergence of other fungal pathogens may occur over time [28, 39–41]. In HIV-infected patients with odynophagia, endoscopy is generally reserved for those situations in which the patient fails to respond to empiric antifungal therapy.

Fluconazole, a triazole antifungal agent, is indicated in HIV-infected patients with mucocutaneous candidiasis who do not respond to topical therapy or ketoconazole [42, 43]. Trials comparing fluconazole to ketoconazole suggest equal or superior efficacy and fewer side effects for fluconazole and similar relapse rates [44–51]. Most (80%) of the drug is excreted unchanged by the kidney. Common side effects include nausea, vomiting, and mild elevation of serum transaminases. A number of

Table 24-1 *Treatment of candidiasis associated with HIV disease*

Type of infection	Treatment
Thrush	Nystatin suspension swish and swallow, 5 ml five times/day
	or
	Clotrimazole troche, 10 mg five times/day
Cutaneous infection	Clotrimazole cream
Vaginitis	Clotrimazole cream or troches
Mucocutaneous infection, refractory to topical therapy	Ketoconazole, 200 mg po qd
	or
	Fluconazole, 50–100 mg po qd
Esophagitis	Ketoconazole, 200–400 mg po qd
	or
	Fluconazole, 100–200 mg po qd
Fungemia or disseminated infection	Amphotericin B, 0.6 mg/kg/day IV

important drug interactions have been reported with fluconazole, including increased serum levels of phenobarbital and cyclosporin, and potentiation of warfarin (Coumadin) and oral sulfonylureas; a decreased serum level of fluconazole has been noted when the agent is given with rifampin [44]. Because its effect on the fetus is uncertain, the use of fluconazole should be avoided during pregnancy. Itraconazole and an experimental triazole, SCH39304, which are similar to fluconazole in their high bioavailability, predominant renal excretion, and low toxicity, are currently undergoing clinical trial evaluation.

Disseminated candidiasis requires treatment with intravenous amphotericin B, a polyene antifungal agent. The optimal duration of therapy is unknown. Its use is associated with significant toxicity, including fever, chills, thrombophlebitis, and renal dysfunction. No evidence has been found that the addition of flucytosine to amphotericin is beneficial in the treatment of disseminated candidiasis in HIV-infected patients.

Prognosis and Prevention

Because the *Candida* species is a commensal organism, mucocutaneous infection can be expected to recur in the immunodeficient patient unless prophylaxis is maintained. However, there are no studies that document the frequency of recurrence or the efficacy of prophylaxis. Two ongoing AIDS Clinical Trials Group protocols compare fluconazole and clotrimazole in the prevention of thrush and evaluate the efficacy of chlorhexidine mouthwash for prevention and treatment of thrush.

Disseminated disease may occur in the context of neutropenia despite prophylaxis. Data are inadequate to determine the impact of prophylaxis on the development of fungal resistance [52, 53]. Nosocomial transmission of fungal pathogens is uncommon. Isolating patients is unnecessary; however, health care workers are urged to employ barrier techniques and thorough hand washing to avoid cross-contamination.

References

1. Baldwin GC, et al. Human immunodeficiency virus causes mononuclear phagocyte dysfunction. *Proc Natl Acad Sci* 87:3933–3937, 1990.
2. Crislip MA, Edwards JE. Candidiasis. *Infect Dis Clin North Am* 3:103–133, 1989.
3. Whelan WL, Kirsch DR, Kwon-Chung KJ, et al. *Candida albicans* in patients with the acquired immunodeficiency syndrome: Absence of a novel or hypervirulent strain. *J Infect Dis* 162:513–518, 1990.
4. Barone R, Ficarra G, Gaglioti D, et al. Prevalence of oral lesions among HIV-infected intravenous drug abusers and other risk groups. *Oral Surg Oral Med Oral Pathol* 69:169–173, 1990.
5. Gottlieb MS, Schroff R, Schanker HM, et al. *Pneumocystis carinii* pneumonia and mucosal candidiasis in previously healthy homosexual men. *N Engl J Med* 305:1425, 1981.
6. Klein RS, Harris CA, Small CB, et al. Oral candidiasis in high-risk patients as the initial manifestation of the acquired immunodeficiency syndrome. *N Engl J Med* 311:354–358, 1984.
7. Murray HW, Godbold JH, Jurica KB, Roberts RB. Progression to AIDS in patients with lymphadenopathy or AIDS-related complex: Reappraisal of risk and predictive factors. *Am J Med* 86:533–538, 1989.
8. Ficarra G, Barone R, Gaglioti D, et al. Oral hairy leukoplakia among HIV-positive intravenous drug abusers: A clinicopathologic and ultrastructural study. *Oral Surg Oral Med Oral Path* 65:421–426, 1988.
9. Greenspan JS, Greenspan D, Winkler JR. Diagnosis and management of the oral manifestations of HIV infection and AIDS. *Infect Dis Clin North Am* 2:373–385, 1988.
10. Walsh TJ, Hamilton SR, Belitsos N. Esophageal candidiasis: Managing an increasingly prevalent infection. *Postgrad Med* 84:193–205, 1988.
11. Centers for Disease Control. Revision of the surveillance case definition for acquired immunodeficiency syndrome. *MMWR* 36 (suppl):1–15, 1987.
12. Carpenter CCJ, Mayer KH, Fisher A, et al. Natural history of acquired immunodeficiency syndrome in women in Rhode Island. *Am J Med* 86:771–775, 1989.
13. Imam N, et al. Hierarchical pattern of mucosal candida infections in HIV-seropositive women. *Am J Med* 89:142–146, 1990.
14. Pena JM, Martinez-Lopez MA, Arnalich F, et al. Esophageal candidiasis associated with acute infection due to human immunodeficiency virus: Case report and review. *Rev Infect Dis* 13:872–875, 1991.

15. Scott GB, Hutto C, Makuch RW, et al. Survival in children with perinatally acquired human immunodeficiency type 1 infection. *N Engl J Med* 321:1791–1796, 1989.
16. Bonacini M, Young T, Laine L. The causes of esophageal symptoms in human immunodeficiency virus infection. *Arch Intern Med* 151:1567–1572, 1991.
17. Agha FP, Lee HH, Nostrant TT. Herpetic esophagitis: A diagnostic challenge in immunocompromised patients. *Am J Gastroenterol* 81:246–253, 1986.
18. Sobel JD. Vaginal infections in adult women. *Med Clin North Am* 74:1573–1602, 1990.
19. Rhoads JL, Wright DC, Redfield RR, Burke DS. Chronic vaginal candidiasis in women with human immunodeficiency virus infection. *JAMA* 257:3105–3107, 1987.
20. Oriba HA, Lo JS, Bergfeld WF. Disseminated cutaneous fungal infection and AIDS. *Cleve Clin J Med* 57:189–191, 1990.
21. Diamond RD. The growing problem of mycoses in patients infected with the human immunodeficiency virus. *Rev Infect Dis* 13:480–486, 1991.
22. Ehni W, Ellison RT. Spontaneous *Candida albicans* meningitis in a patient with the acquired immune deficiency syndrome (letter). *Am J Med* 83:806–807, 1987.
23. Haron E, Feld R, Tuffnell P, et al. Hepatic candidiasis: An increasing problem in immunocompromised patients. *Am J Med* 83:17–26, 1987.
24. Matthews R, Burnie J, Smith D, et al. Candida and AIDS: Evidence for protective antibody. *Lancet* 2:263–266, 1988.
25. Kirpatrick CH. Host factors in defense against fungal infections. *Am J Med* 77:1–12, 1984.
26. Cohen MS, Isturiz RE, Malech HL, et al. Fungal infection in chronic granulomatous disease: The importance of the phagocyte in defense against fungi. *Am J Med* 71:59–66, 1981.
27. Tavitian A, Raufman J, Rosenthal LE. Oral candidiasis as a marker for esophageal candidiasis in the acquired immunodeficiency syndrome. *Ann Intern Med* 104:54–55, 1986.
28. Tavitian A, Raufman J, Rosenthal LE, et al. Ketoconazole-resistant candida esophagitis in patients with acquired immunodeficiency syndrome. *Gastroenterology* 90:443–445, 1986.
29. Devita VT, Broder S, Fauci AS, et al. Developmental therapeutics and the acquired immunodeficiency syndrome. *Ann Intern Med* 106:568–581, 1987.
30. Bonacini MB, Laine L, Gal AA, et al. Prospective evaluation of blind brushing of the esophagus for *Candida* esophagitis in patients with human immunodeficiency virus infection. *Am J Gastroenterol* 85:385–389, 1990.
31. Ellis CA, Spivack ML. The significance of candidemia. *Ann Intern Med* 67:511–522, 1967.
32. Rinaldi MG. Problems in the diagnosis of invasive fungal diseases. *Rev Infect Dis* 13:493–495, 1991.
33. Sugar AM, Alsip SG, Galgiani JN, et al. Pharmacology and toxicity of high-dose ketoconazole. *Antimicrob Agents Chemother* 31:1874–1878, 1987.

34. Lewis JH, Zimmerman HJ, Benson GD, Ishak KG. Hepatic injury associated with ketoconazole therapy: Analysis of 33 cases. *Gastroenterology* 86:503–513, 1984.

35. Duarte PA, Chow CC, Simons F, Ruskin J. Fatal hepatitis associated with ketoconazole therapy. *Arch Intern Med* 144:1069–1070, 1984.

36. Sonino N. Drug therapy: The use of ketoconazole as an inhibitor of steroid production. *N Engl J Med* 317:812–818, 1987.

37. Smith AG. Potentiation of oral anticoagulants by ketoconazole. *Br Med J* 288:188–189, 1984.

38. Safety of terfenadine and astemizole. *Med Letter* 34:9–10, 1992.

39. Sobel JD. Recurrent vulvovaginal candidiasis: A prospective study of the efficacy of maintenance ketoconazole therapy. *N Engl J Med* 315:1455–1458, 1986.

40. Korting HC, Ollert M, Georgii A, Froschel M. *In vitro* susceptibilities and biotypes of *Candida albicans* isolates from the oral cavities of patients infected with human immunodeficiency virus. *J Clin Microbiol* 26:2626–2631, 1988.

41. Powderly WG. Mucosal candidiasis caused by non-albicans species of *Candida* in HIV-positive patients. *AIDS* 6:604–605, 1992.

42. Kauffman CA, Bradley SF, Ross SC, Weber DR. Hepatosplenic candidiasis: Successful treatment with fluconazole. *Am J Med* 91:137–141, 1991.

43. Anaissie E, Bodey GP, Kantarjian H, et al. Fluconazole therapy for chronic disseminated candidiasis in patients with leukemia and prior amphotericin B therapy. *Am J Med* 91:142–150, 1991.

44. Larsen RA. Azoles and AIDS. *J Infect Dis* 162:727–730, 1990.

45. DeWit S, Weerts D, Goossens H, Clumeck N. Comparison of fluconazole and ketoconazole for oropharyngeal candidiasis in AIDS. *Lancet* 1:746–748, 1989.

46. Meunier F, Aoun M, Gerard M. Therapy for oropharyngeal candidiasis in the immunocompromised host: A randomized double-blind study of fluconazole versus ketoconazole. *Rev Infect Dis* 12 (suppl 3):S364–S368, 1990.

47. Laine L, Conteas C, DeBruin M, Multicenter Study Group. A prospective, randomized trial of fluconazole versus ketoconazole for candida esophagitis. *Gastroenterology* 98:A458, 1990.

48. Dismukes WE. Azole antifungal drugs: Old and new. *Ann Intern Med* 109:177–179, 1988.

49. Hay RJ. Overview of studies of fluconazole in oropharyngeal candidiasis. *Rev Infect Dis* 12 (suppl 3):S334–S337, 1990.

50. Robinson PA, Knirsch AK, Joseph JA. Fluconazole for life-threatening fungal infections in patients who cannot be treated with conventional antifungal agents. *Rev Infect Dis* 12 (suppl 3):S349–S363, 1990.

51. Laine L, et al. Fluconazole compared with ketoconazole for the treatment of candida esophagitis in AIDS. *Ann Intern Med* 117:655–660, 1992.

52. Samonis G, Rolston K, Karl C, et al. Prophylaxis of oropharyngeal candidiasis with fluconazole. *Rev Infect Dis* 12 (suppl 3):S369–S373, 1990.

53. Klein RS. Prophylaxis of opportunistic infections in individuals infected with HIV. *AIDS* 3 (suppl 1):S161–S173, 1989.

25 / Conventional Bacterial Infections

Maura A. Fagan, Robert A. Witzburg

Conventional bacterial infections are frequently associated with HIV disease. The occurrence of recurrent, complicated, or severe bacterial infections may be the first clinical evidence of immunodeficiency in HIV-seropositive patients [1]. Bacterial infections may require repeated hospitalization, therapy with potentially toxic antibiotic agents, and, occasionally, surgical intervention. Early recognition and treatment of conventional bacterial infections may result in reduced morbidity and mortality (Table 25-1).

Epidemiology

Rolston and associates [2] reported a rate of 31 bacterial infections per 100 hospitalizations of HIV-infected patients. In this series of predominantly homosexual men, 90 percent of the infections were nosocomial in origin. In a study by Witt and colleagues [3] from Boston City Hospital, bacterial infections developed significantly more often in injection drug users (IDUs) than in homosexual men (58 vs. 14%). In an autopsy series, Nichols and coworkers [4] reported that bacterial infections were present in 83 percent of patients with HIV disease, were more common than opportunistic infections, and were the sole or contributing cause of death in 37 percent of cases. *Staphylococcus aureus* was the most frequently isolated pathogen, with *Streptococcus pneumoniae* and *Haemophilus influenzae* responsible for most of the other bacterial infections.

Pathogenesis

The pathophysiology of bacterial infections in the HIV-infected patient involves abnormalities in cell-mediated, humoral, and nonspecific immunity [5–8]. Quantitative and functional deficits in CD4 lymphocytes, with diminished cytokine production and impaired macrophage

343

Table 25-1 Management guidelines for bacterial infection in HIV disease

1. Recommend HIV antibody testing in patients with bacterial infection who have an HIV risk factor.
2. Obtain blood cultures in all systemically ill-appearing patients with HIV disease. Attempt to identify the source of bacteremia and choose empiric antibiotic therapy based on the pathogens most likely to cause this type of infection.
3. Choose specific antibiotic therapy on the basis of Gram's stain and culture results of body fluids and/or biopsy material.
4. Identify and correct reversible causes of neutropenia.
5. Use appropriate immunizations as early as possible in the course of HIV disease.

activity, predispose to infection with *Salmonella, Listeria,* and *Mycobacteria.* Inadequate production of opsonizing antibodies reduces defense against encapsulated organisms, such as *Strep. pneumoniae* and *H. influenzae* [7, 8]. Neutrophil dysfunction impairs chemotaxis, phagocytosis, and bacterial killing [9]. Loss of integrity of the mucocutaneous barrier in IDUs and in patients undergoing invasive diagnostic and therapeutic procedures increases the risk of aspiration pneumonia and sinusitis (through disruption of the upper respiratory tract) and local and disseminated infection with *Staph. aureus* (through disruption of the skin).

Clinical Syndromes

Common bacterial infections in HIV disease are listed in Table 25-2.

Bacteremia

In a study of community-acquired infections in AIDS patients, Krumholz and associates [10] reported bacteremia as a complication in 5 percent of cases. Among 44 episodes of bacteremia, 10 were secondary to pulmonary infections, 8 were associated with infected intravascular catheters, and 7 resulted from cellulitis. In a series from Boston City Hospital, 34 episodes of bacteremia were described in 16 patients who were predominantly IDUs [3]. Of 25 community-acquired infections, the majority were caused by *Staph. aureus, Strep. pneumoniae,* or other streptococci. All of the *Staph. aureus* bacteremias occurred in IDUs, with endocarditis the most common type of infection. Streptococcal bacteremias were associated with either pneumonia or endocarditis. Recent data indicate that HIV-infected IDUs are also at increased risk for bacteremia with *H. influenzae,* type b [11].

Table 25-2 Common bacterial infections in HIV disease

Infection	Pathogens	Treatment*	Prevention
Bacteremia	Staph. aureus	Oxacillin	Avoid unnecessary intravascular lines
	Gram-negative rods	Third-generation cephalosporin, aztreonam, or aminoglycoside	
Pneumonia	Strep. pneumoniae	Penicillin	Appropriate immunizations
	H. influenzae	Ampicillin, third-generation cephalosporin, or aztreonam	
Periodontitis	Oral anaerobes	Debridement, curettage, antibacterial mouthwash, antibiotics prn	Good preventive dental care
Sinusitis	Strep. pneumoniae	Ampicillin or TMP-SMZ, decongestant, surgical drainage prn	
	H. influenzae		
Gastroenteritis	Salmonella species	Ampicillin, TMP-SMZ, or quinolone	Avoid undercooked meats, raw eggs
	Shigella species		
	Campylobacter species	Erythromycin	
	Clostridium difficile	Metronidazole or oral vancomycin	Avoid unnecessary antibiotics
Skin/soft tissue infections			
Cellulitis/folliculitis	Staph. aureus	Dicloxacillin or first-generation cephalosporin	Good skin hygiene
Bacillary angiomatosis	Rickettsia-like organism	Erythromycin	
Pyomyositis	Staph. aureus	Oxacillin, surgical drainage	

TMP-SMZ = trimethoprim-sulfamethoxazole.
*Choice of specific antibiotic therapy should be based on sensitivity testing and knowledge of the patient's allergy history.

HIV-infected patients with indwelling central venous catheters have an increased rate of bacteremia compared to individuals without HIV infection [12]. In the clinically stable patient, management of catheter-associated infections can be attempted initially with antibiotic therapy alone, leaving the device in place. However, if the patient is acutely ill or has persistent fever or bacteremia, discontinuation of the intravascular catheter is necessary.

Neutropenia is common in HIV disease, and neutrophil counts below $500/mm^3$ have been associated with an increased risk of bacterial infection [13]. Neutropenic patients are prone to infection with staphylococci, enteric gram-negative pathogens, and *Pseudomonas aeruginosa*, as well as fungi [13, 14]. The optimal management of the febrile neutropenic HIV-infected patient is uncertain, but most clinicians elect to use empiric broad-spectrum antibiotic therapy pending culture results. The role of colony stimulating factors in the prevention and treatment of conventional bacterial infections in neutropenic patients has not been established.

As many as 50 percent of HIV-infected patients with bacteremia may have no clinical evidence of systemic toxicity [10, 12]. In one study, the median duration of fever before diagnosis in patients with *Staph. aureus* bacteremia was 6 days [15]. The case fatality rate for community-acquired bacteremia in HIV-infected patients may be as high as 9 percent, with half of deaths attributable to inappropriate empiric therapy directed against opportunistic pathogens [10].

Pneumonia

Bacterial pulmonary infections are common and frequently severe in HIV-infected patients [16–19]. Among hospitalized patients with HIV disease, the frequency of bacterial pneumonia may be as high as 50 percent; in one outpatient methadone program, the incidence of bacterial pneumonia was increased fourfold in HIV-seropositive clients [20]. Schuchat and associates [21] found that advanced immunodeficiency was associated with a higher incidence of complications, including bacteremia and empyema, and increased mortality.

The most common causes of bacterial pneumonia in HIV-infected patients are *Strep. pneumoniae* and *H. influenzae* [4, 10]. Its clinical presentation, including the abrupt onset of fever, productive cough, and pleuritic chest pain, may be accompanied by atypical radiologic findings [17–19, 22]. In patients with advanced HIV disease, the clinical picture may be further complicated by the coexistence of bacterial and opportunistic infections, particularly *Pneumocystis carinii* pneumonia [3].

Evaluation of the patient with suspected bacterial pneumonia includes sputum for microscopic examination and culture, chest radiograph, arterial blood gases, and blood cultures. Diagnosis is made by sputum examination and culture in approximately 75 percent of cases; blood cultures identify the pathogen 20 to 40 percent of the time [17, 18, 22]. The syndrome of fever, purulent sputum, and localized infiltrate on chest x-ray strongly suggests bacterial pneumonia, and additional diagnostic procedures are generally of little value [23].

Upper Aerodigestive Tract Infections

Gingivitis and periodontitis, the result of infection with anaerobic mouth flora, are common and sometimes severe in HIV-infected patients [24]. Management includes local debridement, curettage, antibacterial mouthwash, and antibiotic therapy as needed. Otitis media and sinusitis occur in up to 40 percent of patients with HIV disease and are the presenting illness in 10 percent [25–27]. As in lower respiratory tract infections, the predominant pathogens are *Strep. pneumoniae* and *H. influenzae*, but *Staph. aureus*, anaerobes, enteric gram-negative organisms, mycobacteria, and fungi sometimes play a role [25]. Symptoms of sinusitis range from mild coryza to fever, headache, and nasal discharge, but may be nonspecific or absent. Treatment consists of antibiotic therapy and decongestants. Relapsing or chronic disease is common, often necessitating surgical intervention.

Gastrointestinal Tract Infection

The gastrointestinal (GI) tract is a frequent site of bacterial infection in HIV disease. Dryden and Shanson [28] reviewed causes of diarrhea in 179 HIV-seropositive patients and found nontyphoidal *Salmonella* species in 5 cases, *Campylobacter* species in 4, and *Shigella* species in 1. In a prospective study of 132 AIDS patients with intestinal infection, René and associates [29] reported stool cultures that were positive for *Salmonella* species in 6 patients, *Shigella* species in 1, and *Yersinia* species in 1. Advanced HIV disease does not appear to be a predictor of bacterial diarrhea, but homosexuality may increase the risk [29, 30]. In the United States, residence in the Northeast, minority status, and injection drug use predispose to salmonellosis [31].

Invasive bacterial pathogens of the GI tract, including *Salmonella*, *Shigella*, and *Campylobacter* species, may cause severe and/or prolonged illness in patients with HIV disease. The incidence of salmonellosis is increased 20 to 100-fold in HIV-infected patients [31, 32]. The condition most often presents with fever and constitutional symptoms. Gastrointestinal complaints may be entirely absent, and blood and stool cultures typically grow a nontyphoidal strain of the organism, such as

Salmonella typhimurium or *enteritidis* [31–34]. The source of bacteremia, which is present in up to 50 percent of cases, is frequently not identified [31–33, 35].

Management of *Salmonella* infection, especially recurrent bacteremia, may be problematic. Initial treatment, based on drug sensitivity testing, consists of a 3-week course of ampicillin, trimethoprim-sulfamethoxazole (TMP-SMZ), a third-generation cephalosporin, or a quinolone. However, as many as 50 percent of patients relapse after completion of this regimen, and chronic maintenance antibiotic therapy is generally recommended.

Shigella infection generally manifests as fever, abdominal pain and tenderness, and bloody diarrhea, with symptoms slowly escalating for weeks before presentation [36–39]. Identification of the organism may require multiple stool cultures. Shigellemia, rare in the immunocompetent host, is not uncommon in HIV-infected patients [38, 39]. A 10- to 14-day course of ampicillin, TMP-SMZ, or a quinolone, based on sensitivity testing results, is usually adequate to eradicate the organism. Although relapsing disease has been described, it generally responds to retreatment; maintenance antibiotic therapy is not often necessary [37, 39].

Campylobacter gastroenteritis occurs more frequently in the presence of HIV infection, with annual incidence reported as high as 519 in 100,000 AIDS patients [40]. Clinical features include fever, protracted diarrhea, and weight loss [41, 42]. Although many cases are self-limited, erythromycin is indicated for treatment of protracted or severe disease. Treatment failures and early relapse due to erythromycin resistance have been reported [41, 42]. Lack of clinical response within the first week of treatment or early relapse should prompt a change in therapy to tetracycline or a quinolone.

Clostridium difficile enterocolitis, which may follow the use of any antibiotic agent, appears to occur more frequently in association with HIV disease. Clindamycin, ampicillin, and cephalosporins are the most common precipitants. Management consists of discontinuation of the antibiotic and administration of metronidazole or oral vancomycin.

Skin and Soft Tissue Infections

Bacterial infections of the skin are a source of considerable morbidity in HIV-infected patients. *Staph. aureus*, the most common pathogen, has been implicated in cellulitis, ecthyma, bullous impetigo, hidradenitis suppurativa, folliculitis, bullous impetigo, subcutaneous abscess, and the syndrome of generalized pruritus [43, 44].

Folliculitis presents as multiple, small, erythematous papules and pustules involving the face, trunk, or groin. Staphylococci can be identified on Gram's stain of pus. The condition usually responds to treatment with an oral antistaphylococcal penicillin or cephalosporin; the addition of rifampin may be helpful in refractory cases. Staphylococcal skin infection may occur as a primary event or as a superinfection complicating other skin disorders. In advanced HIV disease, even relatively minor breaks in skin integrity may result in local infection and bacteremia.

Staphylococcal pyomyositis occurs in approximately 1 in 10,000 patients with HIV infection, generally at an advanced stage of disease [45]. The condition presents with fever and localized painful soft tissue swelling, with the large muscles of the legs most commonly involved. Management consists of surgical drainage and prolonged parenteral antibiotic therapy. Relapsing disease has been described.

Bacillary angiomatosis, a poorly understood but apparently infectious disorder, involves the skin and viscera [46, 47]. The condition generally presents with painless, plaque-like skin lesions that may resemble Kaposi's sarcoma. Visceral involvement manifests as fever, abdominal pain, and progressive hepatic failure. Warthin-Starry stained biopsy specimens show bacilli similar to those seen in cat-scratch fever, and DNA studies indicate that the pathogen is a rickettsia-like organism [20]. Diagnosis of bacillary angiomatosis is made on the basis of clinical presentation and histology. Treatment with erythromycin generally results in prompt resolution of skin lesions. Visceral disease may also respond to antibiotic therapy, although relapses have been reported.

Prevention

Primary prevention of infection with some conventional bacteria may be possible with immunization. The Advisory Committee on Immunization Practices recommends the following immunization protocol for all HIV-infected patients [48, 49]: (1) 23-valent pneumococcal vaccine, (2) *H. influenzae* type b (Hib) conjugate vaccine, and (3) tetanus toxoid, adsorbed (Td).

It would appear that immunization early in the course of HIV disease, while the patient is asymptomatic and has a relatively high CD4 lymphocyte count, is most likely to result in a protective immunologic response. However, some patients will show an antigenic response to immunizations even after development of AIDS [5, 6, 50–53].

Patients should be advised to thoroughly cook eggs, chicken, and meat products in order to prevent infection with *Salmonella*, *Campylobacter*, and *Listeria*; unpasteurized dairy products should be avoided. Patients should also be instructed in the proper cleansing of hands, utensils, and cutting boards for food preparation. The effectiveness of conventional "modified reverse precautions" for hospitalized neutropenic HIV-infected patients is unknown. It is uncertain whether eradication of cutaneous staphylococcal colonization is beneficial in preventing invasive disease [54].

References

1. Drucker E, Webber MP, McMaster P, Vermund SH. Increasing rate of pneumonia hospitalizations in the Bronx: A sentinel indicator for human immunodeficiency virus. *Int J Epidemiol* 18:926–933, 1989.
2. Rolston KVI, Radentz S, Rodriguez S. Bacterial and fungal infections in patients with the acquired immunodeficiency syndrome. *Cancer Detect Prev* 14:377–381, 1990.
3. Witt DJ, Craven DE, McCabe WR. Bacterial infections in adult patients with the acquired immune deficiency syndrome (AIDS) and AIDS-related complex. *Am J Med* 82:900–906, 1987.
4. Nichols L, et al. Bacterial infections in the acquired immune deficiency syndrome: Clinicopathologic correlations in a series of autopsy cases. *Am J Clin Pathol* 92:787–790, 1989.
5. Lane HC, Masur H, Edgar LC, et al. Abnormalities of B-cell activation and immunoregulation in patients with the acquired immunodeficiency syndrome. *N Engl J Med* 309:453–458, 1983.
6. Amman AJ, Schiffman G, Abrams D, et al. B-cell immunodeficiency in acquired immune deficiency syndrome. *JAMA* 251:1447–1449, 1984.
7. Muller F, Rollag H, Froland SS. Reduced oxidative burst responses in monocytes and monocyte-derived macrophages from HIV-infected subjects. *Clin Exp Immunol* 82:10–15, 1990.
8. Barat LM, Craven DE, Steinberg JL, et al. A prospective study of documented fever in patients infected with HIV-1: Diagnosis and outcome in a municipal hospital. Seventh International Conference on AIDS, Florence, June 1991.
9. Murphy PM, Lane HC, Fauci AS, Gallin JI. Impairment of neutrophil bactericidal capacity in patients with AIDS. *J Infect Dis* 158:627–630, 1988.
10. Krumholz HM, Sande MA, Lo B. Community-acquired bacteremia in patients with acquired immunodeficiency syndrome: Clinical presentation, bacteriology, and outcome. *Am J Med* 86:776–779, 1989.
11. Casadevall A, et al. *Hemophilus influenzae* type b bacteremia in adults with AIDS and at risk for AIDS. *Am J Med* 92:587–590, 1992.
12. Raviglione MC, Battan R, Pablos-Mendez A, et al. Infections associated with Hickman catheters in patients with acquired immunodeficiency syndrome. *Am J Med* 86:780–786, 1989.
13. Shaunak S, Bartlett JA. Zidovudine-induced neutropenia: Are we too cautious? *Lancet* 2:91–92, 1989.
14. Kielhofner M, et al. Life-threatening *Pseudomonas aeruginosa* infections in patients with human immunodeficiency virus infection. *Clin Infect Dis* 14:403–411, 1992.
15. Jacobson MA, Gellerman H, Chambers H. *Staphylococcus aureus* bacter-

emia and recurrent staphylococcal infection in patients with acquired immunodeficiency syndrome and AIDS-related complex. *Am J Med* 85:172–176, 1988.

16. Murata GH, Ault MJ, Meyer RD. Community-acquired bacterial pneumonias in homosexual men: Presumptive evidence for a defect in host resistance. *AIDS Res* 1:379–393, 1984–85.

17. Stover DE, White DA, Romano PA, et al. Spectrum of pulmonary diseases associated with the acquired immune deficiency syndrome. *Am J Med* 78:429–437, 1985.

18. Polsky B, Gold JWM, Whimbey E, et al. Bacterial pneumonia in patients with the acquired immunodeficiency syndrome. *Ann Intern Med* 104:38–41, 1986.

19. Magnenat JL, et al. Mode of presentation and diagnosis of bacterial pneumonia in human immunodeficiency virus–infected patients. *Am Rev Respir Dis* 144:917–922, 1991.

20. Zuger A. Bacterial infections in AIDS. *AIDS Clinical Care* 4:9 and 10, 1992.

21. Schuchat A, et al. Use of surveillance for invasive pneumococcal disease to estimate the size of the immunosuppressed HIV-infected population. *JAMA* 265:3275–3279, 1991.

22. Levine SJ, White DA, Fels AOS. The incidence and significance of *Staphylococcus aureus* in respiratory cultures from patients infected with the human immunodeficiency virus. *Am Rev Respir Dis* 141:89–93, 1990.

23. Amorosa JK, Nahass RG, Nosher JL, Gocke DJ. Radiologic distinction of pyogenic pulmonary infection from *Pneumocystis carinii* pneumonia in AIDS patients. *Radiology* 175:721–724, 1990.

24. Murray PA, et al. The microbiology of HIV-associated periodontal lesions. *J Clin Periodontol* 16:636–642, 1989.

25. Rothstein SG, Persky MS, Edelman BA, et al. Epiglottitis in AIDS patients. *Laryngoscope* 99:389–392, 1989.

26. Zurlo JJ, et al. Sinusitis in HIV-1 infection. *Am J Med* 93:157–162, 1992.

27. Godofsky EW, et al. Sinusitis in HIV-infected patients: A clinical and radiologic review. *Am J Med* 93:163–170, 1992.

28. Dryden MS, Shanson DC. The microbial causes of diarrhoea in patients infected with the human immunodeficiency virus. *J Infect* 17:107–114, 1988.

29. René E, Marche C, Regnier B, et al. Intestinal infections in patients with acquired immunodeficiency syndrome: A prospective study in 132 patients. *Dig Dis Sci* 34:773–780, 1989.

30. Antony MA, Brandt LJ, Klein RS, Bernstein LH. Infectious diarrhea in patients with AIDS. *Dig Dis Sci* 33:1141–1146, 1988.

31. Levine WC, Buehler JW, Bean NH, Tauxe RV. Epidemiology of nontyphoidal *Salmonella* bacteremia during the human immunodeficiency virus epidemic. *J Infect Dis* 164:81–87, 1991.

32. Celum CL, Chaisson RE, Rutherford GW, et al. Incidence of salmonellosis in patients with AIDS. *J Infect Dis* 156:998–1002, 1987.

33. Glaser JB, Morton-Kute L, Berger SR, et al. Recurrent *Salmonella typhimurium* bacteremia associated with the acquired immunodeficiency syndrome. *Ann Intern Med* 102:189–193, 1985.

34. Fischl MA, Dickinson GM, Sinave C, et al. *Salmonella* bacteremia as manifestation of acquired immunodeficiency syndrome. *Arch Intern Med* 146:113–115, 1986.

35. Nadelman RB, Mathur-Wagh U, Yancovitz SR, Mildvan D. *Salmonella* bacteremia associated with the acquired immunodeficiency syndrome (AIDS). *Arch Intern Med* 145:1968–1971, 1985.

36. Simor AE, Poon R, Borczyk A. Chronic *Shigella flexneri* infection preceding development of acquired immunodeficiency syndrome. *J Clin Microbiol* 27:353–355, 1989.

37. Blaser MJ, Hale TL, Formal SB. Recurrent shigellosis complicating human immunodeficiency virus infection: Failure of pre-existing antibodies to confer protection. *Am J Med* 86:105–107, 1989.

38. Mandell W, Neu HC. Shigella bacteremia in adults. *JAMA* 255:3116–3117, 1986.

39. Baskin DH, Lax JD, Barenberg D. Shigella bacteremia in patients with the acquired immune deficiency syndrome. *Am J Gastroenterol* 82:338–341, 1987.

40. Sorvillo FJ, Lieb LE, Waterman SH. Incidence of campylobacteriosis among patients with AIDS in Los Angeles County. *J AIDS* 4:598–602, 1991.

41. Perlman DM, Ampel NM, Schifman RB, et al. Persistent *Campylobacter jejuni* infections in patients infected with human immunodeficiency virus (HIV). *Ann Intern Med* 108:540–546, 1988.

42. Bernar E, Roger PM, Carles D, et al. Diarrhea and *Campylobacter* infections in patients infected with the human immunodeficiency virus. *J Infect Dis* 159:143–144, 1989.

43. Scully M, Berger TG. Pruritus, *Staphylococcus aureus*, and human immunodeficiency virus infection. *Arch Dermatol* 126:684–685, 1990.

44. Duvic M. Staphylococcal infections and the pruritus of AIDS-related complex. *Arch Dermatol* 123:1217–1220, 1987.

45. Schwartzman WA, Lambertus MW, Kennedy CA, Goetz MB. Staphylococcal pyomyositis in patients infected by the human immunodeficiency virus. *Am J Med* 90:595–600, 1991.

46. Schlossberg D, Morad Y, Krouse TB, et al. Culture-proved disseminated cat-scratch disease in acquired immunodeficiency syndrome. *Arch Intern Med* 149:1437–1439, 1989.

47. LeBoit PE, Egbert BM, Stoler MH, et al. Epithelioid haemangioma-like vascular proliferation in AIDS: Manifestation of cat scratch disease bacillus infection? *Lancet* 1:960–963, 1988.

48. Advisory Committee on Immunization Practices. Immunization of children infected with human T-lymphotrophic virus type III/lymphadenopathy-associated virus. *MMWR* 35:595–598, 603–606, 1986.

49. ACIP. Pneumococcal polysaccharide vaccine. *MMWR* 38:64–76, 1989.

50. Huang KL, Ruben FL, Rinaldo CR, et al. Antibody responses after influenza and pneumococcal immunization in HIV-infected homosexual men. *JAMA* 257:2047–2050, 1987.

51. Poland GA, et al. Routine immunization of the HIV-positive asymptomatic patient. *J Gen Intern Med* 5:147–150, 1990.

52. Janoff EN, Douglas JM, Jr, Gabriel M, et al. Class-specific antibody response to pneumococcal capsular polysaccharides in men infected with human immunodeficiency virus type 1. *J Infect Dis* 158:983–990, 1988.
53. Rhoads JL, Birx DL, Wright DC, et al. Response to vaccination in HIV sero-positive subjects. Third International Conference on AIDS, Washington, DC, 1987.
54. Ganesh R, Castle D, McGibbon D, et al. Staphylococcal carriage and HIV infection. *Lancet* 2:558, 1989.

26/Kaposi's Sarcoma

Timothy P. Cooley

Kaposi's sarcoma (KS) was first described in 1872 by the Hungarian dermatologist Moritz Kaposi, and before the AIDS epidemic it was a rare tumor [1]. Classic, endemic, acquired, and epidemic forms of KS have been described. The "classic" form presents with multiple violaceous skin nodules on the lower extremities. It predominates in elderly men of Mediterranean or Eastern European background, has an indolent course, and is frequently associated with hematologic malignancies [2, 3]. The "endemic" form of KS, found in children and young men in equatorial Africa, is more virulent than the classic form [4]. "Acquired" KS occurs in patients treated with immunosuppressive drugs, especially those individuals who have received organ transplants [5–7]. "Epidemic" KS associated with HIV infection was first observed among young homosexual men in major urban areas in the United States during the early 1980s [8–15]. Although the histopathology of all forms of KS is virtually identical, the clinical manifestations differ remarkably, with the epidemic form exhibiting a more variable and aggressive course [16, 17].

Pathogenesis

Several recent studies have attempted to elucidate the pathogenesis of epidemic KS. There is increasing evidence to support the presence of an unidentified, sexually transmitted cofactor that may induce KS in conjunction with HIV infection [18–21]. Surveillance data from the Centers for Disease Control (CDC) indicate that rates for KS are highest among those who acquire HIV sexually. Kaposi's sarcoma was four times more common in HIV-infected women with bisexual partners than in those who had partners with other risk behaviors [18]. Friedman-Kien and Alvin [19] reported seven cases of KS in HIV-seronegative homosexual men; the serostatus of six was confirmed by polymerase chain reaction and p24 antigen studies, suggesting that KS in homosexual men may be caused by a sexually transmitted agent other than HIV.

Recent studies at the National Cancer Institute (NCI) have established another possible mechanism for the development of KS. Cultured KS cell lines were shown to produce soluble factors promoting the growth of angiogenic lesions in nude mice that were histologically similar to those of KS but genotypically murine [14, 22]. Further studies demonstrated that cultured KS cells produced high levels of basic fibroblast growth factor and interleukin-1-beta, which are angiogenic factors inducing autocrine and paracrine growth effects [23]. These reports suggest that KS develops as a result of the production of these cytokines in proximity to HIV-infected cells, with the tumor cells later becoming independent through the development of growth factors.

Researchers at the University of California at Los Angeles (UCLA) have suggested that the cytokine interleukin-6 (IL-6) may be an important factor in the development of KS [24]. However, although IL-6 does induce growth of KS cells in culture, this effect is not consistent. Subsequent research at the NCI and UCLA has identified oncostatin M, a cytokine produced by activated CD4 lymphocytes, as an important pathogenic factor [25, 26].

Other investigators believe that HIV may play a more direct role in the development of KS. Two recent studies suggest that the HIV transactivating (tat) gene may be important in the induction of KS [27, 28]. Transgenic mice bearing the tat gene develop KS-like lesions. This occurrence correlates with male gender, suggesting hormonal control, and with the expression of tat in the skin of the animals. However, tat is not expressed by KS itself or by the cell lines derived from KS lesions. Another recent study showed that tat protein release into tissue culture by HIV-infected cells promotes the growth of KS [27]. These reports suggest that tat or a tat-induced factor might be released by HIV-infected cells, promoting activation and growth of target cells involved in the pathogenesis of KS.

Epidemiology

Kaposi's sarcoma is 20,000 times more common in patients with AIDS than in the US general population, and the incidence varies greatly among different HIV transmission groups [18, 29]. Approximately 94 percent of epidemic KS has been diagnosed in homosexual or bisexual men; KS develops in 21 percent of homosexual or bisexual men with AIDS [18]. The disease is seen infrequently in AIDS patients with other risk behaviors, occurring in 6 percent of cases from endemic areas, 4 percent of cases related to blood transfusion, and 3 percent of heterosexual injection drug users [18]. Hemophiliacs and women who acquire HIV infection heterosexually have very small risk (<1%) of developing KS [18].

Overall, KS develops in approximately 15 percent of patients with

AIDS at some point during the course of their disease [18, 30]. Analysis of CDC data shows that the percentage of AIDS patients with KS as an indicator disease has declined by 20 percent per year in homosexual men and by 10 percent per year in other HIV risk groups between 1983 and 1988 [18]. A similar study by the San Francisco Department of Health found that the proportion of AIDS patients in whom KS developed declined from 60 to 20 percent between 1981 and 1987 [30]. This finding does not seem to be an artifact of selective underreporting and may reflect changing patterns of behavior among homosexual men, resulting in reduced exposure to a sexually transmitted infectious agent [18, 30, 31].

Clinical Manifestations

Epidemic KS has a variable clinical course, ranging from minimal disease presenting as an incidental finding to explosive tumor growth resulting in death [16, 17, 32]. The distribution of cutaneous lesions is more widespread than in other forms of the disease [8, 16, 17]. Most patients have multiple painless, nonpruritic subcutaneous tumor nodules that vary in size from several millimeters to several centimeters in diameter [8–15] (see Plates 15 and 16). Lesions are usually hyperpigmented, brownish-red to purplish-black, and nonblanching. Less commonly, patients have plaque-like lesions, particularly on the soles of the feet and thighs [33]. Exophytic tumor masses with breakdown of overlying skin are infrequent but may occur in areas exposed to trauma [33]. Lymphedema, particularly in the face, genitalia, and lower extremities, is seemingly out of proportion to the extent of cutaneous disease [34].

Extracutaneous spread of KS is common. Lymph node involvement is found in up to 30 percent of AIDS-related KS, but is not a poor prognostic sign, as it is in African KS [33–35]. Intraoral KS occurs in approximately one third of patients and is the initial site of disease in about 15 percent [36–40] (see Plate 4). Kaposi's sarcoma of the oral cavity affects the mucosa of the hard and soft palates and, less commonly, the gingiva, tonsillar pillars, and pharynx. Complications include superficial ulceration of palatal lesions and dental displacement or bleeding from gingival lesions. The majority of patients with oral involvement have lesions elsewhere in the gastrointestinal tract [41].

Gastrointestinal involvement, most common in the stomach and duodenum, is found in 40 percent of KS cases at the time of initial diagnosis and in almost 80 percent at autopsy [42–44]. Gastrointestinal KS is more likely if extensive cutaneous disease is present but has been reported in patients without skin involvement [41, 42, 45]. Diagnosis is usually made by endoscopic visualization of typical red, raised, nonulcerated lesions that vary in size from 0.5 to 2.0 cm in diameter [33]. Because lesions tend to be submucosal, only a minority of biopsies are positive [42]. Gastrointestinal KS sometimes appears as smooth round masses protruding into the intestinal lumen [43, 44, 46]. While demonstrable on contrast barium studies, they are rarely seen on computed tomographic scans.

The clinical presentation of pulmonary KS is often nonspecific. Dyspnea and a nonproductive cough are nearly universal; fever is common but in most cases related to a concomitant infection [47–50]. Pulmonary KS may cause severe symptoms, including bronchospasm and progressive respiratory insufficiency [49, 51–53]. The chest x-ray may be normal or show diffuse bilateral infiltrates in an alveolar, interstitial, mixed alveolar-interstitial, or nodular pattern, as well as pleural effusions [50, 51, 54–60] (see Fig. 10-3). The presence of violaceous endobronchial lesions on bronchoscopy is diagnostic of pulmonary KS; transbronchial biopsy may result in significant bleeding, and crush artifact can make identification of typical histologic patterns difficult [50–52, 61, 62]. Bronchoscopy fails to provide evidence of KS in up to 30 percent of patients in whom pulmonary involvement is subsequently confirmed by open lung biopsy or autopsy [50, 52, 61, 62]. The majority of patients with pulmonary KS have extensive cutaneous disease at the time of diagnosis [48, 53, 56, 63, 64].

Diagnosis

A 4- to 6-mm punch biopsy of a skin lesion is usually adequate to establish the diagnosis of KS. Fine-needle aspiration biopsy can also be used to evaluate cutaneous, oral mucosal lesions and lymph nodes [65, 66]. Pathologically, KS is characterized by the proliferation of spindle-shaped cells that form slit-like spaces, which may contain extravasated erythrocytes. Mixed with the spindle cells are fibroblasts, endothelial cells, inflammatory cells, and evidence of neoangiogenesis [8, 67–69].

While diagnosis of cutaneous KS is relatively easy, the detection and documentation of extracutaneous sites of disease can be more difficult. Gastrointestinal and endobronchial lesions can be viewed endoscopically, but biopsies have a low yield [33, 42, 50, 51, 55–60]. Recent data show that KS is frequently thallium avid and that sequential gallium and delayed 3-hour thallium scintigraphy represent a potentially useful noninvasive technique for detecting extracutaneous KS, particularly lymphatic and pulmonary involvement [70–72]. Enhanced thallium uptake with negative gallium uptake occurs in areas of biopsy-proven KS, whereas infection is gallium avid and thallium negative, and lymphoma is both thallium avid and gallium avid [71, 73–76].

Prognosis

Until recently, there was no uniform staging system for KS [77]. Studies have shown that early tumor stage and the absence of systemic symptoms correlate closely with increased survival [32, 78–80]. A history of prior opportunistic infection implies a poor prognosis, with median survival of only 7 months [16, 32, 80]. Another important prognostic factor is the CD4 cell count, with an 85 percent one-year survival rate for patients with a CD4 count greater than $300/mm^3$ compared to a 35 percent one-year survival rate for those with a CD4 count less than $100/mm^3$ [32, 80, 81]. In AIDS patients with KS, mortality may occur as a direct result of tumor progression, but is more often related to other complications of HIV disease [33, 82]. A new staging system proposed by the AIDS Clinical Trials Group is intended to be comprehensive and facilitate the evaluation of treatment [82] (Table 26-1). In addition to extent of tumor and presence of constitutional symptoms, this system incorporates immunologic staging reflected by CD4 count.

Management

The choice of therapy in epidemic KS is problematic given the variable natural history of the disease. With the exception of pulmonary or gastrointestinal involvement, KS is rarely life threatening, and the goals of treatment are usually palliative. There are no data to show that the current systemic agents used in the therapy of AIDS-related KS increase survival [16]. However, treatment may result in significant palliation by decreasing the size of cutaneous lesions, alleviating the discomfort associated with edema and ulcerations, and controlling symptoms associated with mucosal or visceral involvement.

Local Modalities

Small localized lesions can be surgically excised or removed by electrodesiccation and curettage. Topical application of liquid nitrogen has been used successfully to treat localized skin lesions [33]. Individual cutaneous and intraoral lesions can be treated with dilute vinblastine injection, achieving response rates of greater than 90 percent [83, 84]. The complications of intralesional chemotherapy include local pain and skin irritation.

Radiation Therapy

Kaposi's sarcoma is a radiosensitive tumor, with response rates of 50 to 85 percent [85]. Radiation therapy is most effective as a palliative mea-

Table 26-1 Staging system for Kaposi's sarcoma

	Good risk (0) (all of the following)	Poor risk (1) (any of the following)
Tumor (T)	Confined to skin and/or lymph nodes and/or minimal oral disease	Tumor-associated edema or ulceration Extensive oral, GI, or other nonnodal visceral KS
Immune system (I)	CD4 cells $\geq$ 200/mm^3	CD4 cells $<$ 200/mm^3
Systemic illness (S)	No history of opportunistic infection or thrush No "B" symptoms Karnofsky performance status $\geq$ 70%	History of opportunistic infection or thrush "B" symptoms present Karnofsky performance status $<$ 70% Other HIV-related illness (lymphoma, neurologic disease)

Source: Adapted from SE Krown, C Metroka, JC Werntz, AIDS Clinical Trials Group Oncology Committee, Kaposi's sarcoma in the acquired immune deficiency syndrome: A proposal for uniform evaluation, response and staging criteria. *J Clin Oncol* 7:1201–1207, 1989.

sure to relieve localized mass effect and pain, particularly in the lower extremities. Optimal dosing schedules have not been established, but doses of 25 to 30 Gray (Gy) generally produce tumor regression [85, 86]. A single fraction of 8 Gy appears to give equivalent results to more prolonged fractionation schedules [87]. Acute radiation toxicity, including mucositis, desquamation, and hyperpigmentation, is often disproportionate to the amount of radiation delivered. Local toxicity in the treatment of oropharyngeal lesions can be so severe that many authorities consider radiation therapy to be a measure of last resort [86, 88, 89].

Interferon

Initial studies of alpha-interferon revealed a clear dose response of tumor regression, with high doses ($>$20 million units) resulting in objective response rates of 10 to 40 percent [90]. Response to interferon correlated with preservation of immune function; nonresponders had a history of previous opportunistic infection and significant constitutional symptoms. Patients with cutaneous KS but no history of opportunistic infection or systemic symptoms have shown tumor response rates of 30 to 50 percent [90, 91]. Common side effects of alpha-interferon include a flu-like syndrome with fevers, chills, and malaise; dose reduction is required in up to one third of patients because of chronic fatigue, malaise, and neutropenia [90].

Alpha-interferon has been shown to have antiviral effects in vitro and in vivo [92, 93]. While zidovudine (ZDV) alone has been shown to have no effect on KS, recent clinical studies have confirmed the in vitro synergistic antiviral and antitumor effects of combined therapy with alpha-interferon and ZDV [94–101]. As with earlier studies, the major dose-limiting toxicity is neutropenia. Fibroblast beta-interferon, which has a substantially higher maximum tolerated dose and less hematologic toxicity than alpha-interferon, has no significant antitumor effect in patients with advanced KS [102].

In an effort to improve the hematologic tolerance of the alpha-interferon/ZDV combination, Krown and associates [103] treated five patients with KS in a phase I trial using recombinant granulocyte/macrophage colony stimulating factor (GM-CSF). All required a reduction in GM-CSF dose because of leukocytosis; no reductions in interferon or ZDV doses were required. A recent phase II study using ZDV, alpha-interferon, and GM-CSF showed significant antitumor response in 50 percent of patients with minimal toxicity [104].

Chemotherapy

Active chemotherapeutic agents for the treatment of KS include doxorubicin, vinblastine, vincristine, bleomycin, and etoposide (VP-16). In general, single-agent therapy has been used in early disease and combination therapy in advanced disease, with response rates varying from 25 to 85 percent [16]. Recent studies using combinations of doxorubicin, bleomycin, and vinblastine or vincristine have shown response rates of 66 to 86 percent [105, 106].

Standard doses of cytotoxic chemotherapy in the treatment of advanced KS are associated with severe myelosuppression and frequent development of opportunistic infections [107]. Contrary to earlier experience with high-dose chemotherapy, the use of marrow-sparing agents, such as vincristine and bleomycin, in combination with low doses of myelosuppressive drugs often results in clinical and functional improvement in patients with aggressive cutaneous or visceral disease. The most effective regimen appears to be ABV (adriamycin at doses of 10–20 mg/m^2, bleomycin, and vincristine), with reported response rates of 45 to 88 percent and a median survival of 9 months [108, 109]. In a recent series of patients with symptomatic pulmonary KS, an overall response rate to ABV of 80 percent was reported [47]. Significant myelosuppression occurs in 40 to 50 percent of patients, with a 30 percent incidence of opportunistic infections when *Pneumocystis carinii* pneumonia prophylaxis is used [109]. Preliminary results from ongoing studies using ABV with ZDV and ABV/ZDV with GM-CSF show improved response rates compared to ABV alone, with acceptable toxicity (unpublished data, AIDS Clinical Trials Group). Planned studies will evaluate ABV in combination with didanosine (ddI) or dideoxycytidine (ddC).

References

1. Albini A, Mitchell CD, Thompson EW, et al. Invasive activity and chemotactic response to growth factors by Kaposi's sarcoma cells. *J Cell Biochem* 36:369–376, 1988.
2. Auerbach HE, Brooks JJ. Kaposi's sarcoma: Observation and a hypothesis. *Lab Invest* 52:44–46, 1985.
3. Beakstead JH, Wood GS, Fletcher V. Evidence of the origin of Kaposi's sarcoma from lymphatic endothelium. *Am J Pathol* 119:294–299, 1985.
4. Brooks JJ. Kaposi's sarcoma: A reversible hyperplasia. *Lancet* 2:1309–1311, 1986.
5. Burgess WH, Maciag T. The heparin binding (fibroblast) growth factor family of proteins. *Annu Rev Biochem* 58:575–606, 1989.
6. Bussolino F, Wang JM, Delfilippi P, et al. Granulocyte and granulocyte-macrophage colony stimulating factors induce human endothelial cells to migrate and proliferate. *Nature* 337:471–473, 1989.
7. Clark SC, Kamen R. The human hematopoietic colony stimulating factors. *Science* 236:1229–1236, 1987.
8. Friedman-Kien AE. Disseminated Kaposi's sarcoma syndrome in young homosexual men. *J Am Acad Dermatol* 5:468–471, 1981.
9. Centers for Disease Control. Kaposi's sarcoma and pneumocystis pneumonia among homosexual men: New York City and California. *MMWR* 30:305–308, 1981.
10. Hymes KB, Cheung TL, Green JB, et al. Kaposi's sarcoma in homosexual men: A report of eight cases. *Lancet* 2:598, 1981.
11. Friedman-Kien AE, Laubenstein LJ, Rubinstein P, et al. Disseminated Kaposi's sarcoma in homosexual men. *Ann Intern Med* 96:693–700, 1982.
12. Marmor M, Laubenstein L, William DC, et al. Risk factors for Kaposi's sarcoma in homosexual men. *Lancet* 1:1084–1086, 1982.
13. Jaffe HW, Keewhan C, Thomas PA, et al. National case control study of Kaposi's sarcoma and *Pneumocystis carinii* pneumonia in homosexual men: Part 1, epidemiologic results. *Ann Intern Med* 99:145–151, 1983.
14. Drew WL, Miner RC, Ziegler JL, et al. Cytomegalovirus and Kaposi's sarcoma in young homosexual men. *Lancet* 2:125–127, 1982.
15. Urmacher C, Myskowski P, Ochoa M, Jr, et al. Outbreak of Kaposi's sarcoma in young homosexual men. *Am J Med* 72:69–75, 1982.
16. Krigel RL, Friedman-Kien AE. Kaposi's Sarcoma. In VT DeVita, S. Hellman, SA Rosenberg (eds), *AIDS: Etiology, Diagnosis, Treatment and Prevention.* Philadelphia: Lippincott, 1988. Pp 245–261.
17. Krown SE. AIDS-associated Kaposi's sarcoma: Pathogenesis, clinical course and treatment. *AIDS* 2:71–80, 1988.

18. Beral V, Peterman TA, Berkelman RL, Jaffe HW. Kaposi's sarcoma among patients with AIDS: A sexually transmitted infection? *Lancet* 335:123–128, 1990.
19. Friedman-Kien AE, Alvin E. Kaposi's sarcoma in HIV-1 seronegative homosexual men (abstract). Sixth International Conference on AIDS, San Francisco, June 1990.
20. Archibald CP, Schechter MT, Craig KJP, et al. Evidence for a sexually transmitted cofactor for Kaposi's sarcoma in a cohort of homosexual men (abstract). Sixth International Conference on AIDS, San Francisco, June 1990.
21. Jacobson LP, Munoz A, Dudlet J, et al. Examination of timing of potential Kaposi's sarcoma cofactor relative to HIV-1 infection (abstract). Sixth International Conference on AIDS, San Francisco, June 1990.
22. Drew WL, Mills J, Levy J, et al. Cytomegalovirus infection and abnormal T lymphocyte subset ratios in homosexual men. *Ann Intern Med* 103:61, 1985.
23. Ensoli B, Nakamura S, Salahuddin SZ, et al. AIDS-Kaposi's sarcoma–derived cells express cytokines with autocrine and paracrine growth effects. *Science* 243:223, 1989.
24. Miles SA, Nezair AR, Salazar-Gonzalez JF, et al. AIDS Kaposi sarcoma-derived cells produce and respond to interleukin 6. *Proc Natl Acad Sci USA* 87:4068–4072, 1990.
25. Nair BC, DeVico AL, Nakamura S, et al. Identification of a major growth factor for AIDS-Kaposi's sarcoma cells as Oncostatin M. *Science* 255:1430–1432, 1992.
26. Miles SA, Martinez-Maza O, Rezai A, et al. Oncostatin M as a potent mitogen for AIDS-Kaposi's sarcoma-derived cells. *Science* 255:1432–1434, 1992.
27. Ensoli B, Barillari G, Salahuddin SZ, et al. *Tat* protein of HIV-1 stimulates growth of cells derived from Kaposi's sarcoma lesions of AIDS patients. *Nature* 345:84–86, 1990.
28. Vogel J, Hinrichs SH, Reynolds RK, et al. The HIV *tat* gene induces dermal lesions resembling Kaposi's sarcoma in transgenic mice. *Nature* 335:606–611, 1988.
29. Des Jarlais DC, Marmor M, Thomas O, et al. Kaposi's sarcoma among four different AIDS risk groups. *N Engl J Med* 310:1119, 1984.
30. Rutherford GW, Schwarz SK, Lemp GF, et al. The epidemiology of AIDS-related Kaposi's sarcoma in San Francisco. *J Infect Dis* 159:569–572, 1989.
31. Polk BF, Munoz A, Fox R, et al. Decline of Kaposi's sarcoma (KS) among participants in MACS (abstract). Fourth International Conference on AIDS, Stockholm, June 1988.
32. Mitsuyasu RT, Taylor JMG, Glaspy J, Fahey JL. Heterogeneity of epidemic Kaposi's sarcoma: Implications for therapy. *Cancer* 57:1657–1661, 1986.
33. Heyer DM, Kahn JO, Volberding PA. HIV Related Kaposi's Sarcoma. In PT Cohen, MA Sande, PA Volberding (eds), *The AIDS Knowledge Base.*

Waltham, MA: The Medical Publishing Group, 1990. Pp 7.1.3.1–
7.1.3.19.

34. Volberding P. Therapy of Kaposi's sarcoma in AIDS. *Semin Oncol* 11:60–
67, 1984.

35. Moskowitz LB, Hensley TG, Gould EW, Weiss SD. Frequency and ana-
tomic distribution of lymphadenopathic Kaposi's sarcoma in the
acquired immunodeficiency syndrome: An autopsy series. *Hum Pathol*
16:447–456, 1985.

36. Lozada F, Silverman S, Migliorate C, et al. Oral manifestations of tumor
and opportunistic infections in the epidemic of acquired immune deficiency syndrome. *Cancer* 45:4646–4648, 1985.

37. Green T, Beckstead J, Lozada-Nur F, et al. Histopathologic spectrum of
oral Kaposi's sarcoma. *Oral Surg* 58:306–314, 1984.

38. Sooy CD. Otolaryngologic manifestations of acquired immunodeficiency syndrome. *West J Med* 141:674, 1984.

39. Gnepp DR, Chandler W, Hyams V. Primary Kaposi's sarcoma of the
head and neck. *Ann Intern Med* 100:107–114, 1984.

40. Keeney K, Abaza NA, Tidwel O, Quinn P. Oral Kaposi's sarcoma in
acquired immune deficiency syndrome. *J Oral Maxillofac Surg* 45:815–
821, 1987.

41. Saltz RK, Kurtz RC, Lightdale CJ, et al. Kaposi's sarcoma. Gastrointestinal
involvement correlation with skin findings and immunologic function.
Dig Dis Sci 29:817–823, 1984.

42. Friedman SL, Wright TL, Altman DF. Gastrointestinal Kaposi's sarcoma
in patients with the acquired immune deficiency syndrome: Endoscopic
and autopsy findings. *Gastroenterology* 890:102–108, 1985.

43. Rose HS, Balthazar EJ, Megibow AJ, et al. Alimentary tract involvement
in Kaposi's sarcoma: Radiographic and endoscopic findings in 25 homosexual men. *Am J Radiol* 139:661–666, 1982.

44. Frager DH, Frager JD, Brandt LJ, et al. Gastrointestinal complications of
AIDS: Radiologic features. *Radiology* 158:597–603, 1986.

45. Barrison IG, Foster S, Harris JW, et al. Upper gastrointestinal Kaposi's sarcoma in patients positive for HIV antibody without cutaneous disease.
Br Med J 296:92–93, 1988.

46. Moon KL, Federle MP, Abrams DI, et al. Kaposi's sarcoma and lymphadenopathy syndrome: Limitations of abdominal CT in acquired immunodeficiency syndrome. *Radiology* 150:479–483, 1984.

47. Gill PS, Alcil B, Colletti P, et al. Pulmonary Kaposi's sarcoma: Clinical
findings and results of therapy. *Am J Med* 87:57–61, 1989.

48. Garay SM, Belenko M, Fazzini E, Schinella R. Pulmonary manifestations
of Kaposi's sarcoma. *Chest* 91:39–43, 1987.

49. Ognibene FP, Steis RG, Macher AM, et al. Kaposi's sarcoma causing pulmonary infiltrates and respiratory failure in the acquired immunodeficiency syndrome. *Ann Intern Med* 102:471–475, 1985.

50. Meduri GU, Stover DE, Lee M, et al. Pulmonary Kaposi's sarcoma in the
acquired immune deficiency syndrome. *Am J Med* 81:11–18, 1986.

51. Kaplan LC, Hopewell PC, Jaffe H, et al. Kaposi's sarcoma involving the

lung in patients with the acquired immune deficiency syndrome. *J AIDS* 1:23–30, 1988.

52. Pitchenik AF, Fischl MA, Saldana MJ. Kaposi's sarcoma of the tracheobronchial tree: Clinical, bronchoscopic and pathologic features. *Chest* 87:122–124, 1985.

53. Kornfeld H, Axelrod JL. Pulmonary presentation of Kaposi's sarcoma in a homosexual patient. *Am Rev Respir Dis* 127:248–249, 1983.

54. Case Records of the Massachusetts General Hospital (Case 1-1990). *N Engl J Med* 322:43–51, 1990.

55. Nyberg DA, Federle MP. AIDS-related Kaposi's sarcoma and lymphoma. *Semin Roentgenol* 22:54–65, 1987.

56. Davis SD, Henschke CI, Chamides BK, Westcott JL. Intrathoracic Kaposi's sarcoma in AIDS patients: Radiographic-pathologic correlation. *Radiology* 163:495–500, 1987.

57. Naidich DP, Tarras M, Garay SM, et al. Kaposi's sarcoma: CT-radiographic correlation. *Chest* 96:723–728, 1989.

58. Sivit CJ, Schwartz AM, Rockoff SD. Kaposi's sarcoma of the lung in AIDS: Radiologic-pathologic analysis. *Am J Radiol* 148:25–28, 1987.

59. Ognibene FP, Shelhamer JH. Kaposi's sarcoma. *Clin Chest Med* 9:459–465, 1988.

60. Kramer EL, Sanger JJ, Garay SM, et al. Gallium scans of the chest in patients with AIDS. *J Nucl Med* 28:1107–1114, 1987.

61. Hanson PJV, Hancourt-Webster JN, Grazzard BG, Collins JV. Fibroscopic bronchoscopy in the diagnosis of pulmonary Kaposi's sarcoma. *Thorax* 42:269–271, 1987.

62. Lau KY, Rubin A, Littner M, Krauthammer M. Kaposi's sarcoma of the tracheobronchial tree: Clinical, bronchoscopic and pathologic features. *Chest* 89:158–159, 1986.

63. Niedt GW, Schinella RA. Acquired immunodeficiency syndrome: Clinico-pathologic study of 56 autopsies. *Arch Pathol Lab Med* 109:727–734, 1985.

64. Bach MC, Bagwell SP, Fanning JP. Primary pulmonary Kaposi's sarcoma in the acquired immunodeficiency syndrome: A cause of persistent pyrexia. *Am J Med* 85:274–275, 1988.

65. Bottles K, McPhaul LW, Volberding P. Fine-needle aspiration biopsy of patients with acquired immunodeficiency syndrome (AIDS): Experience in an outpatient clinic. *Ann Intern Med* 108:42–45, 1988.

66. Hales M, Bottles K, Miller T, et al. Diagnosis of Kaposi's sarcoma by fine-needle aspiration biopsy. *Am J Clin Pathol* 88:20–25, 1987.

67. Reynolds WA, Winkleman RK, Soule EH. Kaposi's sarcoma: A clinico-pathologic study with particular reference to its relationship to the reticuloendothelial system. *Medicine* 44:419–433, 1965.

68. Gottlieb GJ, Ackerman AB. Kaposi's sarcoma: An extensively disseminated form in young homosexual men. *Hum Pathol* 13:882–892, 1982.

69. McNutt NS, Fletcher V, Conant MA. Early lesions of Kaposi's sarcoma in homosexual men: An ultrastructural comparison with other vascular proliferations in skin. *Am J Pathol* 111:62–77, 1983.

70. Lee VW, Rosen MP, Baum A, et al. AIDS-related Kaposi's sarcoma: Findings on thallium-2021 scintigraphy. *Am J Radiol* 151:1233–1235, 1988.

71. Lee VW, Fuller JD, O'Brien MJ, et al. Pulmonary Kaposi sarcoma in patients with AIDS: Scintigraphic diagnosis with sequential thallium and gallium scanning. *Radiology* 180:409–412, 1991.

72. Lee VW, Chen H, Panageas E, et al. Subcutaneous Kaposi's sarcoma: Thallium scan demonstration. *Clin Nucl Med* 15:569–571, 1990.

73. Salvotore M, Canatu L, Porta E. T1-201 as a positive indicator for lung neoplasm: Preliminary experience. *Radiology* 121:487–488, 1976.

74. Tonami N, Shuke N, Yokoyama K, et al. Thallium 201: SPECT in evaluation of suspected lung cancer. *J Nucl Med* 30:997–1004, 1981.

75. Waxman AD, Ramanna L, Said J. Thallium scintigraphy in lymphoma: Relationship to gallium-67 (abstract). *J Nucl Med* 30:915, 1989.

76. Hamada S, Nishimura T, Hayashida K, Uchara T. Intracardiac malignant lymphoma detected by gallium-67 and thallium-201 chloride. *J Nucl Med* 29:1868–1870, 1988.

77. Volberding PA. Moving towards a uniform staging for human immuno-deficiency virus–associated Kaposi's sarcoma. *J Clin Oncol* 7:1184–1185, 1989.

78. Krigel RL, Laubenstein LJ, Muggia FM. Kaposi's sarcoma: A new staging classification. *Cancer Treat Rep* 67:531–534, 1983.

79. Mitsuyasu, RT, Groopman JE. Biology and therapy of Kaposi's sarcoma. *Semin Oncol* 11:53–59, 1984.

80. Mituyasu RT. Clinical variants and staging of Kaposi's sarcoma. *Semin Oncol* 14 (suppl 3):13–18, 1987.

81. Taylor J, Afrasiabi R, Fahey JL, et al. Prognostically significant classification of immune changes in AIDS with Kaposi's sarcoma. *Blood* 67:666–671, 1986.

82. Krown SE, Metroka C, Werntz JC, AIDS Clinical Trials Group Oncology Committee. Kaposi's sarcoma in the acquired immune deficiency syndrome: A proposal for uniform evaluation, response and staging criteria. *J Clin Oncol* 7:1201–1207, 1989.

83. Conant MA, Galzagorry G, Illeman M. Intralesional vinblastine (Velban) treatment of lesions of Kaposi's sarcoma (abstract). Fifth International Conference on AIDS, Montreal, June 1989.

84. Epstein J, Lozade-Nur F, McLeod WA, et al. Oral Kaposi's sarcoma in AIDS: Management with intralesional chemotherapy (abstract). Fifth International Conference on AIDS, Montreal, June 1989.

85. Chak LK, Gill PS, Levine AM, et al. Radiation therapy for acquired immunodeficiency syndrome–related Kaposi's sarcoma. *J Clin Oncol* 6:863–867, 1988.

86. Harris JW, Reed TA. Kaposi's Sarcoma in AIDS: The Role of Radiation Therapy. In JM Veath (ed), *Frontiers of Radiation Therapy and Oncology*. Basel: Karger, 1985. Pp 126–132.

87. Quivey JM, Wara WM, Berson AM. Radiotherapy for the treatment of AIDS-related Kaposi's sarcoma: An updated analysis (abstract). Sixth International Conference on AIDS, San Francisco, June 1990.

88. Epstein JB, Lozada-Nur F, McLeod A, Spinelli J. Oral Kaposi's sarcoma in acquired immunodeficiency syndrome. *Cancer* 64:2424–2430, 1989.
89. Cooper JS, Fried PR, Laubenstein LJ. Initial observations of the effect of radiotherapy on epidemic Kaposi's sarcoma. *JAMA* 252:934–935, 1984.
90. Krown SE. The role of interferon in the therapy of epidemic Kaposi's sarcoma. *Semin Oncol* 14 (suppl 3):27–33, 1987.
91. Groopman JE, Scadden DT. Interferon therapy for Kaposi's sarcoma associated with the acquired immunodeficiency syndrome (AIDS). *Ann Intern Med* 110:335–337, 1989.
92. Ho DD, Hartshorn KL, Rota TR, et al. Recombinant human interferon alpha-A suppresses HTLV-III replication in-vitro. *Lancet* 1:602–604, 1985.
93. Lane HC, Kovacs JA, Feinberg J, et al. Antiretroviral effects of interferon-alpha in AIDS-associated Kaposi's sarcoma. *Lancet* 2:1218–1222, 1988.
94. Hartshorn KL, Vogt MW, Chou TC, et al. Synergistic inhibition of human immunodeficiency virus in vitro by azidothymidine and recombinant alpha A interferon. *Antimicrob Agents Chemother* 31:168–172, 1987.
95. de Wit R, Reiss P, Bakker RJM, et al. Lack of activity of zidovudine in AIDS-associated Kaposi's sarcoma. *AIDS* 3:847–850, 1989.
96. Lane CH, Fallon T, Walker RE, et al. Zidovudine in patients with human immunodeficiency virus (HIV) infection and Kaposi's sarcoma. *Ann Intern Med* 111:41–50, 1989.
97. Krown SE, Gold TWM, Niedzwieck D, et al. Interferon-alpha with zidovudine: Safety, tolerance and clinical and virologic effects in patients with Kaposi's sarcoma associated with the acquired immunodeficiency syndrome (AIDS). *Ann Intern Med* 112:812–821, 1990.
98. Fischl MA. Antiretroviral therapy in combination with interferon for AIDS-related Kaposi's sarcoma. *Am J Med* 90 (suppl 4A):2S–8S, 1991.
99. Fischl M, Reese J, Dearmas L, et al. Phase I study of interferon-alpha and AZT in patients with AIDS-related Kaposi's sarcoma (abstract). Fourth International Conference on AIDS, Stockholm, June 1988.
100. Krown S, Bundow D, Gansbacher B, et al. Interferon-alpha plus zidovudine: A phase I trial in AIDS-associated Kaposi's sarcoma (KS) (abstract). Fourth International Conference on AIDS, Stockholm, June 1988.
101. Kovacs JA, Deyton L, Davey R, et al. Combined zidovudine and interferon-alpha therapy in patients with Kaposi's sarcoma and the acquired immunodeficiency syndrome (AIDS). *Ann Intern Med* 111:280–287, 1989.
102. Miles SA, Wang H, Cortes J, et al. Beta-interferon therapy in patients with poor-prognosis Kaposi's sarcoma related to the acquired immunodeficiency syndrome (AIDS). *Ann Intern Med* 112:582–589, 1990.
103. Krown SE, Paredes J, Bundown D, Flomenbert N. Combination therapy with interferon alpha (IFN-a), zidovudine (AZT, and recombinant granulocyte-macrophage colony-stimulating factor (GM-CSF): A phase I trial in patients with AIDS-associated Kaposi's sarcoma (abstract). Sixth International Conference on AIDS, San Francisco, June 1990.
104. Scadden DT, Bering HA, Levine JD, et al. Granulocyte-macrophage col-

ony-stimulating factor mitigates the neutropenia of combined interferon alpha and zidovudine treatment of acquired immunodeficiency syndrome–associated Kaposi's sarcoma. *J Clin Oncol* 9:802–808, 1991.

105. Gill PS, Deyton L, Rarick M, et al. Results of a prospective trial of adriamycin, bleomycin and vincristine in the treatment of epidemic Kaposi's sarcoma. *Proc Am Soc Oncol* 6:5, 1987.

106. Gelmann EP, Longo D, Lance HC, et al. Combination chemotherapy of disseminated Kaposi's sarcoma in patients with the acquired immunodeficiency syndrome. *Am J Med* 82:456–462, 1987.

107. Laubenstein LJ, Krigel RL, Odajnyk CM, et al. Treatment of Kaposi's sarcoma with etoposide or combination of doxorubicin, bleomycin, and vinblastine. *J Clin Oncol* 2:1115–1120, 1984.

108. Gill PS, Rarick M, McCutchan JA, et al. Systemic treatment of AIDS-related Kaposi's sarcoma: Results of a randomized trial. *Am J Med* 90:427–433, 1991.

109. Gill PS, Rarick MU, Espira B, et al. Advanced acquired immunodeficiency syndrome–related Kaposi's sarcoma: Results of pilot studies using combination chemotherapy. *Cancer* 65:1074–1079, 1990.

27/AIDS-Related Lymphoma

Timothy P. Cooley

In 1985, the Centers for Disease Control included systemic high-grade, B-cell, non-Hodgkin's lymphoma (NHL) in HIV-infected patients as a criterion for the diagnosis of AIDS [1]. Currently, NHL develops in about 5 percent of AIDS patients during the course of their disease, generally as a late manifestation [2–4]. It is anticipated that the incidence of lymphoma in this population will continue to rise as HIV-infected patients live longer [3, 4]. Recent clinical data suggest that patients with symptomatic HIV infection who survive for 3 years on antiretroviral therapy have a high probability of developing NHL [3].

Pathogenesis

Non-Hodgkin's lymphoma has been frequently observed in association with abnormal cell-mediated immunity, such as that occurring with immunosuppressive therapy related to organ transplantation [5, 6]. Circumstantial evidence supports a role for Epstein-Barr virus (EBV) in the etiology of NHL in this setting [7]. Unlike transplant-associated lymphoma but similar to non-African Burkitt's lymphoma, EBV genomes are found in a minority of cases of HIV-related NHL [8].

Although the pathogenesis of HIV-related NHL remains unclear, some of its molecular characteristics have been identified. A wide spectrum of both monoclonal and polyclonal lymphomas have been described in patients with AIDS, similar to lymphomas arising in patients with transplant-associated immunodeficiency [9]. Early data on HIV-related NHL found a high frequency of c-myc translocations, raising speculation that chromosomal translocation with resultant oncogene activation may play a role in the pathogenesis of NHL [10]. However, more recent studies report a high frequency of polyclonal lymphomas with no evidence for c-myc translocation [10]. It is currently hypothesized that AIDS-related NHL may appear as a result of chronic viral antigenic and mitogenic stimulation leading to B-cell overproliferation [10–12].

Epidemiology

Since the beginning of the HIV epidemic, epidemiologic studies have demonstrated an increased frequency of NHL in a population at high risk for HIV infection: never-married men, aged 25 to 54 years, who live in neighborhoods with high AIDS-related mortality [13]. No such increase has been identified among men who have married or in women regardless of marital status. Although never-married men include some heterosexuals, it is assumed that most homosexual men at risk for HIV infection would be in this category.

While the majority of cases of NHL in North America have been reported in homosexual or bisexual men, the disease may occur in patients with any risk behavior [14]. Series from the University of Southern California (USC) and the University of California at San Francisco (UCSF) reported that greater than 90 percent of their patients with NHL were male homosexuals [2, 15, 16]. In contrast, a report from New York University indicated that 19 percent of their cases of lymphoma occurred in patients with a history of injection drug use [17]. In Italy, 64 percent of patients with HIV-related NHL have a history of injection drug use [18]. Lymphoma has also affected hemophiliacs, with a 24-fold increase in incidence compared to expected rates [19].

Clinical Manifestations

The majority of patients with HIV-related NHL have high-grade, B-cell lymphomas of either B-immunoblastic or small noncleaved type, which may be Burkitt or non-Burkitt variants [15, 20–23]. This pathologic spectrum is most unusual when compared to previous series of lymphomas before the AIDS epidemic, in which only 4 to 9 percent were of the B-immunoblastic type and 5 to 7 percent were of the small noncleaved type [23, 24].

Nearly all patients with HIV-related NHL present with widespread disease, and 75 percent report constitutional symptoms [14]. The most characteristic clinical feature is the high frequency of extranodal disease, which is found in up to 85 percent of cases, compared to a 40 percent incidence in NHL not associated with HIV infection [2, 5, 6, 16–18, 25–31]. Common sites of involvement include bone marrow (25%), central nervous system (CNS; 32%), gastrointestinal tract (26%), liver (12%), and kidney (9%) [16, 17, 25–30]. Unusual sites of extranodal disease, such as the myocardium and popliteal fossa, have also been reported [13, 20]. Although primary CNS lymphoma accounts for up to 25 percent of HIV-related NHL, metastatic brain involvement is unusual in patients with systemic lymphoma [32–34].

Diagnosis

Diagnosis is made by excisional lymph node biopsy or biopsy of an involved extranodal site. Routine staging should also include computed tomography (CT) scanning of the head, chest, abdomen and pelvis; gallium scan; lumbar puncture with cytologic analysis of cerebrospinal fluid; and bone marrow examination. Gastrointestinal symptoms should be investigated endoscopically.

Prognosis

In a review of patients followed at USC, shortened survival was associated with a Karnofsky performance status of less than 70 percent, a diagnosis of AIDS before the appearance of NHL, and lymphomatous involvement of bone marrow [29]. The poor prognosis group had a median survival of 4 months, compared to 11 months in the group without these features. A similar analysis performed at UCSF showed that total CD4 count was the most important predictor of survival, with patients who had counts of less than $100/mm^3$ having a median survival of 4.5 months, compared to 24 months in patients with counts greater than $100/mm^3$ [2]. Negative predictors of survival also included a Karnofsky performance status of less than 70 percent and the presence of extranodal disease [2].

Management

Although aggressive combination chemotherapy for high-grade NHL not associated with HIV infection is highly effective, chemotherapy for AIDS-related NHL has been less successful, with complete response rates of only 33 to 60 percent and an overall median survival of 5 to 7 months [17, 25]. Treatment is frequently complicated by opportunistic infections and severe hematologic toxicity. A recent AIDS Clinical Trials Group (ACTG) study using low-dose m-BACOD (methotrexate, bleomycin, doxorubicin, cyclophosphamide, vincristine, and dexamethasone) with CNS prophylaxis and zidovudine (ZDV) maintenance demonstrated a 46 percent complete response rate [35]. A phase I pilot study using adjunctive granulocyte/macrophage colony stimulating factor (GM-CSF) showed that standard doses of m-BACOD could be given with acceptable toxicity [36]. A large-scale ACTG trial is now under way comparing low-dose m-BACOD to standard-dose therapy with GM-CSF.

A randomized trial of CHOP (cyclophosphamide, doxorubicin, vincristine, and prednisone) with or without GM-CSF in 30 patients demonstrated that the severity and duration of neutropenia associated with chemotherapy was significantly reduced in patients who had received GM-CSF [37]. However, in patients receiving GM-CSF, median p24 antigen levels more than doubled from baseline, suggesting stimulation of HIV replication. The overall complete response rate was 67 percent in both groups. Allogeneic bone marrow transplantation with ZDV has been attempted in one patient with AIDS-related NHL, and, although the patient died of tumor relapse 47 days after transplant, analysis of autopsy tissue showed no evidence of HIV by either culture or polymerase chain reaction [38]. Immunologic monitoring showed loss of HIV antibody, suggesting that HIV-infected recipient cells may have been eradicated by ablative chemoradiotherapy and that ZDV may have prevented the establishment of HIV infection in donor cells.

Primary Central Nervous System Lymphoma

Primary CNS lymphoma accounts for up to 25 percent of cases of HIV-related NHL [21, 32, 33, 34, 39]. The prognosis is extremely poor, with a median survival of less than one month from the time the patient first seeks medical attention [32, 33]. The most common symptoms are headache, seizures, cranial nerve palsies, and hemiparesis [32, 33]. However, subtle personality changes and altered mental status may be the only findings on presentation [32].

The clinical and radiologic manifestations of primary CNS lymphoma may be indistinguishable from those of CNS toxoplasmosis [32–34]. On CT and MRI scans, lymphomas appear as isodense or hyperdense space-occupying lesions showing contrast enhancement [33, 40] (see Fig. 15-4). In contrast to CNS toxoplasmosis, lymphomas generally appear as solitary lesions larger than 3 cm involving the cerebrum, cerebellum, basal ganglion, or pons, with varying degrees of edema and mass effect [33, 40]. Definitive diagnosis requires brain biopsy [40]. Pathologic findings are identical to those described in systemic AIDS-related lymphoma [32]. Standard therapy, which consists of whole-brain irradiation with 30 to 35 Gray (Gy) and a 10-Gy boost to the primary lesion, does not appear to improve survival [32, 33].

Hodgkin's Disease

Hodgkin's disease (HD), particularly the mixed cellularity subtype, continues to be reported in patients with HIV infection, with an increased incidence found in homosexual men [41–46]. Hodgkin's disease in

HIV-infected patients is more aggressive than in the general population, usually presenting as stage III or IV disease [41, 47]. The more advanced stage is largely due to the high incidence of bone marrow involvement, which is present at initial diagnosis in 48 percent of HIV-infected patients with HD, compared to 3.5 percent of historical controls [47]. As in HIV-related NHL, other sites of extranodal disease are also common [47]. HIV-related HD is associated with a poor prognosis despite therapy with standard chemotherapeutic regimes such as MOPP (nitrogen mustard, vincristine, procarbazine, and prednisone) or ABVD (doxorubicin, bleomycin, vincristine, and dexamethasone) [47]. The survival rate of historical controls, 80 percent at 9 years, contrasts sharply with the one-year survival rate of 30 percent in HIV-related HD [47, 48]. Poor prognosis appears more closely related to the development of opportunistic infections and profound myelosuppression than to uncontrolled HD [47].

References

1. Centers for Disease Control. Revision of the case definition of acquired immunodeficiency syndrome for national reporting: United States. *Ann Intern Med* 103:402–403, 1985.
2. Kaplan LD, Abrams DI, Feigal E, et al. AIDS associated non-Hodgkin's lymphoma in San Francisco. *JAMA* 261:719–724, 1989.
3. Pluda JM, et al. Development of non-Hodgkin's lymphoma in a cohort of patients with severe human immunodeficiency (HIV) infection on long-term antiretroviral therapy. *Ann Intern Med* 113:276–282, 1990.
4. Moore RD, Kessler, H, Richman DD, et al. Non-Hodgkin's lymphoma in patients with advanced HIV infection treated with zidovudine (abstract). Seventh International Conference on AIDS, Florence, June 1991.
5. Hoover R, Fraumeni JF. Risk of cancer in renal transplant patients. *Lancet* 2:55–57, 1973.
6. Frizzera G, Rosai J, Delner LP, et al. Lymphoreticular disorders in primary immunodeficiencies: New finding based on an up-to-date histologic classification of 35 cases. *Cancer* 46:692–699, 1980.
7. Hanto DW, Frizzera G, Purtilo DT, et al. Clinical spectrum of lymphoproliferative disorders in renal transplant recipients and evidence for the role of Epstein Barr virus. *Cancer Res* 41:4253–4261, 1981.
8. Subar M, Neri A, Inghirami G, et al. Frequent c-myc oncogene activation and infrequent presence of Epstein-Barr virus genome in AIDS-associated lymphoma. *Blood* 72:667–671, 1988.
9. Cleary MI, Nalesnik MA , Shearer WT, Sklar J. Clonal analysis of transplant associated lymphoproliferations based on the structure of the genomic termini of the Epstein Barr virus. *Blood* 72:349–352, 1988.
10. Pelicci PG, Knowles DM, II, Arlin ZA, et al. Multiple monoclonal B cell expansions and c-myc oncogene rearrangements in acquired immune

deficiency syndrome–related lymphoproliferative disorders: Implications for lymphomagenesis. *J Exp Med* 164:2049–2060, 1986.

11. Pahwa S, Pahwa R, Saxinger C, et al. Influence of the human T-lymphotropic virus/lymphadenopathy–associated virus and functions of human lymphocytes: Evidence of immunosuppressive effects and polyclonal B-cell activation by banded viral and lymphocyte preparations. *Proc Natl Acad Sci USA* 82:8198–8202, 1985.

12. Yarchoan R, Redfield R, Broder S. Mechanisms of B cell activation in patients with acquired immunodeficiency syndrome and related disorders: Contribution of antibody producing B cells, of Epstein Barr virus–infected B cells, and of immunoglobulin production induced by human T cell lymphotropic virus, type III/lymphadenopathy–associated virus. *J Clin Invest* 73:439–447, 1986.

13. Kristal AR, Nasca PC, Burkett WS, Mikl J. Changes in the epidemiology of non-Hodgkin's lymphoma associated with epidemic human immunodeficiency virus (HIV) infection. *Am J Epidemiol* 128:711–718, 1988.

14. Levine AM. Reactive and neoplastic lymphoproliferative disorders with HIV infection. In VT DeVita, S Hellman, SA Rosenberg (eds), *AIDS: Etiology, Diagnosis, Treatment and Prevention.* Philadelphia: Lippincott, 1988. Pp 263–275.

15. Levine AM, Meyer PR, Begandy MK, et al. Development of B-cell lymphoma in homosexual men: Clinical and immunologic findings. *Ann Intern Med* 100:7, 1984.

16. Levine AM, Gill PS, Meyer PR, et al. Retrovirus and malignant lymphoma in homosexual men. *JAMA* 254:1921, 1985.

17. Knowles DM, Chamulak GA, Subar M, et al. Lymphoid neoplasia associated with the acquired immunodeficiency syndrome (AIDS). *Ann Intern Med* 108:744–753, 1988.

18. Monfardini S, Vaccher E, Foa R, et al. AIDS associated non Hodgkin's lymphoma in Italy: Intravenous drug users versus homosexual men. *Ann Oncol* 1:203–211, 1990.

19. Rabin CS, et al. Incidence of lymphomas and other cancers in HIV-infected and HIV-uninfected patients with hemophilia. *JAMA* 267:1090–1094, 1992.

20. Levine AM, Gill PS. AIDS-related malignant lymphoma: Clinical presentation and treatment approaches. *Oncology* 1:41–46, 1987.

21. Ziegler JL, Beckstead JA, Volberding PA, et al. Non-Hodgkin's lymphoma in 90 homosexual men. *N Engl J Med* 311:565–570, 1984.

22. Lukes RJ, Collins RD. Immunologic characterization of human malignant lymphoma. *Cancer* 34:1488, 1974.

23. Non-Hodgkin's Lymphoma Pathologic Classification Project: National Cancer Institute sponsored study of classifications of non-Hodgkin's lymphomas: Summary and description of a working formulation for clinical usage. *Cancer* 49:2112, 1982.

24. Lukes RJ, Parker JW, Taylor CR, et al. Immunologic approach to non-Hodgkin's lymphomas and related leukemias: Analysis of results of multiparameter studies of 425 cases. *Semin Hematol* 15:322–351, 1978.

25. Bermudez MA, Grant KM, Rodvien R, Mendes F. Non-Hodgkin's lym-

phoma in a population with or at risk for acquired immunodeficiency syndrome: Indications for intensive chemotherapy. *Am J Med* 86:71–76, 1989.

26. Gill PS, Levine AM, Krailo M, et al. AIDS-related malignant lymphoma: Results of prospective treatment trials. *J Clin Oncol* 5:1322, 1987.

27. Kalter SP, Riggs SA, Cabanillas F, et al. Aggressive non-Hodgkin's lymphomas in immunocompromised homosexual males. *Blood* 66:655–659, 1985.

28. Kaplan MH, Susin M, Pahwa SG, et al. Neoplastic complications of HTLV-III infection: Lymphomas and solid tumors. *Am J Med* 82:389–396, 1987.

29. Levine AM, Loureiro C, Sullivan-Halley J, et al. HIV-related lymphoma: Prognostic factors predictive of survival. *Blood* 72:247a, 1988.

30. Lowenthal DA, Straus DJ, Campbell SW, et al. AIDS-related lymphoid neoplasia: The Memorial Hospital Experience. *Cancer* 61:2325–2337, 1988.

31. Jones SE, Faks Z, Bullm M, et al. Non-Hodgkin's lymphoma IV. Clinico-pathologic correlation of 405 cases. *Cancer* 31:806–823, 1973.

32. Gill PS, Levine MA, Meyer PR et al. Primary CNS lymphoma in homosexual men: Clinical, immunologic and pathologic features. *Am J Med* 78:742–748, 1985.

33. So YT, Beckstead JH, Davis RL. Primary central nervous system lymphoma in acquired immunodeficiency syndrome: A clinical and pathologic study. *Ann Neurol* 20:556–572, 1986.

34. Rosenblum ML, Levy RM, Bredesen DE, et al. Primary central nervous system lymphomas in patients with AIDS. *Ann Neurol* 23 (suppl):S13–S16, 1988.

35. Levine AM. Low dose chemotherapy with CNS prophylaxis and zidovudine (AZT) maintenance for AIDS-related lymphoma: Follow-up data from a multi-institutional trial. *Blood* 74 (suppl 1):239a, 1989.

36. Walsh D, Wernt T, Laubenstein L, et al. Phase I study of m-BACOD with GM-CSF in AIDS-associated non-Hodgkin's lymphoma (NHL): Preliminary results. *Blood* 74 (suppl 1):126a, 1989.

37. Kaplan LD, Kahn JO, Crowe S, et al. Clinical and virologic effects of recombinant human granulocyte-macrophage colony stimulating factor in patients receiving chemotherapy for human immunodeficiency virus–associated non-Hodgkin's lymphoma: Results of a randomized trial. *J Clin Oncol* 9:929–940, 1991.

38. Holland HK, Saral R, Rossi JJ. Allogeneic bone marrow transplantation, zidovudine, and human immunodeficiency virus type 1 (HIV-1) infection. *Ann Intern Med* 111:973–981, 1989.

39. Formenti SC, Gill PS, Lean E, et al. Primary central nervous system lymphoma in AIDS. *Cancer* 63:1101–1107, 1989.

40. Gill PS, Graham RA, Boswell W, et al. A comparison of imaging, clinical and pathologic aspects of space occupying lesions within the brain in patients with acquired immunodeficiency syndrome. *Am J Physiol Imaging* 1:134–139, 1986.

41. Baer D, Anderson ET, Wilkinson LS. Acquired immunodeficiency syn-

drome in homosexual men with Hodgkin's disease. *Am J Med* 80:738–740, 1986.

42. Unger PD, Stranchen JA. Hodgkin's disease in AIDS-related complex patients. *Cancer* 58:821–825, 1986.

43. Roithmann S, Toledano M, Tourani JM, Andrieu JM. HIV-associated lymphomas (HAL): Report of 160 cases from France (abstract). Sixth International Conference on AIDS, San Francisco, June 1990.

44. Tirelli U, Carbone A, Monfardini S, et al. Malignant tumors in patients with immunodeficiency virus infection: A report of 580 cases. *J Clin Oncol* 7:1582–1583, 1989.

45. Hessol NA, Katz MH, Liu JY, et al. Increased incidence of Hodgkin disease in homosexual men with HIV infection. *Ann Intern Med* 117:309–311, 1992.

46. Rubio R, Serrano M, Flores E, et al. Hodgkin's disease in intravenous drug users (IVDU) with HIV infection (abstract). Sixth International Conference on AIDS, San Francisco, June 1990.

47. Ames ED, Conjalka MS, Goldberg AF, et al. Hodgkin's disease and AIDS: Twenty-three new cases and a review of the literature. *Hematol Oncol Clin North Am* 5:343–356, 1991.

48. Colby TV, Hoppe RT, Warnke RA. Hodgkin's disease: A clinicopathologic study of 659 cases. *Cancer* 49:1848–1858, 1981.

IV/Special Topics

28/Antiretroviral Therapy

Kevan L. Hartshorn

Specific therapy to control viral replication has become a cornerstone in the management of HIV-infected patients. Antiretroviral therapy is undergoing continual evolution, and current recommendations will clearly change over time. Currently, three drugs are approved by the Food and Drug Administration (FDA) for the treatment of HIV infection: zidovudine (ZDV) (formerly known as azidothymidine [AZT]), didanosine (ddI), and dideoxycytidine (ddC). Zidovudine has been shown to enhance survival and slow HIV disease progression and is recommended as initial therapy in most patients. Didanosine has been approved in patients who have been on prolonged ZDV therapy, who are intolerant to ZDV, or who have clinical or immunologic evidence of disease progression on ZDV. Dideoxycytidine is recommended for use in combination with ZDV in patients with advanced HIV disease. This chapter reviews these three agents and discusses the direction of current research. In addition, a comprehensive strategy for antiretroviral therapy is presented.

Zidovudine

Mechanism of Action and Pharmacology

Zidovudine is a thymidine analogue utilized by retroviral reverse transcriptases, leading to premature termination of the HIV DNA chain [1]. Mammalian DNA polymerases apparently have greater ability to detect and remove the aberrant nucleotide, accounting for the relatively specific effect of ZDV on viral replication. Zidovudine must be converted into a triphosphate derivative in the host cell before it can become incorporated into DNA. The active antiviral compound is not ZDV itself but rather its triphosphate derivative. Pharmacologically, ZDV has the advantages of high oral bioavailability and central nervous system penetration due to lipid solubility. The serum half-life is approximately one hour. Trough levels achieved with every 4 hour administration exceed the concentration shown to inhibit HIV replication in vitro. The drug is metabolized principally by glucuronidation in the liver, with a lesser contribution (25%) from direct renal excretion of the active compound. The hepatic metabolite is also handled by the kidney, and marked accu-

379

mulation occurs in renal failure [2]. Both ZDV and its hepatic metabolite are incompletely removed by dialysis, and probenecid decreases ZDV excretion substantially, probably by its effect on liver glucuronidation and renal excretion.

Clinical Effects

Clinical benefits of ZDV have been documented with respect to survival and general health status, immunologic status and incidence of opportunistic infections, neurologic status, and HIV-related immune thrombocytopenic purpura (ITP).

The clinical effects of 250 mg ZDV given orally every 4 hours have been studied in a randomized, placebo-controlled trial involving 160 AIDS patients recently recovered from *Pneumocystis carinii* pneumonia (PCP) and 122 AIDS-related complex (ARC) patients considered at high risk for development of AIDS [3]. Despite the relatively short (6 months) duration of the initial trial, a marked improvement in survival was noted in both AIDS and ARC patients who received ZDV; overall, 1 death occurred in the ZDV group, compared to 19 in the placebo group. A significant decrease in the incidence and severity of opportunistic infections was noted in the ZDV group as well. Improved performance status and weight gain were observed, as were increased CD4 lymphocyte counts and regained skin test reactivity. The ZDV-treated ARC group was noted to have a more sustained rise in CD4 cell counts and greater clinical benefit than the AIDS group.

A substantially larger number of patients (4,805) with AIDS diagnosed on the basis of prior PCP received ZDV as part of a compassionate-use protocol before drug licensure [4]. A 73 percent survival rate was noted at 44 weeks, which was significantly higher than that of historical controls. In this study, delay in the onset of ZDV therapy after AIDS diagnosis and lower pretreatment performance status were associated with poorer clinical outcome.

Since these landmark studies, the clinical indications for ZDV have been expanded and refined. An AIDS Clinical Trials Group (ACTG) protocol was performed in which 524 patients with prior PCP were randomized to treatment with 250 mg ZDV orally every 4 hours, versus 200 mg every 4 hours for 4 weeks, followed by 100 mg every 4 hours for the remainder of the study [5]. After a median of 2 years of follow-up evaluation, improved survival and reduced rates of neutropenia and anemia were noted in the low-dose group. The effects on CD4 cell counts and p24 viral antigen levels were similar in both groups. Other studies have confirmed the finding that lower-dose ZDV is as effective as and less toxic than the high-dose regimen in symptomatic HIV-infected patients [6].

Two major studies have established benefits of ZDV treatment in asymptomatic or mildly symptomatic subjects with HIV infection. One trial compared ZDV, 200 mg every 4 hours, to placebo in 711 people with mildly symptomatic HIV infection and CD4 cell counts of $200/mm^3$ or greater [7]. The trial was discontinued after approximately one year because the ZDV group showed a reduced progression to AIDS. In addition, CD4 cell counts remained higher and p24 viral antigen levels lower in the ZDV group. Stratification of patients by CD4 count showed that clinical benefits were confined to the ZDV treatment group with CD4 cell counts between $500/mm^3$ and $200/mm^3$, and were not observed in those with an initial CD4 cell count greater than $500/mm^3$. Another trial randomized 1,338 asymptomatic, HIV-infected subjects with CD4 counts between $500/mm^3$ and $200/mm^3$ to one of three treatment regimens: placebo; ZDV, 300 mg five times a day; or ZDV, 100 mg five times a day [8]. This trial eliminated the nighttime ZDV dose for all subjects to improve compliance. Significant reduction in progression to AIDS or advanced ARC, and increases in CD4 cell counts and reduction of p24 antigen levels, were again observed in the ZDV groups. The low-dose ZDV group experienced equivalent benefits and reduced toxicity compared to the high-dose ZDV group. In fact, the incidence of hematologic toxicity was no different from that observed in control subjects.

In a recent study of symptomatic patients with HIV infection, early treatment with high-dose ZDV delayed progression to AIDS, but did not improve survival and appeared to be associated with greater toxicity than if initiated when the CD4 cell count fell below $200/mm^3$ or when an AIDS-defining diagnosis developed [9]. Because of this, the authors suggested that clinicians might consider delaying the initiation of ZDV therapy in patients with CD4 cell counts between 500 and $200/mm^3$ whose condition is stable. Despite an earlier report that ZDV therapy may not significantly benefit some minorities, recent studies indicate that the drug appears to be effective in women, blacks, Latinos, and drug users [10, 11].

The minimum effective daily dose of ZDV is still uncertain. A pilot study showed that very low dose ZDV (100 mg orally three times a day) had short-term clinical and antiviral effects similar to those of higher-dose regimens in patients with AIDS-related complex [12]. The frequency of dosing is also evolving. Several European studies have employed a regimen of 200 mg ZDV three times a day and found similar efficacy to every 4 hour administration.

Clinical benefits of ZDV have not been confined to enhancement of immunologic function and general health status. In the original placebo-controlled trial, a subset of patients was studied with respect to cognitive function, and significant improvement was noted in the ZDV group, especially among those with AIDS [3]. A smaller pilot study of ZDV in patients with HIV dementia also showed benefit [13]. Three reports have shown a positive effect on platelet counts in individuals with HIV-related thrombocytopenia [14–16].

Toxicity

In general, ZDV is well tolerated. The most frequent complaint among subjects receiving ZDV in clinical trials has been nausea, which occurs in 3 to 10 percent. Headaches, insomnia, rash, and malaise have been described as well, although similar rates of these symptoms have been observed in placebo groups. One case of Stevens-Johnson syndrome, thought to be related to ZDV, has been reported [4]. Seizure activity and a single case of lethal neurotoxicity have been ascribed to ZDV [4, 17, 18]. Two cases of ZDV overdose have been reported, both of which had minimal sequelae [19, 20].

The most common and troublesome toxicities of ZDV are hematologic, most notably anemia and neutropenia. In the original randomized trial, anemia occurred significantly more frequently in ZDV recipients, with 21 percent becoming transfusion dependent, compared to 4 percent in the placebo group. Neutropenia was described in 16 percent of ZDV recipients versus 2 percent of those receiving placebo [3]. Other reports confirm that severe, prolonged marrow hypoplasia may result from ZDV therapy [21]. This effect should be distinguished from the nearly universal development of macrocytosis and megaloblastic erythroid changes in the bone marrow of ZDV recipients. These changes, which probably result from interference of ZDV monophosphate with generation of thymidine triphosphate, generally do not portend hematologic deterioration.

The use of lower doses of ZDV has reduced the frequency of hematologic toxicity (Table 28-1). In addition, it has also become clear that HIV-infected patients with minimal symptoms and CD4 cell counts of greater than $200/mm^3$ have a substantially reduced incidence of anemia and neutropenia. Despite earlier concerns regarding coadministration of acetaminophen with ZDV, the analgesic does not appear to affect significantly either ZDV clearance or production of its glucuronide conjugate [22].

Recombinant erythropoietin and granulocyte/monocyte colony stimulating factor (GM-CSF) have been demonstrated to ameliorate, respectively, the anemia and the neutropenia associated with ZDV administration [23, 24]. Daily subcutaneous erythropoietin has been shown to reduce the transfusion requirement of severely anemic ZDV-treated patients with serum erythropoietin levels of less than 500 mU/ml. Prior studies had indicated that the neutropenia associated with AIDS or with

Table 28-1 *Incidence of anemia[a] and neutropenia[b] in ZDV recipients*

| | Incidence by ZDV dosage (% of patients) | | | |
| | High dose | | Low dose | |
HIV disease stage	Anemia	Neutropenia	Anemia	Neutropenia
AIDS	39	51	29	37
Symptomatic, not AIDS	5	4		
No symptoms	6	6	1	2

[a]Anemia = hemoglobin < 8 grams/deciliter.
[b]Neutropenia = neutrophil count < 0.750×10^9/liter.
Source: Based on data from [5, 7, 8, 17].

ganciclovir treatment for cytomegalovirus infection was improved by GM-CSF administration [25, 26]. Granulocyte colony stimulating factor (G-CSF), unlike GM-CSF, does not appear to enhance HIV replication, and, therefore, may be the preferred agent [27]. Chemotherapy and other drug treatment, such as trimethoprim-sulfamethoxazole or ganciclovir, may necessitate interruption of ZDV therapy. Table 28-2 presents options for managing hematologic intolerance associated with ZDV administration. In some cases, reduction of the ZDV dose to 100 mg orally three times a day may ameliorate toxicity.

Other fairly well-documented adverse events attributable to ZDV include generalized myopathy, cardiomyopathy, and cholestatic hepatitis [28–30]. The incidence of myopathy related to ZDV appears to be highest among patients who have received the drug for 12 months or more and occurs in 1 to 2 percent of those with early HIV infection [17]. Zidovudine myopathy manifests as proximal muscle weakness with an increased level of serum creatine phosphokinase (CPK), and is sometimes severe. Nonsteroidal antiinflammatory agents often improve symptoms, but discontinuation of ZDV or institution of corticosteroid therapy, or both, may be necessary. Histologic examination reveals abnormalities in muscle mitochondria, perhaps resulting from ZDV-induced inhibition of gamma-DNA polymerase, which can be differentiated from the immune-mediated myopathy characteristic of HIV infection itself [31].

Viral resistance to ZDV has been described in patients who have received the drug for 6 months or more [32]. In one study, 93 percent of viral isolates from patients on ZDV for 3 years or more were resistant [33]. However, while the clinical significance of this finding is uncertain, it appears to correlate in some patients with disease progression. Resistance to ZDV does not extend to the dideoxynucleosides, ddI or ddC,

Table 28-2 Management options for patients with ZDV intolerance

Type of intolerance[a]	Treatment options[b]
Anemia requiring transfusion	Administer erythropoietin or change to ddI
Neutropenia (< 500 granulocytes/mm³)	Administer G-CSF, or change to ddI (or ddC)
Nonhematologic	Change to ddI (or ddC)

[a]Whether due to ZDV per se or to the use of necessary, concurrent myelosuppressive agents, such as chemotherapy, ganciclovir, or trimethoprim-sulfamethoxazole.
[b]Dose reduction of ZDV to 100 mg po tid may ameliorate mild hematologic intolerance, but the clinical efficacy of this regimen is unproven.

suggesting that switching to a regimen containing one of these agents might be beneficial after several months to a year of treatment with ZDV. Patients with symptomatic HIV infection receiving ZDV who survive for an extended period of time appear to be at increased risk for development of non-Hodgkin's lymphoma [34]. Whether this trend is related to immunosuppression itself or antiretroviral therapy, or both, is uncertain.

Treatment Recommendations

The currently recommended dose of ZDV is either 100 mg orally five times a day or 200 mg orally three times a day. The effects and toxicity of ZDV in the context of renal failure are not well documented, but, in patients undergoing dialysis, a dose of 100 mg orally three times a day has been proposed [35]. The frequency of follow-up evaluation depends on the stage of HIV disease and preexisting hematologic abnormalities. In addition to careful follow-up of blood counts, periodic electrolyte, liver function tests, and CPK should be performed. The annual cost of ZDV therapy is approximately $2,000. An indigent patient assistance program is available through the Burroughs Wellcome Company (telephone: 1-800-722-9294).

Didanosine

Mechanism of Action and Pharmacology

The mechanism of action of ddI is similar to that of ZDV [1]. Didanosine is converted in the body into dideoxyadenosine, which is then phosphorylated to form the active compound ddATP. Since this nucleotide lacks a hydroxyl group in the 3' position, it, like ZDV and ddC, results in HIV reverse transcriptase inhibition and viral DNA chain termination.

Renal handling of ddI accounts for about 50 percent of total body clearance. It is not yet clear what effect renal or hepatic dysfunction has on the pharmacology or toxicology of ddI, and current recommendations include a proviso that dose reductions should be considered in these settings.

Clinical Effects

Three phase I studies of ddI have now been completed [36–38]. The agent has been shown to have anti-HIV activity in vivo, to increase CD4 lymphocyte counts, and to have early clinical benefit when administered orally once or twice a day. Didanosine appears to be free of hematologic toxicity and, in fact, was associated with a significant elevation in hemoglobin in one trial [37].

Kahn and coworkers [39] recently reported the results of ACTG 116B/117, in which the role of ddI in patients with advanced HIV disease who had previously been treated with ZDV was evaluated. This multicenter, double-blind study involved 913 patients who had received ZDV for at least 16 weeks. Study participants had AIDS, ARC with CD4 cell counts of $300/mm^3$ or less, or asymptomatic HIV infection with CD4 cell counts of $200/mm^3$ or less. Subjects were randomly assigned to receive ZDV, 600 mg per day; ddI, 750 mg per day; or ddI, 500 mg per day. After a mean follow-up period of 55 weeks, significantly more new AIDS-defining events occurred in the ZDV group than in the 500 mg ddI group; death rates in the two groups were comparable. The efficacy of ddI was unrelated to the duration of previous ZDV therapy. Increases in CD4 cell count and decreases in p24 antigen level were more pronounced in both ddI groups than in patients who continued to receive ZDV.

Toxicity

The major dose-limiting toxicities of ddI are pancreatitis and peripheral neuropathy. Pancreatitis occurred in 9 percent of patients in the phase I trials who were receiving the currently recommended dose of ddI. Didanosine-related pancreatitis can be fatal if it is not recognized promptly. If abdominal pain, nausea, vomiting, or significantly elevated serum amylase occurs in association with ddI treatment, the drug should be discontinued pending full clinical assessment. The incidence of pancreatitis is greater (30%) in patients with a history of prior pancreatitis and in those with advanced HIV disease. Patients with alcoholism, hypertriglyceridemia, or concurrent use of intravenous pentamidine may also be more prone to this complication. Peripheral neuropathy, characterized by numbness, tingling, and pain in the feet and hands, occurred in approximately 3 percent of patients in phase I trials who were receiving the currently recommended dose of ddI. In the ACTG 116B/117 trial, neuropathy was no more frequent in the ddI group (approximately 14% incidence) than in the group receiving ZDV [39]. Neuropathic symptoms are reversible if identified early. Evidence of significant neuropathy should result in discontinuation of ddI therapy.

Other toxicities of ddI include elevation of serum uric acid level at higher doses, diarrhea (more frequent with the powder than the tablet preparation), and restlessness. Retinal depigmentation has been reported in pediatric patients, prompting a recommendation for periodic ophthalmologic examinations. One case of fatal hepatic failure related to ddI has been described [40]. Didanosine preparations contain acid-buffering components, and ketoconazole, dapsone, and ciprofloxacin which require gastric acid for absorption, should not be taken within 2 hours of its administration.

Drug resistance has been noted in HIV isolates obtained from patients treated with ddI [41]. Similar to ZDV, ddI resistance results from mutations in viral reverse transcriptase. Of interest, these mutations differ from those conferring ZDV resistance, and in fact, previously ZDV-resistant strains show evidence of greater ZDV sensitivity when ddI resistance is acquired.

Treatment Recommendations

Didanosine is available in buffered 25 and 100 mg tablets, which must be chewed completely or predisolved in water, and powder form. It should be administered on an empty stomach and is dosed in adults according to body weight. In patients 60 kg or more, the dose is 200 mg orally twice a day in tablet form, or 250 mg orally twice a day of powder dissolved in 4 ounces of water. In patients less than 60 kg, the dose is 125 mg orally twice a day in tablet form, or 167 mg orally twice a day of powder dissolved in 4 ounces of water. The approximate annual cost of ddI is $2,500. Bristol-Myers–Squibb offers an assistance program for uninsured patients (telephone: 1-800-788-0123).

Dideoxycytidine

Dideoxycytidine is another dideoxynucleotide that is the subject of active clinical investigation. Initial trials of this agent employed higher doses than are currently being studied or recommended, and a prohibitive incidence of painful, severe peripheral neuropathy was noted, despite significant antiretroviral effect and minimal hematologic toxicity [42]. Recent trials using lower doses have shown that antiretroviral effect is preserved, with reduced neurotoxicity [43]. However, ddC does not penetrate into the spinal fluid as well as ZDV, which may limit its usefulness in the treatment of HIV-related encephalopathy. Recent data indicate that ddC is inferior to ZDV as monotherapy in the initial treatment of HIV infection (unpublished results, ACTG 114). However, patients who are intolerant to ZDV or who have disease progression on ZDV therapy appear to benefit equally from switching to either ddC or ddI (unpublished results, community research study).

Meng and coworkers [44] recently reported on a phase I–II study examining combination therapy with ZDV and ddC in patients with advanced HIV infection. Fifty-six patients with AIDS, or ARC and CD4 cell counts of $200/mm^3$ or fewer, who had not received prior antiretroviral therapy were randomly assigned to one of six treatment groups. These included every 8 hour combination therapy with ZDV, 50 mg, 100 mg, or 200 mg, and ddC dosed at either 0.005 mg/kg or 0.01 mg/kg, and monotherapy with 50 mg ZDV every 8 hours. The median follow-up period was 40 weeks. Neither drug appeared to affect the pharmacokinetic profile of the other. Serious hematologic toxicity did not differ among the regimens. Severe sensory peripheral neuropathy occurred in two patients. One study patient developed markedly abnormal liver function tests and died following a sepsis-like syndrome. The mean maximal increase in CD4 counts was 109 cells/mm^3; a decrease in serum p24 antigen levels was noted in all regimens except ZDV monotherapy.

The recommended dose of ddC is 0.750 mg three times a day given in conjunction with ZDV, 200 mg orally three times a day. Toxicities of ddC include peripheral neuropathy, gastrointestinal intolerance, and mucosal ulcerations [45]. Hoffmann-LaRoche offers a patient assistance program (telephone: 1-800-526-6367).

Future Directions in Antiretroviral Therapy

Current research is focused on development of different classes of reverse transcriptase inhibitors, as well as identification of compounds that might act as inhibitors of other parts of the viral life cycle. Phase I trials of novel reverse transcriptase inhibitors are under way at various centers including Boston City Hospital. While soluble CD4 inhibits HIV replication in vitro by preventing virus attachment to the cell, its effects have been marginal in vivo [46]. Methods of conjugating CD4 to other molecules are being explored [47]. Inhibitors of the HIV protease, antisense DNA, and ribozymes have in vitro activity and may translate into clinically useful compounds. Alpha-interferon administered subcutaneously has been shown to have antiretroviral effect in patients with early HIV infection or Kaposi's sarcoma, although its usual toxicities, including flu-like syndrome and mild bone marrow suppression, have also been observed [48]. There are currently insufficient data to support the use of low-dose oral alpha-interferon for the treatment of HIV infection [49]. Inosine pranobex has been found to significantly delay progression to AIDS in a randomized, placebo-controlled trial [50]. This agent is believed to function as an immunomodulator, although its precise mechanism of action is not well defined [51].

Combination antiretroviral therapy may offer the best hope for control of HIV infection [52]. Alpha- and beta-interferons synergistically inhibit HIV when used in combination with ZDV or other reverse transcriptase inhibitors [53]. Trials have evaluated the clinical efficacy of combination therapy with ZDV and alpha-interferon, and ZDV and acyclovir [54, 55]. Zidovudine and alpha-interferon have been employed successfully in patients with Kaposi's sarcoma. This combination is an attractive alternative to chemotherapy for such patients, although the hematologic toxicity of ZDV is enhanced. High-dose acyclovir was recently reported to confer a survival benefit in patients with advanced HIV disease; the combination of ZDV and acyclovir is currently the subject of a multicenter ACTG trial [56]. At present the most active area of clinical research involves combinations of ZDV, ddI, and ddC, which, given their differing toxicities and mechanisms of HIV resistance, may prove more beneficial than monotherapy with any single agent. A recently completed in vitro study using ZDV, ddI, and nevirapine, a nonnucleoside reverse transcriptase inhibitor, indicates that "convergent" combination chemotherapy may offer an advantage over other regimens [57].

Recommendations for Antiretroviral Therapy

For newly diagnosed patients with HIV infection, assessment of clinical status and CD4 cell count should guide the choice of therapy [58] (Table 28-3). If the patient's CD4 count is greater than $500/mm^3$, no antiretroviral treatment is recommended, but it is advised that follow-up evaluations with repeat CD4 count be given at least every 6 months. If the patient has a CD4 cell count of $500/mm^3$ or below on repeated determinations, ZDV therapy should be initiated. At follow-up visits, complete blood counts should be obtained to monitor for hematologic toxicity; serum CPK levels, liver function tests, and renal function tests should also be checked periodically. All patients with CD4 cell counts of less than $200/mm^3$ should receive both ZDV and PCP prophylaxis.

If drug intolerance develops, the ZDV can be restarted at a reduced dose (100 mg orally three times a day), or ddI (or ddC) can be substituted

Table 28-3 Recommendations for antiretroviral therapy

CD4 cell count/ clinical setting	Treatment	Laboratory monitoring
> 500/mm³	None	CD4 count q6mo
500–200/mm³	ZDV, 100 mg 5×/day or 200 mg tid	CBC q1–3mo, chemistries q3mo, CD4 count q3mo
< 200/mm³	ZDV as above and PCP prophylaxis	CBC q1–3mo, chemistries q3mo, CD4 count q3mo
Disease progression on ZDV	Change to ddI (or ddC) or Combination therapy with ZDV and ddI or ZDV and ddC	See text
ZDV intolerance	See Table 28-2	See Table 28-2

provided the patient has no history of pancreatitis or severe neuropathy. If ZDV is continued and there is evidence of disease progression manifested by the development of significant symptoms and/or decline in CD4 cell count to 200/mm³ or less, ddI (or ddC) should be substituted. Patients who have been on ZDV for more than 16 weeks appear to have a lower risk of developing AIDS if they are switched to ddI as opposed to continuing on ZDV [39]. Combination therapy with ZDV and ddI has been well tolerated in early clinical trials and associated with an increase in CD4 counts [59]. ZDV/ddI and ZDV/ddC combination therapies are generally reserved for patients with disease progression on monotherapy, although their precise roles in antiretroviral treatment await the outcome of an ongoing ACTG trial. Since long-term follow-up study of patients treated with ZDV indicates that mortality is greatest when the CD4 cell count drops below 50/mm³, an important goal of antiretroviral therapy is to keep the count above this level [60].

References

1. Yarchoan R, Mitsuya H, Myers CE, et al. Clinical pharmacology of 3'-azido-2',3'-dideoxythymidine and related dideoxynucleosides. N Engl J Med 321:726–738, 1989.
2. Laskin OL, DeMiranda P, Blum MR. Azidothymidine steady-state pharmacokinetics in patients with AIDS and AIDS-related complex. J Infect Dis 159:8745–8747, 1989.
3. Fischl MA, Richman DD, Grieco MH, et al. The efficacy of AZT in the

treatment of patients with AIDS and AIDS-related complex. *N Engl J Med* 317:185–191, 1987.

4. Kirk TC, Doi P, Andrews E, et al. Survival experience among patients with AIDS receiving zidovudine. *JAMA* 260:3009–3053, 1988.

5. Fischl MA, Parker CB, Pettinelli C, et al. A randomized controlled trial of a reduced daily dose of zidovudine in patients with the acquired immunodeficiency syndrome. *N Engl J Med* 323:1009–1014, 1990.

6. Nordic Medical Research Council's HIV Therapy Group. Double-blind dose-response study of zidovudine in AIDS and advanced HIV infection. *Br Med J* 304:13–17, 1992.

7. Fischl MA, Richman D, Hansen N, et al. The safety and efficacy of zidovudine (AZT) in the treatment of subjects with mildly symptomatic human immunodeficiency virus type 1 (HIV) infection. *Ann Intern Med* 112:727–737, 1990.

8. Volberding PA, Lagakos SW, Koch MA, et al. Zidovudine in asymptomatic human immunodeficiency virus infection. *N Engl J Med* 322:941–949, 1990.

9. Hamilton JD, et al. A controlled trial of early versus late treatment with zidovudine in symptomatic human immunodeficiency virus infection: Results of the Veterans Affairs Cooperative Study. *N Engl J Med* 326:437–443, 1992.

10. Lagakos S, et al. Effects of zidovudine therapy in minority and other subpopulations with early HIV infection. *JAMA* 266:2709–2712, 1991.

11. Easterbrook PJ, et al. Racial and ethnic differences in outcome in zidovudine-treated patients with advanced HIV disease. *JAMA* 266:2713–2718, 1991.

12. Collier AC, Bozzette S, Coombs RW, et al. A pilot study of low dose zidovudine in human immunodeficiency virus infection. *N Engl J Med* 323:1015–1021, 1990.

13. Yarchoan R, Berg G, Brouwers P, et al. Response of HIV associated neurological disease to AZT. *Lancet* 1:132–135, 1987.

14. Hymes KB, Greene JB, Karpatkin S. The effect of azidothymidine on HIV-related thrombocytopenia. *N Engl J Med* 318:516–517, 1988.

15. Gottlieb MS, Wolfe PR, Chafey S. Case report: Response of AIDS-related thrombocytopenia to intravenous and oral azidothymidine (3'-azido-3'-deoxythymidine). *AIDS Res Hum Retrovir* 3:109, 1987.

16. The Swiss Group for Clinical Studies on AIDS. Zidovudine for the treatment of thrombocytopenia associated with HIV. *Ann Intern Med* 109:718–721, 1988.

17. Richman DD, Fischl MA, Frieco MH, et al. The toxicity of AZT in the treatment of patients with AIDS and AIDS-related complex. *N Engl J Med* 317:192–197, 1987.

18. Hagler DN, Frame PT. AZT neurotoxicity. *Lancet* 2:1392–1393, 1986.

19. Spear JB, Kessler HA, Nusinoff-Lehrman S, de Miranda P. Zidovudine overdosage. *Ann Intern Med* 109:76–77, 1988.

20. Pickus OB. Overdose of zidovudine. *N Engl J Med* 318:1206, 1988.

21. Gill PS, Rarick M, Brynes RK, et al. AZT associated bone marrow failure in AIDS. *Ann Intern Med* 107:502–505, 1987.

22. Sattler FR, Ko R, Antoniskis D, et al. Acetaminophen does not impair clearance of zidovudine. *Ann Intern Med* 114:937–940, 1991.
23. Fischl M, Galpin JE, Levine JD, et al. Recombinant human erythropoietin for patients with AIDS treated with zidovudine. *N Engl J Med* 322:1488–1493, 1990.
24. Pluda JM, Yarchoan R, Smith PD, et al. Subcutaneous recombinant granulocyte-macrophage colony-stimulating factor used as a single agent and in an alternating regimen with azidothymidine in leukopenic patients with severe human immunodeficiency virus infection. *Blood* 76:463–472, 1990.
25. Groopman JE, Mitsuyasu RT, DeLeo MJ, et al. Effect of recombinant human granulocyte-macrophage colony-stimulating factor on myelopoiesis in the acquired immunodeficiency syndrome. *N Engl J Med* 317:593–598, 1987.
26. Grossberg HS, Bonnem EM, Buhles WC. GM-CSF with ganciclovir for the treatment of CMV retinitis in AIDS. *N Engl J Med* 320:1560, 1989.
27. Miles SA, Mitsuyasu RT, Moreno J, et al. Combined therapy with granulocyte colony-stimulating factor and erythropoietin decreases hematologic toxicity from ziduvodine. *Blood* 77:2109–2117, 1990.
28. Bessen LJ, Greene JB, Louie E, et al. Severe polymyositis-like syndrome associated with zidovudine therapy of AIDS and ARC. *N Engl J Med* 318:708, 1988.
29. Herskowitz A, et al. Cardiomyopathy associated with antiretroviral therapy in patients with HIV infection: A report of six cases. *Ann Intern Med* 116:311–313, 1992.
30. Dubin G, Braffman MN. Zidovudine-induced hepatotoxicity. *Ann Intern Med* 110:85–86, 1989.
31. Dalakas MC, Illa I, Pezeshkpour GH, et al. Mitochondrial myopathy caused by long-term zidovudine therapy. *N Engl J Med* 322:1098–1105, 1990.
32. Richman DD. Zidovudine resistance of human immunodeficiency virus. *Rev Infect Dis* 12 (suppl):S506–S512, 1990.
33. Land S, et al. Incidence of zidovudine-resistant human immunodeficiency virus isolated from patients before, during, and after therapy. *J Infect Dis* 166:1139–1142, 1992.
34. Pluda JM, et al. Development of non-Hodgkin lymphoma in a cohort of patients with severe human immunodeficiency virus (HIV) therapy on long-term antiretroviral therapy. *Ann Intern Med* 113:276–282, 1990.
35. Deray G, Diquet B, Martinez F, et al. Pharmacokinetics of zidovudine in a patient on maintenance hemodialysis. *N Engl J Med* 319:1606-1607, 1988.
36. Lambert JS, Seidlin M, Reichman RC, et al. 2'3'-dideoxyinosine (ddI) in patients with the acquired immunodeficiency syndrome or AIDS-related complex. *N Engl J Med* 322:1333–1340, 1990.
37. Cooley TP, Kunches LM, Saunders CA, et al. Once-daily administration of 2'3'-dideoxyinosine (ddI) in patients with the acquired immunodeficiency syndrome or AIDS-related complex. *N Engl J Med* 322:1340–1345, 1990.

38. Yarchoan R, Mitsuya H, Thomas RV, et al. In vivo activity against HIV and favorable toxicity profile of 2'3'-dideoxyinosine. *Science* 245:412–415, 1989.
39. Kahn JO, et al. A controlled trial comparing continued zidovudine with didanosine in human immunodeficiency virus infection. *N Engl J Med* 327:581–587, 1992.
40. Lai KK, Gang DL, Zawacki JK, Cooley TP. Fulminant hepatic failure associated with 2',3'-dideoxyinosine (ddI). *Ann Intern Med* 115:283–284, 1991.
41. St. Clair MH, Martin JL, Tudor-Williams G, et al. Resistance to ddI and sensitivity to AZT induced by a mutation in HIV-1 reverse transcriptase. *Science* 253:1557–1559, 1991.
42. Merigen TC, Skowron G, Bozzette SA, et al. Circulating p24 antigen levels and responses to dideoxycytidine in human immunodeficiency virus (HIV) infections. *Ann Intern Med* 110:189–194, 1989.
43. Broder S. Proceedings of a symposium. Dideoxycytidine (ddC): A potent antiretroviral agent for human immunodeficiency virus infection. *Am J Med* 88 (suppl 5B):1S–33S, 1990.
44. Meng TC, et al. Combination therapy with zidovudine and dideoxycytidine in patients with advanced human immunodeficiency virus infection. *Ann Intern Med* 116:85–86, 1992.
45. Indorf AS, Pegram PS. Esophageal ulceration related to zalcitabine (ddC). *Ann Intern Med* 117:133–134, 1992.
46. Schooley RT, et al. Recombinant soluble CD4 therapy in patients with the acquired immunodeficiency syndrome (AIDS) and AIDS-related complex: A phase I–II escalating dosage trial. *Ann Intern Med* 112:247–253, 1990.
47. Finberg RW, Wahl SM, Allen JB, et al. Selective elimination of HIV-1 infected cells with an interleukin-2 receptor specific cytotoxin. *Science* 252:1703–1705, 1991.
48. Lane HC, Davey V, Kovacs JA, et al. Interferon-alpha in patients with asymptomatic human immunodeficiency virus (HIV) infection. *Ann Intern Med* 112:805–810, 1990.
49. US Department of Health and Human Services. *HHS News,* April 28, 1992.
50. Pedersen C, Sandstrom E, Petersen CS, et al. The efficacy of inosine pranobex in preventing the acquired immunodeficiency syndrome in patients with human immunodeficiency virus infection. *N Engl J Med* 322:1757–1763, 1990.
51. Kweder SL, Schnur RA, Cooper EC. Inosine pranobex: Is a single positive trial enough? (editorial). *N Engl J Med* 322:1807–1809, 1990.
52. Groopman JE. The challenge of combination antiretroviral therapy. *Am J Med* 90 (suppl 4A):1S–30S, 1990.
53. Hartshorn KL, Vogt MW, Neumeyer D, et al. Synergistic inhibition of HIV replication in vitro by AZT and recombinant interferon alpha. *Antimicrob Agents Chemother* 31:168–172, 1987.
54. Kovacs JA, Deyton L, Davey R, et al. Combined zidovudine and interferon-alpha therapy in patients with Kaposi sarcoma and the acquired

immunodeficiency syndrome (AIDS). *Ann Intern Med* 111:280–287, 1989.

55. Hollander H, Lifson AR, Maha M, et al. Phase I study of low-dose zidovudine and acyclovir in asymptomatic human immunodeficiency virus seropositive individuals. *Am J Med* 87:628–632, 1989.

56. Youle M, European-Australian Acyclovir Study Group. Double blind, placebo controlled trial of high dose acyclovir for the prevention of cytomegalovirus disease in late stage HIV disease. Eighth International Conference on AIDS, Amsterdam, July 1992.

57. Chow Y-K, et al. Use of evolutionary limitations of HIV-1 multidrug resistance to optimize therapy. *Nature* 361:650–654, 1993.

58. National Institutes of Health. State-of-the-art conference on azidothymidine therapy for early HIV Infection. *Am J Med* 89:335–344, 1990.

59. Yarchoan R, et al. Therapy of AIDS or symptomatic HIV infection with simultaneous or alternating regimens of AZT and DDI. Eighth International Conference on AIDS, Amsterdam, July 1992.

60. Yarchoan R, Venzon DJ, Pluda JM, et al. CD4 count and the risk for death in patients infected with HIV receiving anti-retroviral therapy. *Ann Intern Med* 115:184–189, 1991.

29/Ambulatory Management of HIV Infection

Jon D. Fuller, Howard Libman

Clinical practice begins with the recognition that education to prevent HIV infection should be part of routine health care maintenance. Clinicians who provide an opportunity for patients to ask frank questions about HIV infection will help them to acquire an understanding of behaviors that could place them at risk. Education about the types of casual contact that do not lead to viral transmission will assist them in learning to live and work comfortably with HIV-infected individuals.

HIV Antibody Testing

Some patients seek HIV antibody testing on their own. In other cases, the clinician takes the initiative by recommending HIV antibody testing to patients with historical risks for HIV infection or clinical findings suggestive of the diagnosis [1–7] (Table 29-1).

Pretest and Posttest Counseling

The benefits of early HIV antibody testing include the capacity to receive appropriate medical care and to modify behaviors in order to decrease the risk of transmission to others (Table 29-2). However, testing is also associated with some risks. Receiving a positive result can have devastating personal and social effects. HIV seropositivity may adversely affect one's eligibility for life insurance, health insurance, employment, and housing, and suicide has been reported in asymptomatic persons who have received the news of a positive test result [8–12]. Patients who undergo HIV antibody testing should have a full understanding of its ramifications through pretest and posttest counseling. Antibody testing is contraindicated in patients who cannot provide informed consent; who are unable to understand the implications of test results; who are psychotic, suicidal, or emotionally disturbed; or who lack adequate personal support systems to cope with the stress of receiving a positive result (see Table 29-1).

Table 29-1 *Indications and contraindications for HIV antibody testing*

Historical indications
　　Men who have sex with men
　　Persons with multiple sexual partners
　　Current or past injection drug users
　　Recipients of blood products between 1978 and 1985
　　Persons with current or past sexually transmitted diseases
　　Prostitutes and their sexual partners
　　Women of childbearing age who are at risk through drug use, prostitution,
　　　　unprotected sex
　　Children born to HIV-infected mothers
　　Sexual partners of those at risk for HIV infection
Clinical indications
　　Tuberculosis
　　Syphilis
　　Recurrent shingles
　　Unexplained chronic constitutional symptoms
　　Unexplained chronic generalized adenopathy
　　Unexplained diarrhea or wasting
　　Unexplained encephalopathy
　　Unexplained thrombocytopenia
　　Unexplained thrush or chronic vaginal candidiasis
Contraindications
　　Pretest and posttest counseling unavailable
　　Inability to provide informed consent
　　Acute psychosis or severe emotional disturbance
　　Suicidality
　　Lack of adequate personal support system

Confirmation of Reported Seropositivity

A variety of economic and health care benefits may become available to HIV-infected patients, and several reports in the literature have documented individuals who misrepresent themselves as seropositive in order to take advantage of these. This behavior may also be a manifestation of the Munchausen syndrome, with a characteristic desire to repeatedly undergo unnecessary and often invasive diagnostic procedures [13–15]. For these reasons, it is prudent to confirm a verbally reported positive HIV antibody test result in patients without characteristic manifestations of HIV disease.

Clinical Evaluation in HIV Infection

Because the clinical manifestations of HIV infection are protean, the clinician should be methodical in his or her approach to the history and physical examination.

Table 29-2 *Potential benefits and risks of HIV antibody testing*

Benefits
Individual health
    Antiretroviral therapy
    Prophylaxis for *Pneumocystis carinii* pneumonia
    Screening and prophylaxis for tuberculosis
    Screening for and treatment of syphilis and other sexually transmitted diseases
    Administration of appropriate vaccinations
    Other routine health care maintenance
    Patient education
Public health
    Reduction of high-risk behaviors
    Monitoring of HIV infection epidemiology
Risks
False-positive test result
False-negative test result
Adverse psychological reactions
Loss of confidentiality
Societal discrimination

Medical History

While certain disease manifestations may be seen with a higher incidence in certain subpopulations (e.g., Kaposi's sarcoma [KS] among homosexual men), the manner in which an individual has acquired HIV infection does not generally affect management. However, for the purposes of epidemiologic reporting, it is important to identify the risk behavior(s) that constitute the likely source(s) of infection for each individual. This information also guides the clinician in educating the patient about specific changes in behavior that will be necessary in order to minimize the risk of transmitting HIV to others.

Particular items in the medical history are of significance in managing HIV-infected patients. It is important to establish if the patient has a history of syphilis because of the increased risk of relapse and central nervous system involvement. A history of genital warts or of receptive anal intercourse in both men and women should be carefully sought; human papillomavirus (HPV) infection in association with HIV-induced immune suppression can predispose to cervical dysplasia and cancer, as well as squamous cell carcinoma of the anus [16–19].

Many common skin conditions, including eczema, seborrhea, psoriasis, warts, molluscum contagiosum, and herpes simplex virus (HSV) infection, may be exacerbated by HIV infection. Patients with a history of hepatitis B virus (HBV) infection may experience viral reactivation, leading to clinical hepatitis or reversion to infectious status, or both [20–22]. Since the immune response to HBV infection, and not HBV itself, causes hepatitis, clinical disease may not be apparent until therapy with immunorestorative agents such as zidovudine (ZDV) or alpha-interferon is initiated. A history of tuberculosis exposure is important to obtain, since the risk of developing active disease is significantly increased in HIV-infected individuals [23].

Review of Systems

Since severe weight loss can accompany many of the infectious or neoplastic complications of HIV infection, any significant decrease in weight should prompt a diagnostic evaluation for opportunistic disease. Weight loss may also be an indication for the use of nutritional supplements or megestrol acetate [24, 25]. The presence of chronic, low-grade fever may be the earliest manifestation of infections, such as *Pneumocystis carinii* pneumonia (PCP), mycobacterial disease, or cryptococcosis, or of neoplasia, especially lymphoma. Sweats may result from cytokines released in response to HIV infection; they are also sometimes a marker for infection or neoplasia.

Generalized lymphadenopathy is frequently seen in HIV-infected patients and usually represents a benign, reactive process that may regress with more advanced disease [26]. However, individual nodes or groups of nodes that are bulky, matted, or tender may warrant evaluation for infection or tumor, particularly if constitutional symptoms are present and no specific etiology has been identified [27, 28].

A history of new, pigmented skin lesions should raise the clinician's suspicion for KS (see Plates 15,16). However, cat scratch bacillus can also cause erythematous, nodular lesions resembling KS, making biopsy preferable to empiric diagnosis [29, 30]. Mucocutaneous ulcers may represent infection with HSV cytomegalovirus, *Staphylococcus aureus*, or mycobacteria. Nodular skin lesions may indicate the presence of molluscum contagiosum (see Plate 11) or verruca vulgaris, both of which may grow rapidly.

Human immunodeficiency virus can enter the central nervous system at the time of primary infection, resulting in a variety of neurologic syndromes [31, 32]. Irritability, persistent headaches, mental status changes, memory loss, and inability to concentrate may be manifestations of HIV encephalopathy, which may occur at any stage of the disease, or of opportunistic infection or tumor. Peripheral nerve involvement by HIV may manifest as painful paresthesias, numbness, or weakness. Autonomic neuropathy may produce orthostatic hypotension, nocturia, urinary or fecal incontinence, or gastroparesis.

HIV-related oral manifestations include white patches or plaques on the tongue or buccal mucosa (thrush or hairy leukoplakia), gingival inflammation or swelling (necrotizing gingivitis), ulceration (HSV, cytomegalovirus [CMV], or aphthous stomatitis), and KS of the palate, gingiva, or pharynx (see Plates 1–6). Chronic sinusitis is frequently associated with HIV infection and may cause persistent headaches, nasal discharge, and cough.

Shortness of breath and dyspnea on exertion may be manifestations of PCP or other pulmonary infections, pulmonary KS, lymphoid interstitial pneumonitis (LIP), or HIV-related cardiomyopathy. Retrosternal chest pain with swallowing or odynophagia is characteristic of candidal, HSV, or CMV esophagitis. Posterior pharyngeal discomfort on swallowing may be caused by severe oral candidiasis, aphthous ulcers, or infection with CMV or HSV, while dysphagia is sometimes a manifestation of autonomic neuropathy.

Myalgias and arthralgias may represent, respectively, HIV-induced myositis and arthritis, including Reiter's syndrome and psoriatic arthritis. Myalgias may also indicate myopathy associated with chronic ZDV therapy [33, 34]. The fibromyalgia syndrome—the triad of depression, insomnia, and pain at tendon insertions—has also been described with increased frequency among HIV-infected patients [35].

Physical Examination

Skin
Seborrheic dermatitis may present atypically with a papular or nodular appearance in HIV-infected patients [36] (see Plate 14). This condition often involves the moustache, beard, eyebrows, scalp, forehead, retroauricular skin, nipples, and perianal area. Psoriasis may be exacerbated by HIV infection and improve during ZDV therapy [37–40].

An otherwise rare skin condition known as eosinophilic pustular folliculitis (EPF) has been described in HIV-infected patients and may be mistaken for one of the atypical presentations of seborrheic dermatitis. EPF frequently begins as a pruritic, papular eruption and develops into a weeping, crusting ulcer with a hypertrophic margin and central healing. While the etiology of EPF remains obscure, it may represent a nonspecific response to skin saprophytes [41, 42].

Staphylococcus aureus infection may result in recurrent folliculitis, impetigo (see Plate 12), furuncles, or abscesses. Bacteremia may develop even in patients without intravascular catheters or other predisposing factors [43].

Mycotic infection of the nail bed, onychomycosis, is common and may present as typical "powdery" disintegration or discoloration of the distal nail or as thickening of the nail bed. Patients receiving ZDV frequently develop nail bed dyschromia, which manifests as asymptomatic vertical, and occasionally horizontal, striping [44–46].

Herpes simplex virus infection may cause chronic or recurrent ulceration of the oral, labial, buccal, genital, and perirectal tissues (see Plate 9). Relapse is common and may require chronic suppressive antiviral therapy. If HSV infection is present for more than one month, it constitutes an AIDS-defining diagnosis.

Recurrent shingles (reactivation of varicella-zoster virus [VZV]) is commonly associated with early HIV infection [47] (see Plate 10). Zoster may present as localized or disseminated disease, manifested by a painful or dysesthetic prodrome followed by vesicles, which weep and gradually crust; ophthalmitis and encephalitis rarely occur [48, 49]. Although disseminated VZV infection generally responds well to acyclovir, increased morbidity and mortality have been reported in this population [50].

Kaposi's sarcoma of the skin can present as macules, plaques, or nodules, and may wax and wane without therapy (see Plates 15, 16). While KS lesions are characteristically blue-red or purple, they may become brown with age. Cutaneous KS of the extremities or involvement of regional lymph nodes can lead to lymphatic obstruction and dependent edema. Sites with a particularly high incidence of KS include the lower extremities, tip of the nose, oral cavity (gums, hard palate, posterior pharynx; see Plate 4), and bulbar and palpebral conjunctivae. Kaposi's sarcoma lesions may appear less violaceous on dark-skinned persons and may be mistaken for nevi.

Many localized and disseminated infections may present as nodules, papules, pustules, or plaques. Facial involvement may be mistaken for seborrhea [51]. Any skin lesions that are unresponsive to empiric therapy, especially in the presence of systemic symptoms, should be considered for biopsy and culture.

Lymph Nodes
Generalized lymphadenopathy is common, with intermittent symptoms corresponding to nodal enlargement and involution. Commonly involved sites include the cervical, occipital, axillary, and femoral/inguinal chains. Lymph nodes are typically 1 to 2 cm in diameter, firm, nontender, and nonadherent.

Oropharynx
Thrush or oropharyngeal candidiasis may present in several patterns. In its pseudomembranous form, it is a white, curd-like membrane that can be removed to reveal an erythematous mucosal surface; potassium hydroxide preparation of mucosal scrapings demonstrates budding yeast and pseudohyphae (see Plate 1). Atrophic thrush is slightly tender and appears as an erythematous, smooth, or papular region on mucous membranes, especially the hard palate. Angular cheilitis manifests as fissuring and erythema of the corners of the mouth. Pseudomembranous

thrush may interfere with eating, cause a bad taste in the mouth, or be cosmetically unacceptable.

Hairy leukoplakia is a white, vertical, corrugated lesion usually appearing on the sides or dorsum of the tongue, buccal mucosa, or both (see Plate 3). Epstein-Barr virus can be detected in many biopsy specimens, although other viruses, including HSV and HPV, have also been suggested as causative agents [52–54]. Hairy leukoplakia is not dangerous in itself and rarely causes symptoms, but it is a marker for immune suppression and has been correlated with more rapid HIV disease progression [55]. There is no specific treatment for hairy leukoplakia, although it may regress with antiviral therapy.

Acute necrotizing ulcerative gingivitis (ANUG) manifests as painful, swollen gums associated with an erythematous, horizontal line at the gingivodental border (see Plate 5). ANUG can lead to severe and sometimes rapidly progressive periodontal disease. Patients with obvious or suspected gingival or periodontal pathology should be empirically started on penicillin or clindamycin, and promptly referred to a dentist or oral surgeon [56].

Eyes

Since a variety of opportunistic infections may involve the cornea, conjunctiva, or retina of HIV-infected patients, a careful eye examination, including visualization of the fundus, should be performed regularly. A dilated examination is necessary to visualize the peripheral retina. Lesions of the cornea or conjunctiva may occur with KS, or with VZV or *Microsporidia* infection [57–58]. Retinal lesions may be caused by HIV, CMV, *P. carinii, Toxoplasma gondii,* syphilis, *Candida,* or histoplasmosis [59–63].

Cotton-wool spots, commonly associated with HIV infection, are pale, moderately well-delineated white patches with fluffy or discrete borders (see Plate 7). Usually asymptomatic, they may remain stable over time or disappear in one location while they appear in another. While the etiology of cotton-wool spots is unknown, they may represent an inflammatory response to HIV itself [64].

Cytomegalovirus retinitis is one of the most serious and frequent ophthalmologic complications of HIV infection, occurring in 15 to 40 percent of persons diagnosed with AIDS and often causing monocular or binocular blindness [65]. Cytomegalovirus infection manifests as perivascular yellow or white lesions, usually associated with areas of hemorrhage (see Plate 8). In contrast to the smooth, homogeneous appearance of cotton wool patches, CMV retinitis is patchy or "chunky," and has been described as resembling "scrambled eggs and ketchup." Early CMV disease may be limited to the periphery of the retina and be observable only on indirect, dilated examination. HIV-infected patients who are noted to have any retinal lesions should be evaluated by an ophthalmologist, as should individuals with new visual symptoms, such as "floaters," decreased acuity, or flashing bright lights.

Cardiopulmonary System
While cardiopulmonary examination is often nonspecific, several HIV-related conditions may result in characteristic physical findings [66]. *Pneumocystis carinii* pneumonia may be accompanied by dry basilar rales and is occasionally associated with malar rash and arthropathy. Pulmonary KS may present with pleural effusion, frequently unilateral, manifested by decreased breath sounds and dullness to percussion. Congestive cardiomyopathy can result from HIV infection, antiretroviral agents, or opportunistic infections such as PCP or toxoplasmosis [67, 68]. Bacteremia from intravascular devices occurs with increased frequency in this population [69, 70]. If valvular disease develops as a complication of bacteremia, characteristic signs of endocarditis may be present.

Abdomen
Hepatic tenderness or enlargement may signify infiltration with opportunistic infection or tumor, or the presence of viral hepatitis. Splenomegaly may be due to tumor, bacterial or mycobacterial abscess, or disseminated *P. carinii* infection. Abdominal masses may result from lymphoma, KS, or involvement of mesenteric nodes with *Mycobacterium avium* complex (MAC) or other opportunistic infections.

Rectum
Genital warts and HSV infection are the most frequently encountered perirectal pathology; KS, candidiasis, or psoriasis may also be seen. Anal cancers in this population are generally palpable on digital examination and may be tender and friable. They develop in squamous epithelium between the anal verge and the dentate line.

Genitourinary Tract
Recurrent vaginal candidiasis, HSV infection, and pelvic inflammatory disease (PID) occur with increased frequency in HIV-infected women [71–73]. Candidal and herpetic infections are prone to relapse and may require chronic suppressive therapy. Human papillomavirus infection in the setting of HIV-induced immune suppression can also lead to the development of cervical dysplasia and cancer, which may be more aggressive in this population [74].

Nervous System

During the neurologic examination, particular attention should be paid to the patient's mental status. However, screening mental status examinations may not be sensitive for early HIV encephalopathy. Patients with complaints of decreased concentration or memory may require formal neuropsychological testing. Other neurologic abnormalities may include cranial and peripheral nerve palsies, painful peripheral neuropathy, or focal motor deficits caused by intracranial mass lesions or spinal cord involvement by HIV or CMV [75, 76].

Laboratory Evaluation

Baseline laboratory evaluation is important in screening for systemic disease and monitoring for drug toxicity (Table 29-3).

Complete Blood Count

A complete blood and differential count should be performed on all patients. Cytopenia may occur without symptoms and should prompt appropriate evaluation. Anemia, thrombocytopenia, and/or leukopenia may be caused by HIV-induced marrow suppression, antiviral therapy, or infiltration of the marrow by infection or tumor; thrombocytopenia and leukopenia may also be mediated by autoantibody production.

Liver Function Tests and Hepatitis Serologies

Liver function tests and HBV serologies should be obtained on all patients. Sexually active homosexual men and injection drug users (IDUs) are at increased risk for HBV infection, and many patients require treatment with potentially hepatotoxic drugs. An isolated increased serum alkaline phosphatase may suggest infiltration of the liver by tuberculosis or MAC. Hepatitis C virus (HCV) infection may result in chronic active hepatitis, and antibody to HCV has been identified in many HIV-infected patients [77].

Syphilis Serology

Syphilis may progress more rapidly, be more resistant to standard therapies, be more prone to reactivation, and be more difficult to detect by standard serologic testing in HIV-infected individuals [78–83]. Baseline screening for syphilis and annual retesting are warranted in all patients, and central nervous system involvement should be considered in anyone with a positive syphilis serology.

Tuberculosis Testing

Tuberculosis presents more frequently as extrapulmonary disease in HIV-infected patients [84–86]. Because skin testing depends on intact

Table 29-3 Baseline laboratory evaluation of the HIV-infected patient

Complete blood and differential counts
Liver function tests
Hepatitis B virus serologies
Syphilis serology
PPD and anergy panel
Chest x-ray
Urinalysis
Renal function tests
(?) Toxoplasmosis serology
(?) Serum cryptococcal antigen
Glucose 6-phosphate dehydrogenase
CD4 cell count

cell-mediated immunity, anergy is more common with advanced immunosuppression. For this reason, induration of 5 mm or more in response to an intermediate-strength purified protein derivative (PPD) is considered positive in HIV-infected patients [87]. Since the risk of developing active tuberculosis in this population is greater than that of developing isoniazid hepatitis, a positive PPD is an indication for prophylactic therapy in the previously untreated individual regardless of age and timing of PPD conversion. Isoniazid prophylaxis for one year should also be given to anergic HIV-seropositive patients at high risk for TB, including IDUs, the homeless, prisoners, alcoholics, immigrants from endemic countries, and those with recent TB exposure [88].

Chest X-Ray
A screening chest x-ray may be helpful in detecting the subtle changes of early PCP at a future time. For this reason, it is desirable, especially in the patient with a history of cigarette smoking or injection drug use, to obtain a baseline x-ray. Asymptomatic hilar adenopathy due to MAC, histoplasmosis, tuberculosis, cryptococcosis, or lymphoma may also be detected on screening radiographs.

Urinalysis and Renal Function Tests
HIV-related renal disease, including focal and segmental glomerulosclerosis, may be identified on baseline urinalysis and renal function tests [89, 90]. Many drugs used in the management of HIV disease require dosage adjustment in the presence of renal dysfunction.

Toxoplasma Serology
Some authors have recommended that Toxoplasma antibody titers be obtained as part of the baseline evaluation of HIV-infected patients. This

information may have value in selecting patients for prophylaxis (should this become routine practice) and for identifying patients at risk for developing active disease.

Serum Cryptococcal Antigen
Serum assay for polysaccharide capsule antigens of *Cryptococcus neoformans* has been reported to be 99 percent sensitive in detecting meningitis [91]. However, routine serum antigen screening of asymptomatic individuals is of little clinical utility at present.

Glucose 6-Phosphate Dehydrogenase (G6PD)
Patients for whom dapsone has been prescribed for PCP treatment or prophylaxis should be screened for the presence of G6PD deficiency before initiation of therapy.

HIV Disease Staging

A number of clinical and laboratory variables are useful in staging HIV infection. Staging guides decisions regarding antiretroviral and PCP prophylactic therapies, provides prognostic information, and helps to focus differential diagnosis for specific clinical problems.

Laboratory Tests

CD4 Cell Count
CD4 cell counts are highly correlated with the progression of HIV disease. While the normal CD4 count ranges between $1,300/mm^3$ and $430/mm^3$, it is generally above $800/mm^3$ in healthy persons [92]. CD4 cell counts have been shown to decrease by 50 to 85 cells/mm^3/yr in HIV-infected individuals, although one study has suggested that this decline may be as low as 15 cells/mm^3/yr in IDUs [93–95]. While opportunistic infections do not usually occur with CD4 counts between $800/mm^3$ and $400/mm^3$, HSV, VZV, thrush, and fungal or bacterial infections of the skin may be seen with counts below $400/mm^3$ (Fig. 29-1). A CD4 count of less than $200/mm^3$ indicates severe immune suppression, with increased risk for serious opportunistic infections, such as PCP, toxoplasmosis, and cryptococcal meningitis. Patients with counts of less than $50–100/mm^3$ are also at risk for CMV and MAC infections, and for lymphoma. It is important to remember, however, that many patients with very low CD4 counts may be symptom free for months to a year or more [96].

Some investigators have suggested that the percentage of total lymphocytes that are CD4 cells may provide a more reliable indication of

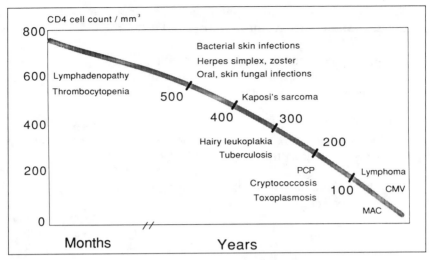

Figure 29-1. *Relationship of CD4 cell count to clinical manifestations of HIV infection.*

immune function than the absolute CD4 cell count [97]. However, current Centers for Disease Control (CDC) recommendations for instituting PCP prophylaxis do not include a CD4 percentage criterion [98].

Obtaining reliable CD4 counts is not always easily accomplished [99]. Since CD4 counts have a diurnal variation in most individuals, serial samples should be obtained at approximately the same time of day. Intercurrent illnesses, especially herpesvirus infections, may cause transient CD4 cell count depression. Since inter- and intralaboratory variation in test results may occur, it is wise to confirm the initial CD4 count and any subsequent values that are grossly different from baseline, especially if such results would lead to new therapeutic interventions.

p24 Antigenemia

The *gag* gene of HIV codes for a nuclear protein of 24 daltons known as the p24 antigen. p24 Antigenemia has been correlated with active viral replication and progression of HIV disease, and a decline in p24 antigen level implies the effectiveness of antiretroviral therapy [100].

β_2-Microglobulin

β_2-Microglobulin is a low molecular weight globulin that forms part of the class 1 histocompatibility complex present on most somatic cells. β_2-Microglobulin levels correlate with increased cell death and reflect the general level of lymphoid activation; they are increased in the presence of viral infections and hematologic malignancies. β_2-Microglobulin levels greater than 5 μg/ml are associated with progression of HIV disease [101, 102]. Despite being a relatively inexpensive assay, β_2-microglobulin testing is not available in many clinical settings. β_2-Microglobulin levels may be elevated among IDUs without HIV infection, decreasing the assay's usefulness in HIV-infected drug users [103].

Neopterin

Macrophages increase their production of neopterin, a metabolite of guanosine triphosphate, under the influence of gamma-interferon secreted from activated T cells. Elevated serum or urinary neopterin levels in HIV-infected patients have a prognostic value that is independent of CD4 cell count [104–106].

Use of Staging Laboratory Tests

In general, CD4 cell counts and percentages are adequate for staging patients. If disease progression appears to occur despite antiretroviral treatment, as assessed by clinical manifestations or decline in CD4 count, p24 antigen, β_2-microglobulin, or neopterin levels may provide useful complementary data.

Clinical Markers of Disease Progression

Information from a number of natural history studies suggests that certain clinical markers may identify patients at risk for disease progression. Being at either end of the age spectrum of HIV disease appears to confer a negative prognosis, as does the presence of systemic symptoms, hairy leukoplakia, thrush, anemia, or leukopenia. Neither VZV infection nor generalized lymphadenopathy suggests a poor prognosis, although previously swollen nodes that involute may signal a decline in immune function. There are conflicting data regarding the prognostic significance of thrombocytopenia [107–114].

Stratified Management of HIV Infection

CD4 Cell Count Greater than 500/mm³

Antiretroviral therapy should only be considered in patients who have constitutional symptoms, encephalopathy, or thrombocytopenia [115] (Table 29-4). Asymptomatic patients should be seen every 3 to 4 months. Although there are few medical interventions to offer, patients may greatly benefit from education about their disease, emotional support, and routine health care maintenance.

Table 29-4 Stratified management of HIV infection

CD4 cell count > 500/mm³
    No specific therapy
    Focus on patient education and health care maintenance issues
    Follow-up visits q3–4mo
    Repeat CD4 counts q6mo
CD4 cell count of 500–200/mm³
    Offer antiretroviral therapy with ZDV
    Follow-up visits q1–2mo
    Repeat CD4 counts q3mo
CD4 cell count of 200–50/mm³
    Add *Pneumocystis carinii* prophylaxis
    Consider switching patients receiving ZDV to another antiretroviral agent
    Close surveillance for opportunistic infections
    Follow-up visits monthly
    Repeat CD4 counts q3mo
CD4 cell count < 50/mm³
    Consider further modification of antiretroviral regimen
    Close surveillance for CMV, MAC, and lymphoma
    Follow-up visits q1–4wk
    Repeat CD4 counts unnecessary

CD4 Cell Count Between 500 and 200/mm³

Patients in this group should be offered ZDV therapy [116]. Follow-up visits should be scheduled at 1- to 2-month intervals, with careful attention to monitoring for antiretroviral drug toxicity.

CD4 Cell Count Less than 200/mm³

This group (recently included in the Centers for Disease Control case definition of AIDS [117]), is at greatest risk for serious opportunistic infections or tumors, and should be seen at monthly intervals. If there is evidence of disease progression on ZDV, consideration should be given to changing the antiretroviral regimen (see following section). Prophylaxis for PCP should be initiated once the CD4 cell count falls below 200/mm³; it is also indicated in patients with a prior history of PCP and in those with counts above 200/mm³ who have thrush or persistent unexplained fever [99].

CD4 Cell Count Less than 50/mm³

Patients in this group are at increased risk for death [118, 119]. They should be monitored carefully for CMV and MAC infections, and for lymphoma. Initiation of rifabutin prophylaxis for MAC infection should be considered (see Chap. 18).

Approach to Antiretroviral Therapy

At present, ZDV is the first-line antiretroviral agent (see Table 28-3). A total daily dose of 500 to 600 mg per day should be administered as one 100-mg capsule five times a day or two capsules three times a day. Headache and nausea, which may occur with initiation of therapy, can be minimized by gradually increasing the dose over a week or more and by using analgesics and antiemetics as needed. Chronic toxicities include bone marrow suppression, myositis, and, rarely, liver function test abnormalities. Patients in whom anemia or neutropenia develops on ZDV can be treated with colony stimulating factors, such as erythropoietin or granulocyte colony stimulating factor (G-CSF), or switched to another agent. Patients receiving ZDV who have evidence of disease progression manifested by the development of an opportunistic infection or decline in CD4 cell count should be considered for other antiretroviral regimens.

The antiretroviral agent didanosine (ddI) has been approved for clinical use based on preliminary evidence showing a rise in CD4 cell counts and symptomatic improvement during short-term use. Results from a recently completed clinical trial indicate that symptomatic patients receiving ZDV benefit from switching to ddI when their CD4 cell count falls to $300/mm^3$ or lower and asymptomatic patients benefit once their CD4 count is $200/mm^3$ or below [120].

Didanosine dosing is calculated by weight (125–200 mg orally twice a day), with all patients taking two tablets at each dose in order to receive an adequate amount of incorporated antacid. Didanosine should be administered 1 hour before or 2 hours after eating to maximize absorption. Tablets must be chewed or predissolved in water but should not be swallowed whole. Didanosine may interfere with absorption of dapsone if the two drugs are taken simultaneously. The principal toxicities of ddI are peripheral neuropathy and pancreatitis, and therapy should be discontinued if either develops. Neuropathy is generally reversible once the agent is stopped and may not recur if it is resumed at a lower dose. Serum amylase or lipase levels should be evaluated periodically to detect asymptomatic pancreatitis.

Although dideoxycytidine (ddC) does not appear to have a role as initial monotherapy for HIV infection, combination therapy with ZDV and ddC has recently been approved for patients who have advanced disease with significant clinical or immunologic deterioration on ZDV alone. This recommendation was based on a study indicating that patients who received both drugs had better CD4 cell count responses than those who received monotherapy with either drug [121]. The principal toxicities of ddC are gastrointestinal ulcerations and dysfunctions, and peripheral neuropathy. When used in combination, the recommended doses are ZDV, 200 mg/ddC, 0.750 mg, each three times a day. Patients who experience anemia or neutropenia should be treated with colony stimulating factors or have their ZDV dose reduced or the drug discontinued; those in whom gastrointestinal dysfunction or peripheral neuropathy develops should have their ddC therapy stopped and reintroduced at a lower dose after symptoms have resolved.

Approach to Pneumocystis *Pneumonia Prophylaxis*

Data continue to accrue regarding the relative efficacy of various prophylactic regimens in different patient populations. Based on the results of a trial comparing trimethoprim-sulfamethoxazole (TMP-SMZ) with aerosol pentamidine (AP) as secondary prophylaxis, the CDC has recommended that oral TMP-SMZ is the drug of choice to prevent PCP [98] (see Fig. 17-3). While TMP-SMZ, one double-strength tablet daily, is suggested, one published series of patients with CD4 counts less than $200/mm^3$ experienced no breakthrough infections using one double-strength tablet three times a week [122]. Patients can be rechallenged with TMP-SMZ if a mild reaction develops, but those with major toxicity should either be treated with AP or desensitized using gradually increasing doses of TMP-SMZ. Patients receiving AP in whom an adverse reaction or breakthrough disease develops should be managed with dapsone, intravenous pentamidine, or Fansidar.

Other Considerations in Clinical Management

Substance Abuse Issues

Many HIV-infected patients have a history of substance abuse involving alcohol, cocaine, crack, or opiates. Clinicians should recognize that the stress of being seropositive or of developing symptomatic disease may lead to substance abuse recidivism. Maintenance of sobriety is a key component of comprehensive care, and, in some situations, substance abuse treatment may be a higher priority than care for HIV infection, since the latter may be impossible or ineffectual in the context of active drug use.

Psychosocial Support

Informing clients about support groups and AIDS service organizations available within the community is another important aspect of primary care. "Buddies" available through many service organizations can provide long-term emotional support that may otherwise be unavailable to patients who have been estranged from family or the community at large.

Personal Finances

Initial assessment of the patient's financial situation and insurance status should also be part of the intake process, with attention given to ascertaining eligibility for entitlement programs for health care, general relief, disability, and housing.

Legal Issues

A variety of legal issues can take on dramatic significance for those with life-threatening HIV disease, especially when the patient is a single parent or involved in a nontraditional relationship such as a long-term homosexual union. Making provision for substituted judgment by executing an advanced directive for health care or durable power of attorney and attending to custody arrangements are important issues that patients face. Many AIDS service organizations provide legal services to help patients draw up legal instruments and deal with custody issues.

Food Safety

Caution in food preparation and handling is important given the vulnerability to infections that accompanies immunosuppression. Using a plastic or glass instead of wooden cutting board may decrease the chance of bacterial contamination. Microwaved foods, especially poultry, should be allowed to stand for a few minutes after cooking to ensure that heat is evenly distributed. Because of the risk of salmonellosis, raw egg products should not be consumed. Raw seafood (sashimi, sushi, oysters) or meat (steak tartare) should also be avoided because of potential transmission of bacterial and protozoal pathogens.

Pet Safety

Pets can be an important source of companionship, affection, and comfort for HIV-infected patients [123]. While a few animals may present a risk for acquiring particular infections, most domestic pets can be cared for safely if common sense guidelines are followed (Table 29-5).

Health Care Maintenance in HIV Infection

The provision of primary care to HIV-infected patients includes routine health care maintenance, as well as vaccination and screening examination protocols adapted to this population. A suggested health care maintenance regimen is presented in Table 29-6.

Table 29-5 Pet care guidelines

General pet hygiene
    Wash hands frequently after animal contact
    Use gloves when changing litter box or cleaning aquarium
    Keep the pet's living and feeding area clean, and control fleas
    Avoid contact with a pet's body fluids
Cats
    Cats can carry toxoplasmosis and transmit it through contact with feces or cat
      litter
    Keep cat litter boxes away from kitchen and eating areas and change the litter
      box daily, using care to avoid inhalation of dust particles
    Disinfect the litter box at least once a month
Preventive veterinary medicine
    Keep vaccinations current
    Take pets in for a routine examination at least once a year
    Contact a veterinarian if the animal shows signs of possible illness
    Have all new pets examined by a veterinarian to screen for diseases and
      parasites
Animal bites
    Tend to any animal bites immediately to help prevent infection by rinsing with
      cold running water
    Disinfect with a preparation such as Betadine solution
    After first aid, always contact your physician

Source: Modified from Pets Are Wonderful Support (PAWS), *Safe Pet Guidelines*. Education Department, PO Box 460489, San Francisco, CA 94146-0489 (telephone: 415-824-4040).

Periodic Physical Examination

Pelvic Examination

As was previously noted, HIV-infected women with HPV infection may be at increased risk for cervical cancer. At least one study has suggested that Papanicolaou smears may be relatively insensitive for the detection of cervical dysplasia in this population, and its authors advocate the routine use of colposcopy [124]. However, this finding has not been confirmed by others, and the CDC currently recommends only annual Pap smears [125]. We suggest Pap smears twice each year to HIV-infected women at our institution, with colposcopic evaluation of any suspicious lesions.

Rectal Examination

Patients with a history of receptive anal intercourse or anogenital condylomas should have surveillance rectal examinations performed regularly.

Table 29-6 HIV routine health care maintenance schedule

Issue	Intake	Semiannually	Annually
Pneumococcal vaccine	X		
Hepatitis B vaccine	X[a]		
Influenza vaccine			X
Haemophilus vaccine	X		
Rectal examination	X		X[b]
Breast examination	X[c]		X[c]
Syphilis serology	X		X
Chlamydia/gonorrhea	X		X
Pap smear	X[c]	X[c]	
Mammography	X[c,d]		X[c,d]
PPD, controls	X		X[e]
Patient education	X	X	
Mental health assessment	X		
Addiction assessment	X		

[a]HBV-seronegative patients.
[b]Patients with a history of receptive anal intercourse and/or HPV infection.
[c]Women only.
[d]Baseline at age 35–40; annually after the age of 40 or 50.
[e]PPD-negative or previously anergic patients with improved CD4 cell counts.

Immunizations

Overview

Ensuring that appropriate immunizations are administered constitutes an important part of routine health care for HIV-infected patients (Table 29-7). Because diminished antibody production in response to vaccination is associated with profound immunosuppression, immunizations should be administered as early in the course of HIV disease as possible.

Questions regarding safety of live-virus vaccines in HIV-infected persons were raised in 1987, when disseminated vaccinia developed in an asymptomatic, seropositive military recruit after the administration of smallpox vaccine [126, 127]. Disseminated mycobacterial disease has also been reported following bacillus Calmette-Guérin (BCG) vaccination in two symptomatic HIV-infected adults [128, 129]. However, these cases appear to represent the only observed serious morbidity from live viral vaccination of HIV-infected patients reported to date.

Influenza Vaccine

Although yearly immunization with influenza vaccine has been recommended for HIV-infected persons, diminished antibody response has been associated with advanced immunosuppression [130]. In one

Table 29-7 Immunization guidelines for HIV-infected patients

Vaccine	Children	Adults
DPT	Yes	Td preparation
OPV	No	No
e-IPV	Yes	No
MMR	Yes	Yes
HbCV	Yes	Yes
Hepatitis B	Yes	Yes
Influenza	Yes	Yes
Pneumococcal	Yes	Yes
BCG	Yes	Yes

DPT = diphtheria-pertussis-tetanus; Td = diphtheria-tetanus; OPV = oral poliovirus vaccine; e-IPV = enhanced inactivated polio vaccine; MMR = measles-mumps-rubella; HbCV = *Haemophilus influenzae* type b conjugate vaccine; BCG = bacillus Calmette-Guérin.
Source: Adapted from DE Craven et al., Immunization of adults and children infected with human immunodeficiency virus. *Infect Dis Clin Prac* 1:330–338, 411–423, 1992; American College of Physicians Task Force on Adult Immunization and Infectious Disease Society of America, *Guide for Adult Immunization* (2nd ed), 1990; Centers for Disease Control, Update of adult immunization: Recommendations of the Immunization Practices Advisory Committee. *MMWR* 40:1–94, 1991; and American Academy of Pediatrics, *Report of the Committee on Infectious Diseases* (22nd ed), 1991.

study, 94 to 100 percent of seronegative control subjects had an adequate antibody response, compared to 52 to 89 percent of asymptomatic seropositive individuals and 13 to 50 percent of those with advanced HIV disease [131].

Pneumococcal Vaccine
Pneumococcal pneumonia and bacteremia have been shown to occur with increased frequency in HIV-infected patients [132, 133]. Pneumococcal vaccine is recommended for persons who are predisposed to bacteremic pneumococcal disease if they are capable of producing an antibody response [134]. Although some studies have described impaired responsiveness to pneumococcal vaccine in symptomatic HIV disease, others have suggested that, at least in asymptomatic seropositive individuals and those with mild HIV-related symptoms, adequate antibody response is achievable [135–137].

Haemophilus Influenzae, *Type B*, Vaccine
Because patients with HIV infection are at increased risk for bacteremia infection with *H. influenzae*, routine use of *H. influenzae* vaccine has been advocated for this population [138].

29. Ambulatory Management of HIV Infection   413

Measles-Mumps-Rubella Vaccine (MMR)

Six fatal cases of measles in unvaccinated HIV-infected children have been reported to the CDC, suggesting that the risk of life-threatening measles in unvaccinated HIV-infected patients appears more likely than the development of disease as a result of vaccination [139]. MMR is given at the usual ages for all asymptomatic HIV-infected children and should be considered in those who are symptomatic.

Polio Vaccine

Oral poliovirus vaccine (OPV) results in shedding of live virus. Although vaccination-related paralytic poliomyelitis is rare (1 in 2.6–4.3 million doses), most recent cases of polio in the United States have resulted from vaccination [140, 141]. Despite this risk, administration of OPV to many HIV-infected children in Europe and the US has not resulted in adverse reactions [142]. Nevertheless, to minimize the possibility of causing active disease, enhanced inactivated polio vaccine (e-IPV) should be used instead of OPV to immunize HIV-infected children and their household contacts [143]. Adults who were not vaccinated as children do not need to be immunized.

Hepatitis B Vaccine

Some decreased responsiveness to antibody production following vaccination with hepatitis B vaccine has been noted in the HIV-infected population [144, 145]. Nevertheless, patients who are hepatitis B surface antigen and antibody negative and remain at risk for acquiring HBV should be considered for vaccination [146].

Tetanus Toxoid

No adverse reactions to the administration of tetanus toxoid have been reported among HIV-infected children or adults. Current recommendations are for children to receive the usual sequence of diphtheria-pertussis-tetanus (DPT) injections; a booster dose (Td) should be administered to adults every 10 years.

References

1. Gabel RH, Barnard N, Norko M, O'Connel RA. AIDS presenting as mania. *Compr Psychiatry* 27:251–254, 1986.
2. Jones GH, Kelly CL, Davies JA. HIV and onset of schizophrenia. *Lancet* 1:982, 1987.
3. Perry S, Jacobsen P. Neuropsychiatric manifestations of AIDS-spectrum disorders. *Hosp Community Psychiatry* 37:135–142, 1986.

4. Maccario M, Scharre DW. HIV and acute onset of psychosis. *Lancet* 2:342, 1987.
5. Berman A, Espinoza LR, Diax JD, et al. Rheumatic manifestations of human immunodeficiency virus infection. *Am J Med* 85:59–64, 1988.
6. Buskila D, Gladman D. Musculoskeletal manifestations of infection with human immunodeficiency virus. *Rev Infect Dis* 12:223–235, 1990.
7. Fuente C, Velez A, Martin N, et al. Reiter's syndrome and human immunodeficiency virus infection: Case report and review of the literature. *Cutis* 47:181–185, 1991.
8. Foreman J. Suicides raise questions on AIDS testing. *The Boston Globe* February 2, 1987.
9. Glass RM. AIDS and suicide. *JAMA* 259:1369–1370, 1988.
10. Goldblum P, Moulton J. AIDS-related suicide: A dilemma for health care providers. *Focus* 2:1–2, 1986.
11. Marzuk PM, Tierney H, Tardiff K, Mann J, et al. Increased risk of suicide in persons with AIDS. *JAMA* 259:1333–1337, 1989.
12. Pierce C. Suicides underscore urgency of HIV test counseling. *Fam Pract News* 17:16, 1987.
13. Tyson E, Fortenberry JD. Fraudulent AIDS: A variant of Munchausen's syndrome. *JAMA* 258:1889–1890, 1987.
14. Evans GA, Gill MJ, Gerhart S. Factitious AIDS. *N Engl J Med* 319:1605–1606, 1988.
15. Levine SS. An AIDS diagnosis used as focus of malingering. *West J Med* 148:337–338, 1988.
16. Daling JR, Weiss NS, Hislop G, et al. Sexual practices, sexually transmitted diseases, and the incidence of anal cancer. *N Engl J Med* 317:973–977, 1987.
17. Enck RE. Squamous cell cancers and the acquired immunodeficiency syndrome. *Ann Intern Med* 106:773, 1987.
18. Overly WL, Jakubek DJ. Multiple squamous cell carcinomas and human immunodeficiency virus infection. *Ann Intern Med* 102:334, 1987.
19. Sonnex C, Mindel A. Sexual practices, sexually transmitted diseases, and the incidence of anal cancer. *N Engl J Med* 318:990, 1988.
20. Bodsworth N, Donovan B, Nightingale BN. The effect of concurrent human immunodeficiency virus infection on chronic hepatitis B: A study of 150 homosexual men. *J Infect Dis* 160:577–582, 1989.
21. Bodsworth NJ, Cooper DA, Donovan B. The influence of human immunodeficiency virus type 1 infection on the development of the hepatitis B virus carrier state. *J Infect Dis* 163:1138–1140, 1991.
22. Vento S, Di Perri G, Luzzati R, et al. Clinical reactivation of hepatitis B in anti-HBs–positive patients with AIDS. *Lancet* 1:332–333, 1989.
23. Selwyn PA, Hartel D, Lewis VA, et al. A prospective study of the risk of tuberculosis among intravenous drug users with human immunodeficiency virus infection. *N Engl J Med* 320:545–550, 1989.
24. Furth PA. Megestrol acetate and cachexia associated with human immunodeficiency virus (HIV) infection. *Ann Intern Med* 110:667, 1989.
25. Von Roenn JH, Murphy RL, Weber KM, et al. Megestrol acetate for treat-

ment of cachexia associated with human immunodeficiency virus (HIV) infection. *Ann Intern Med* 109:840–841, 1988.

26. Gold JWM, Weikel CS, Godbold J, et al. Unexplained persistent lymph-adenopathy in homosexual men and the acquired immune deficiency syndrome. *Medicine* 64:203–213, 1985.

27. Abrams DI. AIDS-related lymphadenopathy: The role of biopsy. *J Clin Oncol* 4:126–127, 1986.

28. Libman H. Generalized lymphadenopathy. *J Gen Intern Med* 2:48–58, 1987.

29. Koehler JE, LeBoit PE, Egbert BM, Berger TG. Cutaneous vascular lesions and disseminated cat-scratch disease in patients with the acquired immunodeficiency syndrome (AIDS) and AIDS-related complex. *Ann Intern Med* 109:449–455, 1988.

30. Marasco WA, Lester S, Parsonnet J. Unusual presentation of cat scratch disease in a patient positive for antibody to the human immunodeficiency virus. *Rev Infect Dis* 11:793–804, 1989.

31. Denning DW, Anderson J, Rudge P, Smith H. Acute myelopathy associated with primary infection with human immunodeficiency virus. *Br Med J* 143–144, 1987.

32. Goudsmit J, De Wolf F, Paul DA, et al. Expression of human immunodeficiency virus antigen (HIV-Ag) in serum and cerebrospinal fluid during acute and chronic infection. *Lancet* 2:177–180, 1986.

33. Dalakas MC, Illa I, Pezeshkpour GH, et al. Mitochondrial myopathy caused by long-term zidovudine therapy. *N Engl J Med* 322:1098–1105, 1990.

34. Arnaudo E, Dalakas M, Shanske S, et al. Depletion of muscle mitochondrial DNA in AIDS patients with zidovudine-induced myopathy. *Lancet* 337:508–510, 1991.

35. Simms RW, Zerbini CAF, Ferrante N, et al. Fibromyalgia syndrome in patients infected with human immunodeficiency virus. *Am J Med* 92:368–374, 1992.

36. Eisenstat BA, Wormser GP. Seborrheic dermatitis and butterfly rash in AIDS. *N Engl J Med* 311:189, 1984.

37. Johnson TM, Duvic M, Rapini RP, et al. AIDS exacerbates psoriasis. *N Engl J Med* 313:1415, 1985.

38. Fuchs D, Hausen A, Reibnegger G, et al. Psoriasis, gamma-interferon, and the acquired immunodeficiency syndrome. *Ann Intern Med* 106:165, 1987.

39. Duvic M, Rios A, Brewton GW. Remission of AIDS-associated psoriasis with zidovudine. *Lancet* 2:627, 1987.

40. Ruzicka T, Froschl M, Hohenleutner U. Treatment of HIV-induced retinoid-resistant psoriasis with zidovudine. *Lancet* 2:1469–1470, 1987.

41. Soeprono FF, Schinella RA. Eosinophilic pustular folliculitis in patients with acquired immunodeficiency syndrome. *J Am Acad Dermatol* 14:1020–1022, 1986.

42. Buchness MR, Lim HW, Hatcher VA, et al. Eosinophilic pustular folliculitis in the acquired immunodeficiency syndrome: Treatment with ultraviolet B phototherapy. *N Engl J Med* 318:1183–1186, 1988.

43. Jacobson MA, Gellermann H, Chambers H. *Staphylococcus aureus* bacteremia and recurrent staphylococcal infection in patients with acquired immunodeficiency syndrome and AIDS-related complex. *Am J Med* 85:172–176, 1988.

44. Furth PA, Kazakis AM. Nail pigmentation changes associated with azidothymidine (zidovudine). *Ann Intern Med* 107:350, 1987.

45. Panwalker AP. Nail pigmentation in the acquired immunodeficiency syndrome (AIDS). *Ann Intern Med* 107:943–944, 1987.

46. Vaiopoulos G, Mangakis J, Karabinis A, et al. Nail pigmentation and azidothymidine. *Ann Intern Med* 108:777, 1988.

47. Friedman-Kien AE, Lafleur FL, Gendler E. Herpes zoster: A possible early clinical sign for development of acquired immunodeficiency syndrome in high-risk individuals. *J Am Acad Dermatol* 14:1023–1028, 1986.

48. Sandor EV, Millman A, Croxson TS, et al. Herpes zoster ophthalmicus in patients at risk for the acquired immunodeficiency syndrome (AIDS). *Am J Ophthalmol* 101:153–155, 1986.

49. Ryder JW, Croen K, Kleinschmidt-DeMaster K. Progressive encephalitis three months after resolution of cutaneous zoster in a patient with AIDS. *Ann Neurol* 19:182–188, 1986.

50. Cohen PR, Beltrani VP, Grossman ME. Disseminated herpes zoster in patients with human immunodeficiency virus infection. *Am J Med* 84:1076–1080, 1988.

51. Perniciaro C, Peters MS. Tinea faciale mimicking seborrheic dermatitis in a patient with AIDS. *N Engl J Med* 314:315–316, 1986.

52. Oral viral lesion (hairy leukoplakia) associated with acquired immunodeficiency syndrome. *MMWR* 34:549–550, 1985.

53. Greenspan JS, Greenspan D, Lennette ET, et al. Replication of Epstein-Barr virus within the epithelial cells of oral "hairy" leukoplakia, an AIDS-associated lesion. *N Engl J Med* 313:1564–1571, 1985.

54. Friedman-Kien AE. Viral origin of hairy leukoplakia. *Lancet* 2:694, 1986.

55. Greenspan D, Greenspan JS, Hearts NG, et al. Relation of oral hairy leukoplakia to infection with the human immunodeficiency virus and the risk of developing AIDS. *J Infect Dis* 155:475–481, 1987.

56. Greenspan JS, Greenspan D, Winkler JR. Diagnosis and management of the Oral Manifestations of HIV Infection and AIDS. In MA Sande, PA Volberding (eds), *The Medical Management of AIDS.* Philadelphia: Saunders, 1988. P 131.

57. Krause PR, Straus SE. Zoster and its complications. *Hosp Pract,* 25:61–76, 1990.

58. Centers for Disease Control. Microsporidian keratoconjunctivitis in patients with AIDS. *MMWR* 39:188–189, 1990.

59. Sneed SR, Blodi CF, Berger BB, et al. *Pneumocystis carinii* choroiditis in patients receiving inhaled pentamidine. *N Engl J Med* 322:936–937, 1990.

60. Cantrill HL, Henry K, Sannerud K, Balfour HH. HIV infection of the retina. *N Engl J Med* 318:1539, 1988.

61. Pomerantz RJ, Kuritzkes DR, De la Monte SM, et al. Infection of the retina by human immunodeficiency virus type 1. *N Engl J Med* 317:1643–1647, 1987.

62. Holland GN, Pepose JS, Pettit TH, et al. Acquired immune deficiency syndrome: Ocular manifestations. *Ophthalmology* 90:859–873, 1983.
63. Mines JA, Kaplan HJ. Acquired immunodeficiency syndrome (AIDS): The disease and its ocular manifestations. *Int Ophthalmol Clin* 26:73–115, 1986.
64. Freeman WR, Chen A, Henderly DE, et al. Prevalence and significance of acquired immunodeficiency syndrome–related microvasculopathy. *Am J Ophthalmol* 107:229–235, 1990.
65. Bloom JN, Palestine AG. The diagnosis of cytomegalovirus retinitis. *Ann Intern Med* 109:963–969, 1988.
66. Acierno LJ. Cardiac complications in acquired immunodeficiency syndrome (AIDS): A review. *J Am Coll Cardiol* 13:1144–1154, 1989.
67. Herskowitz A, et al. Cardiomyopathy associated with antiretroviral therapy in patients with HIV infection: A report of six cases. *Ann Intern Med* 116:311–313, 1992.
68. Calabrese LH, Proffitt MR, Yen-Lieberman B, et al. Congestive cardiomyopathy and illness related to the acquired immunodeficiency syndrome (AIDS) associated with isolation of retrovirus from myocardium. *Ann Intern Med* 107:691–692, 1987.
69. Raviglione MC, Battan R, Pablos-Mendez A, et al. Infections associated with Hickman catheters in patients with acquired immunodeficiency syndrome. *Am J Med* 86:780–786, 1989.
70. Skoutelis AT, Murphy RL, MacDonell KB, et al. Indwelling central venous catheter infections in patients with acquired immune deficiency syndrome. *J AIDS* 3:335–342, 1990.
71. Hankins CA. Issues involving women, children, and AIDS primarily in the developed world. *J AIDS* 3:443–448, 1990.
72. Imam N, Carpenter CCJ, Mayer KH, et al. Hierarchical pattern of mucosal candida infections in HIV-seropositive women. *Am J Med* 89:142–146, 1990.
73. Rhoads JL, Wright DC, Redfield RR, Burke DS. Chronic vaginal candidiasis in women with human immunodeficiency virus infection. *JAMA* 257:3105–3107, 1987.
74. Centers for Disease Control. Risk for cervical disease in HIV-infected women—New York City. *MMWR* 39:846–849, 1990.
75. Petito CK, Navia BA, Cho ES, et al. Vacuolar myelopathy pathologically resembling subacute combined degeneration in patients with the acquired immunodeficiency syndrome. *N Engl J Med* 312:874–879, 1985.
76. Singh BM, Levine S, Yarrish RL, et al. Spinal cord syndromes in the acquired immune deficiency syndrome. *Acta Neurol Scand* 73:590–598, 1986.
77. Sherman KE, Freeman S, Harrison S, Andron L. Prevalence of antibody to hepatitis C virus in patients infected with the human immunodeficiency virus. *J Infect Dis* 163:414, 1991.
78. Tramont EC. Syphilis in the AIDS era. *N Engl J Med* 316:1600–1601, 1987.
79. Berry CD, Hooton TM, Collier AC, et al. Neurologic relapse after benzathine penicillin therapy for secondary syphilis in a patient with HIV infection. *N Engl J Med* 316:1587–1589, 1987.

80. Johns DR, Tierney M, Felsenstein D. Alteration in the natural history of neurosyphilis by concurrent infection with the human immunodeficiency virus. *N Engl J Med* 316:1569–1572, 1987.
81. Hicks CB, Benson PM, Luptom GP, et al. Seronegative secondary syphilis in a patient infected with the human immunodeficiency virus (HIV) with Kaposi's sarcoma: A diagnostic dilemma. *Ann Intern Med* 107:492–495, 1987.
82. Centers for Disease Control. Continuing increase in infectious syphilis—United States. *MMWR* 37:35–38, 1988.
83. Spence MR, Abrutyn E. Syphilis and infection with the human immuno-deficiency virus. *Ann Intern Med* 107:587, 1987.
84. Sunderam G, McDonald RJ, Maniatis T, et al. Tuberculosis as a manifes-tation of the acquired immunodeficiency syndrome (AIDS). *JAMA* 265:362–366, 1986.
85. Centers for Disease Control. Tuberculosis and acquired immunodefi-ciency syndrome—Florida. MMWR 35:587–590, 1986.
86. Chaisson RE, Schecter GF, Theuer CP, et al. Tuberculosis in patients with the acquired immunodeficiency syndrome: Clinical features, response to therapy, and survival. *Am Rev Respir Dis* 136:570–574, 1987.
87. Centers for Disease Control. Purified protein derivative (PPD)-tuberculin anergy and HIV infection: Guidelines for anergy testing and management of anergic persons at risk of tuberculosis. *MMWR* 40:27–33, 1991.
88. Centers for Disease Control. Tuberculosis and human immunodeficiency virus infection: Recommendations of the Advisory Committee for the Elimination of Tuberculosis (ACET). *MMWR* 38:237–238,243–250, 1989.
89. Sreepada TK, Filippone EJ, Nicastri AD, et al. Associated focal and seg-mental glomerulosclerosis in the acquired immunodeficiency syndrome. *N Engl J Med* 310:669–673, 1984.
90. Carbone L, D'Agati V, Chent JT, Appel GB. Course and prognosis of human immunodeficiency virus–associated nephropathy. *Am J Med* 87:389–395, 1989.
91. Chuck SL, Sande MA. Infections with *Cryptococcus neoformans* in the acquired immunodeficiency syndrome. *N Engl J Med* 321:794–799, 1989.
92. Macy EM, Adelman DC. Abnormal T-cell subsets in normal persons. *N Engl J Med* 319:1608–1609, 1988.
93. Moss AR, Bacchetti P, Osmond D, et al. Seropositivity for HIV and the development of AIDS or AIDS related condition: Three year follow-up of the San Francisco General Hospital cohort. *Br Med J* 296:745–750, 1988.
94. Munoz A, Carey V, Saah AJ, et al. Predictors of decline in CD4 lympho-cytes in a cohort of homosexual men infected with human immunodefi-ciency virus. *J AIDS* 1:396–404, 1988.
95. Margolick JB, Munoz A, Vlahov D, et al. Changes in T-lymphocyte subsets in intravenous drug users with HIV-1 infection. *JAMA* 267:1631–1636, 1992.
96. Phillips AN, Lee CA, Elford J, et al. Serial CD4 lymphocyte counts and development of AIDS. *Lancet* 337:389–392, 1991.
97. Kessler HA, Landay A, Pottage JC, Benson CA. Absolute number versus

percentage of T-helper lymphocytes in human immunodeficiency virus infection. *J Infect Dis* 161:356–357, 1990.

98. Centers for Disease Control. Recommendations for prophylaxis against *Pneumocystis carinii* pneumonia for adults and adolescents infected with human immunodeficiency virus. *MMWR* 41(RR-4):1–11, 1992.

99. Hoover DR, et al. Effect of CD4 cell count measurement variability on staging HIV-1 infection. *J AIDS* 5:794–802, 1992.

100. MacDonell KB, Chmiel JS, Poggensee L, et al. Predicting progression to AIDS: Combined usefulness of CD4 lymphocyte counts and p24 antigenemia. *Am J Med* 89:706–712, 1990.

101. Heering P, Arning M. Neopterin and B2-microglobulin as markers for AIDS. *Lancet* 1:281, 1987.

102. Zolla-Pazner S, William D, El-Sadr W, et al. Quantitation of B2-microglobulin and other immune characteristics in a prospective study of men at risk for acquired immune deficiency syndrome. *JAMA* 251:2951–2955, 1984.

103. Davenny K, Buono D, Schoenbaum E, et al. Baseline health status of intravenous drug users with and without HIV infection. Seventh International Conference on AIDS, Florence, June 1991.

104. Davey RT, Lane HC. Laboratory methods in the diagnosis and prognostic staging of infection with human immunodeficiency virus type 1. *Rev Infect Dis* 12:912–930, 1990.

105. Fahey JL, Taylor JMG, Detels R, et al. The prognostic value of cellular and serologic markers in infection with human immunodeficiency virus type 1. *N Engl J Med* 322:166–172, 1989.

106. Polis MA, Masur H. Predicting the progression to AIDS. *Am J Med* 89:701–705, 1990.

107. Eyster ME, Gail MH, Ballard JO, et al. Natural history of human immunodeficiency virus infections in hemophiliacs: Effects of T-cell subsets, platelet counts, and age. *Ann Intern Med* 107:1–6, 1987.

108. Moss AR. Predicting who will progress to AIDS. *Br Med J* 197:1067–1068, 1988.

109. Polk BF, Fox R, Brookmeyer R, et al. Predictors of the acquired immunodeficiency syndrome developing in a cohort of seropositive homosexual men. *N Engl J Med* 316:61–66, 1987.

110. Lefrere JJ, Salmon D, Courouce AM. Evolution towards AIDS in HIV-infected individuals. *Lancet* 1:1220–1221, 1988.

111. Kaplan JE, Spira TJ, Fishbein DB, et al. A six-year follow-up of HIV-infected homosexual men with lymphadenopathy: Evidence for an increased risk of developing AIDS after the third year of lymphadenopathy. *JAMA* 260:2694–2697, 1988.

112. Holzman RS, Walsh CM, Karpatkin S. Risk for the acquired immunodeficiency syndrome among homosexual men seropositive for the human immunodeficiency virus. *Ann Intern Med* 106:383–386, 1987.

113. Kaslow RA, Phair JP, Friedman HB, et al. Infection with the human immunodeficiency virus: Clinical manifestations and their relationship to immune deficiency. *Ann Intern Med* 107:474–480, 1987.

114. Fuchs D, Reibnegger G, Wachter H. Neopterin levels correlating with the

Walter Reed staging classification in human immunodeficiency virus (HIV) infection. *Ann Intern Med* 107:784–785, 1987.

115. Fischl MA, Richman DD, Hansen N, et al. The safety and efficacy of zidovudine (AZT) in the treatment of subjects with mildly symptomatic human immunodeficiency virus (HIV) infection: A double-blind, placebo-controlled trial. *Ann Intern Med* 112:727–737, 1990.

116. Volberding PA, Lagakos SW, Koch MA, Pettinelli C. Zidovudine in asymptomatic human immunodeficiency virus infection: A controlled trial in persons with fewer than 500 CD4 positive cells per cubic millimeter. *N Engl J Med* 322:941–949, 1990.

117. Centers for Disease Control. 1993 revised classification system for HIV infection and expanded surveillance case definition for AIDS among adolescents and adults. *MMWR* 41(RR-17):1–19, 1992.

118. Yarchoan R, Venzon DJ, Pluda JM, et al. CD4 count and the risk for death in patients infected with HIV receiving antiretroviral therapy. *Ann Intern Med* 115:184–189, 1991.

119. Phillips AN, Elford J, Sabin C, et al. Immunodeficiency and the risk of death in HIV infection. *JAMA* 268:2662–2666, 1992.

120. Kahn JO, et al. A controlled trial comparing continued zidovudine with didanosine in human immunodeficiency virus infection. *N Engl J Med* 327:581–587, 1992.

121. Meng TC, et al. Combination therapy with zidovudine and dideoxycytidine in patients with advanced human immunodeficiency virus infection. *Ann Intern Med* 116:85–86, 1992.

122. Ruskin J, LaRiviere M. Low-dose co-trimoxazole for prevention of *Pneumocystis carinii* pneumonia in human immunodeficiency virus disease. *Lancet* 337:468–471, 1991.

123. Haladay J. Animal assisted therapy for PWAs: bringing a sense of connection. *AIDS Patient Care* 3:38–39, February 1989.

124. Tarricone NJ, Maiman M, Vieira J. Colposcopic evaluation of HIV seropositive women. Sixth International Conference on AIDS. San Francisco, June 1990.

125. Centers for Disease Control. AIDS in women—United States. *MMWR* 39:845–846, 1990.

126. Immunization Practices Advisory Committee, Centers for Disease Control. General Recommendations on Immunization. *Ann Intern Med* 98:615–622, 1983.

127. Redfield RR, Wright DC, James WD, et al. Disseminated vaccinia in a military recruit with human immunodeficiency virus (HIV) Disease. *N Engl J Med* 316:673–676, 1987.

128. Centers for Disease Control. Disseminated *M. bovis* infection from BCG vaccination of a patient with acquired immunodeficiency syndrome. *MMWR* 34:227–228, 1986.

129. Tardieu M, Truffot-Pernot C, Carrire JP, et al. Tuberculous meningitis due to BCG in two previously healthy children. *Lancet* 1:440–441, 1988.

130. Immunization Practices Advisory Committee: Prevention and control of influenza. *MMWR* 36:373–387, 1987.

131. Nelson KE, Clements ML, Miotti P, et al. The influence of human immu-

nodeficiency virus (HIV) infection on antibody responses to influenza vaccines. *Ann Intern Med* 109:383–388, 1988.

132. Whimbey E, Gold JWM, Polsky B. Bacteremia and fungemia in patients with the acquired immunodeficiency syndrome. *Ann Intern Med* 104:511–514, 1986.

133. Simberkoff MS, Sadr WE, Schiffman G, Rahal JJ. *Streptococcus pneumoniae* infections and bacteremia in patients with acquired immunodeficiency syndrome, with report of a pneumococcal vaccine failure. *Am Rev Respir Dis* 130:1174–1176, 1984.

134. Health and Public Policy Committee, American College of Physicians. Pneumococcal vaccine. *Ann Intern Med* 104:118–120, 1986.

135. Amman AJ, Schiffman G, Abrams D, et al. B-cell immunodeficiency in acquired immunodeficiency syndrome. *JAMA* 251:1447–1449, 1984.

136. Huang KL, Ruben FL, Rinaldo CR, et al. Antibody responses after influenza and pneumococcal immunization in HIV-infected homosexual men. *JAMA* 257:2047–2050, 1987.

137. Masur H, Michelis MA, Greene JB, et al. An outbreak of community-acquired *Pneumocystis carinii* pneumonia: Initial manifestation of cellular immune dysfunction. *N Engl J Med* 305:1431–1438, 1981.

138. Casadevall A, et al. *Haemophilus influenzae* type b bacteremia in adults with AIDS and at risk for AIDS. *Am J Med* 92:587–590, 1992.

139. Centers for Disease Control. Measles in HIV-infected children, United States. *MMWR* 37:183–186, 1988.

140. Schonberger LB, McGowan JE, Gregg MB. Vaccine-associated poliomyelitis in the United States: 1961–1972. *Am J Epidemiol* 104:202–211, 1976.

141. Immunization Practices Advisory Committee. Poliomyelitis prevention. *MMWR* 31:106, 1982.

142. von Reyn CF, Clements CJ, Mann JM. Human immunodeficiency virus infection and routine childhood immunisation. *Lancet* 2:669–672, 1987.

143. Immunization Practices Advisory Committee. Poliomyelitis prevention: Enhanced-potency inactivated poliomyelitis vaccine—supplementary statement. *MMWR* 36:795–799, 1987.

144. Odaka N, Eldred L, Cohn S. Comparative immunogenicity of plasma and recombinant hepatitis B virus vaccines in homosexual men. *JAMA* 260:3635–3637, 1988.

145. Collier AC, Corey L, Murphy VL, Handsfield HH. Antibody to human immunodeficiency virus (HIV) and suboptimal response to hepatitis B vaccination. *Ann Intern Med* 109:101–105, 1988.

146. Centers for Disease Control. Protection against viral hepatitis: Recommendations of the Immunization Practices Advisory Committee (ACIP). *MMWR* 39:1–26, 1990.

30/HIV Education and Prevention

Robert Carr, Anna Wald, Christopher Shanahan, Douglas Hein

Education is currently the only means to effectively control the AIDS epidemic [1, 2]. However, discussion of sexual behaviors and illicit drug use is often uncomfortable for both physicians and patients. In order to prevent HIV transmission, not only does basic information need to be conveyed to the patient, but support and guidance are essential in clarifying values and developing health promotion skills [3–7].

Primary care physicians play a crucial role in educating their patients [8]. They are in a unique position to reinforce a healthy lifestyle and allay unfounded fears. An assessment of the risk of acquiring HIV infection and provision of basic information regarding HIV transmission and risk reduction are worthwhile for all patients. Unfortunately, results of a recent survey indicate that only 11 percent of physicians routinely ask questions about high-risk behaviors [9].

In taking a sexual history and teaching about risk reduction, the clinician must tailor the encounter to the individual patient. For the "worried well" with a low risk of HIV infection, emphasis should be placed on conveying general information about high-risk behaviors and exploration of patient concerns. For persons at high risk for HIV infection, whether or not their serostatus is known, education should emphasize the need for personal responsibility in protection of self and partner(s).

Risk Assessment for HIV Infection

Although risk assessment for HIV infection is an important component of the medical history, Lewis and Freeman [10], in a study of 1,000 primary care physicians in California, reported that fewer than 4.5 percent documented the sexual orientation of their patients and only 10 percent asked questions about HIV risk behaviors. Since injection drug use, homosexuality, and having multiple sexual partners may be associated with social stigma, it is essential that questioning about high-risk activities be performed in a nonjudgmental manner. Patients are rarely offended by explicit questions if they perceive that the purpose is to improve their health [5, 11–14]. In conducting a risk assessment in patients from different cultural backgrounds, sensitivity must be paid to how sexual and drug use information is obtained. For example, in some Latino and Caribbean cultures, discussions of sex are generally not considered part of family life. Once an accurate risk assessment has been completed, clinicians are in a much better position to offer patients specific and relevant messages about HIV risk reduction.

A variety of studies have attempted to assess the relative risk of acquiring HIV infection through specific sexual behaviors. Hearst and Hulley [13] estimated transmission rates ranging from 1 in 50,000,000 for sex with a low-risk partner using a condom to as high as 2 in 3 for unprotected intercourse with an HIV-infected partner. The seroprevalence rate of sexual partners of HIV-infected individuals ranges from 7.9 to 73.0 percent [15].

Human immunodeficiency virus infection can be transmitted during homosexual and heterosexual activity, but appears to be more easily spread from man to woman than from woman to man [16]. Risk factors for male-to-female transmission include anal sex and older age of the female partner, while those for female-to-male transmission include advanced stage of HIV infection in the index case and sexual contact during menses.

The long-term maintenance of health-motivated risk reduction, be it sobriety from alcohol or drugs, adherence to a diet, or smoking cessation, is often more difficult than the initial phase of behavioral change [15]. For example, an increased rate of unsafe sexual behaviors in homosexual men has recently been reported following several years of improvement in response to the HIV epidemic [17, 18]. For all sexually active patients, factors that encourage relapse to unsafe behaviors include alcohol and drug use, lack of available condoms, pressure from partner(s) who do not want safer sex, and a general sense of low HIV prevalence in the community. Knowledge of one's HIV serostatus may not have a significant effect on sexual risk reduction [19].

Taking a Sexual History

Taking a sexual history can be a difficult exercise for both the physician and patient. However, an accurate detailed description of the patient's sexual behavior is essential to provide meaningful education about HIV risk reduction. In introducing the topic of sexual history, the reason for collecting such information should be clearly stated. For example, one might say, "Understanding your sexual history is important to assess your risk for many diseases including HIV infection. I realize that this information is personal and may be somewhat embarrassing for both of us." Validating the uncomfortable nature of the interview demonstrates understanding and support for the patient.

In discussing the sexual experience of patients, questions should be asked in a nonjudgmental manner, avoiding stereotypical terms, and focusing on behaviors rather than self-identified labels [17, 20]. For example, one might ask, "Do you have sex with women or men or both?" rather than, "Are you gay or heterosexual?" Some patients who have relationships with members of the same sex do not identify themselves as homosexual. Clear language should be used when describing sexual activity. For example, when asking about receptive anogenital contact, one could say, "Does your partner ever put his penis in your rectum?" Colloquial names should be used for body parts and sexual behaviors if patients are not familiar with more formal terms.

Sexual Behavior Risk Reduction

Changes in sexual behavior in response to the HIV epidemic are well documented in the gay community. Behavioral changes in homosexual men have included decreased number of partners, reduction in the practice of swallowing semen, and decreased frequency of oral-anal and anogenital sex [1, 21]. Behavioral changes in heterosexuals and minority populations are not well established [1, 22]. In a survey of 10,000 randomly selected heterosexuals, a substantial proportion at risk for HIV infection never used condoms, including 38 percent of those with multiple partners, 70 percent of those with a high-risk partner, and 75 percent of transfusion recipients [23]. In a Massachusetts study of adolescents, only 15 percent indicated that they had effected changes in sexual behavior as a result of concern about AIDS [1]. These data suggest that safer sex practices are poorly followed in communities that consider themselves to be at low risk for HIV infection.

Physicians should counsel patients about sexual behavior risk reduction during regular office visits. One approach to safe sex education is to identify specific sexual activities, rate them in terms of safety, and explain how risk can be reduced for each (Table 30-1). Exposure of nonintact skin or mucous membranes to blood, bloody vaginal secretions, and/or semen is the mechanism through which HIV infection is spread sexually. Men with advanced HIV disease who are not receiving antiretroviral therapy have the highest rate of detectable virus in their semen and may be at greatest risk for transmission [24].

More uncommon sexual practices should be kept in mind because they may also be part of the heterosexual or homosexual patient's experience. These may include "scat" (sex involving feces); "fisting" (insertion of fingers or fist in anus); sadomasochism, which may involve pierc-

Table 30-1 *Relative risk of sexual behaviors*

Highest risk
Unprotected anal intercourse
Unprotected vaginal intercourse
Oral-anal sex ("rimming")

Moderate risk
Anal intercourse with condom
Vaginal intercourse with condom
Unprotected oral-genital sex

Lower risk
Oral sex with condom or barrier
Deep kissing ("French," "wet")
Mutual masturbation

Lowest risk
Dry kissing
Hugging
Holding hands
Massage

ing, cutting of skin, and/or bondage; and the use of sex toys, which may potentially cause rectal trauma or allergic reactions.

It should be emphasized to patients that, while no form of sexual activity can be guaranteed safe, consistency in safer sexual practices is important in minimizing risk of HIV acquisition. This message is particularly important in injection drug users (IDUs) because there is evidence that this population is less likely to practice safer sex even if significant improvement in drug use behaviors has occurred [1, 4, 11]. In addition, some studies indicate that up to 80 percent of male IDUs have non–drug-using partners [4, 11]. Because some homosexual men and IDUs practice safer sex with casual but not steady partners, the physician should remember to encourage risk reduction in all sexual relationships.

The efficacy of condoms in reducing the risk of HIV transmission has been clearly established [2, 12]. Lubricated latex condoms are recommended for vaginal and anal intercourse; unlubricated latex condoms are suggested for oral sex with a man. Dental dams and other barrier devices have been advocated for oral sex with women, but their effectiveness is uncertain and they have not become popular. Nonoxynol-9, a compound that is viricidal and spermicidal, and enhances protection against other sexually transmitted diseases (STDs), may be a useful adjunct to condoms, although its role is controversial. The recently described "female condom" may be an alternative for women who are unable to convince their partners to wear condoms. Physicians should be aware that in some relationships women who attempt to initiate changes in sexual behavior may place themselves at risk for domestic violence or abandonment.

Injection Drug Use Risk Reduction

Changes in drug use behaviors as a result of concern about AIDS were identified as early as 1984 [1]. These were promoted through media messages, educational campaigns, community-based outreach efforts, and word of mouth among drug users [12]. It is clear to IDUs, recovering addicts, and health care providers that no one strategy is sufficient. Increased access to drug treatment, clear and consistent messages about sharing drug paraphernalia, and social programs and support groups are all important [25]. Communication in the drug-using culture is predominantly verbal. Programs designed to foster behavioral change among IDUs have demonstrated that, in order to be effective, risk reduction messages must be heard repeatedly from multiple sources, and face-to-face encounters have the greatest impact [11].

The critical message from physicians should be for active IDUs to seek treatment. Unfortunately, access to drug treatment is limited in many parts of the United States. Information on how to obtain or clean "works" (needles and syringes) and protect sexual partners should also be included in patient visits. If available, referral to HIV antibody testing and drop-in counseling services specifically targeted to IDUs should be offered.

Health care providers should draw from the experience of other IDUs. The most important factor in behavioral change in an IDU is the perception that other users are also altering behaviors [4]. Because in some cases the addict may not trust the physician, direct counseling may not be as effective as hearing about behavioral change from friends or recovering addicts. Physicians should reinforce the notion that to stop sharing needles works, or to clean them effectively is a way to show "solidarity" with other users and to take care of each other. This message is designed to shift significance away from needle sharing, which has traditionally been a sign of trust and companionship in the drug-using culture. Information about drug use risk reduction should always include a discussion of the consequences of HIV infection in sexual partners and children. However, focusing on the personal consequences of developing AIDS is probably not as effective an intervention in that IDUs live with a clear awareness of the threat of death through drug use [11].

"Shooting galleries," where drug users rent space and paraphernalia, have been more commonly associated with the use of intravenous cocaine. Some IDUs ignore the potential risk and share needles with strangers out of convenience or economy, or both. The short half-life of cocaine, whether intravenous, smoked freebase, or as "crack," necessitates more frequent dosing and, therefore, is associated with an increased risk of HIV exposure [26]. Use of intravenous cocaine has also been related to an increased prevalence of STDs, especially syphilis, in heterosexual drug users [27]. Ulcerative STDs have been shown to be independent risk factors for HIV seroconversion [28, 29].

HIV Antibody Test Counseling

The process involved in HIV counseling and testing presents an important opportunity for the clinician to discuss risk reduction strategies. The objective of pretest counseling is to share information so that the patient can make an informed decision about the test. The objective of posttest counseling is to provide interpretation of test results and to discuss their implications. It is important to remember that HIV antibody testing is rarely an "emergency" and is best offered in a setting that facilitates continuity of care. Early linkage of seropositive patients with medical care and clinical trials is essential. Major issues to be addressed in pretest and posttest counseling sessions are outlined in the following section. Indications and contraindications for HIV antibody testing are presented in Chap. 29.

Major Issues in Pretest Counseling

- Ask the patient to identify ways in which he/she is at risk for HIV infection. When time is limited, this can help focus the session more quickly. Patients should never be compelled to reveal risk behaviors.
- Exposure means that a person has come into contact with HIV but has not necessarily been infected with the virus. Infection means that HIV has entered the person's blood system.
- Tell the patient how the testing process works and what the test means. The test is for antibodies to HIV, not for AIDS. There is a potential 6-month "window period" between infection and development of detectable antibody. This is counted from the last time the patient feels that he/she could have had significant exposure to HIV.
- A negative test result means that antibody was not found or has not yet been produced by the immune system. A negative test does not mean a person is immune to HIV. A person who tests negative but has practiced unsafe behaviors during the window period may be infected with HIV and be infectious to others.
- A positive test result means that a person is infected and infectious, but does not mean a person has AIDS.

- An indeterminate result means that antibody other than HIV may be registering on the test. A person who is in the process of seroconverting may also have an indeterminate result. It is recommended that a patient with indeterminate results have a second antibody test 6 to 8 weeks later.
- It is important to determine whether the patient has adequate personal supports in place. To ascertain this information:

  1. Ask the patient if anyone knows that he/she is having the test
  2. Find out if the patient has anyone to talk to during the waiting period for results
  3. Encourage the patient to utilize existing support systems, such as 12-step programs, recovery groups, psychotherapy, pastoral counseling, peer support groups (including Alcoholics Anonymous and Narcotics Anonymous), or friends
  4. Make referrals for additional support if necessary

- Ask the patient to consider bringing a support person when he/she comes for the test results. In some cases, the patient's spouse or partner may not be the best choice given their own risk for infection. It is important for the patient to choose someone who can realistically be a resource if a crisis develops.
- Ask the patient what it would mean for him/her to get a negative or positive test result. Some reactions of people who test negative may include (1) profound relief, (2) a feeling of immunity to HIV, (3) a confirmation of the need to practice safer sexual and drug use behaviors, or (4) survivor guilt by virtue of being part of a discordant couple or separated from the people in their life who are HIV positive. Establish a plan with the patient to outline what he/she will do if the test result is negative.
- As you discuss a potential positive result, explain to the patient that you can provide information about support groups, medical and mental health referrals, and partner notification programs. Establish a plan to outline what he/she will do if the test result is positive.

Major Issues in Posttest Counseling

- Use the posttest session to review answers to pretest questions.
- Posttest counseling is most effective when it is tailored to the patient's reasons for undergoing testing and his/her risk behavior. Negative results do not mean that a person can stop practicing safer sex and needle use.
- Common reactions from patients who test seropositive include periods of silence, sadness, crying, anger, resentment, fear of illness, and con-

cern for partners and family members. After hearing such bad news, patients may be unable to absorb much additional information.

- Help the seropositive patient make a plan for the next 24 hours and assist him/her in ways to get support from physicians and/or family members.
- Assess the patient for risk of suicide. Because of this possibility, immediate access to trained mental health clinicians is essential.
- Refer the patient for primary care, where the benefits of early medical intervention and availability of clinical trials will be reviewed.
- Assess with the patient the need for HIV testing of children and/or partners.

References

1. Becker MH, Joseph JG. AIDS and behavioral change to reduce risk: a review. *Am J Public Health* 78:394–410, 1988.
2. Cleary PD. Education and the prevention of AIDS. *Law, Medicine, and Health Care* 16:267–273, 1988.
3. Brandt AM. AIDS in historical perspective: Four lessons from the history of sexually transmitted diseases. *Am J Public Health* 78:367–371, 1988.
4. DesJarlais DC, Friedman SR. The psychology of preventing AIDS among intravenous drug users: A social learning conceptualization. *Am Psychol* 43-11:865–870, 1988.
5. Jones LH. AIDS, education, and the community health nurse. *J Community Health Nurs* 5:159–165, 1988.
6. Moran TA, et al. Informational needs of homosexual men diagnosed with AIDS or AIDS-related complex. *Oncol Nurs Forum* 15:311–314, 1988.
7. Pinching AJ. Current issues in the management of AIDS patients. *J AIDS* 1:583–592, 1988.
8. Northfelt DW, Hayward RA, Shapiro MF. The acquired immunodeficiency syndrome is a primary care disease. *Ann Intern Med* 109:773–775, 1988.
9. Ferguson KJ, Stapleton JT, Helms CM. Physician's effectiveness in assessing risk for human immunodeficiency virus infection. *Arch Intern Med* 151:561–564, 1991.
10. Lewis CE, Freeman HE. The sexual history taking and counseling practices of primary care physicians. *West J Med* 147:165–167, 1987.
11. Friedman SR, DesJarlais DC, Sotheran JL. AIDS health education for intravenous drug users. *Health Educ Q* 13:383–393, 1986.
12. Ginzburg HM, et al. Health education and knowledge assessment of HTLV-III disease among intravenous drug users. *Health Educ Q* 13:373–382, 1986.
13. Hearst N, Hulley SB. Preventing the heterosexual spread of AIDS: Are we giving our patients the best advice? *JAMA* 259:2428–2432, 1988.

14. Johnson JA, et al. A program using medical students to teach high school students about AIDS. *J Med Educ* 63:522–530, 1988.
15. DeGruttola V, Seage GR, Mayer KH, Horsburgh CR. Infectiousness of HIV between male homosexual partners. *J Clin Epidemiol* 42:849–856, 1989.
16. European Study Group on Heterosexual Transmission of HIV. Comparison of female to male and male to female transmission of HIV in 563 stable couples. *Br Med J* 304:809–813, 1992.
17. Ekstrand M, Stall R, Frutchey C, Christen P. Averting disaster: Addressing relapse and ongoing AIDS prevention programs for self-identified gay and bisexual men of all colors. Produced by the San Francisco AIDS Foundation and the Center for AIDS Prevention Studies, University of California, San Francisco.
18. Van Griensven GJP, et al. Effect of human immunodeficiency virus antibody knowledge on high risk sexual behavior with steady and non-steady sexual partners among homosexual men. *Am J Epidemiol* 129:596–603, 1989.
19. Zenliman JM, et al. Effect of HIV posttest counseling on STD incidence. *JAMA* 267:843–845, 1992.
20. Russell M. Impediments to accessing services for black gay and bisexual men who choose not to be "gay identified." Sixth International Conference on AIDS, San Francisco, June 1990.
21. McCusker, et al. Effects of HIV antibody test knowledge on subsequent sexual behaviors in a cohort of homosexually active men. *Am J Public Health* 78:462–467, 1988.
22. Peterson JL, Marin G. Issues on the prevention of AIDS among black and Hispanic men. *Am Psychol* 11:871–877, 1988.
23. Cantania JA, et al. Prevalence of AIDS-related risk factors and condom use in the United States. *Science* 258:1101–1106, 1992.
24. Anderson DJ, et al. Effects of disease stage and zidovudine therapy on the detection of human immunodeficiency virus type 1 in semen. *JAMA* 267:2769–2774, 1992.
25. Board of Trustees Report. Drug abuse in the United States. *JAMA* 265:2102–2107, 1991.
26. Chaisson RE, Bacchetti P, Osmond D, et al. Cocaine use and HIV infection in intravenous drug users in San Francisco. *JAMA* 261:561–565, 1989.
27. Centers for Disease Control. Relationship of syphilis to drug use and prostitution—Connecticut and Philadelphia, Pennsylvania. MMWR 37:755–758, 764, 1988.
28. Greenblatt RM, Lukehart SL, Plummer FA, et al. Genital ulceration as a risk factor for human immunodeficiency virus in Kenya. Third International Conference on AIDS, Washington DC, 1987.
29. Katzenstein DA, Latif A, Bassett MT, et al. Risks for heterosexual transmission of HIV in Zimbabwe. Third International Conference on AIDS, Washington, DC, 1987.

31/Infection Control and Risk Reduction for Health Care Workers

Robert A. Burke, Gail M. Garvin, Carol A. Sulis

The potential for occupational transmission of HIV is a serious concern among health care workers (HCW) [1–4]. In 1988, the Centers for Disease Control (CDC) estimated a 0.42 percent risk of infection following occupational exposure to HIV-infected blood or bloody body fluids [5]. As of February 1993, 102 cases of occupationally acquired HIV infection in HCW had been reported in the United States (Table 31-1). In 33 instances, HCW had a negative baseline HIV test at the time of exposure (C Ciesielski, CDC, personal communication). Most were the result of needlestick or other sharps injuries. The timing and source of acquisition of HIV infection for the other 69 HCW are not well documented (B Garza, CDC, personal communication). In addition to percutaneous injuries, a small number of HIV seroconversions following mucous membrane or nonintact skin occupational exposure have also been reported [5–16]. Factors that are believed to influence the risk of occupational HIV transmission include the type and extent of exposure and the immunologic characteristics of both the source ("donor") and recipient [5–30] (Table 31-2).

Universal Precautions/Body Substance Isolation

Health care workers can reduce their risk of exposure to blood and body fluids through the use of basic safety measures, barrier precautions, and technologically safer instruments [6, 11–25, 30–44]. In 1987, the CDC issued a set of infection control guidelines designed to prevent or minimize the risk of occupational exposure to blood-borne pathogens [11]. These guidelines, known as "universal precautions," are reflected in a series of regulations enacted by the Occupational Safety and Health Administration (OSHA) [22, 35] (Table 31-3).

Universal precautions are based on the premise that all patients are potentially infectious. Recommendations include the use of protective

432

Table 31-1 *Occupationally acquired HIV infection in US health care workers*

Clinical status	No.	Type of exposure	No.	Occupation	No.
		Documented Seroconversion[a]			
AIDS	7	Percutaneous	28	Laboratory worker	13
HIV infection	26	Mucocutaneous	4	Nurse	12
		Both	1	Physician	4
				Other	4
		Presumed Seroconversion[b]			
HIV infection	69	Not available		Not available	

[a]Requires a baseline negative HIV antibody test.
[b]Includes HCW with HIV infection who have not reported other risk factors and who describe a history of occupational exposure to blood, body fluids, or HIV-infected laboratory material but for whom seroconversion after exposure was not documented (B Garza, personal communication).
Data reported to the Centers for Disease Control as of 2/93 (B Garza, personal communication).

clothing and equipment, and special techniques to prevent contamination of mucous membranes and skin with potentially infectious body fluids or laboratory preparations. HIV has been isolated from blood; semen; vaginal secretions; amniotic fluid; cerebrospinal, synovial, pleural, peritoneal, and pericardial fluids; and organs for transplant [22, 24, 45]. The risk of transmission of HIV from feces, nasal secretions, sputum, saliva, sweat, tears, urine, or vomitus is very low unless they contain visible blood [22]. However, some institutions have incorporated the CDC recommendation of universal precautions into an expanded policy called "body substance isolation," which requires that protective clothing or barrier devices be used whenever skin or mucous membrane exposure to *any* body fluid, tissue, or culture can be anticipated [44].

A comprehensive program of universal precautions is burdensome, difficult to implement, and expensive, and not all of the procedures are equally effective [34, 36–38, 43, 46–57]. Compliance with universal precautions may reduce the incidence of skin and mucous membrane exposures, but may also promote a false sense of security [36–38, 47, 50–53, 55–57]. Most sharp devices, including disposable needle/syringe combinations, winged steel needle intravenous sets, intravenous catheter stylets, scalpels, and suture needles, can cause injuries, which often occur during recapping or disposal [36, 43, 46]. Despite implementation of aggressive infection control education programs and engineering controls, such as sharps disposal systems, some investigators have recently reported a significant increase in occupational injuries [36, 55].

Table 31-2 Factors in assessing significance of HCW exposure to HIV

Risk factor	Commentary
Number of exposures	Single vs. multiple
Type of exposure	Percutaneous Mucosal Cutaneous
Type of fluid	Concentrated virus (e.g., tissue culture) Blood Other body fluid Age of fluid (e.g., fresh sample)
Severity of injury or exposure	Depth of wound (superficial vs. deep) Size of wound Duration of contact (brief vs. prolonged) Evident infectious material introduced? How much?
Source (donor) characteristics	Stage of HIV disease Presence of viremia Presence of antigenemia Use of antiretroviral medication
HCW characteristics	Hygiene First aid procedure following exposure Skin integrity Use of barriers at the time of exposure Immunologic status Use of prophylactic agents

Because percutaneous exposures account for 80 percent of occupationally acquired HIV infection, more emphasis needs to be placed on measures to reduce sharps injuries [41, 47]. OSHA requires that health care institutions purchase devices with incorporated safety features if available; design changes could eliminate 85 to 95 percent of injuries [35, 43]. Safety design modifications should be automatic and not depend on the interest or cooperation of the user. Examples include needleless systems and needles that recess or resheathe spontaneously [33]. Institutions should attempt to prevent sharps-related injuries in all areas, including the operating room [36, 37, 43, 50].

The procedures listed below are recommended when performing invasive procedures or when handling blood, body fluids, or contaminated equipment [11, 22, 41]. OSHA requires that employers document HCW compliance with these measures [35].

1. Hand washing (10-second scrub with hand soap) should be performed before and after patient contact. If intact skin is contami-

Table 31-3 *Methods to reduce the risk of nosocomial infection*

Procedure*	Precautionary measure
Any direct patient contact	10-sec hand wash before and after patient contact
Handling blood or body fluid, or equipment contaminated with blood or body fluid	Wear gloves; remove immediately after task, and wash hands
If soiling of clothes or arms is likely	Wear a fluid-resistant gown or apron; discard or launder after use
If splash to the face is likely	Wear a mask and protective eyewear
Direct contact with a lesion, rash, or mucous membrane	Wear gloves; remove immediately after, and wash hands
Phlebotomy, insertion of intravenous catheter	Wear gloves; do not recap, bend, or cut needle; discard all needles and sharps in a puncture-resistant container located at the point of use
Arterial puncture or cannulation	Wear gloves, mask, and protective eyewear
Aerosolized medication treatment in an immunosuppressed patient	Treat patient in a booth or room with negative pressure and external exhaust; HCW entering room or providing direct care during or immediately after treatment should wear snugly fitting 1- to 5-μ filtration mask or particulate respirator
Reusable equipment and devices	
Device enters the bloodstream or normally sterile body cavity	Wash thoroughly and sterilize
Device touches intact mucosa but does not penetrate the body	Wash thoroughly and perform high-level disinfection at a minimum
Device touches only intact skin	Clean with a hospital-grade disinfectant

*In all cases, sterile equipment should be used with aseptic technique.

nated with blood or body fluid, the area should be washed immediately. Health care workers with exudative lesions or weeping dermatitis should not perform direct patient care or invasive procedures [25].

2. Gloves should be worn whenever blood or body fluid is handled. No differences have been reported in permeability between *intact* latex and vinyl gloves [22]. Gloves should be worn for a single pro-

cedure and removed carefully to avoid skin contamination. Hands should be thoroughly washed after removing gloves. Some institutions require several pairs of gloves or cotton liners for extra protection during certain procedures. If maximum tactile sensation is not essential, steel mesh gloves that can be sterilized are available for procedures that present a high risk of cuts or punctures.

3. Needles, scalpels, and other sharp instruments should be handled carefully to prevent injuries. Whenever possible, open needles should be replaced with devices that include a safety feature to prevent accidental puncture of the user. A list of acceptable devices is being prepared jointly by the CDC, Food and Drug Administration, and OSHA. Although injuries that occur during recapping or disposal have been recognized for years, HCW compliance with safety measures is difficult to achieve [46, 47, 55, 56]. *Needles should never be recapped, bent, broken, or removed from syringes by hand.* Needles and sharps should be disposed of immediately after use in a puncture-resistant container, located at the point of use. Availability of containers may significantly decrease injuries related to disposal, but they must be designed to avoid jamming and be maintained and emptied or replaced by properly trained personnel on a regular basis [33, 36].

4. Surgical procedures that require blind manipulations and hand-held sharps should be modified whenever possible [25].

5. A fluid-resistant gown or protective apron should be worn if soiling is anticipated, and it should be discarded after a single use.

6. Protective eyewear and a mask should be worn if a blood or body fluid splash to the mouth, nose, or eyes is anticipated.

7. To avoid mouth-to-mouth resuscitation, barrier devices or resuscitation bags should be strategically located in areas where the need for resuscitation is predictable.

8. Surgical procedures should include appropriate barrier precautions. For some subspecialties, universal precautions require additional or enhanced precautions. For example, the US Public Health Service recommends the use of protective wear and barrier devices to prevent transmission of blood-borne organisms during dental and oral surgical procedures [19]. Other examples include the use of face shields during orthopedic surgery with electric saws and vacuum devices to recover flume during cautery [37, 40, 50, 53].

9. Postmortem procedures for all patients should include complete protective wear for any HCW at risk for fluid or tissue contamination. All cadavers should be considered potentially infectious, as should all surfaces and equipment that were contaminated during autopsy.

10. All HCW should receive mandatory annual education about infection control and safe work practices [2, 33, 35, 55].

The HIV-Infected Health Care Worker

Following an investigation of a cluster of HIV infections among patients of a Florida dentist, there has been great public concern about HIV-infected HCW performing invasive procedures [58, 59, 60]. In response, the CDC has recommended that HCW who perform exposure-prone procedures know their HIV status and voluntarily refrain from performing these procedures unless they have sought counsel from an expert review panel [25]. Extensive debate has failed to produce either a list of "exposure-prone" procedures or a consensus on the means to enforce this recommendation [6, 25, 61–65]. Each institution should develop policies and resources for retraining, counseling, medical care, and disability compensation of HIV-infected personnel.

Cleaning and Disinfection

Reusable instruments and equipment used in patient care should be appropriately cleaned, and then disinfected or sterilized. All practices related to cleaning and reprocessing of equipment should be rigorously monitored [35]. Equipment and devices that enter the bloodstream or body cavities should be sterilized [66]. Equipment and devices that touch intact mucous membranes but do not penetrate the body should at least undergo high-level disinfection or be sterilized if possible. Equipment and devices that only touch intact skin should be cleaned with a detergent or as indicated by the manufacturer [11].

Once outside the human body, HIV is sensitive to heat and light, and is easily killed by many hospital-grade and some "household" disinfectants [11, 41, 67–70]. Germicides that are effective against HIV on pre-cleaned, environmental surfaces usually have Environmental Protection Agency labels that include directions for use [67]. Hospital-grade chemical disinfectants that have been shown to deactivate HIV include quaternary ammonium chloride, 0.3% hydrogen peroxide, 50% ethanol, 35% isopropanol, paraformaldehyde, phenolic sodium hypochlorite, and 50 ppm sodium hypochlorite, which is equivalent to household bleach diluted 1 : 100 with water [21, 68–70]. Spills of blood or body fluids should be cleaned immediately. The HCW should wear heavy-duty rubber gloves, wipe up the spill with absorbent material, and wash the area with a hospital-grade disinfectant. Disposable cleaning material that is grossly soiled with blood should be discarded as hazardous infectious waste [11, 22, 35, 42]. Operators of machines used in specimen preparation, such as a centrifuge, must be trained to clean the equipment thoroughly and safely should breakage or accidental contamination with blood or body fluids occur.

Detergent and hot-water washing (160°F) of dishes and laundry is adequate decontamination for HIV [17, 31]. Laundry that is soiled with blood or body fluids should be transported in leak-proof bags and handled as little as possible. It should be washed for 25 minutes with detergent and hot water (160°F). If a low-temperature water cycle is used, detergents that are suitable for this type of washing should be employed [11].

Protection of Ancillary Staff

Specimen Preparation

All fluid and tissue specimens should be considered potentially infectious. Specimens should be placed in a tightly closed container, which in turn is sealed within a leak-proof transport bag labeled with an easily recognizable biohazard warning [18, 35]. Requisition forms attached to the outside of the bag need not contain any reference to the patient's HIV status, since universal precautions or body substance isolation procedures should be used by all laboratory personnel.

Hazardous/Infectious Waste Disposal

All needles and sharps should be placed in a puncture-resistant container immediately after use, and containers handled in accordance with federal, state, and local regulations. Material that is grossly contaminated with blood must be discarded in bags or containers colored or marked according to applicable health authority regulations. Some local regulators allow the disposal of bulk blood and blood products directly into the municipal sewerage system [17]. However, in most laboratory areas, any fluid that could contain HIV or hepatitis B virus (HBV) may be poured into the sanitary sewer system only after a disinfectant is added [42]. Gloves should be worn, as well as protective eyewear and a mask, if splashing can be anticipated.

While there has been a great deal of public concern over the environmental impact of medical waste, there is no evidence to suggest that it is any more infectious than community waste. Viruses such as HIV require living cells for survival and are not likely to endure long enough to become a significant environmental health problem [41, 71].

Management of Accidental Exposures

Occupational exposure to HIV through accidental needlesticks is common and often unreported by residents and medical students [72]. Every institution should have a protocol that clearly defines the procedure to be followed in the event that an HCW is exposed to blood or bloody body fluid [35]. The protocol should be easily accessible to HCW and consistently followed. Routine care, including thorough washing and clinical evaluation of injury, should be performed immediately after a percutaneous or mucous membrane exposure. The HCW supervisor and employee health service should be informed, and the institution's protocol for potential HBV/HIV exposure followed [22, 26, 35, 73]. The source patient should be assessed to determine the likelihood of HIV/HBV infections. If there is no record of a recent negative serologic test, the patient should be tested for HBV infection and asked to consent to HIV antibody testing. If the source patient is HIV seronegative, follow-up evaluation may be unnecessary [74]. If the source patient cannot be identified, refuses testing, or is HIV infected, further evaluation of the exposed HCW should begin immediately. A baseline HIV antibody or antigen test should be performed as soon as possible, with follow-up tests at 6 weeks, 3 months, and 6 months [5, 6, 11, 24]. While the risk of seroconversion for exposed HCW is very low, the CDC suggests following Public Health Service recommendations for reducing HIV transmission, such as practicing safe sex and refraining from blood or organ donation, during the follow-up period [24, 75, 76].

Reporting of potentially significant exposures should be encouraged [55]. Information must be confidential and not used in a punitive manner. Epidemiologic data about such injuries are sparse [6, 36, 37]. Within an individual institution, such data could be used to assure that the "blood and body fluid exposure" protocol is being implemented consistently, while providing an opportunity to change unsafe practices. On a national level, better information might permit more rational design and implementation of prevention programs.

Many health care institutions now offer antiretroviral chemoprophylaxis with zidovudine (ZDV) to HCW who have potentially been exposed to HIV. There are no compelling data to support or discourage the use of ZDV for preventive purposes [24]. In general, the ZDV dose administered is 200 mg orally every 4 hours for 6 weeks; recipients must be monitored regularly for hematologic toxicity. Health care workers who have suffered a significant parenteral or mucous membrane exposure should weigh the potential risks and benefits of postexposure chemoprophylaxis [24, 30, 77–80].

Other Infections that Require Additional Precautionary Measures

Varicella-Zoster Virus

Persons who are susceptible to varicella-zoster virus may contract chickenpox by direct, unprotected contact with a zoster patient. Health care workers who provide direct care to patients with zoster should wear gloves. Because zoster may disseminate more readily in the immunocompromised individual, HIV-infected patients should be isolated in a private negative-pressure room with external venting for the duration of their illness. Nonimmune HCW should avoid entering the room.

Mycobacterium tuberculosis Infection

Although the annual incidence of M. tuberculosis infection in the US is 9 in 100,000, the rate among HIV-infected patients is much higher. Tuberculosis (TB) may occur in early HIV disease and differ in clinical presentation from TB in an immunocompetent host [81–86]. Clinicians must maintain a high index of suspicion for TB in all HIV-infected patients with pulmonary symptoms. Strict respiratory isolation precautions should be used for patients with suspected or confirmed pulmonary TB. Because of the increased prevalence of multidrug-resistant TB among AIDS patients, isolation precautions should be continued until clinical and bacteriologic response to therapy is documented or until three successive sputum smears are negative for acid-fast organisms (AFB) [85, 86]. Infectious patients should not be discharged to residential facilities, such as nursing homes, hospices, and correctional institutions, unless appropriate AFB precautions can be implemented [86].

Techniques that reduce the number of air-borne droplet nuclei should be used. Examples include requesting that patients cover the nose and mouth when coughing or sneezing, and placing patients in a private room with the door closed. The room should have negative pressure and external venting with five to six air exchanges per hour. Some authorities recommend ultraviolet irradiation of the air in the upper part of the room. Persons entering the room should wear 1- to 5-μ filtration particulate respirators or filtered masks [35, 85].

Sputum induction and aerosol pentamidine treatments that induce cough may facilitate transmission of TB [87]. These procedures should be performed in a negative-pressure room or booth with external venting. Health care workers who provide direct care during or immediately after such treatments should wear filtration particulate respirators or filtered masks and use appropriate barrier precautions [82, 85–87].

All HCW who have potential exposure to TB should participate in an organized screening program and have at least one purified protein derivative (PPD) skin test every year. Each institution should rigorously monitor compliance, and data should be analyzed to evaluate the effectiveness of infection control practices [85, 86].

Other Opportunistic Diseases

AIDS-indicative diseases that do not require special infection control precautions include extrapulmonary TB, atypical mycobacterial infection, candidiasis, coccidioidomycosis, cryptosporidiosis, cryptococcosis, histoplasmosis, toxoplasmosis, Kaposi's sarcoma and other malignancies, and progressive multifocal leukoencephalopathy [88].

References

1. Brennan TA. Transmission of the human immunodeficiency virus in the health care setting: Time for action. N Engl J Med 324:1504–1509, 1991.
2. Hayward RA, Shapiro MF. A national study of AIDS and residency training: Experiences, concerns, and consequences. Ann Intern Med 114:23–32, 1991.
3. Granich R. Students' attitudes about AIDS (letter). Ann Intern Med 114:1066, 1991.
4. Singh V, Hamadeh R. AIDS and residency training (letter). Ann Intern Med 114:605–606, 1991.
5. Marcus R, CDC Cooperative Needlestick Surveillance Group. Surveillance of health care workers exposed to blood from patients infected with human immunodeficiency virus. N Engl J Med 319:1118–1123, 1988.
6. Bell DM. Human immunodeficiency virus transmission in health care settings: Risk and risk reduction. Am J Med 91 (suppl 3B):294S–300S, 1991.
7. Weiss SH, Saxinger WC, Rechtman D, et al. HTLV-III infection among health care workers: Association with needlestick injuries. JAMA 254:2089–2093, 1985.
8. McCray E, CDC Cooperative Needlestick Surveillance Group. Special Report: Occupational risk of the acquired immunodeficiency syndrome among health care workers. N Engl J Med 314:1127–1132, 1986.
9. Gerberding JL, Bryant-LeBlanc CE, Nelson, K, et al. Risk of transmitting the human immunodeficiency virus, cytomegalovirus, and hepatitis B virus to health care workers exposed to patients with AIDS and AIDS-related conditions. J Infect Dis 156:1–8, 1987.
10. Centers for Disease Control. Update: Human immunodeficiency virus

infections in health care workers exposed to blood of infected patients. *MMWR* 36:285–289, 1987.

11. Centers for Disease Control. Recommendations for prevention of HIV transmission in health-care settings. *MMWR* 36 (suppl 2):3–18, 1987.

12. Centers for Disease Control. Update: Acquired immunodeficiency syndrome and human immunodeficiency virus infection among health care workers. *MMWR* 37:229–239, 1988.

13. Klein RS, Phelan JA, Freeman K, et al. Low occupational risk of human immunodeficiency virus infection among dental professionals. *N Engl J Med* 318:86–90, 1988.

14. Gerberding JL. Occupational health issues for providers of care to patients with HIV infection. *Infect Dis Clin North Am* 2:321–328, 1988.

15. Henderson DK, Fahey BJ, Willy M, et al. Risk for Occupational transmission of human immunodeficiency virus type 1 (HIV-1) associated with clinical exposures: A prospective evaluation. *Ann Intern Med* 133:740–746, 1990.

16. Beekmann SE, Fahey BJ, Gerberding JL, Henderson DK. Risky business: Using necessarily imprecise casualty counts to estimate occupational risks for HIV-1 infection. *Infect Control Hosp Epidemiol* 11:371–379, 1990.

17. Centers for Disease Control. Recommendations for preventing transmission of infection with T-lymphotropic virus type III/lymphadenopathy-associated virus in the workplace. *MMWR* 34:682–686, 691–695, 1985.

18. Conte JE. Infection with human immunodeficiency virus in the hospital. *Ann Intern Med* 105:730–736, 1986.

19. Centers for Disease Control. Recommended infection-control practices for dentistry. *MMWR* 35:237–242, 1986.

20. Kuhls TL, Viker S, Parris NB, et al. Occupational risk of HIV, HBV, and HSV-2 infections in health care personnel caring for AIDS patients. *Am J Public Health* 77:1306–1309, 1987.

21. McCray E, Martone W. Infection Control Considerations in HIV Infection. In: G Wormser, R Stahl, E Bottone (eds), *AIDS and Other Manifestations of HIV Infection*. Park Ridge, NJ: Noyes Publications, 1987. Pp 950–974.

22. Centers for Disease Control. Update: Universal precautions for prevention of transmission of human immunodeficiency virus, hepatitis B virus, and other bloodborne pathogens in health-care settings. *MMWR* 37:377–388, 1988.

23. Centers for Disease Control. Guidelines for prevention of transmission of human immunodeficiency virus and hepatitis B virus to health-care workers and public safety workers. *MMWR* 38 (suppl 6):1–37, 1989.

24. Centers for Disease Control. US Public Health Service statement on management of occupational exposure to human immunodeficiency virus (HIV), including considerations regarding zidovudine post-exposure use. *MMWR* 39(RR-1):1–14, 1990.

25. Centers for Disease Control. Recommendations for preventing transmission of human immunodeficiency virus and hepatitis B virus to patients during exposure-prone invasive procedures. *MMWR* 40:(RR 8):1–9, 1991.

26. Sullivan MT, Williams AE, Fang CT, et al. Transmission of human T-lym-

photropic virus types I and II by blood transfusion: A retrospective study of recipients of blood components (1983 through 1988). *Arch Intern Med* 151:2043–2048, 1991.

27. Gaughwin MD, Gowans E, Ali R, Burrell C. Bloody needles: The volumes of blood transferred in simulations of needlestick injuries and shared use of syringes for injection of intravenous drugs. *AIDS* 5:1025–1027, 1991.

28. Colebunders R, Ryder R, Francis H, et al. Seroconversion rate, mortality, and clinical manifestations associated with the receipt of a human immunodeficiency virus–infected blood transfusion in Kinshasa, Zaire. *J Infect Dis* 164:450–456, 1991.

29. Hagan MD, Meyer KB, Kopelman RI, Pauker SG. Human immunodeficiency virus infection in health care workers: A method for estimating individual occupational risk. *Arch Intern Med* 149:1541–1544, 1989.

30. Henderson DK, Gerberding JL. Prophylactic zidovudine after occupational exposure to the human immunodeficiency virus: An interim analysis. *J Infect Dis* 160:321–327, 1989.

31. *Guidelines for Handwashing and Hospital Environmental Control, 1985.* Hospital Infections Program, CDC, US Government Printing Office.

32. Infection control measures for all patients. *AIDS Policy and the Law* July 15, 1987:3.

33. Special report and product review: Needlestick prevention devices. *Health Devices* 20:154–167, 1991.

34. Klein RS. Universal precautions for preventing occupational exposures to human immunodeficiency virus type 1 (editorial). *Am J Med* 80:141–144, 1991.

35. Department of Labor. Occupational Safety and Health Administration. 29 CFR Part 1910.1030. Occupational exposure to bloodborne pathogens. *Federal Register* 56:64004–64182, December 6, 1991.

36. McCormick RD, Meisch MG, Ircink FG, Maki DG. Epidemiology of hospital sharps injuries: A 14-year prospective study in the pre-AIDS and AIDS eras. *Am J Med* 91 (suppl 3B):301S–307S, 1991.

37. Panlilio AL, Foy DR, Edwards JR, et al. Blood contacts during surgical procedures. *JAMA* 265:1533–1537, 1991.

38. Wong ES, Stotka JL, Chinchilli VM, et al. Are universal precautions effective in reducing the number of occupational exposures among health care workers? A prospective study of physicians on a medical service. *JAMA* 265:1123–1128, 1991.

39. US Department of Labor. OSHA instruction CPL 2-2.44B, February 1990.

40. AAOS Task Force on AIDS and Orthopedic Surgery. *Recommendations for the Prevention of Human Immunodeficiency Virus (HIV) Transmission in the Practice of Orthopedic Surgery.* Park Ridge, IL:American Academy of Orthopedic Surgeons, 1989.

41. Becker CE, Cone JE, Gerberding J. Occupational infection with human immunodeficiency virus (HIV): Risks and risk reduction. *Ann Intern Med* 110:653–656, 1989.

42. Agent summary statement for human immunodeficiency viruses (HIVs) including HTLV-III, LAV, HIV-1, and HIV-2. *MMWR* 37 (suppl 4):1–17, 1988.

43. Jagger J, Hunt EH, Brand-Elnaggar J, Pearson RD. Rates of needle-stick injury caused by various devices in a university hospital. *N Engl J Med* 319:284–288, 1988.

44. Lynch P, Jackson MM, Cummings MJ, Stamm WE. Rethinking the role of isolation practices in the prevention of nosocomial infections. *Ann Intern Med* 107:243–246, 1987.

45. Erice A, Rhame FS, Heussner RC, et al. Human immunodeficiency virus infection in patients with solid-organ transplants: Report of five cases and review. *Rev Infect Dis* 13:537–547, 1991.

46. Willy ME, Dhillon GL, Loewen NL, et al. Adverse exposures and universal precautions practices among a group of highly exposed health professionals. *Infect Control Hosp Epidemiol* 11:351–356, 1990.

47. Becker MH, Janz NK, Band J, et al. Noncompliance with universal precautions policy: Why do physicians and nurses recap needles? *Am J Infect Control* 18:232–239, 1990.

48. Kelen GD, DiGiovanna TA, Celentano DD, et al. Adherence to universal (barrier) precautions during interventions on critically ill and injured emergency department patients. *J AIDS* 3:987–994, 1990.

49. Doebbeling BN, Wentzel RP. The direct costs of universal precautions in a teaching hospital. *JAMA* 264:2083–2087, 1990.

50. Gerberding JL, Littell C, Tarkington A, et al. Risk of exposure of surgical personnel to patients' blood during surgery at San Francisco General Hospital. *N Engl J Med* 322:1788–1793, 1990.

51. Kelen GD, Green GB, Hexter DA, et al. Substantial improvement in compliance with universal precautions in an emergency department following institution of policy. *Arch Intern Med* 151:2051–2056, 1991.

52. Popejoy SL, Fry DE. Blood contact and exposure in the operating room. *Surg Gynecol Obstet* 172:480–483, 1991.

53. Gerberding JL, Schecter WP. Surgery and AIDS: Reducing the risk (editorial). *JAMA* 265:1572–1573, 1991.

54. Samuels ME, Koop CE, Hartsock PI. Single use syringes (letter). *N Engl J Med* 324:996–997, 1991.

55. Mangione CM, Gerberding JL, Cummings SR. Occupational exposure to HIV: Frequency and rates of underreporting of percutaneous and mucocutaneous exposures by medical housestaff. *Am J Med* 90:85–90, 1991.

56. Gerberding JL. Does knowledge of human immunodeficiency virus infection decrease the frequency of occupational exposure to blood? *Am J Med* 91 (suppl 3B):308S–311S, 1991.

57. Fahey BJ, Koziol DE, Banks SM, Henderson DK. Frequency of nonparenteral occupational exposures to blood and body fluids before and after universal precautions training. *Am J Med* 90:145–153, 1991.

58. Centers for Disease Control. Possible transmission of human immunodeficiency virus to a patient during an invasive dental procedure. *MMWR* 39:489–493, 1990.

59. Centers for Disease Control. Update: Transmission of HIV infection during an invasive dental procedure—Florida. *MMWR* 40:21–33, 1991.

60. Ciesielski C, et al. Transmission of human immunodeficiency virus in a dental practice. *Ann Intern Med* 116:798–805, 1992.

61. New York Academy of Medicine. The risk of contracting HIV infection in the course of health care. *JAMA* 265:1872–1873, 1991.
62. Danila RN, MacDonald KL, Rhame FS, et al. A look-back investigation of patients of an HIV-infected physician. *N Engl J Med* 325:1406–1411, 1991.
63. Gostin L. The HIV-infected health care professional. Public policy, discrimination, and patient safety. *Arch Intern Med* 151:663–665, 1991.
64. Lowenfels AB, Wormser G. Risk of transmission of HIV from surgeon to patient (letter). *N Engl J Med* 325:888–889, 1991.
65. Cowen DN, Brundage JF, Pomerantz RS, et al. HIV infection among members of the US Army Reserve components with medical and health occupations. *JAMA* 265:2826–2830, 1991.
66. Marcus R, Favero MS, Banerjee S, et al. Prevalence and incidence of human immunodeficiency virus among patients undergoing long-term hemodialysis. *Am J Med* 90:614–619, 1991.
67. Environmental Protection Agency. Clarification of HIV (AIDS virus) labeling policy for antimicrobial pesticide products. *Federal Register* 54:6288–6290, 1989.
68. Resnick L, Veren K, Salahuddin SZ, et al. Stability and inactivation of HTLV-III/LAV under clinical and laboratory environments. *JAMA* 255:1887–1891, 1986.
69. Sattar SA, Springthorpe VS. Survival and disinfectant inactivation of the human immunodeficiency virus: A critical review. *Rev Infect Dis* 13:430–447, 1991.
70. Rutala WA. APIC guideline for selection and use of disinfectants. *Am J Infect Control* 18:99–117, 1990.
71. Keene JH. Medical waste: A minimum hazard. *Infect Control Hosp Epidemiol* 12:682–685, 1991.
72. O'Neill TM, et al. Risk of needlesticks and occupational exposures among residents and medical students. *Arch Intern Med* 152:1451–1456, 1992.
73. Centers for Disease Control. Hepatitis B virus: A comprehensive strategy for eliminating transmission through universal childhood vaccination: recommendations of the Immunization Practices Advisory Committee (ACIP). *MMWR* 40(RR-13):1–25, 1991.
74. Imagawa DT, Lee MH, Wolonsky SM, et al. Human immunodeficiency virus type 1 infection in homosexual men who remain seronegative for prolonged periods. *N Engl J Med* 320:1458–1462, 1989.
75. Centers for Disease Control. Additional recommendations to reduce sexual and drug abuse–related transmission of human T-lymphotropic virus type III/lymphadenopathy-associated virus. *MMWR* 35:152–155, 1986.
76. Centers for Disease Control. Provisional public health service interagency recommendations for screening donated blood and plasma for antibody to the virus causing acquired immunodeficiency syndrome. *MMWR* 34:1–5, 1985.
77. Allen UD, Guerriere M, Read SE, Detsky AS. Percutaneous injuries among health care workers: The real value of human immunodeficiency virus testing of "donor" blood. *Arch Intern Med* 151:2033–2040, 1991.

78. White AC, Miller SM. HIV infection after needlesticks (letter). *Ann Intern Med* 114:253, 1991.

79. Durand E, LeJeunne C, Hugues FC. Failure of prophylactic zidovudine after suicidal self-inoculation of HIV-infected blood (letter). *N Engl J Med* 324:1062, 1991.

80. Henderson DK. Postexposure chemoprophylaxis for occupational exposure to human immunodeficiency virus type 1: Current status and prospects for the future. *Am J Med* 91 (suppl 3B):312S-319S, 1991.

81. DesPrez RM, Heim CR. *Mycobacterium tuberculosis*. In GL Mandell, RG Douglas, JE Bennett (eds), *Principles and Practice of Infectious Diseases* (3rd ed). New York: Churchill Livingstone, 1990. Pp 1879-1880.

82. Centers for Disease Control. Tuberculosis and human immunodeficiency virus infection: Recommendations of the Advisory Committee for the Elimination of Tuberculosis (ACET). *MMWR* 38:236-238, 243-250, 1989.

83. Centers for Disease Control. Tuberculosis and acquired immunodeficiency syndrome—New York City. *MMWR* 36:785-790,795, 1987.

84. US Dept. of Health and Human Services, *Core Curriculum on Tuberculosis* (2nd ed). Document 00-t 5763, April 1991. P 11.

85. Centers for Disease Control. Guidelines for preventing the transmission of tuberculosis in health-care settings, with special focus on HIV-related issues. *MMWR* 39(RR-17):1-29, 1990.

86. Centers for Disease Control. Nosocomial transmission of multidrug-resistant tuberculosis to health-care workers and HIV-infected patients in an urban hospital—Florida. *MMWR* 39:718-722, 1990.

87. Centers for Disease Control. *Mycobacterium tuberculosis* transmission in a health clinic—Florida, 1988. *MMWR* 38:256-264, 1989.

88. Centers for Disease Control. CDC Guidelines for Isolation Precautions in Hospitals. US Dept of Health and Human Services, 1986.

32/The Homosexual/Bisexual Patient

Jon D. Fuller

Despite the recent increase in AIDS cases acquired through injection drug use in the United States, homosexual and bisexual men remain the single largest group infected with HIV. Familiarity with the special needs of this population is important in the provision of medical care.

Before the AIDS epidemic, the training of health care workers in the treatment of gay and bisexual patients emphasized those medical conditions to which they were more prone than the general public. After the American Psychiatric Association removed homosexuality as a diagnostic category from its *Diagnostic and Statistical Manual* in 1973, increased attention was drawn to the presence of long-term, stable relationships among gay men and women, and clinicians began to focus on the promotion of healthy lifestyles for those who appeared to be constitutionally homosexual [1–3]. When the gay community was first affected by the AIDS epidemic in the early 1980s, other issues became prominent as well. These included incorporating a homosexual patient's partner into the medical decision-making process; recognizing the psychological effect of persistent, heavy losses on the gay community; and anticipating the need for a substitute decision maker by identifying a health care proxy.

Since men account for the vast majority of homosexual persons infected with HIV, this chapter focuses primarily on the care of gay and bisexual men. However, consideration of HIV transmission and disease is also relevant to lesbian health care [4]. Although lesbians as a group have a very low prevalence of HIV infection, the virus is found in cervical secretions and can be spread from woman to woman [5–8]. Some lesbians have a history of sexual relations with heterosexual or bisexual men, and health care providers should not make broad assumptions about sexual behavior based solely on self-described sexual orientation [9, 10].

Health Care Concerns Before the AIDS Epidemic

Knowing that a male patient is homosexual or bisexual is important in considering the differential diagnosis for certain clinical problems. This has been particularly well appreciated for sexually transmitted infectious diseases. For example, since approximately 20 percent of pharyngeal or rectal gonococcal infections among homosexual men may be asymptomatic, regular cultures of the throat, urethra, and rectum have been suggested as part of the health care maintenance of sexually active gay and bisexual men [11, 12].

In order to take an adequate medical history and evaluate a patient's risk for specific medical conditions, clinicians need to be comfortable with inquiring in a nonjudgmental manner about sexual orientation and activities, including the use of toys or instruments and exposure to urine or feces. Oral-anal intercourse may lead to infection with bacterial pathogens, parasites, chlamydia, hepatitis A virus, or herpes simplex virus. Oral-penile exposure may lead to gonococcal pharyngitis, and rectal intercourse predisposes to gonococcal, chlamydial, and herpetic proctitis, as well as condyloma acuminatum (human papillomavirus infection). Exposure to blood or semen may result in acquisition of hepatitis B, cytomegalovirus (CMV), or HIV infections [13–15]. Noninfectious complications of anal intercourse include prolapsed hemorrhoids, nonspecific proctitis, anal fistulas and fissures, rectal ulcers and tears, and foreign bodies [16].

Health Care Concerns Since the AIDS Epidemic

Identifying the means by which a patient has become infected with HIV can help focus education about reducing the risk of viral transmission to others. In addition, because some HIV-related conditions occur with increased frequency among homosexual and bisexual men, knowledge of an individual's sexual orientation should prompt the clinician to monitor for specific diseases, including Kaposi's sarcoma (KS), shigellosis, and squamous cell carcinoma of the rectum.

Kaposi's Sarcoma

In the early years of the HIV epidemic, KS was reported as the initial AIDS-defining diagnosis in 30 to 40 percent of homosexual and bisexual men, in only 3 to 4 percent of heterosexual men, and very rarely in hemophiliacs; greater than 90 percent of all epidemic KS occurs among gay men [17–20]. Although the reason for this epidemiologic disparity is not known, at least three explanations have been offered. First, CMV may serve as a cofactor in the development of KS following HIV infection. Supporting this hypothesis is the finding of CMV DNA in some KS tumor specimens and the observation of a high incidence of CMV infection ($> 90\%$) among homosexual men [21–24]. Secondly, amyl nitrate inhalants ("poppers"), which are used by some homosexual men to produce a "rush" and relaxation of the anal sphincter, may also predispose to the development of KS [25–28]. Since education in the gay community has stressed avoidance of the exchange of body fluids and counseled against the use of poppers, the incidence of KS as a presenting AIDS diagnosis has decreased to approximately 10 percent [29–31]. The third suggestion, that an unidentified sexually transmitted agent may be a cofactor in development of KS, derives from the observation that KS has occasionally been reported from HIV-seronegative homosexual men, but virtually never from seropositive recipients of infected blood products. Additionally, most women and children who have been diagnosed with AIDS-related KS come from well-delineated geographic areas. Taken together, these data imply that a virus that is sexually transmitted but not spread through blood products may be necessary or even sufficient in itself to lead to the development of KS [32].

Shigellosis

Individuals who have had oral-anal contact with a *Shigella* carrier are at risk for acquiring shigellosis [10]. Oral-anal contact may lead to bacteremia with or without gastrointestinal symptoms.

Rectal Carcinoma

Aggressive squamous cell carcinoma of the rectum has been reported among HIV-infected individuals who have had prior exposure to human papillomavirus [33, 34]. Persons at risk for this tumor include men and women with a history of receptive anal intercourse, as well as those who have condyloma acuminatum. Since these cancers develop in the rectal squamous epithelium below the dentate line, they are usually within reach of the examining finger. They are generally tender and friable on palpation. Because these tumors can grow quite rapidly and treatment is more successful for early disease, patients at risk may benefit from surveillance rectal examinations performed as part of health care maintenance.

Sexual Identity

Many studies before the AIDS era reported that homosexual and bisexual persons were reluctant to share their sexual identity with health care providers and that providers frequently presumed a heterosexual identity of their patients. However, there is also evidence that homosexual persons believe that their quality of care is enhanced when their sexual identity is known [35–37]. While simply knowing that a patient is homosexual or bisexual is medically useful, it is also critical that providers move beyond the "gay" identifier in order to understand the individual's development as a person. Just as there is no "typical" heterosexual person or lifestyle, it is important to recognize that a gay patient's lifestyle, sexual activity, or psychological development may not fit one's preconceived notions of homosexuality.

Kinsey and associates [38] reported that 25 percent of the adult American white male population had at least incidental homosexual experience for at least 3 years between the ages of 16 and 55, and estimated that only 10 percent were predominantly homosexual. Since Kinsey demonstrated that the vast majority of persons have a combination of homo-erotic and hetero-erotic feelings, a patient's brief self-reporting of sexual orientation will generally not provide a full understanding of his or her sexual behavior.

Gay Latino and black men tread an even more difficult path in adjusting to a homosexual life than do their white counterparts, since gay persons appear to be even less accepted within minority communities than in the general culture. Some homosexual persons of color may feel that they have been forced to choose between identifying with their minority community or the largely white, "high-profile" gay community [39].

The goal for the clinician is to understand the patient's sexuality as it is experienced by that individual. Relevant aspects of a homosexual man's personal life include some sense of how comfortable he is with his identity and, if he has "come out," how long he has so self-identified. To what degree is he considered gay by his natural family, and what has been their response? Does his family know his HIV status? If they do not know of his HIV status, or do know and are uncomfortable with the fact, what is the impact of this on his life, and how does he cope with it? Is he in a relationship at present, and, if so, for how long? What is the HIV serostatus of his partner, and what effect has HIV disease had on their relationship? Is he sexually active, and, if so, are risk reduction techniques understood and employed? What is his level of support and connection within the larger gay community? What has been his experience with the AIDS epidemic to date; has he lost many friends or previous partners? How does his personal experience affect his anticipation of the future? [40–42].

Substitute Decision Making

An especially important issue for health care providers to discuss with their homosexual patients is substitute decision making in the event of incompetence resulting from deterioration of their medical condition. If no special arrangements have been made, a homosexual man's natural family is often given authority as next of kin and may countermand the wishes of the patient's life partner, even to the extent of forbidding visiting privileges. In many states, a durable power of attorney for health care may be executed to allow for transfer of decision making to an individual of the patient's choosing. Health care providers should make a special effort to anticipate such eventualities and to discuss with the patient his wishes for resuscitation and substitute decision making early in the course of HIV disease.

Suicidality

While all HIV-infected persons face the burden of an uncertain future, some studies have suggested that this may be borne especially heavily by members of the gay community, with cumulative grief and resultant despair translating into an increased risk of suicide. Multiple losses related to AIDS and intimate involvement with another who has died of AIDS are suicide risk factors for HIV-infected patients. Others may include (1) having recently been informed of a positive HIV test result, (2) having a personal history of losses related to homophobia, (3) living with an unsettled sexual identity, (4) experiencing increased physical pain from disease, and (5) undergoing a loss of physical autonomy and the capacity to control one's bodily functions [43–46].

Health Care Provider Attitudes Toward Homosexuality

Although concerns about disease transmission account for much of the anxiety that has been noted among health care providers toward HIV-infected patients, some may also reflect underlying discomfort in working with homosexual and bisexual individuals [47–49]. Since the American Medical Association has recognized that providers may transfer the care of patients whom they do not feel qualified to treat, remaining untrained may provide a convenient excuse for physicians who do not wish to provide care for homosexual or HIV-infected patients [50]. However, given that there are more than one million HIV-infected Americans and that the majority are homosexual or bisexual men, most primary care physicians will need to become familiar with the health and social concerns of this population [51].

References

1. McWhirter DP, Mattison AM. *The Male Couple.* Englewood Cliffs, NJ: Prentice-Hall, 1984.

2. Council on Scientific Affairs, American Medical Association. Health care needs of a homosexual population. *JAMA* 248:726–739, 1982.
3. Owen WF. The clinical approach to the homosexual patient. *Ann Intern Med* 93:90–92, 1980.
4. White J, Levinson W. Primary care of lesbian patients. *J Gen Intern Med* 8:41–47, 1993.
5. Blaser MJ. Isolation of human immunodeficiency virus from cervical secretions during menses. *Ann Intern Med* 106:912, 1987.
6. Archibald DW, Witt DJ, Craven DE, et al. Antibodies to human immunodeficiency virus in cervical secretions from women at risk for AIDS. *J Infect Dis* 156:240–241, 1987.
7. Marmor M, Laubenstein L, William DC, et al. Possible female-to-female transmission of human immunodeficiency virus. *Ann Intern Med* 105:969, 1986.
8. Monzon OT, Capellan JMB. Female-to-female transmission of HIV. *Lancet* 2:40–41, 1987.
9. Cochran SD, Mays VM. Disclosure of sexual preference to physicians by black lesbian and bisexual women. *West J Med* 149:616–619, 1988.
10. Johnson SR, Guenther SM, Laube DW, Keettel WC. Factors influencing lesbian gynecologic care: A preliminary study. *Am J Obstet Gynecol* 140:20–28, 1981.
11. Dritz S. Medical aspects of homosexuality. *N Engl J Med* 302:463–464, 1980.
12. Sohn N, Robilotti JG. The gay bowel syndrome: A review of colonic and rectal conditions in 200 male homosexuals. *Am J Gastroenterol* 67:478–484, 1977.
13. Corey L, Holmes KK. Sexual transmission of hepatitis A in homosexual men: Incidence and mechanism. *N Engl J Med* 302:435–438, 1980.
14. Owen WF. Sexually transmitted diseases and traumatic problems in homosexual men. *Ann Intern Med* 92:805–808, 1980.
15. Weller IVD. The gay bowel. *Gut* 26:869–875, 1985.
16. Rompalo AM, Stamm WE. Anorectal and enteric infections in homosexual men. *West J Med* 142:647–652, 1985.
17. Centers for Disease Control. Kaposi's sarcoma and *Pneumocystis carinii* pneumonia among homosexual men—New York City and California. *MMWR* 30:305–308, 1981.
18. Centers for Disease Control. Epidemiologic aspects of the current outbreak of Kaposi's sarcoma and opportunistic infections. *N Engl J Med* 306:248–252, 1982.
19. Haverkos HW, Pinsky PF, Drotman DP, Bregman J. Prevalence of Kaposi's sarcoma among patients with AIDS. *N Engl J Med* 312:1518, 1985.
20. Des Jarlais DC, Marmor M, Thomas P, et al. Kaposi's sarcoma among four different AIDS risk groups. *N Engl J Med* 310:1119, 1984.
21. Brodie HR, et al. Prevalence of Kaposi's sarcoma in AIDS patients reflects differences in rates of cytomegalovirus infection in high risk groups. *AIDS Memorandum* 1:12, 1984.
22. Collier AC, Meyers JD, Corey L, et al. Cytomegalovirus infection in homosexual men: Relationship to sexual practices, antibody to human immu-

nodeficiency virus, and cell-mediated immunity. *Am J Med* 82:593–601, 1987.
23. Giraldo G, Beth E. The involvement of cytomegalovirus in acquired immune deficiency syndrome and Kaposi's sarcoma. *Prog Allergy* 37:319–331, 1986.
24. Mintz L, Drew WL, Miner RC, Braff EH. Cytomegalovirus infections in homosexual men: An epidemiologic study. *Ann Intern Med* 99:326–329, 1983.
25. Marmor M, Laubenstein L, William DC, et al. Risk factors for Kaposi's sarcoma in homosexual men. *Lancet* 1:1083–1086, 1982.
26. Haverkos HW, Pinsky, PF, Drotman, P, Bregman, DJ. Disease manifestations among homosexual men with acquired immunodeficiency syndrome: A possible role of nitrites in Kaposi's sarcoma. *Sex Transm Dis* 12:203–208, 1985.
27. Durack DT. Opportunistic infections and Kaposi's sarcoma in homosexual men. *N Engl J Med* 305:1465–1467, 1981.
28. Jorgensen KA, Lawesson SO. Amyl nitrite and Kaposi's sarcoma in homosexual men. *N Engl J Med* 307:893–894, 1982.
29. Rutherford GW, Schwarcz SK, Lemp GF, et al. The epidemiology of AIDS-related Kaposi's sarcoma in San Francisco. *J Infect Dis* 159:569–572, 1989.
30. Des Jarlais DC, Stoneburner R, Thomas P. Declines in proportion of Kaposi's sarcoma among cases of AIDS in multiple risk groups in New York City. *Lancet* 2:1024–1025, 1987.
31. Drew WL, Mills J, Hauer LB, et al. Declining prevalence of Kaposi's sarcoma in homosexual AIDS patients paralleled by fall in cytomegalovirus transmission. *Lancet* 1:66, 1988.
32. Beral V, Peterman TA, Berkelman RL, Jaffe HW. Kaposi's sarcoma among persons with AIDS: A sexually transmitted infection? *Lancet* 335:123–128, 1990.
33. Daling JR, Weiss MS, Hislop G, et al. Sexual practices, sexually transmitted diseases, and the incidence of anal cancer. *N Engl J Med* 317:973–977, 1987.
34. Leichman L, Nigro N, Vaitkevicius VK, et al. Cancer of the anal canal. *Am J Med* 78:211–215, 1985.
35. Smith EM, Johnson SR, Guenther SM. Health care attitudes and experiences during gynecologic care among lesbians and bisexuals. *Am J Public Health* 75:1085–1087, 1985.
36. Dardick L, Gradey KE. Openness between gay persons and health professionals. *Ann Intern Med* 93:115–119, 1980.
37. McGhee RD, Owen WF. Medical aspects of homosexuality. *N Engl J Med* 303:50–51, 1980.
38. Kinsey AC, Pomeroy WB, Martin CE. *Sexual Behavior in the Human Male.* Philadelphia: Saunders, 1948. Pp 610–666.
39. Mays VM, Cochran SD. Black gay and bisexual men coping with more than just a disease. *Focus* 4:1–3, 1988.
40. Nichols SE. Psychosocial reactions of persons with the acquired immunodeficiency syndrome. *Ann Intern Med* 103:765–767, 1985.

41. Cassens BJ. Social consequences of the acquired immunodeficiency syndrome. *Ann Intern Med* 103:768–771, 1985.
42. Forstein M. The psychosocial impact of the acquired immunodeficiency syndrome. *Semin Oncol* 11:77–82, 1984.
43. Samuelson MC. Heavy losses. *Phoenix* September 30, 1988. Pp 4–14.
44. Goldblum P, Moulton J. AIDS-related suicide: A dilemma for health care providers. *Focus* 2:1–2, 1986.
45. Goldblum P. Suicide: Clinical aspects. *Focus* 2:2–4, 1986.
46. Marzuk PM, Tierney H, Tardiff K, et al. Increased risk of suicide in persons with AIDS. *JAMA* 259:1333–1337, 1988.
47. Mathews WC, Booth MW, Turner JD, Kessler L. Physicians attitudes toward homosexuality: Survey of a California county medical society. *West J Med* 144:109–110, 1986.
48. Douglas CJ, Kalman CM, Kalman TP. Homophobia among physicians and nurses: An empirical study. *Hosp Community Psychiatry* 36:1309–1311, 1985.
49. Kelly JA, St. Lawrence JS, Smith S, et al. Stigmatization of AIDS patients by physicians. *Am J Public Health* 77:789–791, 1987.
50. AMA stresses doctors duty to AIDS patients. *Med World News* December 14, 1987. Pp 40–41.
51. Northfelt DW, Hayward RA, Shapiro MF. The acquired immunodeficiency syndrome is a primary care disease. *Ann Intern Med* 109:773–774, 1989.

33/The Drug-Using Patient

Alan A. Wartenberg

In the past, interaction between the health care system and injection drug users (IDUs) was relatively limited, and acute medical issues, such as cellulitis, pneumonia, and drug overdose, predominated. Once treatment was initiated, and often before it was completed, the IDU would leave the hospital or emergency room, as soon as he or she was physically able. Little thought was given to management of chronic medical problems by either the physician or the IDU. The HIV epidemic has dramatically changed this situation [1, 2].

Increasing numbers of individuals have either switched to or initiated drug use with cocaine in the form of freebase or "crack." With increasing heroin purity, many users are "snorting" the drug. Alcohol, benzodiazepine, barbiturate, and oral opiate use are also very prevalent. Disinhibited sexual behavior associated with these agents may enhance HIV transmission. However, since sharing of injection equipment remains the dominant drug-related risk behavior for acquiring HIV infection, the IDU is used as the paradigm for the drug-using patient.

Injection drug users with HIV disease are entering into primary care in increasing numbers and, to the surprise of many physicians, have demonstrated considerable compliance [3]. Health care professionals must learn to deal with the patient who has drug problems in a way that reduces mutual animosity rather than escalating it. Five basic concepts are involved in this effort:

1. Understanding addiction as a process and the addict as someone with a disease
2. Understanding how to deal with difficult behaviors and set limits for the patient
3. Developing a knowledge base to recognize and manage the common medical complications of drug use, particularly withdrawal syndromes
4. Understanding treatment options and how they can be accessed
5. Recognizing the special health care issues of the drug user with HIV disease

455

Addiction as a Process and the Addict as Patient

Chemical dependency is not universally accepted as a disease [4, 5]. The repetition of self-destructive behaviors, whether involving the ingestion of substances or pathologic gambling, is understood by some as poor decision making that is socially conditioned rather than a disease manifestation. However, intoxication, withdrawal, and medical complications of drug addiction clearly fit a disease model; the addiction process has a natural history with a characteristic pattern of behavior and response to interventions. The "moral" or criminalization model that prevailed before the medical model led to preventable deaths in "drunk tanks," to an abysmal record of prison drug treatment programs, and perhaps to the current therapeutic nihilism regarding the addict [6].

The attitude of the health professional toward the IDU has an impact on the quality of care provided. Development of a nonjudgmental posture and the use of positive interpersonal skills, such as empathy, legitimization, respect, support, and partnership, are important [7]. The clinician should attempt to understand the language and culture of the addict. Physicians or nurses who do not comprehend this jargon should ask rather than perpetuate misunderstanding; a dictionary of street drug use is available [8].

If the health care provider maintains a professional and nonjudgmental attitude toward the IDU, treats him or her with the same respect accorded other patients, and creates an atmosphere of caring and concern for the individual's well-being, a positive outcome is more likely. Perpetuation of stereotypes fostered by previous negative experiences must be avoided.

Limit Setting and Dealing with Difficult Behaviors

The responsibilities of the clinician and IDU should be delineated early in the relationship. The tone of conversation should be professional, calm, and reassuring; anger and hostility are counterproductive. The rules of the clinic or inpatient unit should be clearly stated and include absolute intolerance of drug use in the health care setting. Violence, threats of violence, and abusive or threatening language are not acceptable and should lead to sanctions, including discharge from care, if warranted. The health care team, including the physician, nurse, and social worker, must collaborate in determining appropriate regulations and responses, and be unified in their approach to the patient.

Guidelines should be considered in advance for psychoactive drugs, including analgesics, anxiolytics, hypnotics, and antidepressants. When possible, drugs that do not produce significant mood alteration and are less addicting are preferred. Examples include the use of nonsteroidal antiinflammatory drugs for pain, buspirone for long-term anxiety, and low-dose sedating antidepressants for sleep. When possible, nonpharmacologic treatments, such as relaxation tapes, physiotherapy, acupuncture, local heat, and biofeedback, should be used to control symptoms. Patients should be informed in advance if urine toxicology screens will be obtained, and care should be taken to assure that the patient provides a legitimate specimen [9]. Limitations of toxicology studies include failure to detect drugs with short half-lives; specimen substitution or adulteration, or both; and false-positive tests [10]. When properly used, screening for drug use in a timely fashion may serve as a deterrent to repetition of this behavior in the health care setting.

The health care team must decide in advance how it will respond to negative behaviors. If the patient refuses to cooperate after the limits have been set and understood, or repeatedly violates the treatment contract, consideration should be given to discharging the patient from care as soon as medically feasible. If a patient uses drugs in the hospital setting or is involved in behavior that is dangerous to self or others, discharge may be necessary even if the patient has a serious continuing medical condition. Every effort should be made to prevent this outcome, but, if necessary, such an action must be taken without anger and recrimination. The patient should be informed that it is the consequence of his or her violation of the contract [11].

Understanding the motivation of the "hateful patient" can result in a more professional response by the health care provider [12]. A positive urine toxicology screen or other evidence of recent drug use should lead to a discussion with the patient about the factors that precipitated the incident. In some cases, drug use or other negative behaviors may indicate that detoxification is not proceeding properly and that the patient is either being overtreated, which may produce disinhibition, or undertreated, with resultant craving, anxiety, and agitation.

Medical Evaluation and Treatment

In addition to the general medical history, a complete history of drug use is necessary. Specific questions regarding use of opiates, cocaine, alcohol, sedative-hypnotics, and inhalants should be asked, with particular regard to quantity, duration, and last use. Heroin is sold in "bags," with 10 bags to a "bundle." A bag may cost $10 to $20 and contains from 2 to 15 mg heroin, but cost and purity are highly variable. An average bag in New England presently contains 5 to 8 mg heroin. Cocaine is sold in fractions of an ounce, with "eighths," "sixteenths," and "quarters" being common sizes. An eighth contains approximately 3.5 gm of 50 to

80% cocaine but may vary considerably in purity; currently, cocaine costs approximately $50 to $75 per gram. A patient on a cocaine binge or "run" may use more than $500 of cocaine in 1 to 3 days.

Determining the patient's prior experience with drug withdrawal is extremely important [13]. If alcohol or sedatives are being used regularly, abstinence may result in a withdrawal syndrome requiring aggressive medical treatment [13–15]. Opiate withdrawal, while not life threatening, may be very symptomatic and lead to drug-seeking behavior. Methadone is the treatment of choice, although clonidine and high-dose benzodiazepines have been advocated as alternative therapies [16–19]. In general, the initial oral dose of methadone is 5 to 10 mg; intramuscular methadone is almost twice as potent as the oral preparation, and the dose should be adjusted accordingly. If the patient has objective signs of withdrawal, such as piloerection, mydriasis, rhinorrhea, or lacrimation, 10 to 20 mg methadone can be given initially. The starting dose of methadone should not exceed 40 mg per day unless the patient has clearly been receiving the equivalent dose of other opiates; overtreatment may lead to respiratory depression and aspiration. Nonsteroidal antiinflammatory agents, antispasmodics, and sedatives can be used on a short-term basis to control the pain, abdominal cramps, diarrhea, and insomnia of opiate withdrawal.

If a patient attends a methadone treatment program, the dose level should be confirmed. If this is not possible, 40 mg methadone is generally sufficient to cover the first couple of days of hospitalization for individuals receiving higher doses. If a patient is unable to take anything by mouth, the total daily dose of methadone should be reduced approximately 30 to 50 percent and given intramuscularly in three to four divided doses per day. Patients who need narcotic analgesics for pain should receive an appropriate agent; drug tolerance may require a 50 to 100 percent increase over the usual dosage. The maintenance dose of methadone will not provide analgesia for patients with significant pain. Mixed agonist-antagonists, such as pentazocine, butorphanol, and nalbuphine, may precipitate a withdrawal syndrome and should be avoided. If a patient is being discharged from an inpatient setting, the staff of the methadone program should be notified in advance, so that they can plan readmission to their facility.

If naloxone is used to treat respiratory depression, it may produce an abrupt withdrawal syndrome. Following acute treatment with bolus naloxone, a continuous infusion with 4 mg naloxone in 1,000 ml 5% dextrose in water (D5W) at 100 ml per hour can be titrated to maintain adequate ventilation without precipitating significant withdrawal [20]. In severe overdose, large doses of naloxone (2 mg) may be necessary, with repeated administration every 20 to 40 minutes. If the patient is taking methadone or propoxyphene, up to a 4-mg bolus of naloxone may be required to reverse respiratory depression.

Cocaine craving and post-cocaine depression may be severe. Anti-craving agents such as bromocriptine and tricyclic antidepressants, particularly desipramine, have been used with some success in the treatment of post-cocaine symptoms [21, 22]. An initial dose of bromocriptine, 1.25 mg orally, can be given, and, if tolerated, 2.5 to 5.0 mg every 8 to 12 hours may be effective. Desipramine is given orally as 25 to 50 mg initially, increasing the dose by 25 to 50 mg every 2 or 3 days until 100 to 150 mg per day is attained. Other antidepressants can be used in equivalent doses if desipramine is not tolerated. Some of these agents, such as desipramine and fluoxetine, are stimulating and should be given early in the day, whereas others, such as amitryptiline, nortryptiline, and doxepin, are sedating and should be given in the evening or at bedtime. Bromocriptine should be continued until the antidepressant begins to work or cocaine craving has spontaneously subsided.

The optimal duration of antidepressant therapy in this setting is unknown, but 3 months appears adequate. Tricyclic antidepressants may have serious toxicity in some patients, including cardiac dysrhythmias and seizures, and their efficacy in the treatment of post-cocaine symptoms has not been definitively established. The judicious use of short-term anxiolytic agents is warranted in the presence of severe anxiety. Psychotic symptoms can be managed with neuroleptics, but these agents sometimes worsen post-cocaine craving and depression.

General care of all patients with a history of drug or alcohol abuse should include adequate nutrition, as well as the provision of thiamine and multivitamins. Physical or occupational therapy, or both, may also be beneficial. The ability of the health care professional to spend time with the patient and to project reasonable optimism regarding the future is important for a successful outcome. However, while a caring clinician may facilitate behavioral change in the addict, the addict must take primary responsibility for these efforts.

Referral To Drug Treatment

An understanding of treatment options and how to access them is attainable by all health care professionals. If the patient has a supportive social structure and no serious medical or psychiatric disabilities, outpatient treatment may be appropriate. For those with extensive opiate use, methadone detoxification with evaluation for maintenance should be considered [16, 23]. If the patient is placed on methadone in the hospital, it should be with a rapid detoxification (5–10 days), unless there has been consultation with an approved methadone program that agrees to maintain the patient after discharge.

If hospital detoxification is warranted, methadone should be given orally in a single daily dose, preferably in liquid form, and the patient should swallow the entire dose under observation. In general, the dose can be decreased by 2.5 to 5.0 mg per day. Clonidine may be useful in patients being detoxified from short-acting opiates or for those receiving lower-dose methadone (40 mg or less) [17, 18]. In general, an initial dose of 0.1 mg clonidine can be given if the systolic blood pressure is 100 mm Hg or greater, followed by 0.1 to 0.2 mg every 2 to 4 hours, titrating the dose based on clinical response and blood pressure. The optimal daily dose should be maintained for 24 to 48 hours and then tapered over the next 7 to 10 days. Clonidine transdermal patches may be better tolerated in some patients. An initial 0.1-mg patch is placed, and the dose doubled every 2 days until symptomatic improvement occurs; 0.4 to 0.6 mg may be required. Patients may require oral clonidine for the first 24 to 48 hours as the blood levels produced by the patch rise. Use of nonsteroidal antiinflammatory agents, antispasmodics, antidiarrheal agents, and hypnotics is usually required as part of clonidine detoxification.

In patients with less extensive opiate histories, or with primary cocaine or other drug problems, referral to a drug-free program is appropriate. If the patient does not live in a supportive setting or if outpatient therapy has failed, residential treatment is preferred. Such programs are readily available to those with health insurance, but may be harder to find for those receiving medical assistance or those without the capacity to pay. The hospital social work staff or clinic managers should be familiar with local programs.

Self-help programs, such as Narcotics Anonymous, Cocaine Anonymous, and Alcoholics Anonymous, are almost universally available, and patients should be encouraged to attend meetings, join a group, and obtain a sponsor [24, 25]. Programs for family members and significant others, including Nar-Anon and Al-Anon, are often invaluable. Involvement of family and significant others in the treatment program may increase the chance of success [26]. For patients who have difficulty with the "spiritual" nature of these programs, others, such as Rational Recovery and Women in Sobriety, may be acceptable alternatives.

In patients in whom less restrictive treatment has failed, therapeutic communities (long-term residential programs that offer highly structured programs) may be the best option [27]. Communities that are members of Therapeutic Communities of America adhere to accepted standards of care and are preferred. Success rates in highly structured residential programs are better than 90 percent abstinence at 1 year and 70 percent abstinence 3 years after treatment [27].

If immediate placement in a treatment program is not available, referral to self-help groups, family referral, outpatient detoxification using clonidine, and/or other symptomatic measures should be offered. Temporizing measures may be successful until more appropriate treatment options become available.

In well-motivated patients, treatment with naltrexone may be effective in reducing or eliminating illicit opiate use [28]. Naltrexone should be prescribed only for those patients who have been detoxified from opiates, preferably with clonidine. If naltrexone is given to a patient who is still dependent on opiates, it may precipitate a severe and long-lasting withdrawal syndrome. The dose is 50 mg orally once a day; in supervised programs, patients may receive 100 mg on Mondays and Wednesdays and 150 mg on Fridays. Liver function studies should be monitored periodically.

If treatment is refused, the clinician should continue to educate, persuade, and support the patient, while promoting appropriate options at each visit. Improvement in behavior may be gradual, and the clinician may need to accept relatively modest changes over time [29]. Treatment should be viewed as an ongoing process rather than as an isolated event. It may be possible to refer family members into counseling and self-help groups; the reduction in "enabling behaviors" may prompt a previously resistant patient to seek treatment. Cultural and ethnic sensitivity is important; patients may be more likely to accept treatment in self-help groups if they are composed of people of similar backgrounds and/or have a counselor who is linguistically and culturally appropriate.

Special Considerations for the Drug User with HIV Infection

Clinicians who deal with IDUs and other drug-using populations should be familiar with the medical complications that may occur with such use (Table 33-1); several excellent reviews are available [30–35]. The IDU spends much, if not most, of his or her time securing drugs, making it difficult for the actively using patient to devote sufficient time or energy to health promotion. Similarly, the IDU who is trying to recover will be expending most of his or her energy on staying clean and in treatment. HIV antibody testing may increase risk of relapse or increased drug use in IDUs and may increase depression and suicidal ideation, particularly if the patient has preexisting neuropsychological dysfunction [36–38]. HIV testing should be performed with appropriate pretest and posttest counseling; mental health or substance abuse treatment facilities must be available in case a crisis develops [39]. It is important to delay HIV testing in the patient who is emotionally or behaviorally unstable.

In the IDU with known HIV infection, every effort should be made to

Table 33-1 *Medical complications in the drug-using patient*

Bacterial infections
  Pneumonia
  Endocarditis
  Skin and soft tissue infections
  Osteomyelitis/septic arthritis

Tuberculosis

Sexually transmitted diseases
  Syphilis
  Gonorrhea
  Chlamydia
  Herpes simplex virus
  Human papillomavirus

Hepatitis
  Viral hepatitis (A, B, C, delta)
  Alcoholic

Central and peripheral nervous system diseases

Retroviral infections
  HIV infection and its medical complications
  HTLV-I
  HTLV-II

Malignancies
  Lymphoma
  Solid tumors (oropharynx, larynx, lungs)

Miscellaneous
  Constitutional symptoms
  Lymphadenopathy
  Renal disease

Source: Adapted from PA Selwyn, PG O'Connor, Diagnosis and treatment of substance users with HIV infection. *Primary Care* 19:119–156, 1992.

keep the patient in drug treatment, since continued drug use threatens both the individual's health and medical compliance. Because a patient has declined treatment on one occasion does not mean that it should not be offered again at every opportunity; involvement of the patient's family or significant other or the enlistment of counselors may improve the likelihood of acceptance. However, the clinician should be cognizant of confidentiality requirements of federal and state laws regarding substance abuse [40].

The treatment of pain, anxiety, and depression in a population with a history of abusing mood-altering drugs presents special problems for the clinician. In general, pain should be managed in accordance with recognized principles [41, 42]. Initially, salicylates or acetaminophen can be given; if the patient has chronic pain, these agents should be prescribed on a continuing basis. Nonsteroidal antiinflammatory agents are an acceptable alternative and may be better tolerated by some patients. If pain is severe, short-acting opiates, such as codeine, hydrocodone, or oxycodone, can be added to the nonnarcotic analgesics already given. Oral opiates are equally effective in equipotent doses, but codeine tends to cause more nausea and pruritus than other agents.

In general, it is better to avoid fixed combinations of salicylates or acetaminophen with an opiate, since the patient may end up taking toxic doses of the nonnarcotic agent to provide adequate doses of the opiate. If pain cannot be controlled with four or five daily doses of a medication, consideration should be given to switching to a longer-acting opiate such as methadone or sustained-action morphine sulfate (MS-Contin). If methadone is used, patients should be dosed every 6 to 8 hours for analgesic effect; once-daily dosing is usually not effective. Doses of 5 to 10 mg methadone are generally sufficient for pain control, as is 30 to 60 mg MS-Contin every 8 to 12 hours. Patients should be started at a lower dose and titrated upward.

Anxiety may be situational or part of a phobic, panic, or generalized anxiety disorder [43]. Situational anxiety is best treated with reassurance and counseling. Phobic disorders may respond to desensitization therapy, and panic disorder to antidepressants. Generalized anxiety can be treated with buspirone, which is nonaddicting, but takes 2 to 3 weeks to be effective. Depression, whether unipolar or bipolar, is treated in standard fashion, although patients with advanced HIV disease may have difficulty with side effects such as dry mouth and orthostatic hypotension [44, 45]. Many psychiatric disorders, including bipolar and personality disorders, are overrepresented in this population, and posttraumatic stress disorder may occur in combat veterans or patients with a history of childhood sexual trauma.

Patients whose conditions have been stable on mood-altering drugs, even those that produce dependency, need not be switched to other agents. If there is evidence of dose escalation, concomitant abuse of alcohol, or frequent abuse or intoxication, the clinician should proceed with gradual detoxification and substitution of a safer agent or therapy. Patients should be informed in advance that prescriptions for analgesics and mood-altering drugs will not be refilled before the appropriate time interval; prescriptions that are "lost," "stolen," "fell in the toilet," or "were eaten by the dog" are the patient's responsibility. The clinician should, however, provide medication in dose and quantity sufficient to last until the next appointment. It may be preferable to give prescriptions that are to be refilled several times, rather than a 2- or 3-month supply. An agreement to use only one pharmacy is often a helpful part of the therapeutic contract.

Conclusion

HIV-infected patients with a history of drug use can be successfully managed by primary care physicians. Enhancement of one's knowledge base, use of interpersonal skills, and appreciation of approaches to drug treatment are all important. Interested health care providers may find it useful to rotate on a specialized drug treatment unit, particularly one where medical and psychiatric problems are comanaged [46]. Improved attitudes, skills, and behaviors of health professionals who provide care for drug-using patients are essential for the management of HIV disease.

References

1. Schoenbaum EE, et al. Risk factors for human immunodeficiency virus infection in intravenous drug users. *N Engl J Med* 321:874–879, 1989.
2. Chaisson RE, Bachetti P, Osmond D, et al. Cocaine use and HIV infection in intravenous drug users in San Francisco. *JAMA* 261:561–565, 1989.
3. Selwyn PA, et al. Primary care for patients with human immunodeficiency virus (HIV) infection in a methadone maintenance treatment program. *Ann Intern Med* 111:761–763, 1989.
4. Fingarette H. *Heavy Drinking: The Myth of Alcoholism as a Disease.* Berkeley: University of California Press, 1988.
5. Peele S. *Diseasing of America: Addiction Treatment Out of Control.* Lexington, MA: Lexington Books, 1989.
6. Senay EC. The Treatment of Drug Abuse. In S Aneti (ed), *American Handbook of Psychiatry.* New York: Basic Books, 1976.
7. Novack DH. Therapeutic aspects of the clinical encounter. *J Gen Intern Med* 2:346–355, 1987.
8. Johnson NP, Davis CW, Michels PJ. *Dictionary of Street Alcohol and Drug Terms.* Columbia: University of South Carolina Press, 1989.
9. Mackenzie RG, Cheng M, Haftel AJ. The clinical utility and evaluation of drug screening techniques. *Pediatr Clin North Am* 34:423–437, 1987.
10. Verebey K, Martin DM, Gold MS. Interpretation of drug abuse testing: Strengths and limitations of current methodology. *Psychiatr Med* 3:287–297, 1987.
11. Quill TE. Partnerships in patient care: A contractual approach. *Ann Intern Med* 98:228–234, 1983.
12. Groves JE. Taking care of the hateful patient. *N Engl J Med* 298:883–887, 1978.
13. Wartenberg AA. Detoxification of the chemically dependent patient. *RI Med J* 42:451–456, 1989.
14. Sullivan JT, Sellers EM. Treating alcohol, barbiturate and benzodiazepine withdrawal. *Rational Drug Ther* 20:1–9, 1986.
15. Wartenberg AA, Nirenberg TD, Liepman MR, et al. Detoxification of alco-

holics: Improving care by symptom-triggered sedation. *Alcohol Clin Exp Res* 14:71–75, 1990.

16. Cooper JR. Methadone treatment and acquired immunodeficiency syndrome. *JAMA* 262:1664–1668, 1989.

17. Washton AM, Resnick RB. Clonidine for opiate detoxification: Outpatient clinical trials. *Am J Psychiatry* 137:1121–1122, 1980.

18. Kleber HD, et al. Clonidine in outpatient detoxification from methadone maintenance. *Arch Gen Psychiatry* 42:391–394, 1985.

19. Drummond DC, Turkington D, Rahman MZ, et al. Chlordiazepoxide versus methadone in opiate withdrawal: A preliminary double-blind trial. *Drug Alcohol Depend* 23:63–71, 1989.

20. Goldfrank LR, Bresnitz EA. Opioids. In Goldfrank, Flomenbaum, Lewin, Weisman (eds), *Toxicologic Emergencies: A Comprehensive Handbook in Problem Solving*. New York: Appleton-Century-Crofts, 1986. Pp 126–127.

21. Tennant FS, Jr, Saherian AA. Double-blind comparison of amantadine and bromocriptine for ambulatory withdrawal from cocaine maintenance. *Arch Intern Med* 147:109–112, 1987.

22. Gawin FH, et al. Desipramine facilitation of initial cocaine abstinence. *Arch Gen Psychiatry* 46:117–121, 1989.

23. Novick DM, et al. Absence of antibody for human immunodeficiency virus in long-term socially rehabilitated methadone maintenance patients. *Arch Intern Med* 150:97–99, 1990.

24. Bean MH. Alcoholics anonymous. *Psychiatr Ann* 5:7–61, 1975.

25. Zweben JE. Recovery orientated psychotherapy: Facilitating the use of 12-step programs. *J Psychoactive Drugs* 19:243, 1987.

26. Usher ML, Jay J, Glass DR. Family therapy as a treatment modality for alcoholism. *J Stud Alcohol* 43:927–938, 1982.

27. Rosenthal MS. Therapeutic communities: A treatment alternative for many but not all. *J Subst Abuse Treatment* 1:55–58, 1984.

28. O'Brien CP. A new approach to the management of opioid dependence: Naltrexone. *J Clin Psychiatry* 45:57–58, 1984.

29. Goldstein MG, Guise BJ, Ruggiero L, et al. Behavioral medicine strategies for medical patients. In A Stoudemire (ed), *Clinical Psychiatry for Medical Students*. Philadelphia: Lippincott, 1990. Pp 609–629.

30. Selwyn PA. Issues in the clinical management of intravenous drug users with HIV infection. *AIDS* 3 (suppl 1):S201–S208, 1989.

31. Cushman P. The major medical consequences of opioid addiction. *Drug Alcohol Depend* 5:239–254, 1980.

32. Wartenberg AA, Liepman MR. Medical Complications of Substance Abuse. In Lerner, Barr (eds), *Handbook of Hospital Based Substance Abuse Treatment*. New York: Pergamon Press, 1990. Pp 45–65.

33. Stein MD. Clinical review: Medical complications of intravenous drug use. *J Gen Intern Med* 5:249–257, 1990.

34. Selwyn PA. Issues in the clinical management of intravenous drug users with HIV infection. *AIDS* 3 (suppl):S201–S208, 1989.

35. Selwyn PA, O'Connor PG. Diagnosis and treatment of substance users with HIV infection. *Primary Care* 19:119–156, 1992.

36. Ostrow DG. Psychiatric consequences of AIDS: An overview. *Int J Neurosci* 29:1–3, 1986.
37. Marzuk PM, Tierney H, Tardiff K. Increased risk of suicide in persons with AIDS. *JAMA* 259:1333–1337, 1988.
38. Perry SW. Organic mental disorders caused by HIV: Update on early diagnosis and treatment. *Am J Psychiatry* 147:696–710, 1990.
39. AIDS and Chemical Dependency Committee, American Medical Society on Alcoholism and Other Drug Dependencies. *Guidelines for Facilities Treating Chemical Dependency Patients at Risk for AIDS and HIV Infection.* New York, 1988.
40. Blume SB, American Medical Society on Alcoholism and Other Drug Dependencies and the National Council on Alcoholism. *Confidentiality of Patients Records in Alcoholism and Drug Treatment Programs.* New York, 1987.
41. Portnoy RK. Drug treatment of pain syndromes. *Semin Neurol* 7:139–149, 1987.
42. Amadio P, Jr, Cummings DM, Amadio P. A framework for the management of chronic pain. *Am Fam Physician* 38:155–160, 1988.
43. Roth M, Argyle N. Anxiety, panic and phobic disorders: An overview. *J Psychiatr Res* 22 (suppl 1):333–354, 1988.
44. Dilsaver SC, Votolato N, Coffman S. Depression in medical practice. *Am Fam Physician* 38:117–124, 1988.
45. Liepman MR, Nirenberg TD, Porges R, Wartenberg A. Depression Associated with Substance Abuse. In OG Cameron (ed), *Presentations of Depression.* New York: Wiley, 1987. Pp 131–167.
46. Dans PE, Matricciani RM, Otter SE, Reuland DS. Intravenous drug abuse and one academic health center. *JAMA* 263:3173–3176, 1990.

34/HIV Infection in Women

Gladys Gibbs, Beth Zeeman

The greatest increase in reported AIDS cases in the United States is among women. The threat that HIV poses to women's health is formidable, and perinatal transmission of the virus is an increasing problem worldwide. Despite these trends, the impact of HIV infection on the female population is perhaps the most inadequately studied aspect of the epidemic. Relatively little has been written about its medical, psychological, and social consequences. Small numbers of HIV-infected women have been involved in clinical trials, and the risks and benefits of therapeutic interventions are uncertain.

Epidemiology

Ellerbrock and Rogers [1] at the Centers for Disease Control (CDC) have described the epidemiology of AIDS in women compared to heterosexual men in the US. Affected women are, in general, younger than men and less likely (51 vs. 70%) to be injection drug users (IDUs). Thirty percent of women with AIDS are sexual partners of persons with high-risk behaviors; 52 percent are black and 21 percent Latino, and cumulative incidence rates for AIDS in these groups are 13 and 8 times those of white women, respectively [1, 2]. In female IDUs, there is evidence that intravenous cocaine use is an especially high-risk behavior [3].

In 1989, seroprevalence surveys of neonatal cord blood indicated that 1.5 per 1,000 women who gave birth in the US were HIV infected. Even higher rates have been reported in New York (5.8 per 1,000), the District of Columbia (5.5 per 1,000), New Jersey (4.9 per 1,000), and Florida (4.5 per 1,000) [4]. In 1987, Donegan, Edelin, and Craven [5] found that 1.8 percent of cord blood samples at Boston City Hospital were positive for HIV antibody; more recent data from the same institution indicate the seroprevalence rate to be greater than 3 percent [6].

Outside of the US, the epidemiology of HIV infection is quite different. Approximately 80 percent of HIV-infected women worldwide reside in sub-Saharan Africa, where they comprise approximately 50 percent of all AIDS cases. In this region, heterosexual and perinatal transmission of the virus predominate. The World Health Organization estimates that 2.5 million women in sub-Saharan Africa are HIV infected [7]. Several studies suggest that transfer of HIV from men to women occurs more easily than from women to men [8, 9]. Rehmet and associates [10] described a fourfold higher rate of HIV spread from men to women and the time period after first becoming sexually involved with a partner as presenting the greatest risk for transmission.

Factors that appear to increase the rate of sexual transmission of HIV include the presence or a history of genital ulcers, the practice of anal intercourse, and intercourse with an infected partner at an advanced stage of HIV disease [11–14]. Other risk factors for female partners of HIV-infected men include nonmenstrual bleeding during intercourse, nonwhite race, failure to use condoms, and increased number of sexual exposures. Factors that are thought not to increase the risk of HIV transmission include age, duration of the relationship, intercourse during menstruation (which may be a risk factor for transmission from women to men), number of sexually transmitted diseases by history, and circumcision status of the partner [13, 15]. The estimated risk of becoming HIV infected after several years of unprotected sex with the same infected partner ranges from 10 to 45 percent [16]. Vaginal transmission of HIV from women to men and, in one instance, from a woman to another woman, possibly through oral sex, has been documented [17, 18].

Barriers to Care for HIV-Infected Women

With the advent of zidovudine (ZDV) and prophylaxis for *Pneumocystis carinii* pneumonia (PCP), progression to AIDS has slowed and survival has been prolonged [19, 20]. However, many HIV-infected women do not engage in primary care. It is unclear whether this problem represents a lack of awareness of their therapeutic options or an inability or unwillingness to access care. Common impediments to health care for HIV-infected women include ongoing drug use, lack of available treatment programs, child care responsibilities, and psychological barriers such as guilt over HIV transmission to children. Recruitment strategies that can be utilized to deal with these issues include use of neighborhood outreach workers; establishment of clinic day care and food pantry facilities; coordination of HIV, obstetrics-gynecology, and pediatrics care; and improved social services.

Natural History of HIV Infection in Women

Knowledge of the natural history, prognosis, and treatment of HIV infection is based on studies of predominantly male populations, and may not be applicable to women. A study of Rhode Island women found that candidal esophagitis was the most common AIDS-defining illness (38%), and 23 of 24 HIV-infected patients evaluated had candidal infection, with vaginitis the most frequent type [21]. In contrast, another study found PCP to be the most common AIDS-defining disease in women [22].

Moore and associates [23] found that 2-year survival was less for women than men with AIDS in a Maryland study; 53 percent of men with AIDS received ZDV compared to 33 percent of women. Rothenberg and colleagues [24] examined 5,833 AIDS cases in New York City and reported that women survived a mean of 298 days after diagnosis compared to 374 days for men. Female gender remained an independent risk factor for shortened survival even after race, age, and risk behavior were controlled. It is uncertain whether decreased survival in these studies was related to a gender difference in the natural history of HIV infection, greater delay in women seeking primary care, or delayed recognition of HIV disease in women [25]. More recent data have confirmed that the median survival for women following AIDS-defining diagnosis is still reduced (13.4 months) compared to that of men (17 months) [26].

Selected Genital Diseases in HIV-Infected Women

Chronic Vaginal Candidiasis

Candida albicans is a normal colonizer of the female genital tract. While recurrent candidal vaginitis is common in healthy women, it may also be a presenting symptom in women who are HIV infected [27]. Downs and Wallace [28] concluded that refractory candidal vaginitis was a marker for HIV infection. Either topical antifungal therapy (e.g., clotrimazole) or an oral imidazole (e.g., ketoconazole or fluconazole) is generally effective for vulvovaginal candidiasis. However, relapse is common after cessation of these agents, and intermittent or continuous prophylactic therapy may be necessary [29].

Pelvic Inflammatory Disease and Genital Ulcer Disease

Several studies have shown that a significant percentage of women (6.7–17.0%) who require hospitalization for pelvic inflammatory disease (PID) are HIV seropositive [30]. HIV-infected women may be at increased risk for the development of PID, and the inflammation associated with PID may potentiate transmission of HIV [31].

Past or present genital ulcer disease is an independent risk factor for HIV transmission. In addition, HIV infection increases the rate of recurrence of and/or susceptibility to genital ulcer disease and venereal warts (condyloma acuminatum), especially in patients with advanced immunosuppression [32]. Patients with syphilis have been shown to be an important reservoir of HIV, and *Trichomonas* infection may also be involved in the passive transfer of the virus [33, 34].

Human Papillomavirus and Cervical Dysplasia

Human papillomavirus (HPV) causes venereal warts and is a risk factor for cervical squamous intraepithelial lesion (SIL; also known as cervical intraepithelial neoplasia [CIN]), a precursor to cervical cancer. Early information about HPV and altered host immunity obtained from studies of renal transplant patients suggested that the course of cervical disease was more aggressive than usual and patients did not respond well to conventional therapy [35]. Kloser and associates [36] examined 30 HIV-infected women for the prevalence of seven HPV serotypes in a New Jersey clinic. Twenty-seven percent were infected with HPV, 50 percent with intermediate-risk serotypes and one quarter with high-risk serotypes. Vermund and colleagues [37] compared 72 HIV-infected women, 50 percent of whom were asymptomatic, with 60 high-risk HIV-negative women. In the absence of detectable HPV, no association was found between HIV and cervical SIL, whereas when HPV was present, symptomatic HIV-infected women were at greater risk for SIL than asymptomatic HIV-infected women.

Evidence continues to evolve concerning the risk of cervical neoplasia in HIV-infected women. In 1988, Provencher and colleagues [38] demonstrated a strong association between abnormal Papanicolaou smears and HIV seropositivity, identifying abnormal cytology in 67 percent of HIV-positive women compared to 5 percent of seronegative control subjects. Tarricone, Maiman, and Vieira [39] prospectively evaluated 32 HIV-infected women with cytology and colposcopic biopsies; 41 percent had CIN, 47 percent had chronic cervicitis, and only 16 percent had normal histologic cervical biopsies, but Pap smears were abnormal in only 3 (9%) patients. In addition, the presence of CIN strongly correlated with progressive impairment of cellular immunity. Carpenter and associates [40] found that women who acquired HIV infection from drug use were more likely to have SIL than those who contracted HIV heterosexually.

Maiman and associates [41] investigated 37 women under the age of

50 with documented invasive cervical cancer and 77 women referred for evaluation of abnormal Pap smears. They found that HIV-seropositive women with cervical carcinoma presented with a more advanced stage of disease, had more persistent and recurrent disease, and had a shorter interval to recurrence or death. In the group evaluated by colposcopy, HIV-positive women had more extensive, frequently multifocal lesions. In contrast to Maiman's group, Rogo and Kavoo-Linge [42] reported that cervical cancer patients in sub-Saharan Africa were no more likely to be HIV positive than the general population.

While acknowledging a possible association between HIV infection and cervical disease in women, the CDC cautions against premature conclusions from these studies, given their small sample size and methodologic problems [43]. The CDC currently recommends only annual Pap smears for HIV-infected women. However, Tarricone, Maiman, and Vieira [39] have suggested the use of colposcopy as part of the routine gynecologic evaluation, and there is little consensus in this area. In the Boston City Hospital AIDS program, Pap smears are recommended for women twice a year, with colposcopy for any suspicious lesions. There are no contraindications to standard treatment modalities for SIL/CIN in HIV-infected women. The CO_2 laser, surgery, and topical 5-flurorouracil have been used for extensive or resistant disease [38, 44].

Other Gynecologic Problems

In a case-control study, 41 percent of HIV-positive women compared to 24 percent of control subjects had menstrual abnormalities, including amenorrhea or bleeding between periods [45]. Stein and colleagues [46] noted that in HIV-infected women abnormal gynecologic findings were disproportionately frequent compared to complaints. Rates of spontaneous abortions in HIV-positive IDUs have been found to be higher than in control subjects [47]. Severe and persistent sexual dysfunction has also been described in HIV-infected women [48].

Family Planning

The CDC and American College of Obstetricians and Gynecologists (ACOG) recommend HIV antibody testing for women of reproductive age who are at high risk. They also suggest that HIV testing be offered to all pregnant women regardless of risk. However, knowledge of HIV serostatus may not have a significant impact on the decision to terminate a pregnancy. Selwyn and associates [49] reported that, among patients in a methadone clinic, HIV-positive patients were no more likely to have an elective abortion than seronegative ones; Johnstone and colleagues [50] found similar results.

For couples with discordant HIV serostatus, attempts to achieve pregnancy mean exposing the uninfected partner to the virus. The probability that an HIV-infected man will transmit the virus to an uninfected woman during a single episode of vaginal intercourse is estimated to be 0.2 percent [51]. HIV transmission through artificial insemination with washed semen from an HIV-positive husband to an HIV-negative spouse has been documented, although preliminary results using processed semen have been encouraging [52, 53]. HIV has been detected in the spermatozoa of patients with AIDS, and HIV replication may occur in the male germ cell [54].

Certain contraceptives may pose specific health hazards for the HIV-infected woman (Table 34-1). Increased mortality in some animal species from protozoan infections has been documented as a result of depression of cellular immunity by estrogen [55]. In addition, estrogen in oral contraceptive pills (OCP) increases cervical ectropion and may predispose to acquisition of HIV. Simonsen and associates [56], in a study of 418 prostitutes in Nairobi, found OCP use to be an independent risk factor for HIV infection. Because of this, use of OCP in HIV-infected women should be viewed with caution. The intrauterine contraceptive device (IUD) may also be a poor family planning choice for HIV-infected women, as the IUD string may serve as a nidus for ascending infection or cause penile abrasions, which increase the risk of HIV transmission. While latex condoms and nonoxynol-9 have both been shown to provide protection from HIV transmission, neither is ideal. Impediments to condom use include lack of perceived risk, partner rejection, the perception that condoms are unpleasant and unreliable, expense, and religious objections [57, 58]. Spermicides may not adequately coat all susceptible tissues [59]. Concern has also been raised that nonoxynol-9 and contraceptive sponges may enhance HIV transmission through irritation of the vaginal mucosa [60–62].

HIV Infection in Pregnancy

The issue of HIV infection in women is complicated by the fact that approximately 85 percent of women with AIDS are in their childbearing years [43]. Providing clinical care to the HIV-infected pregnant woman is a challenging endeavor. Practitioners are limited by a paucity of clinical trials involving pregnant women and by a general reluctance to use drugs whose safety has not been established in pregnancy. As the incidence of HIV infection in women rises, so does the number of HIV-infected infants. Up to 1 in 57 US women delivering babies in inner-city hospitals are HIV infected [4]. In sub-Saharan African cities, as many as 10 percent of infants born are seropositive [63].

The treatment of pregnant HIV-infected women is often complicated by psychosocial problems, such as poverty, homelessness, drug use, domestic violence, and isolation. Realistic goals in treating HIV-infected pregnant women include:

1. Provision of up-to-date statistics about the risks of maternal-fetal transmission and possible effects of pregnancy on maternal health
2. Education in methods to prevent adult transmission
3. Clinical staging and assessment of the risks and benefits of antiretroviral and PCP prophylaxis therapies
4. Provision of prenatal services with an emphasis on nutrition, as well as monitoring for and treatment of opportunistic diseases
5. Provision of psychological and social support
6. Access to drug treatment programs

Normal pregnancy alters immune status, causing a change in lymphocyte response to infection and a decrease in CD4 lymphocyte counts [64]. These effects could potentially result in a more rapid progression of HIV infection during pregnancy, although this has not been demonstrated to be the case with early disease [65].

Transmission of HIV from mother to fetus is well established, with transplacental transfer believed to be the predominant mode. Exposure to infected maternal blood or vaginal secretions at the time of delivery (perinatal acquisition) is another theoretical mode of transmission. HIV has been isolated from breast milk, and postnatal acquisition of HIV through breast feeding has been reported [66, 67]. The overall transmission rate from an HIV-infected mother to fetus is 15 to 40 percent [68–70]. There is evidence that transmission rates are higher among symptomatic HIV-infected women and those with more advanced disease [63, 68, 70]. In addition, early infant gestational age (< 34 weeks) appears to correlate independently with increased risk of HIV transmission [70].

Initial studies assessing the effect of HIV infection on pregnancy outcome revealed higher rates of preterm labor and low birth weight infants, and more frequent prematurely ruptured membranes [71, 72]. However, more recent reports from both the US and sub-Saharan Africa have shown a higher incidence of sexually transmitted diseases in HIV-infected women, but no difference, when controlled for substance abuse, in rates of prematurely ruptured membranes, gestational age, Apgar scores, congenital abnormalities, or stillbirths [73, 74].

Table 34-1 *The use of contraceptives in HIV infection*

Method of contraception	Typical failure rate (%)	Benefits	Risks	Comments
Sterilization	0.4 (female) 0.15 (male)		Provides no HIV protection	Useful in conjunction with condoms and spermicides
Oral contraceptive	3	50% reduction in hospitalization for PID Decreases time and amount of menstrual flow (decreases exposure of blood to partner) Thickened cervical mucus may provide protection for upper genital tract	Estrogen inhibits cell-mediated immune responses with theoretical risk of accelerated disease progression	Concern about use in this setting because of potential risks
IUD	3		Increases risk of PID String serves as a wick for ascending bacterial infection String may cause penile abrasions	Poor choice

Method	Failure rate	Benefits	Disadvantages	Notes
Latex condom	12	Protects penis from vaginal secretions Protects anus and vagina from semen Provides protection during vaginal or anal intercourse	Significant failure rate as contraceptive method Success depends on acceptance by male partner	
Diaphragm cervical cap	18	Protects cervix and upper female genital tract	Leaves lower vagina and penis unprotected Potential cause of vaginal abrasions	
Sponge	28 (multiparous) 18 (nulliparous)	Adequate spermicidal protection Provides physical barrier to upper female genital tract	Potential cause of vaginal abrasions	Best when used in conjunction with condoms
Nonoxynol-9	21	Inactivates HIV at concentrations present in most spermicidal preparations When used with condoms protects transmission from vaginal or anal intercourse	Significant failure rate as contraceptive method May enhance HIV transmission through irritation of vaginal mucosa	Best when used in conjunction with condoms

Antepartum Care

Human immunodeficiency virus antibody counseling and testing should be offered routinely to all women seeking prenatal care. Special attention should be paid to psychosocial issues that may affect pregnancy. In women with or at risk for HIV infection, history and physical examination should be directed toward the diagnosis of HIV-related diseases. Many of the "normal" complaints of pregnancy, such as fatigue, may mimic symptoms of HIV infection. Screening for tuberculosis, syphilis, chlamydia, gonorrhea, and viral hepatitis should be done routinely, and antibody titers to cytomegalovirus and *Toxoplasma* should also be obtained. CD4 lymphocyte counts should be performed at least each trimester and more frequently in patients with counts near 500/mm^3 and 200/mm^3.

Serum alpha-fetoprotein testing should be offered to all patients at the appropriate gestational age. However, amniocentesis is associated in theory with the risk of HIV transmission to the fetus. Antepartum testing to assure fetal well-being should be performed for the usual obstetric indications, recognizing that many of the risk factors for HIV infection may independently affect pregnancy. Complete clinical guidelines for the management of HIV infection in pregnancy have been published elsewhere [75-77].

Intrapartum and Postpartum Care

It has been clearly demonstrated that HIV transmission can occur transplacentally throughout pregnancy [78, 79]. Fetal scalp blood samples and scalp electrodes should be avoided if possible, and, after birth, fetal skin should be thoroughly cleansed before blood drawing. There is no evidence that HIV transmission is reduced by cesarean section [72]. However, routine use of antibiotic and anticoagulant therapy may significantly decrease postoperative morbidity in HIV-infected patients undergoing cesarean section [80].

Both the CDC and the ACOG recommend bottle feeding for children of HIV-infected women in areas where safe alternatives to breast feeding exist [81, 82]. During the first postpartum visit with the patient, a barrier contraceptive method should be recommended and health maintenance issues for the mother and newborn discussed.

Antiretroviral Therapy

Although it has been shown that ZDV crosses the placenta, antiretroviral therapy in pregnancy has not been evaluated in controlled studies [83]. Rabbit and rat fertility are diminished with very high doses of ZDV, but teratogenic effects have not been demonstrated [84]. Small studies have suggested that ZDV produces minimal toxicity in pregnant women, no teratogenicity, and a reduced rate of vertical transmission [85, 86]. In a recent multicenter survey of ZDV use in 43 HIV-infected pregnant women, no teratogenic abnormalities were noted in any of the 12 infants with first-trimester exposure, and only 2 of 43 mothers experienced dose-limiting drug toxicity [87].

Until more data are available, most authorities recommend that HIV-infected pregnant women receive ZDV if they have AIDS or if their CD4 count is below 200/mm^3. Patients whose counts are between 200/mm^3 and 500/mm^3 should be offered ZDV, but the risk/benefit profile in this population is uncertain. Some clinicians delay antiretroviral therapy until the second trimester, when fetal organogenesis is complete. Patients who elect to take ZDV should be monitored closely with complete blood counts. No data are available on the use of other antiretroviral agents in pregnancy.

Pneumocystis carinii *Prophylaxis*

Pregnant women with HIV infection appear to be at the same risk for PCP as nonpregnant women. Until more data are available, PCP prophylaxis guidelines followed for other HIV-infected persons should be applied to pregnant women [20]. Trimethoprim-sulfamethoxazole (TMP-SMZ), the drug of choice for PCP prophylaxis, has been reported to cause fetal malformations in rats, and the sulfa moiety is associated with kernicterus in the newborn when administered during the third trimester. TMP-SMZ can also cause anemia and leukopenia. However, Ocho [88] studied the drug in pregnancy and found no increase in fetal abnormalities. Although the safety and efficacy of aerosol pentamidine have not been tested in pregnancy, very little is systemically absorbed, and its risk to the fetus is probably small.

Treatment of Serious Opportunistic Infections

Many of the opportunistic infections associated with HIV disease are severe and life threatening. It is imperative to diagnose and treat these infections rapidly in pregnant women. A pregnant woman's health should never be compromised in an effort to protect the fetus from potentially harmful therapies. In fact, fetal well-being is generally best served by optimal medical management of the mother.

Candidal infection of the pharynx or vagina should be treated initially with topical therapy such as nystatin or clotrimazole. Recurrent infection can be managed with oral ketoconazole or fluconazole, although the safety of these agents in pregnancy is unproven. Amphotericin B, the drug of choice for invasive candidiasis, has not been shown to cause fetal damage, although it has only been studied in a small number of pregnant women [89].

Pneumocystis carinii pneumonia should be treated with TMP-SMZ or pentamidine. The theoretical risks of teratogenicity and kernicterus associated with TMP-SMZ are small compared with the risk of hypoxemia and death from untreated PCP. Patients should initially receive parenteral therapy since absorption of oral medications is unpredictable in pregnancy.

Toxoplasmosis should be managed with pyrimethamine/sulfadiazine and folinic acid. While the perinatal risks of these drugs are uncertain, one large study failed to demonstrate adverse effects in fetuses of mothers treated during pregnancy [90].

Acyclovir is indicated for the treatment of mucocutaneous herpes simplex and varicella-zoster infections. The drug appears to be safe in pregnant women, but no controlled studies have been performed.

Treatment of tuberculosis (TB) should not be delayed because of pregnancy. Isoniazid, ethambutol, and rifampin are probably safe for use in this setting; pyrazinamide has not been evaluated [91]. The decision as to whether to delay TB chemoprophylaxis in a pregnant HIV-infected patient who is anergic and at high risk for TB or who has a positive purified protein derivative (PPD) should be individualized.

Ganciclovir or foscarnet is indicated for the treatment of cytomegalovirus retinitis or systemic disease. No data are available regarding the safety of either of these drugs in pregnant women.

References

1. Ellerbrock T, Rogers M. Epidemiology of human immunodeficiency virus infection in women in the United States. *Obstet Gynecol Clin North Am* 17:523–544, 1990.
2. Guinan ME, Hardy A. Epidemiology of AIDS in women in the United States. *JAMA* 257:2039–2042, 1987.
3. Chaisson RE, et al. Cocaine use and HIV infection in intravenous drug users in San Francisco. *JAMA* 261:561–565, 1989.
4. Hoff R, et al. Seroprevalence of human immunodeficiency virus among childbearing women: Estimation by testing samples of blood from newborns. *N Engl J Med* 318:525–530, 1988.
5. Donegan SP, Edelin KC, Craven DE. HIV seroprevalence rate at the Boston City Hospital (letter). *N Engl J Med* 319:653, 1988.
6. Donegan SP. Personal communication, 1992.
7. Chin J. Current and future dimensions of the HIV/AIDS pandemic in women and children. *Lancet* 336:221–224, 1990.
8. Wenstrom KD, Gall SA. HIV infection in women. *Obstet Gynecol Clin North Am* 16:627–643, 1989.

9. Padian NS, et al. Female-to-male transmission of human immunodeficiency virus. *JAMA* 266:1664–1667, 1991.

10. Rehmet S, Staszewski S, Helm EB, et al. Cofactors of HIV transmission in heterosexual couples. Seventh International Conference on AIDS, Florence, June 1991.

11. Kreiss JK, et al. AIDS virus infection in Nairobi prostitutes: Spread of the epidemic in East Africa. *N Engl J Med* 314:414–418, 1986.

12. Centers for Disease Control. Sexually transmitted diseases treatment guidelines. *MMWR* 38:58, 1989.

13. Padian NS, Shiboski SC, Jewell NP. The effect of number of exposures on the risk of HIV transmissions. *J Infect Dis* 161:883–887, 1990.

14. Laga M, et al. Risk factors for HIV infection in homosexual partners of HIV infected Africans and Europeans. Fourth International Conference on AIDS, Stockholm, June 1988.

15. Padian N, Greenblatt R, Glass S, Dull I. Clinical and immunological correlates of heterosexual transmission of HIV. 28th Interscience Conference on Antimicrobial Agents and Chemotherapy. American Society for Microbiology, 1988.

16. Wofsy CB. Human immunodeficiency virus in women. *JAMA* 257:2074–2076, 1987.

17. Fischl MA, et al. Evaluation of heterosexual partners, children, and household contacts of adults with AIDS. *JAMA* 257:640–644, 1987.

18. Monzon OT, Copellan JM. Female-to-female transmission of HIV. *Lancet* 2:40, 1987.

19. Fischl M, et al. The efficacy of AZT in the treatment of patients with AIDS and ARC. *N Engl J Med* 317:185–198, 1987.

20. Centers for Disease Control. Recommendations for prophylaxis against *Pneumocystis carinii* pneumonia for adults and adolescents infected with human immunodeficiency virus. *MMWR* 41(RR-4):1–11, 1992.

21. Carpenter CCJ, et al. Natural history of acquired immunodeficiency syndrome in women in Rhode Island. *Am J Med* 86:771–775, 1989.

22. Chu SY, Buchler JW, Berkelman RL. Impact of the human immunodeficiency virus epidemic on mortality in women of reproductive age, United States. *JAMA* 264:225–229, 1990.

23. Moore RD, et al. Zidovudine and the natural history of AIDS. *N Engl J Med* 324:1412–1416, 1991.

24. Rothenberg R, et al. Survival with the acquired immunodeficiency syndrome. *N Engl J Med* 317:1297–1302, 1987.

25. Schoenbaum E, Webber M. Underdetection of HIV infection in females seeking care at an inner city emergency room in the Bronx, New York City. Seventh International Conference on AIDS, Florence, June 1991.

26. Lemp GF, et al. Survival for women and men with AIDS. *J Infect Dis* 166:74–79, 1992.

27. Rhoads JL, Wright CW, Redfield RR, Burke DS. Chronic vaginal candidiasis in women with human immunodeficiency virus infection. *JAMA* 257:3105–3107, 1987.

28. Downs J, Wallace JJ. A review of Papanicolaou (PAP) smears in HIV-pos-

itive vs. HIV-negative women in a drug treatment program. Seventh International Conference on AIDS, Florence, 1991.

29. Sobel D. Recurrent vulvovaginal candidiasis: A prospective study of the efficiency of maintenance ketoconazole therapy. *N Engl J Med* 315:1455–1458, 1986.

30. Allen MH. Primary care of women infected with the human immunodeficiency virus. *Obstet Gynecol Clin North Am* 117:557–569, 1990.

31. Jones, Wentz (eds), *Novak's Textbook of Gynecology*. Baltimore: Williams & Wilkins, 1988.

32. Malele B, et al. The impact of HIV infection on the incidence of STD in high risk women. Seventh International Conference on AIDS, Florence, June 1991.

33. Levine WC, et al. HIV seropositive and drug use among patients with syphilis attending sexually transmitted disease clinics in Georgia. Seventh International Conference on AIDS, Florence, June 1991.

34. Dolei A, et al. *In vitro* interactions between HIV and *Trichomonas vaginalis*. Seventh International Conference on AIDS, Florence, June 1991.

35. Silman FH, Sedlis A. Anogenital papilloma virus infection and neoplasia in immunodeficient women. *Obstet Gynecol Clin North Am* 14:537–558, 1987.

36. Kloser PC, et al. Human papilloma virus (HPV) and risk of cervical intraepithelial neoplasia in HIV-1–infected inner city women. Sixth International Conference on AIDS, San Francisco, 1990.

37. Vermund SH, et al. Risk of human papillomavirus (HPV) and cervical squamous intraepithelial lesions (SIL) highest among women with advanced HIV disease. Sixth International Conference on AIDS. San Francisco, June 1990.

38. Provencher D, et al. HIV status and positive Papanicolaou screening: Identification of a high-risk population. *Gynecol Oncol* 31:184–188, 1988.

39. Tarricone NJ, Maiman M, Vieira J. Colposcopic evaluation of HIV seropositive women. Sixth International Conference on AIDS, San Francisco, June 1990.

40. Carpenter CCJ, et al. Distinctive features of HIV infection in 200 North American women. Seventh International Conference on AIDS, Florence, June 1991.

41. Maiman M, et al. Human immunodeficiency virus infection and cervical neoplasia. *Gynecol Oncol* 38:377–382, 1990.

42. Rogo KO, Kavoo-Linge. Human immunodeficiency virus seroprevalence among cervical cancer patients. *Gynecol Oncol* 37:87–92, 1990.

43. Centers for Disease Control. AIDS in women. *MMWR* 39:845–846, 1990.

44. Krebs H. The use of topical 5-fluorouracil in treatment of genital condylomas. *Obstet Gynecol Clin North Am* 14:559–568, 1987.

45. Warne PA, et al. Menstrual abnormalities in HIV+ and HIV− women with a history of intravenous drug use. Seventh International Conference on AIDS, Florence, June 1991.

46. Stein J, et al. Gynecologic findings in an HIV-positive outpatient population. Seventh International Conference on AIDS, Florence, June 1991.

47. Casolati E, et al. Sexual behavior in HIV-positive intravenous drug abuser women. Seventh International Conference on AIDS, Florence, June 1991.
48. Brown GR, et al. Psychiatric morbidity in early HIV infection in women: Results of a 3.5 year prospective study. Seventh International Conference on AIDS, Florence, June 1991.
49. Selwyn PA, et al. Prospective study of human immunodeficiency virus infections and pregnancy outcomes in intravenous drug users. JAMA 261:1289–1294, 1989.
50. Johnstone FD, et al. Women's knowledge of their HIV antibody state: Its effect on their decision whether to continue the pregnancy. Br Med J 300:23–24, 1990.
51. Hearst W, Halley SB. Preventing the heterosexual spread of AIDS: Are we giving our patients the best advice? JAMA 259:2428–2432, 1988.
52. Semprini AE, et al. Insemination of HIV-negative women with processed semen of HIV-positive partners. Lancet 340:1317–1319, 1992.
53. Centers for Disease Control. HIV-1 infection and artificial insemination with processed semen. MMWR 39:249–252, 1990.
54. Baccett B, et al. HIV particles detected in spermatozoan of patients with AIDS. Seventh International Conference on AIDS, Florence, June 1991.
55. Grossman C. Interactions between the gonadal steroids and immune system. Science 277:257–261, 1985.
56. Simonsen JN, et al. HIV infection among lower socioeconomic strata prostitutes in Nairobi. AIDS 4:139–144, 1990.
57. Ehrhardt A, et al. Barriers to safer heterosexual sex for women from high HIV prevalence communities. Seventh International Conference on AIDS, Florence, June 1991.
58. Mehryar M, et al. Acceptability and use of condoms in sub-Saharan Africa: A review. Seventh International Conference on AIDS, Florence, June 1991.
59. Stein Z. HIV prevention: The need for methods women can use. Am J Public Health 80:460–462, 1990.
60. Niruthisard S, et al. A randomized comparative trial of mucosal irritation of N-9 and placebo. Seventh International Conference on AIDS, Florence, June 1991.
61. Brown RC, Brown JE. The use of intra-vaginal irritants as a risk factor for the transmission of HIV infection in Zairian prostitutes. Seventh International Conference on AIDS, Florence, June 1991.
62. Kreiss J, et al. Efficiency of nonoxynol-9 contraceptive sponge use in preventing heterosexual acquisition of HIV in Nairobi prostitutes. JAMA 268:477–482, 1992.
63. Ryder RW, et al. Perinatal transmission of the human immunodeficiency virus type I to infants of seropositive women in Zaire. N Engl J Med 320:1637–1642, 1989.
64. Strelkankas AJ, et al. Longitudinal studies showing alterations in the levels and functional response of T and B lymphocytes in human pregnancy. Clin Exp Immunol 32:531–539, 1978.
65. Berrebi A, et al. Influence of pregnancy on HIV disease. Seventh International Conference on AIDS, Florence, June 1991.

66. Zeigler JB, et al. Breast feeding and transmission of HIV from mother to infant. Fourth International Conference on AIDS, Stockholm, June 1988.
67. Thiry L, et al. Isolation of AIDS virus from cell free breast milk of three healthy virus carriers. *Lancet* 2:892, 1985.
68. European Collaborative Study. Mother-to-child transmission of HIV infection. *Lancet* 2:1039–1043, 1988.
69. Blanche S, et al. A prospective study of infants born to women seropositive for human immunodeficiency virus type I. *N Engl J Med* 32:1643–1648, 1989.
70. European Collaborative Study. Risk factors for mother-to-child transmission of HIV-1. *Lancet* 339:1007–1012, 1992.
71. Gloeb J, et al. Human immunodeficiency virus infection in women. *Am J Obstet Gynecol* 159:756–761, 1988.
72. Minkoff H, et al. Pregnancies resulting in infants with acquired immunodeficiency syndrome or AIDS-related complex. *Obstet Gynecol* 69:285–287, 1987.
73. Minkoff HL, et al. Pregnancy outcomes among mothers infected with human immunodeficiency virus and uninfected control subjects. *Am J Obstet Gynecol* 163:1598–1604, 1990.
74. Braddock MR, et al. Impact of maternal HIV infection on obstetrical and early neonatal outcome. *AIDS* 4:1001–1005, 1990.
75. Holman S, et al. Prenatal HIV counseling and testing. *Clin Obstet Gynecol* 32:445–455, 1989.
76. Nanda D. Human immunodeficiency virus infection in pregnancy. *Obstet Gynecol Clin North Am* 3:617–626, 1990.
77. Minkoff H. Care of pregnant women infected with human immunodeficiency virus. *JAMA* 258;2714–2717, 1987.
78. Hill WC, et al. Isolation of acquired immunodeficiency syndrome virus from the placenta. *Am J Obstet Gynecol* 157:10–11, 1987.
79. Lapointe W, et al. Transplacental transmission of HTLV-III virus. *N Engl J Med* 312:1325–1326, 1985.
80. Grossi E, et al. HIV seropositivity and caesarean section. Seventh International Conference on AIDS, Florence, June 1991.
81. American College of Obstetricians and Gynecologists. Prevention of HIV infection and AIDS. ACOG Committee Statement, 1987. Pp 1–8.
82. Centers for Disease Control. Recommendations for assisting in the prevention of perinatal transmission of human lymphotrophic virus type III/lymphadenopathy associated virus and acquired immune deficiency syndrome. *MMWR* 34:681–699, 1985.
83. Jashvant U, et al. Transplacental transfer of zidovudine. Fifth International Conference on AIDS, Montreal, 1989.
84. Maha M. Conference Presentation on Pregnancy and Treatment. National Conference of Women and HIV Infection. Washington, DC, 1990.
85. Ferrazin A, et al. Zidovudine therapy of HIV infection during pregnancy: Assessment of the effect on the newborns. Seventh International Conference on AIDS, Florence, June 1991.
86. Carcassi C, et al. A study of 9 infants born from HIV-1 positive mothers

who continued treatment with AZT during pregnancy. Seventh International Conference on AIDS, Florence, June 1991.

87. Sperling RS, et al. A survey of zidovudine use in pregnant women with human immunodeficiency virus infection. *N Engl J Med* 326:857–861, 1992.
88. Ocho P. Trimethoprim and sulfamethoxazole in pregnancy. *JAMA* 217:1244, 1971.
89. *Physicians Desk Reference,* 1991. Amphotericin B.
90. Daffos F, et al. Prenatal management of 746 pregnancies at risk for congenital toxoplasmosis. *N Engl J Med* 318:271–275, 1988.
91. Snider, DE, Jr, et al. Treatment of tuberculosis during pregnancy. *Ann Rev Respir Dis* 122:65–79, 1980.

35/Overview of Pediatric HIV Infection

Anne Marie Regan, Tina Schwartz, Ellen R. Cooper,
Stephen I. Pelton

The medical and psychosocial implications of HIV disease frequently involve the entire family. Most HIV-infected women are of childbearing age, and the number of children affected by this disease continues to grow. The purpose of this chapter is to present an overview of pediatric HIV infection for the adult health care practitioner.

Epidemiology

AIDS was not described in children until 1982. Widespread recognition of pediatric AIDS was delayed because of difficulty in differentiating it from other congenital immunodeficiencies. As of October 1991, 4,130 children and adolescents in the United States had AIDS, but the number of children infected with HIV who do not meet the case definition of AIDS may be 10 times greater [1]. Approximately 50 percent of children with AIDS have died. Although children represent only 2 percent of all cases of AIDS reported to the Centers for Disease Control (CDC), it is expected that this disease will be among the five leading causes of death in 1- to 4-year-olds in the US by 1995 [1].

Human immunodeficiency virus can be transmitted to children perinatally, through transfusion of contaminated blood products, through the use of shared needles, and sexually. Approximately 80 percent of children under the age of 13 with AIDS were infected perinatally, and 15 percent through blood products. In Massachusetts, anonymous cord blood screening indicates that 2.5 of 1,000 newborns have HIV-infected mothers. However, this rate varies considerably with patient population [2]. For example, at Boston City Hospital, 2.5 to 3.0 of 100 newborns are born to HIV-seropositive mothers. Transfusion-related transmission has become rare since the advent of routine HIV screening of blood products in 1985, but children infected before that time are still being identified. Needle sharing and sexual transmission, principally of concern in adolescents, have also been described in younger children [3–5].

Current estimates of the rate of maternal-fetal transmission are between 13 and 43 percent; most prospective studies indicate it to be 25 to 30 percent [6, 7]. Women who have previously given birth to an HIV-infected child may be at greater risk of the same outcome with subsequent pregnancies. Vertical transmission may also be increased in mothers who have more advanced disease, have a higher plasma HIV titer, or develop primary HIV infection during or just before pregnancy.

The precise timing of HIV transmission from mother to fetus is not well established. The virus has been demonstrated in fetal tissue from first- and second-trimester abortuses [8]. Some investigators believe that a significant proportion of children are infected during the intrapartum period. Data supporting transmission during the birth process include the disparity in infection rate between first and second twins (twin A being infected 50% more frequently than twin B) and the detection of HIV-specific immunoglobulin M (IgM) between 6 and 12 weeks after birth [7, 9]. Postnatal transmission by breast feeding has been documented in a small number of cases, leading to the recommendation that HIV-infected women abstain from this practice if a suitable alternative exists [10].

Natural History and Prognosis

Early recognition and treatment of pediatric HIV infection has affected its clinical course. Data suggest that the latency period following transfusion-acquired infection is significantly shorter in children than in adults (24 vs. 54 months) [11]. The duration of the latency period appears to be inversely related to the age of seroconversion [12]. Recent studies suggest that the latency period for perinatally acquired HIV infection can often be 3 and perhaps as long as 8 years [13, 14].

In the US, there seems to be a subpopulation of children in whom HIV infection presents early in life and progresses quickly. Opportunistic infections are the cause of death in over 60 percent of patients, and 75 percent of children in whom an opportunistic infection develops do not survive longer than one year [15, 16]. Of 172 children diagnosed with symptomatic HIV infection in Miami, Florida, 18 percent died before one year of age [17]. The median survival time for children in whom symptoms of clinical disease appeared before their first birthday was 24.8 months, while the median survival for children who were asymptomatic was 6 years. A more recent study that includes asymptomatic HIV-infected children found the median survival to be 8 years [18].

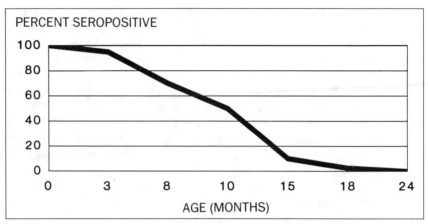

Figure 35-1. *Decay of antibody to HIV in uninfected children born to HIV-infected mothers. (Adapted from European Collaborative Study, Children born to women with HIV-1 infection: Natural history and risk of transmission.* Lancet 337:253–260, 1991.)

Diagnosis of HIV Infection in Children

The diagnosis of HIV infection is complicated by the passive transfer of HIV antibody from infected mothers to their newborn infants. The presence of antibody to HIV detected by enzyme-linked immunosorbent assay (ELISA) and Western blot techniques may not be diagnostic of HIV infection in children under 24 months of age, unlike adults and older children. The CDC has used the classification "P0" to designate an asymptomatic infant less than 15 months of age born to an HIV-infected mother [19]. The CDC case definition for AIDS in children differs from that in adults by its inclusion of multiple or recurrent serious bacterial infections and lymphoid interstitial pneumonitis (LIP) [20].

Figure 35-1 illustrates the decay in ELISA and Western blot activity in children of HIV-infected women who are eventually found to serorevert [6]. Ten months of age represents the time at which 50 percent of uninfected children revert to seronegativity; 24 months of age appears to represent the maximum age at which seroreversion may occur. Children who remain ELISA and Western blot seropositive after 15 months of age meet the CDC criteria for HIV infection.

Culture of peripheral white blood cells for HIV, polymerase chain reaction (PCR) testing, and IgA-specific HIV antibody assays have been evaluated for their ability to distinguish asymptomatic HIV-infected from HIV-uninfected infants. In studies performed by Comeau and colleagues in conjunction with Boston City Hospital and the Massachusetts State Laboratory, viral culture and PCR testing during the first 6 months

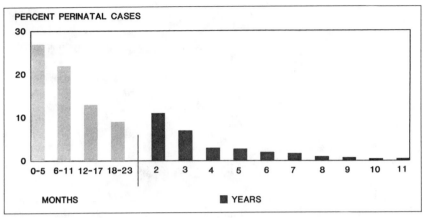

Figure 35-2. Pediatric HIV infection age at diagnosis. (Reprinted with permission of MJ Oxtoby, Perinatally Acquired HIV Infection. In PA Pizzo, CM Wilfert [eds], Pediatric AIDS. Copyright 1991, the Williams & Wilkins Co., Baltimore.)

of life successfully identified the majority of children subsequently proved to be HIV infected [21]. Immunoglobulin A–specific antibody to HIV had limited sensitivity during the first 12 weeks of life. However, after this time, IgA antibody testing was very sensitive, with 26 of 27 HIV-infected children showing positive results. All three of these techniques were quite specific, and there were no false-positive tests. Other reports have confirmed the usefulness of PCR testing and IgA antibody assays in the early diagnosis of HIV infection in children [22–25].

Clinical Manifestations

The onset of clinical manifestations of perinatally acquired HIV infection is extremely variable. Over 80 percent of HIV-infected children have symptoms and signs of disease before 24 to 36 months of age; approximately 10 percent remain asymptomatic for as long as 4 to 10 years [6, 26] (Fig. 35-2). Clinical manifestations of HIV disease in children are often nonspecific (Fig. 35-3). Oral candidiasis, generalized lymphadenopathy, organomegaly, poor weight gain, and developmental delay occur in approximately 40 percent [17]. As many as 10 percent of children have recurrent episodes of invasive bacterial disease, including sepsis, pneumonia, meningitis, and sinusitis. Opportunistic infections, including *Pneumocystis carinii* pneumonia (PCP) and candidal esophagitis, may also be early disease manifestations [17].

Lymphoid interstitial pneumonitis, a chronic, progressive interstitial pulmonary disease, is sometimes the initial complication [27]. It is char-

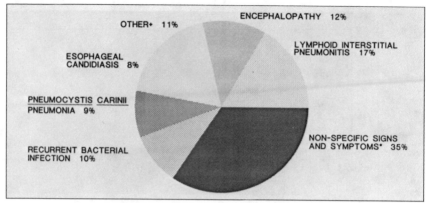

Figure 35-3. Clinical presentations in children with HIV infection. * = Oral candidiasis, poor weight gain, hepatomegaly, splenomegaly, lymphadenopathy, developmental delay; + = other AIDS-defining conditions, such as disseminated herpes simplex, cytomegalovirus disease. (Adapted from GB Scott, et al, Survival in children with perinatally acquired HIV-1. N Engl J Med 321:1791–1796, 1989.)

acterized by tachypnea, absence of fever and cough, interstitial densities on chest x-ray, elevated serum immunoglobulins, and, occasionally, digital clubbing, adenopathy, and parotid swelling. Lung pathology shows diffuse alveolar infiltration with lymphocytes, plasma cells, plasmacytoid lymphocytes, and immunoblasts.

Encephalopathy may also be an early manifestation of HIV disease [28]. Acquired microcephaly with or without cerebral calcification detected by computed tomography, delayed development or loss of already achieved milestones, and/or signs of pyramidal tract disease, such as increased tonicity and hyperreflexia, have all been described.

Heart disease may manifest as myocarditis, cardiomyopathy with or without congestive failure, pericardial effusion, or sudden death [29]. Early cardiac disease is most often asymptomatic, evident only by abnormalities on electrocardiography or echocardiography. Renal disease may present as nephrotic syndrome, acute nephritis, acute renal failure, renal tubular dysfunction, or recurrent urinary tract infection [30]. Electrolyte and acid-base abnormalities are common, frequently precipitated by rapid fluid shifts associated with vomiting or diarrhea. Pancreatitis, hepatitis, unusual skin conditions (especially chronic fungal infections), and hematologic abnormalities have also been described.

Organ System Approach to Clinical Care

Human immunodeficiency virus infection in children is a multisystem problem that requires comprehensive care by a multidisciplinary team.

The management plan should address the medical needs of the child, coordination of care for family members with HIV infection, and attention to the psychosocial needs of the child and family. An organ system approach to selected medical issues is presented in the following sections.

Gastrointestinal/Nutrition

Nutritional assessment is of critical importance in the management of pediatric HIV infection. Assessments should include a detailed nutritional history, evaluation of growth parameters and anthropometric measurements, and selected laboratory studies, including serum albumin, iron, and ferritin. Each visit should include an evaluation of the child's diet and growth. Failure to maintain growth along the child's standard curve requires prompt intervention. HIV-infected children often need some type of nutritional support. This may range from multivitamin supplements to a high-calorie, high-protein, nutrient-dense formula or food regimen. Enteral feeding via gastrostomy tube has proved to be a successful technique when caloric supplements and nutritional counseling have not resulted in adequate weight gain. Total parenteral nutrition may be necessary during enteric infections or acute illness when oral or enteral feedings are not tolerated.

Central Nervous System/Neurodevelopment

Children with HIV infection require frequent monitoring for central nervous system disease and neurodevelopmental abnormalities. A neurologic examination and neurodevelopmental assessment should be obtained as part of the initial evaluation. Computed tomography or magnetic resonance imaging of the head is performed in children with neurologic development abnormalities. Reevaluation of neurodevelopment at regular intervals is important for monitoring disease progression. Individualized treatment strategies should be developed for each child. Ongoing assessment for early intervention services, including home-based occupational therapy, physical therapy, and speech therapy, is an important aspect of care.

Pulmonary

Careful respiratory assessment is an important part of the clinical evaluation. Because of an increased risk of tuberculosis, a skin test (purified protein derivative [PPD]) with control panel should be performed every 6 months in HIV-infected children who previously tested negative or are anergic. Early identification of pulmonary disease is facilitated by monitoring chest radiographs, pulse oximetry, and pulmonary function tests.

Cardiovascular

Myocardial dysfunction may first be identified during periods of acute illness, when anemia, hypoxemia, or sepsis produces cardiac decompensation. HIV-infected children with acute illness or chronic pulmonary disease require especially close monitoring of cardiac function. Electrocardiographic screening should be performed in these settings; children with dysrhythmias may require holter monitoring. Echocardiography is useful to detect ventricular or valvular dysfunction, hypertrophy or dilation of heart chambers, and pericardial effusion.

Renal

Because of the increased risk of renal disease and urinary tract infection, baseline and follow-up blood pressure measurements, urinalysis, and renal function tests and electrolytes should be obtained in HIV-infected children. Use of nephrotoxic drugs should be carefully monitored.

Hematologic

Initial and follow-up measurements of the complete blood count to identify hematologic abnormalities are an essential component of care. Anemia, neutropenia, and lymphopenia may be caused by progression of HIV disease or drug-induced bone marrow suppression.

Other Organ Systems

Routine ophthalmologic examinations are important to facilitate early identification and prompt treatment of cytomegalovirus (CMV) retinitis. Hearing evaluation should be performed in the child who has a history of recurrent otitis media. Routine dental care is important for the early diagnosis of oral lesions and dental decay, as is close inspection of skin for infectious, neoplastic, or drug-induced eruptions.

Common Diagnostic Issues

Fever

An acute febrile illness in an HIV-infected child may represent a serious bacterial infection, a life-threatening opportunistic infection, or a self-limited condition. HIV infection is associated with both cellular and humoral immune defects, and vaccines may fail to provoke protective levels of antibody. HIV-infected children suffer serious bacterial infections, including sepsis, meningitis, pneumonia, visceral abscess, urinary tract infection, and cellulitis. As in other children, encapsulated bacteria, such as *Haemophilus influenzae* type b and *Streptococcus pneumoniae*, are frequent pathogens; gram-negative enteric bacilli may also cause invasive disease [31]. HIV-infected children are at risk for recurrent typical childhood infections, including otitis media, sinusitis, and purulent nasopharyngitis [32]. Common opportunistic diseases to which they are prone include mucocutaneous candidiasis, tuberculosis, PCP, and CMV infection.

The initial evaluation of the HIV-infected child with fever should have three goals: to assess the severity of illness, to identify a likely focus of infection, and to determine its microbiologic etiology. The majority of bacteremic episodes are not associated with focal infection and are manifested by nonspecific findings, such as decreased feeding, lethargy, or irritability [16].

Special attention is given to the head and neck, skin, respiratory, and gastrointestinal examinations. Identification of oral thrush generally indicates poor cellular immune function and increases suspicion of esophageal candidiasis if vomiting, anorexia, or painful swallowing is present. Tachypnea and abnormal auscultatory findings suggest a respiratory focus, such as bacterial pneumonia, PCP, or LIP. Vomiting and abdominal pain may be associated with hepatitis or pancreatitis related to HIV infection or drug therapy. Urinary tract infection is frequently manifested by nonspecific symptoms such as abdominal pain and diarrhea.

Initial laboratory evaluation consists of complete blood count, blood cultures, and urinalysis and culture. Oximetry and chest x-ray are indicated when respiratory symptoms or signs are present. Additional diagnostic tests, such as lumbar puncture, esophagoscopy, or needle aspiration, are individualized based on findings on history and physical examination.

If the child is clinically stable, has a normal white blood cell count and baseline oxygenation, and the family can reliably observe him or her, initial outpatient management is appropriate. In the absence of specific focal findings, following appropriate cultures, a single dose of ceftriaxone (50–75 mg/kg) or other age-appropriate antibiotic can be administered, and a return visit arranged within 48 hours.

When unusual pathogens are suggested by history or physical examination, meningitis is suspected because of irritability or lethargy (even in the face of a normal cerebrospinal fluid analysis), or a fever occurs in the presence of a permanent intravascular catheter, hospitalization is necessary. Empiric therapy consists of a parenteral antistaphylococcal penicillin or vancomycin in combination with a third-generation cephalosporin. Despite earlier concerns, acetaminophen is now considered safe for the treatment of febrile episodes in patients receiving zidovudine (ZDV) [33]. Response of bacterial diseases to antimicrobial therapy in HIV-infected children should be carefully monitored. One report described the failure of amoxicillin in more than 50 percent of symptomatic children with otitis media, despite in vitro sensitivity of pathogens to the drug [34].

Respiratory Symptoms

Children with HIV infection are at risk for common respiratory pathogens, including respiratory syncytial virus, adenovirus, parainfluenza virus, *Bordetella pertussis*, *S. pneumoniae*, and *H. influenzae*. They are also susceptible to PCP, CMV, tuberculosis, *Mycobacterium avium* complex infection, candidiasis, and LIP. When an HIV-infected child has respiratory symptoms, initial laboratory evaluation should include a chest x-ray, oximetry, and blood cultures. An interstitial pattern on chest x-ray in the presence of hypoxemia, tachypnea, and increased serum lactate dehydrogenase suggests PCP but does not exclude other diagnoses. A nasal wash or deep tracheal aspirate should be obtained for viral and bacterial cultures, as well as silver stain or fluorescent antibody evaluation for PCP.

Age-appropriate antimicrobial therapy, such as ceftriaxone, 50 mg/kg/day, should be empirically started. In addition, trimethoprim-sulfamethoxazole (TMP-SMZ) should be administered if clinical or radiologic findings suggest PCP. If the etiology remains unclear after 24 to 48 hours and the child's condition does not improve significantly, plans should be made to perform bronchoscopy or open lung biopsy. Clinically active LIP, marked by tachypnea and hypoxia, is an indication for corticosteroid therapy. The dose of oral prednisone is 2 mg/kg/day, which is gradually tapered to alternate-day therapy after clinical improvement.

Common Therapeutic Issues

Mucocutaneous Candidiasis

Mucocutaneous candidiasis is one of the most common manifestations of pediatric HIV infection. Initial treatment of oropharyngeal candidiasis includes the use of nystatin suspension or clotrimazole troches. Systemic therapy with ketoconazole or fluconazole is necessary for recalcitrant disease or esophageal involvement documented by endoscopy. Cutaneous candidiasis may present as diaper dermatitis or inflammation in skin fold areas. Treatment requires meticulous hygiene and frequent diaper changes in addition to a topical antifungal agent.

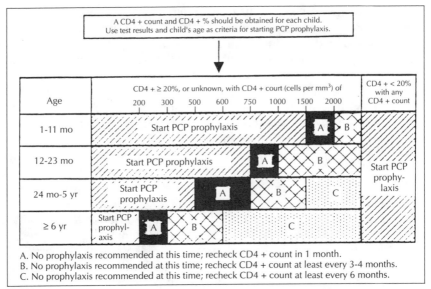

A CD4 + count and CD4 + % should be obtained for each child.
Use test results and child's age as criteria for starting PCP prophylaxis.

A. No prophylaxis recommended at this time; recheck CD4 + count in 1 month.
B. No prophylaxis recommended at this time; recheck CD4 + count at least every 3-4 months.
C. No prophylaxis recommended at this time; recheck CD4 + count at least every 6 months.

Figure 35-4. *Nomogram for initiation of PCP prophylaxis. (Reprinted from Centers for Disease Control, Guidelines for prophylaxis against* Pneumocystis carinii *pneumonia for children infected with human immunodeficiency virus. MMWR 40(RR-2):1–13, 1991.)*

Pneumocystis *Prophylaxis*

Pneumocystis carinii pneumonia was diagnosed in 39 percent of pediatric AIDS cases through 1990 and was the initial diagnosis in 8 to 12 percent [35]. In adults, the relationship between CD4 cell counts and risk for PCP has been firmly established, with the vast majority of patients having CD4 lymphocyte counts of less than 200/mm^3. However, determination of appropriate indications for PCP prophylaxis has been problematic in children because CD4 cell counts are higher than in adults and decrease with advancing age.

The CDC bases its PCP prophylaxis recommendations for children on a compilation of 71 cases from six references. The following are age-adjusted guidelines for the initiation of PCP prophylaxis in HIV-infected children [35] (Fig. 35-4): (1) CD4 count of less than 1,500/mm^3 for children 1 to 11 months, (2) CD4 count of less than 750/mm^3 for children 12 to 23 months, (3) CD4 count of less than 500/mm^3 for children 24 to 71 months, and (4) CD4 count of less than 200/mm^3 for children 72 months and older. In addition, PCP prophylaxis is recommended in children with a CD4 : total lymphocyte ratio of less than 20 percent, regardless of the absolute cell count, and in those with a prior history of PCP [36].

Because of its safety profile, efficacy, and ease of administration, TMP-SMZ is the drug of choice. If rash or neutropenia occurs, the drug should be discontinued for 2 weeks and the patient rechallenged. Complete blood and differential counts should be performed monthly to monitor for hematologic toxicity. Neutropenia has been a frequent observation in children taking TMP-SMZ as chemoprophylaxis, especially when it is prescribed concurrently with ZDV. Aerosol pentamidine in children over 5 years of age and oral dapsone are alternative regimens for those who are intolerant to TMP-SMZ.

Intravenous Immunoglobulin

Children with HIV infection often have recurrent serious bacterial infections caused by encapsulated organisms. Although the majority of HIV-infected children have hypergammaglobulinemia, their response to immunizations is usually impaired [37]. Intravenous immunoglobulin (IVIG) has been advocated by some authorities for use in children with AIDS or symptomatic HIV disease to prevent recurrent bacterial infections [38, 39].

In January 1991, the National Institute of Child Health and Development terminated a randomized, double-blind, controlled trial of IVIG in 372 children with symptomatic HIV disease after demonstrating that subjects receiving IVIG who had CD4 counts of $200/mm^3$ or greater had a significantly prolonged period of time free from serious bacterial infection [40]. IVIG was found to be most effective against invasive pneumococcal disease and acute pneumonia, but no improvement in survival could be demonstrated. Recently, viral and minor bacterial infections affecting the ears, skin, soft tissue, and upper respiratory tract have also been found to be reduced in IVIG recipients [41].

The American Academy of Pediatrics task force on pediatric AIDS recommends IVIG treatment for children with symptomatic HIV infection and a CD4 cell count of $200/mm^3$ or greater [42]. The dose of IVIG that is most frequently used to treat HIV-infected children is 400 mg/kg/month infused intravenously at a slow rate. Adverse reactions are generally mild. Patients who experience toxicity from IVIG infusions may benefit from pretreatment with antihistamines or antipyretics, or both.

Antiretroviral Therapy

Zidovudine, dideoxycytidine (ddC), and didanosine (ddI) have all been approved by the Food and Drug Administration (FDA) for treatment of HIV disease. Surrogate markers of disease activity, including p24 antigenemia and CD4 cell count, are followed in conjunction with clinical parameters to determine therapeutic response. Clinical markers of a favorable therapeutic response include weight gain, increase in neuro-developmental scores, and a decrease in the size of lymph nodes and organomegaly [43]. Antiretroviral drug levels, which are affected by patient age and drug interactions, can also be monitored [44].

Zidovudine

Studies of ZDV in pediatric patients were initiated in 1986 after preliminary results from adult protocols demonstrated efficacy in delaying the onset of opportunistic infections [45, 46]. The first study in children involved intravenous administration of ZDV, with the majority of subjects showing increased appetite and weight, reduction in immunoglobulin levels, and increased CD4 cell counts [45]. Neurodevelopmental abnormalities also improved on ZDV therapy. The largest study of ZDV in children evaluated the efficacy of oral ZDV in patients with AIDS or symptomatic HIV disease. The majority of subjects increased or maintained their weight, demonstrated a reduction in p24 antigen levels, and had a rise in mean CD4 cell counts [47].

Current indications for ZDV therapy in children recommended by a national survey of pediatric specialists include symptomatic HIV infection and asymptomatic infection with a CD4 cell count of less than 500/mm^3 [48]. The most commonly prescribed dose of ZDV is 180 mg/m^2/dose four times a day. However, there is considerable disagreement regarding the optimal regimen, and an ongoing AIDS Clinical Trials Group (ACTG) study is comparing high-dose (180 mg/m^2) and low-dose (90 mg/m^2) therapy. Dosing of infants aged 3 months or younger should be adjusted for age-related renal function. In children under 1 month of age, 2 mg/kg/dose, and in infants 1 to 3 months of age, 3 mg/kg/dose, give blood levels of ZDV that are comparable to 180 mg/m^2/dose in children over 3 months of age [49]. Children receiving ZDV therapy in whom viral resistance develops are at increased risk for poor clinical outcome [50].

The major toxicity associated with ZDV administration in children has been myelosuppression. At the dose of 180 mg/m^2, as many as 26 percent of children have significant anemia or neutropenia that requires dosage adjustment or temporary discontinuation of the drug [47]. Children should have a complete blood count every 2 weeks during the initial 8 weeks of ZDV therapy and monthly thereafter. Dose reduction to 120 mg/m^2 is necessary if there is evidence of significant hematologic toxicity.

Dideoxycytidine

Dideoxycytidine was first studied at the National Cancer Institute (NCI) in 15 children with symptomatic HIV infection [51]. During this 8-week trial, antiretroviral activity was demonstrated by increased CD4 counts in 8 of 15 subjects and by a decrease in p24 antigenemia in 6 of 9. In addition, 2 of 3 children with neurodevelopmental delay improved on ddC. At this time, the ACTG is conducting a trial of two doses of ddC in children with symptomatic HIV infection who are intolerant of ZDV and/or demonstrate disease progression while receiving ZDV. In the NCI study, no children developed peripheral neuropathy; mouth sores and rashes occurred when higher doses were used.

Possible indications for the use of ddC in children with HIV infection include ZDV intolerance or a history of disease progression evidenced by lack of clinical or laboratory improvement after 6 months of ZDV therapy. The current dose of ddC under investigation by the ACTG is 0.005 mg/kg or 0.01 mg/kg orally every 8 hours. Dideoxycytidine is supplied as a raspberry-flavored syrup in a concentration of 0.1 mg/ml. It is recommended that ddC be administered directly into the child's mouth without dilution. If mixture with food is necessary, ddC can be combined with applesauce, in which it is known to be stable.

Didanosine
Experience with ddI in HIV-infected children has been limited. Investigators at the NCI have published results of a study involving the use of ddI in 43 children with symptomatic HIV infection [52]. Antiretroviral activity was demonstrated after 20 to 24 weeks of therapy by significant improvement in CD4 cell counts and p24 antigenemia. The ACTG is currently conducting a trial of two doses of ddI in symptomatic HIV-infected children who are intolerant of and/or unresponsive to ZDV. The number enrolled in the NCI study was small, but the drug was well tolerated in these children. Peripheral neuropathy was not observed, but pancreatitis, which resolved following discontinuation of ddI, developed in two children.

Didanosine has been approved by the FDA for use in HIV-infected children over 6 months of age who demonstrate ZDV intolerance or disease progression after 6 months of treatment with ZDV. The current recommended dose is 200 mg/m^2/day in divided doses every 12 hours. Didanosine is unstable in gastric acid. Oral formulations contain buffering agents to provide maximal absorption. The drug should be taken on an empty stomach, and food should not be eaten one hour before or two hours after its administration.

Immunizations

The efficacy and safety of immunizations in HIV-infected children have been questioned because live-virus vaccination of immunosuppressed persons is associated with the potential risk of viral replication. In order to evaluate the frequency of serious adverse effects after administration of live vaccines, a retrospective review of vaccination histories in 200 HIV-infected children was performed by the New York City Department of Health [53]. No serious sequelae were identified following administration of oral polio (OPV) and measles-mumps-rubella (MMR) vaccines. Many unanswered questions persist regarding the ability of HIV-infected children to mount a protective antibody response. While inactivated vaccines are generally not considered to be harmful for immunosuppressed persons, concern has been expressed by some authorities that their stimulatory effect may accelerate deterioration in immune function [54]. At this time, there are insufficient data to support this hypothesis.

Based on currently available information, the Advisory Committee on Immunization Practice (ACIP) recommends routine immunization of HIV-infected children [55] (see Table 29-7). Previous ACIP recommendations did not include MMR vaccine in symptomatic children because of the potential risk associated with live vaccines. However, several reports of severe measles in unimmunized HIV-infected children resulted in modification of these recommendations. In general, MMR should be administered to HIV-infected children at 15 months of age. In areas where the likelihood of measles exposure is high, children 6 to 11 months of age should be immunized with monovalent measles vaccine, followed by MMR vaccine at 15 months.

The inactive poliovirus (IPV) vaccine is recommended by the ACIP for all HIV-infected children. In addition, any child who lives in a household with an HIV-infected individual should receive IPV. Poliovirus may be excreted in the stool of the recipient for 6 weeks, thereby placing an immunocompromised household contact at risk for vaccine-related polio.

In addition to the routine childhood immunizations, pneumococcal vaccine is recommended for all HIV-infected children at 2 years of age. Influenza vaccine is suggested annually for HIV-infected children older than 6 months and should also be considered for other members of the household. The need for hepatitis B vaccine in HIV-infected children is individualized based on serologic results.

Despite strict adherence to immunization schedules, the possibility exists that HIV-infected children will remain unprotected against infectious diseases commonly seen in the community. Once it has been determined that a child with HIV infection has had a significant exposure to varicella, measles, hepatitis B, or tetanus, appropriate postexposure prophylaxis should be initiated [42].

Psychosocial Care

The diagnosis of a child with HIV infection often identifies an entire family at risk. Parents are immediately faced not only with their child's diagnosis of a chronic progressive illness, but also the likelihood of infection in themselves and other family members. Additionally, they are burdened by concerns for the future care of their family. Parents may experience shock, denial, fear, anger, and guilt. They may be physically and emotionally stressed by their own illness and often experience significant guilt for their role in transmitting the virus to their child. The social stigma associated with HIV disease promotes feelings of isolation and fear of family and community abandonment.

In addition to dealing with the stress of medical illness, families often must cope with the lack of basic social support. Social service assessment is essential. Home-based services, including a visiting nurse and homemaker, are helpful to reduce the stress and demands of everyday care. Families may need advocacy related to school and legal issues. Crises frequently occur with disease progression or death of a parent and may require that extended family or the welfare system assume care and custody of the child.

A psychosocial assessment of the strengths, stressors, losses, coping abilities, and concrete needs of the family is important. Many children and families require mental health services for support, bereavement counseling, and crisis intervention. Provision of appropriate counseling in an environment that meets the family's needs should be available. Children with HIV infection often endure frequent blood drawing, intravenous therapies, and invasive diagnostic tests and need honest preparation, explanation, and support. Play therapy has been useful in helping them work through fears and pain related to their medical care.

References

1. Novello AL, Wise PH, Willoughby A, Pizzo P. Final report of the United States Department of Health and Human Services Secretary's Work Group on pediatric HIV infection and disease: Content and implications. *Pediatrics* 84:547, 1989.
2. Massachusetts Newborn Screening Program, Massachusetts Department of Public Health. Theobald Smith Research Institute, Boston, MA.
3. Gutman LT, St. Claire KK, Weedy C, et al. The epidemiologic intersection in children of sexual abuse and AIDS. In the American Pediatric Society and the Society for Pediatric Research Abstracts. Anaheim, CA: 1990. P 172A.

4. St. Louis ME, et al. Human immunodeficiency virus infection in disadvantaged adolescents. *JAMA* 266:2387–2391, 1991.
5. Centers for Disease Control. Selected behaviors that increase risk for HIV infection among high school students—United States, 1990. *MMWR* 41:231–240, 1992.
6. European Collaborative Study Group. Children born to women with HIV-1 infection: Natural history and risk of transmission. *Lancet* 337:253–260, 1991.
7. Johnson JP, Nair P, Hines SE, et al. Natural history and serologic diagnosis of infants born to human immunodeficiency virus–infected women. *Am J Dis Child* 143:1147–1153, 1989.
8. Sprecher S, Soumenkoff G, Puissant F, et al. Vertical transmission of HIV in 15-week fetus. *Lancet* 2:288–289, 1986.
9. Goedert JJ, Duliege AM, Amos CI, et al. High risk of HIV-1 infection for first-born twins. *Lancet* 338:1471–1475, 1991.
10. Zregler JB, Stewart GJ, Penny R, et al. Breastfeeding and transmission of HIV from mother to infant. Fourth International Conference on AIDS, Stockholm, June 1988.
11. Rogers MF, Thomas PA, Starcher ET, et al. AIDS in children: Report of the CDC national surveillance 1982–1985. *Pediatrics* 79:1008–1014, 1987.
12. Medley GF, Anderson RM, Cox DR, et al. Incubation period of AIDS in patients infected via blood transfusions. *Nature* 328:719–721, 1987.
13. Centers for Disease Control. Revision of the CDC surveillance case definition for AIDS. *MMWR* 36 (suppl 15):3–15, 1987.
14. MaWhinney S, Pagano M. Incubation time for vertically infected AIDS. Seventh International Conference on AIDS, Florence, June 1991.
15. Lampert R, Milben J, O'Donnell R, et al. Life table analysis of children with AIDS. *Pediatr Infect Dis* 5:374–375, 1986.
16. Krasinski K, Borkowsky W, Bork S, et al. Bacterial infection in HIV-infected children. *Pediatr Infect Dis* 7:323, 1988.
17. Scott GB, Hutto C, Makuch RW, et al. Survival in children with perinatally acquired HIV-1. *N Engl J Med* 321:1791–1796, 1989.
18. Tovo PA, et al. Prognostic factors and survival in children with perinatal HIV-1 infection. *Lancet* 339:1249–1253, 1992.
19. Centers for Disease Control. Classification system for HIV infection in children under 13 years of age. *MMWR* 36:225–236, 1987.
20. Centers for Disease Control. Revision of CDC surveillance case definition for acquired immunodeficiency syndrome. *MMWR* 36:3S–15S, 1987.
21. Comeau AM, Harris JS, McIntosh K, et al. Polymerase chain reaction in detecting HIV infection among seropositive infants: Relation to clinical status and age and to results of other assays. *J AIDS* 5:271–278, 1992.
22. Cassol SA, et al. Diagnosis of vertical HIV-1 transmission using the polymerase chain reaction and dried blood spot specimens. *J AIDS* 5:113–119, 1992.
23. Comeau AM, et al. Polymerase chain reaction in detecting HIV infection among seropositive infants: Relation to clinical status and age and to results of other assays. *J AIDS* 5:271–278, 1992.

24. Quinn TC, et al. Early diagnosis of perinatal HIV infection by detection of viral specific IgA antibodies. *JAMA* 266:3439–3442, 1991.
25. Landesman S, et al. Clinical utility of HIV-IgA immunoblot assay in the early diagnosis of perinatal HIV infection. *JAMA* 266:3443–3446, 1991.
26. Oxtoby MJ. Perinatally Acquired HIV Infection. In PA Pizzo, CM Wilfert (eds), *Pediatric AIDS: The Challenge of HIV Infection in Infants, Children and Adolescents.* Baltimore: Williams & Wilkins, 1991.
27. Conner EM, Marquis I, Oleske JM. Lymphoid Interstitial Pneumonitis. In PA Pizzo, CM Wilfert (eds), *Pediatric AIDS: The Challenge of HIV Infection in Infants, Children and Adolescents.* Baltimore: Williams & Wilkins, 1991.
28. Brouwers P, Belman AL, Epstein LG. Central Nervous System Involvement: Manifestations and Evaluation. In PA Pizzo, CM Wilfert (eds), *Pediatric AIDS: The Challenge of HIV Infection in Infants, Children and Adolescents.* Baltimore: Williams & Wilkins, 1991.
29. Kavanaugh-McHugh A, Ruff AJ, Rowe SA, et al. Cardiovascular Manifestations. In PA Pizzo, CM Wilfert (eds), *Pediatric AIDS: The Challenge of HIV Infection in Infants, Children and Adolescents.* Baltimore: Williams & Wilkins, 1991.
30. Salcedo JR, Conner EM, Oleske JM. Renal Complications. In PA Pizzo, CM Wilfert (eds), *Pediatric AIDS: The Challenge of HIV Infection in Infants, Children and Adolescents.* Baltimore: Williams & Wilkins, 1991.
31. Bernstein LT, Krieger BZ, Novick B, et al. Bacterial infection in the acquired immunodeficiency syndrome of children. *Pediatr Infect Dis* 4:472–475, 1985.
32. Barnett ED, Klein JO, Pelton SI, Luginbuhl LM. Otitis media in children born to HIV infected mothers. *Pediatr Infect Dis* 11:360–364, 1992.
33. Steffe EM, King JH, Inciardo JK, et al. The effect of acetaminophen on zidovudine metabolism in HIV-infected patients. *J AIDS* 3:691–694, 1990.
34. Principi N, Marchisio P, Tornaghi R, et al. Acute otitis media in human immunodeficiency virus–infected children. *Pediatrics* 88:566–571, 1991.
35. Centers for Disease Control. Guidelines for prophylaxis against *Pneumocystis carinii* pneumonia for children infected with human immunodeficiency virus. *MMWR* 40 (RR-2):1–13, 1991.
36. Rutstein RM. Predicting risk of *Pneumocystis carinii* pneumonia in human immunodeficiency virus–infected children. *Am J Dis Child* 145:922–924, 1991.
37. Berkman SA, Lee ML, Gale RP. Clinical uses of intravenous immunoglobulins. *Ann Intern Med* 112:278–292, 1990.
38. Calvell TA, Rubinstein A. Intravenous gamma-globulin in infant acquired immunodeficiency syndrome. *Pediatr Infect Dis* 5 (suppl):S207–S210, 1986.
39. Gupta A, Novick BE, Rubinstein A. Restoration of suppressor T-cell functions in children with AIDS following intravenous gamma globulin treatment. *Am J Dis Child* 140:143–146, 1986.
40. The National Institute of Child Health and Human Development Intravenous Immunoglobulin Study Group. Intravenous immune globulin for the prevention of bacterial infections in children with symptomatic human immunodeficiency virus infection. *N Engl J Med* 325:73–80, 1991.

41. Mofenson LM. Prophylactic intravenous immunoglobulin in HIV-infected children with CD4 counts of 0.20 × 10^9/L or more. *JAMA* 268:483–488, 1992.
42. American Academy of Pediatrics. Report of the Committee on Infectious Diseases (22nd ed), 1991.
43. Pizzo PA, Wilfert C. Treatment Considerations for Children with HIV Infection. In PA Pizzo, CM Wilfert (eds), *Pediatric AIDS: The Challenge of HIV Infection in Infants, Children and Adolescents*. Baltimore: Williams & Wilkins, 1991.
44. Balis FM, Blaney SM, Poplack DG. Antiretroviral drug development and clinical pharmacology. *Pediatr Infect Dis* 10:849–857, 1991.
45. Pizzo PA, Eddy J, Falloon J, et al. Effect of continuous intravenous infusion of zidovudine in children with symptomatic HIV infection. *N Engl J Med* 319:889–896, 1988.
46. McKinney PE, Pizzo PA, Scott GB, et al. Safety and tolerance of intermittent intravenous and oral zidovudine therapy in human immunodeficiency virus infected pediatric patients: A phase I study. *J Pediatr* 116:641–647, 1990.
47. McKinney RE, Jr, Maha MA, Connor EM, et al. A multicenter trial of oral zidovudine in children with advanced human immunodeficiency virus disease. *N Engl J Med* 324:1018–1025, 1991.
48. Kline MW, Shearer WT. A national survey on the care of infants and children with human immunodeficiency virus infection. *J Pediatr* 118:817–821, 1991.
49. Boucher FD, Mudlin JA, Ruff A, et al. A phase one evaluation of zidovudine administered to infants exposed at birth to the human immunodeficiency virus. *J Pediatr* 122:137–144, 1993.
50. Tudor-Williams G, et al. HIV-1 sensitivity to zidovudine and clinical outcome in children. *Lancet* 339:15–19, 1992.
51. Pizzo PA, Butler K, Balis F, et al. Dideoxycytidine alone and in an alternating schedule with zidovudine in children with symptomatic HIV infection. *J Pediatr* 117:799–808, 1990.
52. Butler KM, Husson RN, Balis FM, et al. Dideoxyinosine in children with symptomatic human immunodeficiency virus infection. *N Engl J Med* 323:137–144, 1991.
53. McLaughlin M, Thomas P, Onorato I, et al. Live virus vaccines in human immunodeficiency virus–infected children: A retrospective survey. *Pediatrics* 82:229–233, 1988.
54. Advisory Committee on Immunization Practice. Immunization of children infected with human T-lymphotropic virus type III/lymphadenopathy-associated virus. *MMWR* 35:595–606, 1986.
55. Advisory Committee on Immunization Practice. General recommendations on immunization. *MMWR* 38:205–228, 1989.

36 / HIV Infection in Communities of Color

John A. Rich

This chapter addresses the problem of HIV infection in communities of color.* Persons of color, including African-Americans, Haitian-Americans, and Latinos account for a disproportionate share of AIDS cases in the United States, and their numbers continue to grow. Many from these groups are also burdened by poverty, discrimination, and limited access to medical care. Though the diversity among people of color makes it impossible to make valid broad generalizations, this chapter examines possible reasons for the high prevalence of AIDS in communities of color and highlights issues that may be important in the prevention and primary care of HIV infection in these groups.

Epidemiology

Black and Latino persons make up 12.5 and 7 percent, respectively, of the United States population. However, among AIDS patients, 29 percent are black and 16 percent are Latino [1] (Fig. 36-1). This translates into a risk of AIDS that is three times greater for black men than for white men, and risks for Latino and black women that are, respectively, 8 times and 13 times greater than those of their white counterparts [2]. Though early studies showed that black and Latino persons also had shorter survival times following an AIDS-defining diagnosis, more recent data fail to confirm this difference [3]. Studies of US military recruits have documented a rate of HIV seroprevalence that is 3.9 in 1,000 for black persons, compared to 0.9 in 1,000 for white persons [4]. However, since enlistment in the military may be influenced by a number of

*The term communities of color refers to persons of African, Caribbean, Haitian, and Latin American origin and is used here in preference to the term minority. Many of the data presented in the following sections, however, were gathered using the terms black, Hispanic, and white. Black is understood to include not only African-Americans but also Caribbean-Americans and Haitian-Americans. The terms Hispanic and Latino include individuals from Puerto Rico, Dominican Republic, and other islands with Spanish-speaking populations, as well as persons from Central and South America.

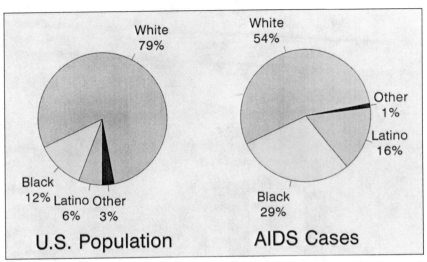

Figure 36-1. *Comparison of ethnic composition of the US population and reported AIDS cases. (Data from Centers for Disease Control, HIV/AIDS Surveillance Report, September 1991.)*

social factors, such studies may be subject to bias and not be generalizable to the population at large.

As of 1991, 76 percent of white men with AIDS acquired HIV infection through sex with another man and only 8 percent via injection drug use, whereas 39 percent of black and 40 percent of Latino men acquired the disease through drug use, and only 36 and 40 percent, respectively, through sex with another man [1] (Fig. 36-2). Also of note is the fact that a relatively greater proportion of men of color with AIDS identify themselves as bisexual (30% for blacks, 20% for Latinos, and 14% for whites), as opposed to exclusively homosexual. This factor may contribute to the higher reported rate of heterosexual HIV transmission in communities of color.

Women of color are strikingly overrepresented among the population with AIDS [1]. Blacks constitute 52 percent of AIDS cases in women, and Latinas comprise 20 percent. For all women with AIDS, regardless of ethnicity, the most common risk factor is injection drug use. For black and Latina women, heterosexual contact with an injection drug user ranks second. Children of color predominate among AIDS patients less than 12 years of age, with black and Latino children comprising 53 and 23 percent of cases, respectively. Almost all of these children were born to HIV-infected mothers [1].

A number of reasons have been cited for the disproportionate prevalence of HIV disease in persons of color. While drug abuse is a problem in white communities as well as communities of color, injection drug use

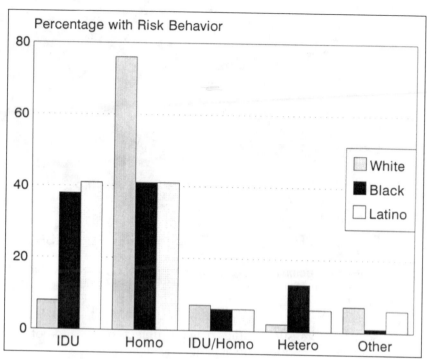

Figure 36-2. *Comparison of HIV risk behaviors for white, black, and Latino men. IDU = injection drug use; Homo = homosexual behavior; Hetero = heterosexual behavior. (Data from Centers for Disease Control, HIV/AIDS Surveillance Report, September 1991.)*

appears to be more common in urban areas plagued by despair and economic uncertainty. Data gathered by the Drug Abuse Warning Network of the National Institute on Drug Abuse show that more than 80 percent of persons presenting to selected emergency rooms throughout the nation with cocaine- or heroin-related complaints are black or Latino [5]. Since these drugs are frequently injected and, by their very nature, may alter judgment with regard to sexual behavior, they are important contributors to the acquisition of HIV infection. This risk may be further enhanced by the practice of using "shooting galleries," proprietary inner-city locations where injection drug users (IDUs) gather and may rent syringes and other apparatus ("works") from the gallery's operator. Needle sharing and the use of contaminated syringes are common in this setting.

Other drugs such as crack cocaine and alcohol may also enhance the risk of HIV infection. Crack has been directly linked to an increased risk of HIV infection through its well-known ability to enhance sexual arousal and inhibit climax [6]. High levels of sexual activity have been reported in "crack houses" (locations where crack users gather for the sale and use of the drug), and the direct exchange of sex for drugs is common. Anthropologists working in the inner city as "crack ethnographers" have observed that some users, when lighting their pipe, may draw in the flame. This, in turn, may singe the lips and cause fissures or small cracks [7]. Since desperate drug users may engage in prostitution, most frequently oral sex, to support their habit, these lip lesions could hypothetically serve as a portal of entry for HIV.

Other factors may also play a role in the increased risk of HIV infection in specific ethnic groups. It is possible that, since a significant number of African-American and Latino men have been involved with the penal system, some may have had homosexual experiences while incarcerated. It is also well known that the presence of genital lesions, such as those resulting from herpes simplex virus infection and syphilis, may facilitate the transmission of HIV infection, and both diseases are endemic in inner-city, low-income communities.

Despite these possible explanations for the higher prevalence of HIV in persons of color, it is important to note that they do not seem to account for all of the increased risk observed. Several studies have noted that even among IDUs, HIV infection is more prevalent among blacks and Latinos than among whites, even when controlled for needle sharing [6, 8]. Similarly, black homosexual and bisexual men have a higher prevalence of HIV infection than their white counterparts [9]. Far from suggesting any biologic or genetic predisposition to HIV infection, Selik and associates [2] concluded that

the wide range of relative risks of AIDS in Blacks and Hispanics for different exposure categories, and the variation in these relative risks by geographic area of residence, support the view that the higher risks of AIDS in Blacks and Hispanics are due primarily to behavioral and perhaps environmental differences between racial/ethnic groups, rather than genetic differences.

Etiology: Cultural Versus Sociopolitical

It has long been assumed that disparities between rates of disease for persons in different ethnic groups reflect differences in culture. More recently, however, emphasis has been placed on sociopolitical issues, which may have an important impact on behaviors and attitudes. Framing differences in behavior as manifestations of cultural differences is problematic since, as De La Cancela [10] points out, cultural explanation "creates the image of minorities as having certain static, exotic, racial or ethnic features that serve as barriers to their accepting an AIDS prevention message." This problem extends also to the care of patients with AIDS. Such cultural characterizations have led to stereotyped notions about taboos concerning discussions of sexuality among Latino families or the reluctance to use condoms among African-Americans. Notions of "machismo" and fatalism have been applied to Latinos regardless of their country of origin [10].

It is perhaps more useful to view the problem of AIDS in communities of color in the context of the complex economic, social, and political realities of the inner city. For example, as Mays and Cochran [11] point out, an economically oppressed woman of color in the inner city may determine that her insistence that her partner use a condom could endanger the relationship itself. Given the low ratio of "available" men to women (75 men to 100 women for African-Americans) and the fact that women may depend on their partners for both emotional and financial support, the wisdom of potentially endangering this relationship is questionable at best. Important interpersonal decisions appear related to economic and political realities rather than to cultural issues [10]. Such circumstances need to be considered in the education of persons with or at risk for HIV infection.

Similarly, Dalton [12] notes that homophobia in the African-American community may stem more from the unequal ratio of men to women and less from a strict cultural bias. He argues that men who are perceived as having "chosen" homosexuality in the midst of a paucity of available heterosexual African-American men due to incarceration and homicide may be resented for their sexual orientation. Certainly, the strong presence of the church in African-American and Latino communities and its general opposition to homosexuality also adds to the perceived intolerance of gay or bisexual men.

Attitudes about HIV/AIDS in Communities of Color

Much has been written about the difficulties of addressing HIV in communities of color and their seeming reluctance to "own the issue of AIDS" [12]. Clearly, one of the strongest influences is racism. With regard to AIDS, this was exemplified in the minds of many African-Americans and Latinos by the delayed response to the epidemic on the part of federal officials at a time when it was clearly growing among inner-city drug users. Skepticism and mistrust grew further when some scientists insisted that HIV had originated in Africa and when Haitians were labeled as a distinct risk group [13]. These incidents were interpreted by many as an attempt to hold people of color responsible for AIDS. To make matters worse, HIV-infected IDUs and homosexual/bisexual men were often portrayed by the media as being less "innocent" than afflicted infants and recipients of tainted blood products.

Seemingly more extreme are the persistent feelings in some communities of color that HIV infection represented a conspiracy of biologic engineering designed to eliminate those who are less valued by society. Such a view was based on the precedent of the Tuskegee syphilis experiment, wherein African-American men were observed without treatment for syphilis, despite the availability of penicillin, in order to define the natural history of the disease [14]. Theories of a conspiracy to infect Africans with HIV have been advanced by a number of authors and are prevalent in the US and abroad [15]. These speculations undoubtedly play a role in distrust for the health care system.

The inner city is awash with other issues that compete with AIDS as prime concerns. Economic instability has spawned what sociologist William Julius Wilson [16] has termed the "underclass," a group of persons in the inner city who are increasingly set apart from the surrounding community by lack of training and skills, unemployment, involvement in street crime, prolonged periods of poverty, and welfare dependence. Contact with the criminal justice system is common as evidenced by a recent study, which found that 24 percent of black men aged 20 to 29 are in jail, on probation, or on parole [17]. In addition, 300,000 blacks are incarcerated in the US, representing 47 percent of the total prison population [18]. Violence in the inner city is widespread; 1 of 30 black men now living will die as a victim of homicide. Access to medical care is limited, exacerbating problems of sexually transmitted diseases and infant mortality. High dropout rates from school and lack of economic opportunity may lead to involvement with the illicit economies of drug trafficking and prostitution, despite their attendant dangers. All of these factors contribute to a general sense of powerlessness and hopelessness in the inner city. HIV infection, in contrast, may seem to some an abstract and distant risk given its long latency. Effective strategies are needed that foster empowerment around a broad spectrum of health and socioeconomic issues in these communities [19].

Issues for Health Care Providers

Family and Community Support

Health care providers must be sensitive to the previously mentioned issues in managing HIV disease in patients of color. Many of these patients, regardless of route of infection, depend heavily on family and friends for support. However, given the ongoing stigma that accompanies homosexuality and drug use within communities, patients may fear acknowledgment of such behaviors, and HIV infection may alienate families at a critical time. The situation in communities of color is thus different from that in the white gay community, where there are often better-established means of group support. The lack of an advocacy system for HIV-infected persons of color makes it all the more important that health care providers attempt to identify and foster available social supports [20].

Substance Abuse Treatment

Substance abuse should always be regarded as a separate diagnosis. Active and untreated drug use will undoubtedly compromise medical compliance and likely increase morbidity and mortality. However, the choice of drug treatment should be individualized depending on the patient's needs and preferences, which may be influenced by community attitudes. Methadone, although effective for many patients, has been viewed by some communities as simply substituting one addiction for another. This preference for "drug-free" programs is reflected in the difficulties that city and state public health officials have faced in finding sites for methadone treatment. Such an attitude was apparent in the resistance of New York City residents to a needle exchange program [12].

This opposition, largely on the basis of community residents feeling excluded from the process of development and institution of the program, exemplifies the complex relationship that inner-city communities have with drug use and abuse. As Harlan Dalton [13] so aptly points out:

We as a community have a complex relationship with drug abuse. On the one hand, we are scared to even admit the dimensions of the problem for fear that we will all be treated as junkies and our culture viewed as pathological. On the other, we desperately want to find solutions. For us, drug abuse is a curse far worse than you can imagine. Addicts prey on our neighborhoods, sell drugs to our children, steal our possessions, and rob us of hope. We despise them. We despise them because they hurt us and because they **are** us. They are a constant reminder of how close we all are to the edge. And "they" are "us" literally as well as figuratively; they are our sons and daughters, our sisters and brothers. Can we possibly cast out the demons without casting out our own kin? (From "AIDS in Blackface." Reprinted by permission of *Daedalus*, Journal of the American Academy of Arts and Sciences, from the issue entitled, "Living with AIDS: Part II," Summer 1989, Vol. 118, No. 3.)

Other important considerations in the choice of a drug treatment program include residential versus outpatient and behavioral versus insight oriented. Individuals who live in settings where there is ongoing drug use and trafficking are probably best served by a program that removes them from such an environment. Residential programs are more costly and, therefore, tend to be more difficult to find. Programs with a strong behavior modification component may be particularly helpful for crack/

cocaine users, for whom the presence of any drug-associated images may evoke strong cravings. Such stimuli may include the site where drugs were purchased, money itself, and even drug prevention commercials that feature drug use symbols or paraphernalia. Usually, these programs exist in conjunction with insight-oriented programs, such as Cocaine Anonymous or Narcotics Anonymous, which are crucial supports to recovering drug users.

The Role of the Church

The church, both Catholic and Protestant denominations, is a strong institution in African-American and Latino communities. Much has been written about the opposition of the church to education about sexual issues, condom distribution, and acceptance of members of the gay community. Nevertheless, some congregations have been active and successful in providing counseling and support to HIV-infected persons, and these resources should not be overlooked. Furthermore, a number of church-affiliated drug treatment programs rely heavily on religious principles in rehabilitation. Many of these programs have been particularly receptive to HIV-infected clients. Drug rehabilitation programs are most successful when they are culturally specific and linguistically appropriate.

Other Issues

Maintaining access to medical care for economically disadvantaged, inner-city, HIV-infected patients is essential. This requires that primary care providers, nurses, and social workers be well versed in financial assistance programs, such as general relief, Social Security Disability Insurance, and Medicaid, as well as sources of support and assistance from local community and charitable agencies. For those who are still able to work, job referrals can be an important source of income and a way to maintain independence and self-esteem.

Many individuals from inner-city communities of color have had unpleasant interactions with the health care system and may be very apprehensive and distrustful of providers in an AIDS clinic [20]. The nature of the disease itself and fears about breaches in confidentiality may deepen this distrust. Development of a safe and trusting environment is therefore crucial to providing good medical care. This may require repeated explanations to patient, family, and partner(s) about the side effects of medications, prognosis of the disease, and methods of risk reduction. However, skepticism on the part of patients should not lead providers to abandon efforts to institute effective therapy or fail to consider enrollment in clinical trials. The building of a trusting patient-doctor relationship, even for IDUs, traditionally considered difficult patients, can lead to improved medical compliance and broad acceptance of diagnostic and treatment modalities.

Discussion of preventing the spread of HIV infection is also an important part of the encounter. Language that suggests the patient to be a "vector" of disease is counterproductive and alienating. Many HIV-infected patients have stable sexual partners and are concerned about spreading the virus to others. For those not in monogamous relationships, emphasis on protection from potentially morbid infections such as herpes simplex and syphilis, in addition to protecting others, may be useful in encouraging condom use and limiting unprotected sexual encounters.

Providers should be aware of the potent stigma associated with HIV infection in communities of color [21]. Some men of color, because of their denial about homosexuality, may not identify with words such as "gay," "bisexual," or "homosexual," or may attribute their infection to another risk behavior. Use of more neutral phrases, such as "sex with another man," may be more acceptable. Many AIDS patients, already affected by racial discrimination, find themselves further alienated by health care workers who may treat them differently because of their diagnosis. Hospital and clinic staff should be educated about the transmission of HIV infection in order to allay fears. Non–English-speaking persons may be further estranged by their language. The use of appropriate interpreters or, ideally, polylingual providers, is essential in this setting.

Finally, any maneuver that can enhance medical compliance should be explored. Recent data suggest that a history of injection drug use does not predict poor compliance with zidovudine, and all eligible patients should be offered this option [22]. Such simple devices as a pill-box with a built-in alarm can be very effective in improving compliance.

HIV Prevention Efforts

Attempts to prevent HIV infection must focus on reducing high-risk behaviors. Within communities of color, such efforts should target the modes of transmission that are the most prevalent, including injection drug use with needle sharing, unprotected sex between men, and heterosexual sex with IDUs. To date, the major strategies for prevention have concentrated on HIV education and protective measures such as condoms. However, recent studies have demonstrated that, among African-Americans and Latinos, levels of knowledge are already quite high [23]. Unfortunately, rates of condom use remain discouragingly low, even among those who know about the specifics of viral transmission. Some studies have suggested that levels of knowledge about HIV are significantly lower among Asians and other recent immigrants [24].

It is clear that knowledge alone is insufficient to alter complex behaviors, particularly in the face of alcohol or other drug use. It is also evident that behavior modification programs must be multifaceted and intensive to attain desired results. A recent study of a New York program for adolescent runaways showed that behavioral change in this population was related to the number of intensive counseling sessions and that increases in consistent condom use required 15 or more sessions [25]. While this population of largely minority youths has special issues and problems, the study indicates that inducing behavioral change is a difficult challenge and requires a powerful, sustained effort.

Future prevention programs will need to employ strategies that empower individuals to act on the knowledge they possess. This may be as simple as teaching a person both how to use a condom and how to discuss using a condom with an indifferent partner. Other programs have used peer educators in an attempt to break through social norms regarding multiple sexual partners or condoms. The courageous revelation by former Los Angeles Laker guard Earvin "Magic" Johnson that he is HIV positive and is devoting his life to increasing awareness about AIDS may have a profound impact on the acceptability of safe sex and condoms, especially among young men of color who view him as a hero and role model. In his own words,

I didn't know that **half** of the Americans currently suffering with this disease are either black or Hispanic. Like most other blacks, I was denying that AIDS was spreading through our community like wildfire while we ignored the flames. . . . My doctors have told me that there are more than 1 million people in the U.S.—many of them black—who are infected with the AIDS virus but don't know because they refuse to get tested. Maybe that will change soon, even though I haven't even begun my crusade . . . [26]

Magic Johnson's story reinforces the notion that anybody can get HIV disease and HIV-infected individuals may appear healthy and well. Such realizations are important to adolescents and adults who continue to believe that they can choose "clean" partners and avoid exposure to HIV infection.

Conclusion

Communities of color are disproportionately affected by HIV disease. Persons of color, particularly those from the inner city, are confronted with a number of difficult economic and political issues. Such factors may account for the high prevalence of HIV infection and necessitate innovative strategies for prevention and treatment. An understanding of community perceptions about disease, drug abuse, and the health care system is critical to the provision of primary care. Individuals with limited previous experience with the health care system can be managed successfully for HIV infection in clinics and community health centers.

References

1. Centers for Disease Control. HIV/AIDS Surveillance Report, September 1991.
2. Selik RM, Castro KG, Pappaiouanou M. Racial/ethnic differences in the risk of AIDS in the United States. Am J Public Health 78:1539–1545, 1988.
3. Rothenberg R, et al. Survival with the acquired immunodeficiency syndrome: Experience with 5833 cases in New York City. N Engl J Med 317:1297–1302, 1987.
4. Leads from the MMWR. Human T-lymphotrophic virus type III/lymphadenopathy-associated virus antibody prevalence in U.S. military recruit applicants. JAMA 356:975–977, 1986.
5. National Institute on Drug Abuse Statistical Series: Data from Drug Abuse Warning Network Series 1, No. 7. DHHS Publication No. ADM 88-1584, 1987.
6. Chaisson RE, Bacchetti P, Osmond D, et al. Cocaine use and HIV infection in intravenous drug users in San Francisco. JAMA 261:561–565, 1989.
7. Holden C. News and Comment: Street-wise crack research. Science 246:1376–1381, 1989.
8. Brown LS, Murphy DL, Primm BJ. Needle sharing and AIDS in minorities (letter). JAMA 258:1474–1475, 1987.
9. Samuel M, Winkelstein W. Prevalence of human immunodeficiency virus infection in ethnic minority homosexual and bisexual men (letter). JAMA 257:1901–1902, 1987.
10. De La Cancela V. Minority AIDS prevention: Moving beyond cultural perspectives toward sociopolitical empowerment. AIDS Educat Prevent 1:141–153, 1989.
11. Mays VM, Cochran SD. Issues in the perception of AIDS risk reduction activities by black and Hispanic/Latino women. Am Psychol 43:949–957, 1988.
12. Dalton H. AIDS in blackface. Daedalus 118:205–227, 1989.
13. Chirimuita R. AIDS, Africa and Racism. London: Free Association Books, 1989.
14. Jones J. Bad Blood: The Tuskegee Syphilis Experiment. New York: New York Free Press, 1981.
15. Madhubuhti HR. Black Men: Obsolete, Single, Dangerous? Chicago: Third World Press, 1990.
16. Wilson WJ. The Truly Disadvantaged. Chicago: The University of Chicago Press, 1987. P 8.

17. *Young Black Men and the Criminal Justice System: A Growing National Problem.* Washington, DC: The Sentencing Project, 1990.
18. Bureau of Justice Statistics, Department of Justice. Correctional Populations in the United States, 1986.
19. Braithwaite RL, Lythcott N. Community empowerment as a strategy for health promotion for black and other minority populations. *JAMA* 261:282–283, 1989.
20. Mays VM, Cochran SD. Acquired immunodeficiency syndrome and black Americans: Special psychosocial issues. *Public Health Rep* 102:224–231, 1987.
21. Peterson JL, Marin G. Issues in the prevention of AIDS among black and Hispanic men. *Am Psychol* 43:871–877, 1988.
22. Samet JH, Libman H, Steger KA, et al. Compliance with zidovudine therapy in patients infected with human immunodeficiency virus, type 1: A cross-sectional study in a municipal hospital clinic. *Am J Med* 92:495–502, 1992.
23. Hardy A. AIDS knowledge and attitudes for April–June 1989. Advance Data from the Vital and Health Statistics of the National Center for Health Statistics. 179:1–7, 1989.
24. Hingson RW, Strunin L, Grady M, et al. Knowledge beliefs and behavioral risks for human immunodeficiency virus 1 infection of Boston public school students born outside the United States mainland. Presented at the American Public Health Association 118th Annual Meeting: School Health Education and Services Section, October 1, 1990.
25. Rotheram-Borus MJ, Koopman C, Haignere C, Davies M. Reducing HIV sexual risk behaviors among runaway adolescents. *JAMA* 226:1237–1241, 1991.
26. *Sports Illustrated*, November 18, 1991. Pp 19, 25–26.

37/Legal Issues Regarding HIV Infection

Leonard H. Glantz

Unlike any other disease, HIV infection has resulted in a large amount of legal commentary and action. This has occurred for a variety of reasons. First, AIDS has primarily afflicted homosexual men and injection drug users, groups that have historically been the victims of discrimination. Second, AIDS is communicable and fatal. Finally, the AIDS epidemic evolved after the concepts of individual and civil rights had been firmly rooted in the social values and law of the United States. All of these factors have contributed to the development of laws designed to avoid or alleviate the stigmatization associated with HIV infection.

For the most part AIDS has produced few new legal issues. Concerns about confidentiality of medical information, informed consent for medical procedures, and discrimination against people with disabilities predated the AIDS epidemic. However, AIDS has compelled us to reexamine our approach to these issues and has raised questions as to whether existing laws have been vigorously enforced.

AIDS has led to the development of many specific state statutes and regulations, which are in a constant process of revision. Because of this, it is not possible to write a complete or definitive chapter on the legal aspects of HIV infection. Should questions arise in practice regarding the rights or obligations of a particular patient or practitioner, it is essential to obtain the advice of an attorney who is knowledgeable about applicable state laws and policies regarding HIV infection. This chapter discusses many of the general legal issues presented by AIDS and describes how a variety of state and federal laws have attempted to address them.

Testing for HIV

One of the earliest controversies to come out of the AIDS epidemic was the testing of persons to determine their serologic status. Health care practitioners, prisons, mental health facilities, employers, insurance companies, and others presented arguments supporting the need to know the HIV status of individuals with whom they dealt. On the other hand, advocates for patients, employees, and insurance policy holders argued that no individual should undergo HIV antibody testing without informed consent because (1) testing could have adverse emotional effects in those identified as HIV positive, in that they would be learning of a potentially life-threatening condition, and (2) testing could result in discrimination against them, with devastating social and financial consequences. As a result of these strong arguments, a number of states, including New York, Massachusetts, California, Illinois, and Maine, have required that persons may not be tested for HIV without their fully informed consent [1-3].

The potential impact on the life of a person being tested for HIV is so great that general rules regarding informed consent probably require that it be provided before testing, even in the absence of a specific state statute. The potential risks and benefits of HIV testing and alternatives should be communicated, as should information that testing is voluntary and confidential. Public health authorities have stated that HIV antibody testing should never be done in the absence of appropriate pretest and posttest counseling, and several states have made counseling a prerequisite to testing [1].

Some states have legislated exceptions to the above rules and permit mandatory testing in certain defined circumstances [1]. Testing may be mandated for persons arrested for prostitution and persons who are indicted or convicted of sexual assault or rape. Additionally, some states permit involuntary testing when a health care worker can document "significant exposure" to blood or infectious bodily fluids during the performance of his or her occupation. However, these statutes have significant procedural requirements. For example, in Rhode Island, the health care worker who is concerned about a "significant exposure" to a patient must do the following:

1. Complete an incident report within 48 hours of the exposure, describing the events in question
2. Submit to a baseline HIV test within 72 hours, with the results being negative
3. Demonstrate that there has been a "significant puncture or mucous membrane exposure" of a type and in sufficient concentration to result in transmission of the AIDS virus
4. Have an exposure evaluation group made up of three impartial health care providers determine that a "significant exposure" has occurred and that the patient has refused to grant informed consent

Once these steps are taken, if a sample of the patient's blood is available, it may be tested for the presence of HIV antibody. If no sample of blood is available, the health care worker may petition the superior court for an order mandating the test [4]. This complex procedure, which is indicative of the importance placed on voluntary testing, is an attempt to balance the rights of patients with the need for information by exposed workers.

Confidentiality

All modern courts that have dealt with this issue have held that the information a physician possesses about a patient is confidential and may not be divulged without consent [5–7]. This legal rule is derived from a long history of medical ethics and practice, licensing statutes, and the contractual obligations that are implied in the doctor-patient relationship. The purpose of the rule assuring patients that information they share with their physicians will remain confidential is to make them secure in disclosing very sensitive facts about themselves that may be needed to make diagnostic and treatment decisions. Information related to the diagnosis of HIV infection would certainly be considered in this realm of protection.

However, confidentiality of medical information is not absolute, and courts and legislatures have made exceptions to the general rule. For example, all states have statutes that require physicians to report suspected cases of child abuse [8]. Similarly, all states require reporting an AIDS diagnosis to public health authorities, similar to the regulations pertaining to other communicable diseases [9]. Such requirements have never been legally challenged, and, if they were, would no doubt be upheld as originating from the public health powers of the state, so long as the information was protected from general disclosure [10].

A number of states have statutes that specifically ensure that HIV antibody test results are confidential [3]. New York includes in its definition of confidential HIV-related information not just the fact that a person "has HIV infection" or an "HIV-related illness," but also the fact that a person has been the subject of an HIV test [11]. States with such confidentiality protections usually require that HIV-related information not be released without written authorization of the patient. These authorizations generally need to specifically identify to whom the disclosure is being made, the purpose for the disclosure, and the time period during which such disclosure can be made [3, 12]. General forms used to authorize the release of other types of medical information are usually insufficient to meet the demands of these specific statutes.

The purpose of these statutes is to limit the disclosure of HIV-related information outside the hospital, not to impede the transfer of information among clinicians involved in the care of a specific patient. However, health care workers and institutions must be very careful to limit this highly sensitive information to only those who have "a need to know." As an example, in a recent case, a physician was diagnosed as having AIDS when he was a patient in the hospital in which he practiced. This information was widely disseminated in the health care community, causing his patients and staff to desert him. A court held that this was sufficient grounds to demonstrate that the hospital did not act appropriately to protect his confidentiality [13]. Similarly, when police officers disclosed to neighbors that a person they were arresting had AIDS, the court held that the officers violated that individual's rights and also found the town that employed the officers liable for failing to adequately train them about AIDS [14].

As important as confidentiality is for people with HIV infection, their right to keep this information secret is not absolute. For example, a number of state statutes permit disclosure to health care workers who have been exposed to a risk of infection [9]. Similarly, there are statutes that give emergency care providers or "first responders," such as emergency medical technicians, paramedics, fire fighters, lifeguards, and police officers, access to a patient's HIV status if they have been significantly exposed to blood or other bodily fluids.

Individual states have different procedures regarding how the first responder gains access to this confidential information. In some cases, a committee or physician must certify the seriousness of the exposure. In Massachusetts, an exposed first responder must file an exposure report form with the facility to which the patient was delivered. If the facility knows the patient's HIV status, it may be disclosed to the exposed first responder without the patient's name [15]. It is the obligation of the first responder who learns of the HIV status of a particular patient not to disclose this information to another person. Given the complexity and specificity of state laws, health care practitioners who are in the position of making decisions regarding the release of HIV-related information need to be knowledgeable about the regulations of their individual state.

Partner Notification

There has been a good deal of professional and scholarly speculation about the duty to warn sexual or needle-sharing partners of patients who are HIV infected [16, 17]. Many practitioners who deal with HIV disease believe that it is their ethical or professional obligation to ensure that others are not placed at risk unknowingly. Before determining if there is a duty to warn, a physician clearly has other obligations to reduce the risk of HIV transmission. The patient should be informed about the ways in which HIV infection is acquired and means to reduce the risk of transmission, including safer sexual practices and avoidance of needle sharing. Also part of the discussion should be the *patient's* obligation to disclose his or her status to partners. Failure to provide such information would constitute a breach of good medical practice, similar to a failure to caution an epileptic about the dangers of driving [18].

Having taken these steps, the question still remains of whether there is a duty to warn known sexual or needle-sharing partners of the patient's HIV serostatus and the potential danger to them. The traditional route to partners at risk of contracting sexually transmitted diseases has been public health officers who engage in contact tracing. It has not been the individual physician's responsibility to serve this role.

The argument that physicians have a "duty to warn," which means that failure to do so could result in liability, is usually based on the California case, *Tarasoff v. The Regents of the University of California* [19]. In this case, a student told a psychologist working for the student health clinic that he intended to kill his girlfriend. The psychologist and the psychiatrist colleagues with whom he had consulted believed that the threat was real, but did little to protect the intended victim. After the murder of the girlfriend, her parents brought suit, arguing that the psychologist should have committed his dangerous patient to a mental hospital. This argument was rejected by the court because of a California law that forbids lawsuits on this basis. The parents then argued that the psychologist should have warned the potential victim of the danger so that she could have taken steps to protect herself. While ultimately decided as a duty-to-warn case, the court's decision did not focus on warning alone. Rather, it held that once a therapist in fact determines that

> . . . a patient poses a serious danger of violence to others, he bears *a duty to exercise reasonable care to protect the foreseeable victim* of that danger [emphasis added]. While the discharge of this duty will necessarily vary with the facts of each case, in each instance the adequacy of the therapist's conflict must be measured against the traditional negligence standard of the rendition of reasonable care under the circumstances.

The duty, then, according to *Tarasoff*, is the exercise of reasonable care to protect potential victims. In most cases, providing the HIV-infected person with the information described above will be all the "reasonable care" necessary to protect sexual partners. In contrast to *Tarasoff*, which is about a mentally deranged, homicidal man, there is no reason to believe that a typical HIV-infected person desires to harm his or her partners. *Tarasoff* was meant to deal with the unusual case, not to obliterate confidentiality for all psychiatric patients, and applies to a victim who could in no way know she was in any danger. Such a description would not pertain to injection drug users who share needles with others. In summary, *Tarasoff* should not be interpreted as a mandate to transform every physician into a public health officer.

It is notable that there are no cases charging that a physician has failed to warn an HIV-infected patient's sex or needle-sharing partner. Furthermore, no state statute *requires* physicians to warn partners that they are at risk. Several states have adopted statutes that permit, but do not require, physicians to make certain disclosures to a known partner. Once again, it is essential to know the specifics of these statutes and what they permit. For example, in Connecticut, a physician may disclose HIV-related information to a partner if both the partner and the HIV-infected person are patients. Before informing the partner, the physician must believe that there is a significant risk of transmission and must have counseled the HIV-infected person to notify the partner. The physician must reasonably believe that no such notification will occur and must tell the infected person of his or her plans to inform the partner. Alternatively, the physician may request a public health officer to contact the partner. However, neither the physician nor the public health officer is permitted to disclose the identity of the original patient [20].

In states with strong confidentiality laws that contain no exceptions to the requirement of patient consent for release of HIV-related information, such disclosures may not be made if they would expose the nature of the patient's condition to others. Furthermore, it should be remembered that when a statute permits or requires obtaining information for a particular purpose, it may not be used for another aim. For example, under New York law, AIDS cases are reported to the state Department of Health for epidemiologic and statistical purposes. Disclosure by the Department of Health of a child's report to a school board was deemed to constitute a violation of that law [21].

Discrimination

Confidentiality of a person's HIV serostatus is considered important because knowledge of it could lead to discriminatory practices by employers, landlords, schools, and even health care practitioners. Whether or not discrimination is prohibited depends on the specific scope of the antidiscrimination law in question. For example, while the federal Rehabilitation Act of 1973 has been instrumental in protecting the jobs of handicapped people, it only applies to federal employees, federal contractors, and programs receiving federal financial assistance

[22, 23]. In addition to their presence in federal laws, antidiscrimination regulations may also be part of state statutes and city ordinances.

The complexity of antidiscrimination law can be demonstrated by posing the question of whether physicians have an obligation to treat patients with HIV infection. Strong ethical and policy arguments have been made arguing that physicians have such an obligation [24]. In 1988, the American Medical Association (AMA) took the position that a physician may not ethically refuse to treat a patient solely because he or she is HIV infected [25]. This position is notable because Principle VI of the 1980 AMA Principles of Medical Ethics states that, except in emergencies, a physician is "free to choose whom to serve . . ." However, the 1988 position argues that this principle does not permit "categorical discrimination." While the AMA's position does not set a legal requirement, it does establish a professional standard of care for the medical community. Some medical licensing boards, including those in New Jersey and Massachusetts, have taken the position that physicians may not categorically refuse to treat AIDS patients [26].

As a general matter of law, physicians do have the right to choose whom they wish to treat with some exceptions. For example, patients who come to an emergency room have a legal right to care, and, because of this, health care providers who work there have an obligation to provide it. Furthermore, once a physician has established a relationship with a patient, the physician must continue to provide necessary care or be liable for abandonment. A provider may terminate a relationship with a patient, but only if the patient has been given adequate notice so that alternative care can be arranged.

A number of antidiscrimination laws prohibit discrimination by "public accommodations." There has been controversy as to whether a physician's office is a public accommodation for purpose of these laws. However, a sweeping federal law enacted in July 1990, the Americans with Disabilities Act (ADA), prohibits discrimination based on disability "in the full and equal enjoyment of the . . . services, facilities, privileges, advantages, or accommodations of any place of public accommodation . . ." [27]. The term *public accommodation* includes both hospitals and the "professional office of a health care worker" [28]. While these provisions of the ADA have not yet been interpreted by a court, it is likely that this section would be found to prohibit discrimination by health care providers.

The laws prohibiting discrimination against people with handicaps or disabilities tend to define these terms expansively, so that the maximum number of individuals can benefit from them. Thus, the ADA, like the earlier federal Rehabilitation Act of 1973, defines the term *disability* to mean (1) a physical or mental impairment that substantially limits one or more major life activities and (2) a situation in which the person has a *record* of such an impairment or is *regarded* as having such an impairment [29]. Therefore, one need not be impaired at all to be "disabled" but need only be treated as a disabled person to be protected by the law. Thus, there is no question that a person with AIDS is disabled, and even an asymptomatic HIV-positive person might be considered "disabled" for purposes of this and other antidiscrimination laws.

The fact that a person is protected by antidiscrimination laws does not mean that person is entitled to a job. The individual must still be able to perform the essential functions that the position requires. Thus, in a landmark Supreme Court case, in which a teacher with tuberculosis was fired from her job, the court found that she was a "handicapped individual" under the federal Rehabilitation Act and, therefore, protected against discrimination [30]. However, to maintain her position she would also need to be "otherwise qualified" to perform the functions of her job. The court found that if a person poses a "significant risk" of communicating an infectious disease to others in the workplace and, if "reasonable accommodations" would not eliminate the risk, that person is not "otherwise qualified." As the court said, "The Act would not require a school board to place a teacher with active, contagious tuberculosis in a classroom with elementary school children" [30]. The court ruled that a finding regarding the presence of a significant risk should be "based on reasonable medical judgment" about (1) how the disease is transmitted, (2) the duration of the risk, (3) the severity of the potential harm if the disease is transmitted, and (4) the probability of transmission.

The ADA takes a similar approach. Otherwise protected individuals can be excluded from the workplace if they pose a "direct threat" to the health or safety of others. To be a direct threat, a person must present a high probability of substantial harm. Mere fear of harm is not enough to exclude people from their jobs. As a result of these types of policies and laws, schoolchildren who are HIV positive can continue to attend school, teachers who are HIV positive can continue to teach, and employees in schools for the mentally retarded cannot be forced to take an HIV antibody test as a condition of employment because they do not present a significant risk of harm to anyone [20, 30, 31, 32].

Ironically, it appears that when health care practitioners are HIV infected the courts seem to give their employers the most flexibility in excluding these individuals from the workplace. In one case, a person was diagnosed as having AIDS, and the hospital in which this occurred knew that one of its nurses, Kevin Leckelt, was a homosexual and had been this patient's roommate for 8 years [33]. The hospital demanded that Leckelt be tested for HIV or disclose the results of a test he had previously obtained himself, both of which he refused to do. The hospital fired him for insubordination, which was upheld by the US Court of Appeals. The court acknowledged that the risk of transmission of HIV from a nurse to a patient is "extremely low and can be minimized by the use of universal precautions," which Leckelt regularly employed. However, the court apparently believed that, since the potential harm—death—was so serious, the extremely low risk was irrelevant. This court's analysis is generally viewed as incorrect in that failure to assess the probability of harm violates antidiscrimination laws.

Similarly, a hospital in New Jersey suspended the privileges of a surgeon who was diagnosed with AIDS in June 1987. The physicians on various hospital committees concluded that the risk of transmission of HIV from the surgeon to a patient was so low that he should be able to continue his work and did not need to disclose this very minimal risk as part of informed consent. The hospital's president and lawyer disagreed with this finding because of "legal and social conditions." Ultimately, the hospital trustees concurred with the president, and the doctor never practiced again. Once again, a court upheld this hospital's action, failing to evaluate adequately the low probability of harm to patients [13].

There are several explanations for these outcomes. First, the disclosure that a dentist in Florida appears to have infected five of his patients with HIV has shaken many people's ability to assess the low probability of this risk [34]. Second, reactions from both the Centers for Disease Control and AMA have made it appear that even the most minimal risks of transmission need to be avoided [35, 36]. Finally, no legal cases have yet been decided solely on the basis of the antidiscrimination laws discussed earlier. For example, Nurse Leckelt was not fired for having AIDS but for being insubordinate. How courts will ultimately decide cases of HIV-infected health care workers based on antidiscrimination laws is unknown. However, it is likely that they will rely to a great extent on how medical and public health authorities define and present the risks of HIV transmission.

Death and Dying

The high mortality of AIDS requires a discussion of the rights of dying patients. Unlike many areas of the law that apply to HIV-infected patients, there is a good deal of uniformity among the states regarding the rights of patients to refuse treatment.

Since the Karen Quinlan case was decided in 1976, a large and consistent body of law has developed that recognizes the rights of individuals to decline life-prolonging treatment [37]. Courts are unanimous that competent people can reject any type of medical intervention, including amputation, resuscitation, assisted ventilation, dialysis, and artificial means of nutrition. A patient's refusal of such interventions does not constitute suicide but is rather the decision to let a disease take its natural course.

Whether or not to accept medical treatment is seen by the courts as an option a patient is free to exercise, rather than an obligation. If a patient is able to understand the nature and consequences of a decision to refuse treatment, then he or she is competent; that is, a patient must be capable of understanding that he or she has an illness or condition, that treatment is available, and the consequences if a treatment is accepted or declined [38]. Competence is a factual issue in each case that does not necessarily require consultation with a mental health expert. If a patient has a relationship with a physician or nurse, that person may be well suited to determine the ability of the patient to understand the issues relevant to competence.

The most difficult and controversial treatment decisions arise when a patient is incompetent. This is because it may be difficult to identify an appropriate surrogate to make life-and-death decisions on behalf of another person. In the case of AIDS, decisions on behalf of incompetent patients may be even more difficult than in other situations because traditional family members who are called on to make proxy decisions may be unavailable or inappropriate.

However, the crisis situation of having to make a treatment decision on behalf of an incompetent AIDS patient is virtually always avoidable. It is crucial for physicians to talk to HIV-infected patients about end-of-life treatment decisions while the patient is competent. By doing so, the patient will be more comfortable knowing that the physician understands and supports his or her decisions, and the physician will not be left guessing what the patient would have wanted done.

Every state has a law authorizing the use of living wills, in which persons can state their treatment directives, and/or durable power of attorney or health care proxy laws, in which one person designates another to make health care decisions for him/her if he/she is incompetent. If a person decides to write a living will, it should be as detailed as possible. It should deal explicitly with matters such as resuscitation, ventilation, use of antibiotics, and artificial nutrition. It is in the area of withholding or withdrawing artificial nutrition that the courts have been most insistent on knowing the patient's actual desires.

It is also advisable for AIDS patients to identify a health care proxy. For example, if a homosexual patient has a long-term companion, that person may well have no legal standing to make health care decisions, particularly in the face of family opposition. Designating the companion as health care proxy grants him or her sole legal authority to make such decisions. It is the joint obligation of health care practitioners and patients to ensure that these matters are attended to while the patient is competent. Legal difficulties that arise at the end of life are generally predictable and preventable.

Conclusion

Just as the AIDS epidemic has necessitated changes in the practice of medicine, it has also required legal innovations. In some instances, it has meant new applications of old laws, and in others, the development of entirely new legislation. For the most part, these rules have been designed to protect the dignity and social well-being of those afflicted with HIV infection. Physicians owe it to themselves and their patients to be aware of the relevant laws and policies in this rapidly changing area.

References

1. Field M. Testing for AIDS: Uses and abuses. *Am J Law Med* 16:34–106, 1990.
2. Mass. Rev. St. Title 5, Section 19230-A.1.
3. Mass. Gen. Laws, Chap. 111, Section 70F.
4. RI Gen. Laws 23-6-14.
5. *Horne v. Patton*, 287 So 2d 824 (Ala., 1974).
6. *Alberts v. Devine*, 395 Mass. 59, 1985.
7. Annas GJ. *The Rights of Patients*. Carbondale: Southern Illinois University Press, 1989.
8. Mnookin R, Weisberg D. *Child, Family and State*. Boston: Little, Brown, 1988. P. 299.
9. Edgar H, Sandomire H. Medical privacy issues in the age of AIDS: Legislative options. *Am J Law Med* 16:155–222, 1990.
10. *Whalen v. Roe*, 429 US 589, 1977.
11. NY Pub. Health Law Section 2780(7).
12. NY Pub. Health Law Section 2780(9).
13. *Estate of Behringer v. The Medical Center at Princeton*, 592 A 2d 1251, (Superior Ct. NJ 1991).
14. *Doe v. Borough of Barrington*, 729 F Suppl 377, (D, NJ, 1990).
15. Mass. Gen. Laws, Chap. 111, Section 111c.
16. Dickins B. Legal limits of AIDS confidentiality. *JAMA* 259:3449–3451, 1988.
17. Gostin L, Curren W. AIDS screening, confidentiality, and the duty to warn. *Am J Public Health* 77:361–365, 1987.
18. *Freese v. Lemmon*, 210 NW 2d 576 (Iowa, 1973).
19. *Tarasoff v. The Regents of the University of California*, 551 P 2d 334, 1976.
20. Conn. Gen. Stat. Sec. 19a—584(a)(b).
21. *District 27 Comm. School v. Board of Educ.*, 502 NYS 2d 325 (Sup., 1986).
22. 29 USC Section 701, et seq.

23. Leonard A. AIDS in the Workplace. In HL Dalton, S Burris (eds), *AIDS and the Law*. New Haven: Yale University Press, 1987. Pp 109–125.
24. Emanuel E. Do physicians have an obligation to treat patients with AIDS? *N Engl J Med* 318:1686–1690, 1988.
25. Council on Ethical and Judicial Affairs. Ethical issues involved in the growing AIDS crisis. *JAMA* 259:1360–1361, 1988.
26. Annas GJ. Not saints, but healers: The legal duties of health care professionals in the AIDS epidemic. *Am J Public Health* 78:844–849, 1988.
27. 42 USC 12182(a).
28. 42 USC 12181(7).
29. 42 USC 12102(2).
30. *School Board of Nassau County v. Arline*, 107 S Ct 1123, 1987.
31. *Chaulk v. US District Court*, 840 F 2d 701, (9th Cir., 1988).
32. *Glover v. Eastern Nebraska Community Office of Mental Retardation*, 686 F Suppl 243 (D, Neb., 1988).
33. *Leckelt v. Board of Commissioners of Hospital District 1*, 909 F 2d 820 (5th Cir., 1990).
34. Ciesielski C, et al. Transmission of human immunodeficiency virus in a dental practice. *Ann Intern Med* 116:798–805, 1992.
35. Centers for Disease Control. Recommendations for preventing transmission of human immunodeficiency virus and hepatitis B virus to patients during exposure-prone invasive procedures. *MMWR* 40:1–9, 1991.
36. Glantz L, Mariner W, Annas G. Risky business: Setting public health policy for HIV-infected health care professionals. *Milbank Quar* 70:43–79, 1992.
37. In the matter of *Quinlan*, 355 A 2d 647 (NJ, 1976).
38. *Lane v. Candura*, 376 NE 2d 1232 (Mass. App., 1978).

Index

Index

Note: Page numbers followed by f indicate figures; those followed by t indicate tables.

Anxiety
  in drug-using patient, 463
  management of, 227
  in psychiatric syndromes, 224
Aphthous ulcerations, 80
ARC. *See* AIDS-related complex
Arterial blood gases, 43–44
  in *Pneumocystis carinii,* 126–127,
    235
Arteriopathy, HIV, 210
Arthralgia, 187, 398
  management of, 195
Arthritis, 188–190
  psoriatic, 189
    management of, 195
  septic, 190
    management of, 195
Aspergillosis
  cerebral, 207
  pulmonary, 133
Atovaquone, 245–246
Atrophic thrush, 399
Autonomic neuropathy, 215
Azidothymidine. *See* Zidovudine
Azithromycin
  for MAC infection, 131, 270
  for toxoplasmosis, 288
AZT. *See* Zidovudine

B lymphocyte, dysregulation of, 160
Bacillary angiomatosis, 104, 209, 349
  clinical manifestations of, 104
  dermatologic manifestations of,
    95t
  differential diagnosis of, 104–105
  evaluation of, 105
  laboratory data on, 104
  management of, 105
Bacillus Calmette-Guérin (BCG)
    vaccination, 412
Bacteremia, 344–346
Bacterial infections
  clinical syndromes, 344–349
  diarrhea with, 148
  differential diagnosis of, 58
  epidemiology of, 343

fever with, 57–58
oral, 79–80
pathogenesis of, 343–344
prevention of, 349–350
pulmonary, 124–128
of skin, 101–105
Barbiturates, abuse of, 455
Barrier precautions, 436
Basal caloric requirements, 68. *See
    also* Nutritional assessment
Bell's palsy, 214
Benzathine penicillin G, 297–298,
    299
Benzodiazepines
  abuse of, 455
  for anxiety, 227
Beta-interferon, 326
Biliary tract disease, 157–158
Bilirubin levels, 38
Biochemical evaluation, 37–39
Bisexuality
  AIDS risk with, 7–8
  Kaposi's sarcoma and, 355–356
Black communities. *See*
    Communities of color
Bleomycin, 360
Blood gases. *See* Arterial blood gases
Body fat content, 66
Body fluid isolation, 432–437
Bone marrow
  cellularity of in HIV infection,
    160–161
  dysplasia of, 41
  examination of, 41
  hypocellularity of, 41
Brain. *See also* Central nervous
    system
  biopsy of, 211, 285, 324
  disorders of, 199–215
  lymphoma of, 209
Bromocriptine, 459
Bronchoalveolar lavage, 44
  for *Pneumocystis carinii*
    pneumonia, 127, 237
Bronchoscopy, 44–45
  for fungal pulmonary infections,
    132–133

Bronchoscopy (*cont.*)
  for *Pneumocystis carinii*
    pneumonia, 237–238
  for respiratory symptom diagnosis,
    138–139
Bullous impetigo, 348

Cachectin, 66
Caloric requirements, calculation of,
  68
Campylobacter infection
  diarrhea with, 148
  gastroenteritis due to, 348
  of GI tract, 347–348
  prevention of, 349–350
Candida, colonization sites of, 336
Candida albicans, 207
  dermatologic manifestations of,
    95t
  in female genital tract, 469
  retinitis with, 89
Candidal encephalitis, 207
Candidiasis
  chronic vaginal, 469
  clinical manifestations of, 336–337
  diagnosis of, 75, 337–338
  disseminated
    hematogenously, 337
    treatment of, 339
  epidemiology of, 336
  esophageal, 153
  genital, 401
  mucocutaneous, 100–101, 336–
    337
    in children, 492
    clinical manifestations of, 100
    management of, 101
    treatment of, 338–339, 492
  oral, 74–76. *See also* Thrush
    in children, 487
  pathogenesis of, 336
  prognosis and prevention of, 339–
    340
  pulmonary, 133
  treatment of, 75–76, 338–339
  in HIV-infected pregnant
    women, 477–478
Carbamazepine, 227

Carcinoma
  oral lesions with, 79
  rectal, 449
Cardiac catheterization, 119
Cardiac disease, 109. *See also* Heart
    disease; *specific conditions*
  endocardial, 117–120
  myocardial, 113–117
  pericardial, 109–113
Cardiac tamponade, 109
  evaluation of, 111–113
  manifestations of, 110
Cardiomegaly, 110
Cardiomyopathy, dilated, 113–117
  management of, 117
Cardiopulmonary system
    examination, 401
Cardiovascular assessment, in HIV-
    infected children, 490
Cat scratch bacillus, 397
Cats, toxoplasmosis in, 288
Cauda equina syndrome, 214–215
CBC. See Complete blood count
CD4 cell count, 4, 39–40, 404–405
  declining, 11, 30–31, 33, 124, 306,
    381
  in determining therapy, 388–389
  didanosine and, 385
  in HIV classification and staging,
    13
  in management of HIV infection,
    406–407
  as prognostic factor in Kaposi's
    sarcoma, 358
  rising, 380
CD4 lymphocytes, deficits and
    bacterial infection, 343–344
CD3 markers, 33
Ceftriaxone
  in children, 492
  for syphilis, 298
Cell-mediated immunity, defective,
    336
Cellulitis, 348
Central nervous system. *See also*
    Brain
  cytomegalovirus infection in, 307–
    308

Clinical markers in HIV infection, 406

Clinical syndromes. *See specific conditions*

Clofazimine, 131, 269–270

Clonidine transdermal patches, 460

Clostridium difficile
    enterocolitis, 348
    titer assay of, 45

Clotrimazole
    for candidal infection in pregnancy, 477
    for candidiasis, 75–76, 101, 492
    efficacy of, 339–340

CMV. *See* Cytomegalovirus infection

CNS lymphoma, 371. *See also* Central nervous system

Cobblestone mucosa, 337–338

Cocaine. *See also* Crack cocaine
    craving for, 459
    intravenous, 428
    sale of, 457–458

Cocaine Anonymous, 460, 509

Coccidioidomycosis, disseminated, 132–133

Cold sore. *See* Herpes labialis

Colitis, cytomegalovirus, 308–309

Colonoscopy, 45

Colposcopy, 411

Communities of color
    attitudes about HIV/AIDS in, 506–507
    HIV infection in, 502–512
        epidemiology of, 502–505
        etiology of, 505–506
        health care provider issues in, 507–510
        prevention efforts in, 510–512

Community support, 507–508

Competence, legal, 523

Complete blood count, 402

Computed tomography, 46–47
    for endocarditis, 119
    for myocardial disease, 116

Condoms
    education about, 511
    efficacy of, 426, 468, 472

Condyloma acuminatum, 449

Confidentiality, 33, 516–517

Conjunctivitis, 84
    infectious, 86

Contraceptives, 472
    in HIV infection, 474–475t

Corticosteroids
    Kaposi's sarcoma and, 247
    for lymphoid interstitial pneumonitis, 136
    neuropsychiatric side effects of, 221t
    for pericardial disease, 113
    for *Pneumocystis carinii* pneumonia, 128, 246–249
    for toxoplasmosis, 287

Cotton-wool spots, 84–85, 400

Counseling
    for HIV antibody testing, 32–33, 394
    post-HIV antibody testing, 429–430
    pre-HIV antibody testing, 428–429

Cowdry type A intranuclear inclusions, 322

Crack cocaine
    in communities of color, 504–505
    increasing use of, 455

Creatinine phosphokinase, 192

Cryotherapy, 107

Cryptococcal antigen assay, 42, 404

Cryptococcal antigen latex agglutination test, 277–278

Cryptococcal infection
    chest roentgenography for, 43
    diagnosis of, 47
    pulmonary, 132

Cryptococcal meningitis, 206
    in immunocompromised patient, 59

Cryptococcosis, 275–281
    clinical manifestations of, 276
    diagnosis of, 276–278
    epidemiology of, 275
    maintenance therapy for, 280
    management of, 278–281

resistance to, 311
for retinitis, 88–89, 478
toxicity of, 312–313
Gastroenteritis, 147
  Campylobacter, 348
Gastrointestinal disorders, 146
  with abdominal pain, 153–154
  bacterial, 347–348
  biliary tract, 157–158
  with cytomegalovirus infection,
    308–309
  diarrheal, 146–153
  hepatic, 154–156
Gastrointestinal examination, in
    HIV-infected children, 489
Gastrointestinal studies, 45–46
Gay bowel syndrome, 151
Gay community, 447
Gay identifier, 450
Genital disease, in HIV-infected
    women, 469–471
Genital ulcer disease, 469–470
Genital warts, 401
Genitourinary tract, physical
    examination of, 401
Geotrichosis, oral lesions with, 76
Germicides, 437
Giardia lamblia, diarrhea with, 151
Giemsa staining, 127
Gingivitis, 79–80, 347
  acute necrotizing ulcerative
    (ANUG), 400
Gingivostomatitis, 76
Glomerulosclerosis, focal,
    segmental, 171, 173–174, 177
Gloves, as universal precaution,
    435–436
Glucose 6-phosphate
    dehydrogenase, 40
  deficiency of, 404
GM-CSF. *See* Granulocyte/
    macrophage colony
    stimulating factor
Gonococcal pharyngitis, 448
G6PD. See Glucose 6-phosphate
    dehydrogenase
Granulocyte colony stimulating
    factor, 164–165

Granulocyte/macrophage colony
    stimulating factor, 164–165
  for AIDS-related lymphoma, 370–
    371
Granulocyte/monocyte colony
    formation, decreased, 161
Granulocyte/monocyte colony
    stimulating factor, 382–383
Granuloma, 161
  bone marrow, 41
Guillain-Barré syndrome, 215

Haemophilus influenzae
  bacteremia, 344
  incidence of, 343
  lower respiratory tract infection,
    347
  pneumonia, 346
  type B, vaccine for, 413
Hair graying, premature, 97t
Haloperidol, 226–227
HAN. *See* Nephropathy, heroin-
    associated
Hand washing, 434–435
Hazardous/infectious waste
    disposal, 438–439
Health care maintenance, 410–414
  routine schedule for in HIV-
    infected patient, 412t
Health care proxy, 523–524
Health care workers
  ancillary staff, 438–439
  attitudes of toward
    homosexuality, 451
  cleaning and disinfection
    procedures for, 437–438
  and communities of color, 507–
    510
  factors in assessing HIV exposure
    of, 434t
  HIV-infected, 437
  HIV status disclosure to, 517
  infection control and risk
    reduction in, 432–441
  management of accidental
    exposures in, 439–440
  Mycobacterium tuberculosis
    infection and, 440–441

Health care workers (*cont.*)
opportunistic diseases and, 440–441
varicella-zoster virus and, 440
Hearing evaluation, in HIV-infected children, 490
Heart disease. *See also* Cardiac disease; *specific conditions*
in children, 488
Hematologic assessment, in HIV-infected children, 490
Hematologic disorders, 160–166
pathophysiology of, 161–162
Hematology studies, 39–40
Hematopoietic progenitor cells, 161
Hemophiliacs, 7
Hemorrhage
adrenal gland, 309–310
ocular, 84
with thrombocytopenia, 165
Hepatic disease, 154–156
Hepatic studies, 45–46
Hepatitis
diagnosis of, 46
peliosis, 156
viral, 154
serological testing of, 41–42, 402
Hepatitis B core antibody (HBcAb), 41
Hepatitis B surface antigen (HBsAg), 41
Hepatitis B virus, 154
accidental exposure to, 439
history of, 396–397
serology for, 402
vaccine for, 414
Hepatitis C virus, 154
antibody, 41–42
Hepatobiliary disease, 155t
with cytomegalovirus infection, 309
Heroin
sale of, 457
snorting of, 455
Heroin-associated nephropathy, 171–173, 184

Herpes labialis, 76, 323
Herpes simplex pneumonitis, 132
Herpes simplex virus
clinical manifestations of, 98–99, 322–323
dermatologic manifestations of, 94t, 398–399
diagnosis of, 323–324
diarrhea with, 148–149
differential diagnosis of, 99
encephalitis, 47, 203
epidemiology of, 321
evaluation of, 99
laboratory data on, 99
management of, 99
oral lesions with, 76–77
pathogenesis of, 322
pericarditis, 111
prevention of, 326
primary infection of, 322–323
reactive infection of, 323
recurrent, 401
refractory mucocutaneous, 59
retinitis with, 89
seborrheic dermatitis and, 96t, 398–399
treatment of, 324–326
in pregnancy, 478
Herpesvirus infections, pulmonary, 132
Herpetic "whitlow," 322
Hidradenitis suppurativa, 348
Histoplasma capsulatum, 90
Histoplasmosis
diagnosis of, 38
disseminated, 132
oral lesions with, 76
HIV. *See* Human immunodeficiency virus
HIV-2 infection, 6
HIV-1, isolation of, 25
HIV antibody testing, 394
clinical use of, 31–32
counseling for, 394, 428
indications and contraindications for, 395t
legal issues of, 514–516

Human immunodeficiency virus
(*cont.*)
natural history of, 9–13
neurologic manifestations of, 199–215
ocular manifestations of, 84–90
oral manifestations of, 74–81
persons at risk for, 32t
predictors of progression of, 12t
prognosis of, 11–12
psychological manifestations of, 219–228
pulmonary manifestations of, 124–139
renal manifestations of, 171–184
rheumatologic manifestations of, 187–196
risk
assessment for, 423–424
reduction, for health care workers, 432–441
seroprevalence data on, 7–8
spectrum of disease of, 10–11
staging of, 404–406
stratified management of, 406–407
structure of, 25–26
syphilis and, 292–299
toxoplasmosis in, 283–288
transmission of, 8–9, 473
perinatal, 467–468, 484–485
varicella-zoster virus in, 326–329
weight loss and malnutrition in, 65–72
WHO clinical stages for, 18, 19t
in women
barriers to care and recruitment of into treatment, 468–469
epidemiology of, 467–468
family planning for, 471–472
natural history of, 469
in pregnancy, 472–478
selected genital diseases in, 469–471
Hyperkalemia, 180
Hyperkeratotic nodules, 98–99
Hypersplenism, 162
Hypertransmitters, 8

Hypoglycemia, pentamidine-induced, 241
Hyponatremia, 180
Hypotension, pentamidine-induced, 240

Idoxuridine, 326
IDUs. *See* Injection drug users
IFA. *See* Immunofluorescent antibody testing
Imidazole, 75
Immune system
cytomegalovirus and function of, 306
in normal pregnancy, 473
Immunizations, 412–414
for bacterial disease, 349
in children, 496–497
Immunocompromise, 59
Immunofluorescent antibody testing, 29
Immunoglobulin A (IgA) antibody assays, 487
Immunoglobulin G (IgG) assay, anti-CMV, 310–311
Immunoglobulin M (IgM) assay, anti-CMV, 310–311
Immunoglobulins, intravenous, in children, 494
Immunologic function, enhancement of, 380–381
Immunoperoxidase stains, 211
Immunosuppression, live-virus vaccination in, 496–497
Impetigo, 398
Incident report, 515
Infectious waste disposal, 438–439
Influenza vaccine, 412–413
INH. *See* Isoniazid
Injection drug users
AIDS-related lymphoma in, 369
bacterial infections in, 343
in communities of color, 503–505
fever in, 60
with HIV infection, 455–464
risk reduction in, 427–428
sexual behavior of, 426
women, 471

Non-Hodgkin's lymphoma
  clinical manifestations of, 369
  diagnosis of, 370
  epidemiology of, 369
  incidence of, 368
  management of, 370–371
  ocular manifestations of, 86
  oral lesions with, 79
  pathogenesis of, 368
  prognosis of, 370
  pulmonary symptoms of, 134–135
Nonsteroidal antiinflammatory
    agents
  for chronic pain in drug-using
      patient, 463
  for pericardial disease, 113
  for ZDV toxicity, 383
Nontreponemal tests, 103
Nortriptyline, 226
Nosocomial infection, risk reduction
    from, 435t
Nuclear lung scans, 236
Nutrition management strategies,
    69–72
Nutritional assessment, 67–68
  in HIV-infected children, 489
Nutritional support, 68–69
Nutritional therapy, 65
  for diarrhea, 153
Nystatin, 75, 477

Ocular hemorrhage, 84
Ocular palsies, 86
Ocular symptoms. See Eyes, disease
    of
Odynophagia, 153
Oligoarthritis, nonspecific, 189
  management of, 195
Oncostatin M, 355
Ophthalmologic examination, 490
Opiates
  abuse of, 455
  for chronic pain in drug-using
      patient, 463
  for pain, 227
  withdrawal from, 458
    treatment for, 461

Opium, deodorized tincture of, 153
Opportunistic infections. See also
    specific diseases
  in pediatric AIDS, 485
  treatment of in HIV-infected
      pregnant women, 477–478
Orabase, 80
Oral-anal intercourse, 425
  infections with, 448
Oral cavity
  hygiene of, 70
  lesions of, 74, 80–81
    bacterial, 79–80
    fungal, 74–76
    HIV-related, 397–398
    neoplastic, 78–79
    viral, 76–78
  nutrition management with
      disorders of, 70
Oral contraceptives, 472
Oral-penile exposure, 448
Oral rehydration therapy, 151–153
Organ system assessment, in HIV-
    infected children, 488–490
Oropharynx, physical examination
    of, 399–400
Otitis media, 347
"Owl's eye" cells, 310

p24 antigen, 30
  appearance of, 33
  decreased level of, 385
  measurement of, 40
p24 antigenemia, 30, 405
Pain
  chronic, 225
    management of, 227
    in drug-using patient, 462–463
Pancreatitis, 154
  with didanosine, 385
Papanicolaou smear, 49
  abnormal and HIV seropositivity,
      470, 471
  for herpes simplex virus, 324
  periodic, 411
Papillary stenosis, 157
Papilledema, 85

with *Candida albicans,* 89
cytomegalovirus, 87–89, 306–307,
    400–401
with herpes simplex and varicella-
    zoster viruses, 89
with *Toxoplasma gondii,* 89
Rheumatologic disorders, 187
    clinical evaluation of, 194–195
    clinical manifestations of, 187–192
    laboratory data on, 192–194
    management of, 195–196
Rhodococcus equi infection, 125
Rifabutin, 131, 270
Rifampin
    for MAC infection, 131, 269–270
    for *Mycobacterium tuberculosis,*
        265
    for tuberculosis in pregnancy, 478
Right to die, 522–524
Risk assessment, 423–424
Risk group trends, 7–8
Risk reduction, 424
    in communities of color, 510–511
    in health care workers, 432–441
    and injection drug use, 427–428
    and sexual behavior, 425–427
Rochalimaea quintana, 104
Roentgenographic studies, 194. *See
    also* Chest x-ray
RPR. *See* Rapid plasma reagin test

Sadomasochism, 425–426
Salicylates, 462–463
Salmonella infection, 59, 344
    diarrhea with, 148
    GI tract, 347–348
    management of, 348
    prevention of, 349–350
Scabies, 96t
"Scat," 425
Sclerosing cholangitis, 157, 309
Seborrheic dermatitis, 96t, 105, 398
    clinical manifestations of, 105
    differential diagnosis of, 106
    evaluation of, 106
    laboratory data on, 105
    management of, 106
Seizure disorder, 211

Self-help programs, 460–461
Septic arthritis, 190
    management of, 195
Seroconversion, febrile illness
    associated with, 57
Serologic response, 33
Serologic testing, 41–42
    for cytomegalovirus, 310–311
    for hepatitis, 402
    for meningoencephalitis, 211
    for rheumatologic disorders, 192
    for syphilis, 294, 402
    Toxoplasma, 403–404
Seropositive response, 429–430
Seroprevalence surveys, 7–8
Serum
    lactate dehydrogenase levels, 38
    transaminases, 38
Serum assay
    cryptococcal antigen, 404
    for malnutrition, 67–68
Sexual behavior
    in drug users, 455
    relative risk of, 426t
    risk reduction for, 425–427
Sexual exposure, unprotected, 9
Sexual history taking, 424–425
Sexual identity, 449–450
Sexually transmitted diseases
    HIV infection and, 9
    increased risk for, 59
    with intravenous cocaine use, 428
    susceptibility of in HIV-infected
        patients, 292
Shigella infection, 148, 347–348
Shigellosis, 449
Shingles. *See* Varicella-zoster virus
"Shooting galleries," 427–428, 504
SIADH. *See* Syndrome of
        inappropriate antidiuretic
        hormone secretion
Sigmoidoscopy, 45
Sinusitis, 347
Sjögren's-like syndrome, 190–191
    management of, 196
Sjögren's syndrome, 191t
Skin
    bacterial infections of, 348–349

Skin (*cont.*)
  biopsy of, 48
  disorders of. *See* Dermatologic
      disorders; *specific conditions*
  history of conditions of, 396–397
  physical examination of, 398–399
  ulcerations of, 293–294
Sleep disorders, 225
Slim disease, 66
Slit-lamp examination, 86–87
Sodium wasting, 37
Soft tissue infections, bacterial, 348–
    349
Specimen preparation, 438
Spermicides, 472
Spinal cord syndromes, 211–213
Splenomegaly, 401
Spondyloarthropathy, 189
Sputum analysis, 44
  for *Pneumocystis carinii*
      pneumonia, 236, 237–238
  for respiratory symptom diagnosis,
      137–138
Squamous cell carcinoma
  oral lesions with, 79
  rectal, 449
Staging, 404–406
Staphylococcus aureus, 59
  in bacteremia, 344–346
  clinical manifestations of, 101–102
  differential diagnosis of, 102
  evaluation of, 102
  folliculitis with, 398
  incidence of, 343
  laboratory data on, 102
  in lower respiratory tract
      infections, 347
  management of, 102
  pericarditis, 111
  reduced defense against, 344
  in septic arthritis, 190
  skin infection, 96t, 348–349
STDs. *See* Sexually transmitted
    diseases
Stereostatic technique, 211
Stool
  examination of in diarrhea, 146

occult blood test, 45, 146
  studies of, 45
Stratified management, 406–407
Streptococcal infection, bacteremia,
    344
Streptococcus pneumoniae, 59, 346
  incidence of, 343
  in lower respiratory tract
      infections, 347
Stress, in HIV-infected children, 498
Stroke syndrome, 210
  with *Mycobacterium tuberculosis,*
    207
Strongyloides, pulmonary symptoms
    of, 133–134
Strongyloides stercoralis, 149
Substance abuse
  issues of, 409
  treatment of in communities of
      color, 508–509
Substitute decision making, 450–451
Suicide risk factors, in homosexual
      patient, 224–225, 451
Sulfadiazine, nephrotoxicity of, 180–
    181
Sulfadiazine-pyrimethamine. *See*
      Pyrimethamine-sulfadiazine
Surgical gown as universal
      precaution, 436
Surgical procedures, 436
Surrogate markers, 40
Syndrome of inappropriate
      antidiuretic hormone
      secretion, 37, 180
Synovial biopsy, 193
Synovial fluid evaluation, 193
Syphilis, 103
  clinical manifestations of, 103, 293
  clinical presentation of, 293–295
  dermatologic manifestations of,
      95t
  diagnosis of, 211, 295–296
  differential diagnosis of, 103
  epidemiology of, 292
  evaluation of, 103
  in eye disease, 87
  laboratory data on, 103

Trimethoprim-sulfamethoxazole
in children, 492
for diarrhea, 148–149
effectiveness of, 251–252
for GI tract infection, 348
in HIV-infected pregnant women, 477
initial therapy with, 242–243
nephrotoxicity of, 180–181
neuropsychiatric side effects of, 221t
with pentamidine, 243–244
for *Pneumocystis carinii* pneumonia
in pregnancy, 478
prophylaxis, 248–249, 252–253, 409, 493–494
treatment, 127–128, 241–244
side effects of, 242
Trimetrexate, 128, 246
Trypanosoma cruzi, focal encephalitis with, 209
Tube feedings, 70
Tuberculosis
distribution of, 263
hepatic involvement in, 155–156
HIV-related, 263–267
incidence of, 129
multidrug-resistant, 130
prevention of, 130–131
skin test for, 263–264
testing for, 402–403
treatment of, 129–130
in HIV-infected pregnant women, 478
Tuboreticular inclusions, 174
Tumor necrosis factor
increased production of, 162
levels of, 66
Tzanck smear, 324
herpes simplex virus diagnosis by, 76
for varicella-zoster virus, 328

Ulcerations
aphthous, 80
cytomegalovirus, 308–309
Ulex europaeus agglutinin, 107

Universal precautions, 432–437
Urinalysis, 37–39, 403
Urine toxicology screens, 457
Uveitis, anterior, 86–87

Vacuolar myelopathy, 212–213
Vaginal candidiasis, 401
Vaginal transmission, 467–468
Valproic acid, 227
Vancomycin, 348
Vanishing bile duct syndrome, 157–158
Varicella-zoster virus, 321, 326–328
clinical manifestations of, 98–99, 327–328
dermatologic manifestations of, 94t
diagnosis of, 328
differential diagnosis of, 99
epidemiology of, 327
evaluation of, 99
immune globulin (VZIG), 329
laboratory data on, 99
management of, 99
meningoencephalitis, 203
multidermatomal, 9
ophthalmicus, 86
oral lesions with, 77
pathogenesis of, 327
pneumonia, 132
precautionary measures for health care workers against, 440
prevention of, 329
recurrent, 399
retinitis with, 89
treatment of, 325t, 328–329
in pregnancy, 478
Vasculitis, 191–192
management of, 196
VDRL testing, 103, 208, 295–296
Villous atrophy, 147
Vinblastine
for Kaposi's sarcoma, 107, 358
neuropsychiatric side effects of, 221t
Vincristine
for Kaposi's sarcoma, 360
neuropsychiatric side effects of, 221t

Violence, 507
Viral infections
diarrhea with, 148–149
oral, 76–78
pulmonary, 131–132
of skin, 93–100
Vitrectomy, 90
Vitreitis, 87
Vomiting, management of, 70
VZV. See Varicella-zoster virus

Warthin-Starry silver stains, 103–104
Warts, 94t
Waste disposal procedures, 438–439
Wasting syndrome, 18
diagnosis of, 67
WB testing. See Western blot
Weight loss
with diarrhea, 71
differential diagnosis of, 66–67
evaluation of, 67–68
factors contributing to, 67t
pattern of, 66
Western blot, 28–29
in children, 486
false-positive rate of, 29
White blood cell count, 193
Women
barriers to care and recruitment of
into treatment programs,
468–469
HIV infection in, 467–478
risk factors in, 468
Women in Sobriety, 460

Xeroderma, 96t
Xerostomia, 80–81

Yellow nails, 97t
Yersinia, 347

ZDV. *See* Zidovudine
Zidovudine
for AIDS-related lymphoma, 370–371
anemia with, 163
approval of, 4
clinical effects of, 380–382
versus dideoxycytidine, 387
erythropoietin and, 40–41
future research on, 388
for prophylaxis in health care
workers, 439–440
for HIV-associated nephropathy,
178–179
for HIV encephalopathy, 202, 226
for idiopathic thrombocytopenic
purpura, 165–166
for Kaposi's sarcoma, 360
mechanism of action and
pharmacology of, 379–380,
408–409
for myocarditis, 117
myopathy
evaluation of, 193, 194–195
management of, 195–196
myositis and, 190
neuropsychiatric side effects of,
221t
for viral infection of mouth, 77
in pediatric HIV patients, 495
for *Pneumocystis carinii*
pneumonia, 251, 252, 494
during pregnancy, 476–477
progression of HIV infection with,
11
recommendations for, 384, 388–389
survival
prolonged with, 468
rates with, 12
toxicity of, 382–384
use with acyclovir, 326
viral resistance to, 383–384